P9-CLF-826

The Dental Hygienist's Guide to Nutritional Care

The Dental Hygienist's Guide to Nutritional Care

Judi Ratliff Davis, MS, CNSD, RD, LD

Cynthia A. Stegeman, RDH, MEd, RD, LD

W. B. SAUNDERS COMPANY

A Division of Harcourt Brace & Company

Philadelphia London Toronto Montreal Sydney Tokyo

W.B. SAUNDERS COMPANY
A Division of Harcourt Brace & Company

The Curtis Center
Independence Square West
Philadelphia, Pennsylvania 19106

Library of Congress Cataloging-in-Publication Data

Davis, Judi Ratliff.
    The dental hygienist's guide to nutritional care / Judi Ratliff Davis, Cynthia A.
Stegeman.
      p. cm.
   ISBN 0-7216-5014-7
    1. Nutrition. 2. Dental hygiene. 3. Mouth—Diseases—Nutritional
aspects. 4. Dental caries—Nutritional aspects. 5. Dental
hygienists. I. Stegeman. Cynthia A. II. Title.
    [DNLM: 1. Oral Health. 2. Nutritional Requirements. 3. Dental
Hygienists. WU 113 D262d 1998.]
  QP141.D365 1998
  617.6′01—dc21
  DNLM/DLC   97-31211

The Dental Hygienist's Guide to Nutritional Care   ISBN 0-7216-5014-7

Printed in the United States of America.

Last digit is the print number: 9 8 7 6 5 4 3 2 1

To My Late Husband:
Thanks for supporting me in my writing and allowing me
to dedicate so many hours to this task.

Judi

To My Husband and Young Son:
Thanks for your constant encouragement
and the countless hours of "quiet time."

Cyndee

Acknowledgments

Because of the diversity of subjects presented in a general nutrition textbook, a compilation of the work of many people, whether direct or indirect, it is necessary to present up-to-date information. Whether the aid was in the area of a research study, verbal, or written communications, each person's help and support is truly appreciated.

Our sincere thanks to Barbara Altshuler, Clinical Assistant Professor, Caruth School of Dental Hygiene, Baylor School of Dentistry, who saw the need for a nutrition textbook for dental hygienists, and took her dream to W.B. Saunders pursuing their backing for this text. Although she was unable to complete this long project with us, she proved invaluable in providing many of the pictures which are an essential part of the learning process to assess oral status.

Special thanks to the dental hygiene faculty at Raymond Walters College, University of Cincinnati, for their expertise, provision of research, and use of many clinical forms. The numerous references in this textbook to colleagues is very much appreciated.

Many thanks to Texas College of Osteopathic Medicine for their superb collection of medical journals and monographs, and especially for the use of the MiniMEDLINE, which was invaluable in accessing the latest medical research.

We would especially like to extend appreciation to Judi's daughter, Debbie Brutsché, and Vikki Tomlinson, who performed superbly at secretarial tasks and computer input during some of the rough pressured times. We are greatly indebted to the late Frank Davis for keeping the computer functioning and always forcing us to update the computer to "speed up" this time-consuming process. Besides those listed, there are countless other friends and relatives to whom we wish to express our gratitude for your encouragement and support.

Objective critiques from reviewers are invaluable to a good publication. We do appreciate the insight, perspective, words of encouragement, and valuable ideas of the following reviewers:

Nancy L. Shearer, RDH, BS, MEd

Elaine Satin, RDH, MS

Elizabeth P. Browne, RD, DSc

Wanda Cloet, MS, BHS

Riva Tougher-Decker, PhD, MS, BS

We also wish to thank the many persons at W.B. Saunders Company who worked so tirelessly in the various phases of planning and producing this book. We are especially grateful to the staff at W.B. Saunders, especially Selma Kaszczuk, Senior Editor, Health-Related Professions for her helpful ideas and for seeing us through this project. We also appreciate the invaluable input, assistance, and encouragement of Rachael Kelly, Assistant Developmental Editor, Health-Related Professions who had to pick up the pieces on numerous occasions to keep us on track.

Judi Ratliff Davis, MS, CNSD, RD, LD, received her BS from the University of Texas at Austin, her MS in nutrition from Texas Woman's University in Denton, and completed a dietetic internship at Indiana University Medical Center in Indianapolis. She has had a variety of experiences in the field of nutrition, including teaching, clinical dietitian, and consultant. She has taught various nutrition and food service courses at Tarrant County Junior College in Fort Worth, Texas. Her roles as a clinical dietitian include Home-Based Community Support, Tarrant County Mental Health Mental Retardation; Rehabilitation Hospital of North Texas, Arlington, Texas; Fort Worth State School, Fort Worth, Texas; Rex Hospital in Raleigh, North Carolina; and Baptist Memorial Hospital in San Antonio, Texas. She has also worked as a nutrition consultant for nursing homes and mental health facilities in western Virginia, San Antonio, and the Dallas-Fort Worth area, for the Greenhouse, a health spa in Arlington, Texas, and for the Sugar Association.

Cyndee Stegeman, RDH, MEd, RD, LD, attended the Dental Hygiene Program at Raymond Walters College, University of Cincinnati where she received an Associate of Applied Science degree, followed by a Bachelor of Science in Public Health Dental Hygiene from Indiana University in Indianapolis. She practiced dental hygiene in general and periodontal private practices for nearly ten years before returning to the University of Cincinnati for her Master of Nutrition Education and completing a comprehensive dietetic internship at The Christ Hospital in Cincinnati. Currently, she is a Consulting Dental Hygienist in the Dental Hygiene Program at Raymond Walters College and has taught Nutrition and Health Education for the past six years. She also practices clinical dietetics at The St. Luke Hospitals in Northern Kentucky with emphasis in cardiac rehabilitation, diabetes education, eating disorders, and weight loss. In addition, she speaks to numerous community and professional groups on nutrition and dentistry. On occasion, she can be found substituting for dental hygienists in private practice.

Preface

The study of nutrition can be an interesting and rewarding subject for dental hygiene students, not only for client education, but also for their own health. This book is designed to show dental hygiene students how to apply sound nutrition principles in assessing, diagnosing, planning, implementing, and evaluating total care of clients and to help the student contribute to the nutritional well-being of clients. The American Dietetic Association recognizes that nutrition is an integral component of oral health. The dental hygienist should assess the oral cavity in relation to the client's nutrition and overall health status and dietary habits. A holistic approach to dietary management of a disease by all members of the health care team is especially appropriate to coordinate managed healthcare.

Since the subject of nutrition is a top priority in today's society, the public faces the challenge of understanding nutritional information. As the health professional that clients may see most often, dental hygienists may be expected to knowledgeably and authoritatively discuss nutritional practices with their clients.

Nutrition information in this book is compiled clearly and concisely to provide an understanding of the therapeutic value of foods in the normal diet. Using the *Objectives* as a guide, both the student and instructor know the important information to be gained from each chapter. Questions in *Student Readiness* at the end of each chapter help students determine their comprehension of the subject. *Test Your NQ* (nutrition quotient) is a brief true-false pretest to stimulate interest in the reading assignment. Answers are located in Appendix E. Learning is also challenged by *Case Applications* in each chapter. *Dental Hygiene Considerations* provide practical information about how this information can affect the client's care or nutritional status; tips in *Nutritional Directions* help the student realize what the client should know or be taught. The *Dental Hygiene Process in Action* in each chapter describes a situation and is followed by the five-step care plan so students can see how to "pull it all together." *Health Applications,* presented in most chapters in Sections I and II, provide updates on "hot topics" in nutrition. These sections contain information on how a vegetarian can obtain an adequate balance of nutrients, causes and treatment of obesity, use of vitamin and mineral supplements, and many other relevant topics. A basic menu introduced in Chapter 1 is used as a basis for modified menus so students can realize types of changes in food choices necessary to meet the dietary restrictions.

Section I, "Orientation to Basic Nutrition," deals with basic principles of nutrition. An understanding of basic nutrition facts is required for a dental hygienist to evaluate the flood of new information available, to make wise judgments about eating habits, and to counsel clients about dietary changes needed. Nutrient deficiencies and excesses are addressed in sections entitled *Hyper-* and *Hypo-,* terms that are more congruent with real life occurrences. Chapters addressing vitamins and minerals are arranged to cover the specific nutrients involved in oral calcified structures or oral soft tissues separately.

Problems specifically involved in application of basic nutrition principles through the lifespan and with ethnic groups are presented in Section II so the dental hygienist can recognize that food choices different from his/her own food patterns may actually be very good. By incorporating any necessary modifications with sensitivity and respect, clients are more likely to make necessary changes. Alterations in nutritional requirements and eating patterns affected by various stages of life are discussed.

"Nutritional Aspects of Oral Health," Section III, includes factors involved in oral problems and nutritional treatment of these problems. In Section III chapters, *Dental Hygiene Considerations* provide specific information established during an *assessment* (physical and dietary), *interventions* or factors that need to be considered in caring for the client, some suggestions for *evaluation* of dental hygiene care of the client's nutritional status, and educational information in *Nutritional Directions*. A nutritional assessment is a basic essential for the nutritional well-being of all clients; this involves performing a physical assessment, evaluating dietary intake/history, and counseling clients about recommended changes in food choices. Many conditions or their outcome are improved by encouraging clients to eat well or to make minor changes in food choices to improve their health.

The Appendix contains reference material. Food composition tables are not included. The authors encourage instructors to make arrangements to have nutritional software for students or to make arrangements for students to have access to the latest issue of USDA Home and Garden Bulletin Number 72, "Nutritive Value of Foods" for students to reference. Nutrition software that is frequently updated usually has nutritional values of many processed foods, fast foods, and the newest low-fat products available. Tables that are important in nutritional assessments are included.

With a better understanding of the importance of food choices, the entire health care team can complement each other and provide optimal care for the client. While specific amounts of nutrients are mentioned, much of this information is presented so dental hygiene students can have a relative idea of amounts for various nutrients, not for prescriptive use.

Contents

Color Plates

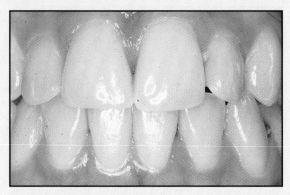

COLOR PLATE 1 Normal gingiva.
(Courtesy of Barbara D. Altshuler, BSDH, MS; Clinical Assistant Professor; Caruth School of Dental Hygiene; The Texas A&M University System; Baylor College of Dentistry; Dallas, TX.)

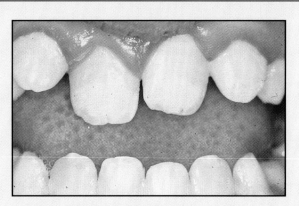

COLOR PLATE 2 Mild fluorosis.
(Courtesy of Alton McWhorter, DDS, MS; Associate Professor Pediatric Dentistry; The Texas A&M University System; Baylor College of Dentistry Dallas, TX.)

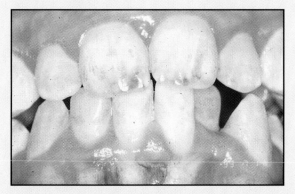

COLOR PLATE 3 Moderate fluorosis.
(Courtesy of Alton McWhorter, DDS, MS; Associate Professor Pediatric Dentistry; The Texas A&M University System; Baylor College of Dentistry; Dallas, TX.)

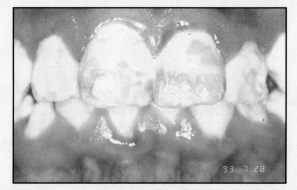

COLOR PLATE 4 Severe fluorosis.
(Courtesy of Alton McWhorter, DDS, MS; Associate Professor Pediatric Dentistry; The Texas A&M University System; Baylor College of Dentistry; Dallas, TX.)

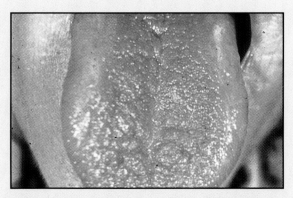

COLOR PLATE 5 Glossitis associated with thiamin deficiency.
(From American Dental Association Council on Dental Therapeutics. Oral Manifestations of Metabolic and Deficiency Changes. Chicago, IL.)

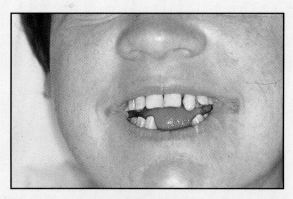

COLOR PLATE 6 Angular cheilitis.
(Courtesy of Barbara D. Altshuler, BSDH, MS; Clinical Assistant Professor; Caruth School of Dental Hygiene; The Texas A&M University System; Baylor College of Dentistry; Dallas, TX.)

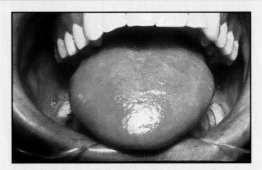

COLOR PLATE 7 Glossitis.
Associated with severe riboflavin deficiency.
(From American Dental Association Council on Dental Therapeutics. Oral Manifestations of Metabolic and Deficiency Changes. Chicago, IL.)

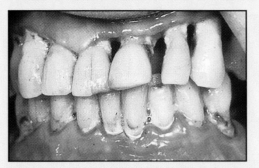

COLOR PLATE 8 Folic acid deficiency.
Chronic peridontitis with loosening of the teeth.
(From American Dental Association Council on Dental Therapeutics. Oral Manifestations of Metabolic and Deficiency Changes. Chicago, IL.)

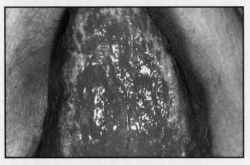

COLOR PLATE 9 Folic acid deficiency.
Fiery red tongue completely devoid of papillae.
(From American Dental Association Council on Dental Therapeutics. Oral Manifestations of Metabolic and Deficiency Changes. Chicago, IL.)

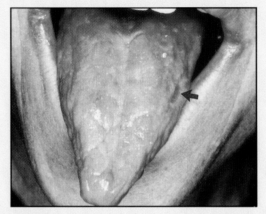

COLOR PLATE 10 Pernicious anemia.
(From Ibsen OAC, Phelan JA. *Oral Pathology for the Dental Hygienist,* 2nd ed. Philadelphia: W.B. Saunders, 1996.)

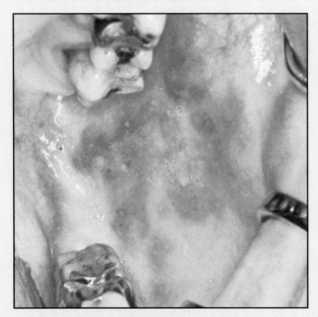

COLOR PLATE 11 Pernicious anemia.
(From Pindborg JJ. *Atlas of Diseases of the Oral Mucosa,* 5th ed. Philadelphia: W.B. Saunders, 1993.)

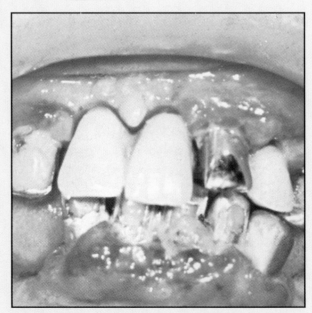

COLOR PLATE 12 Ascorbic acid deficiency.
(From Pindborg JJ. *Atlas of Diseases of the Oral Mucosa,* 5th ed. Munksgaard: W.B. Saunders, 1993, pg 165.)

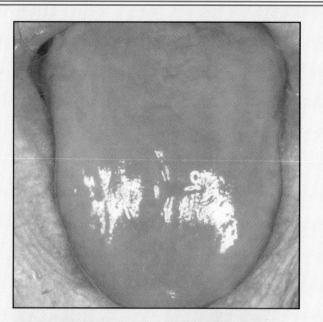

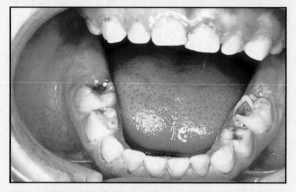

COLOR PLATE 13 Dental caries.

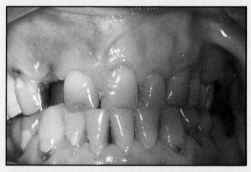

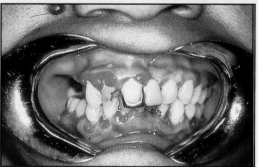

COLOR PLATE 15 Gingival pallor due to anemia.

COLOR PLATE 16 Severe gingivitis with hyperplasia
and inflammation and recession of gingival tissue as
a result of diabetes mellitus.

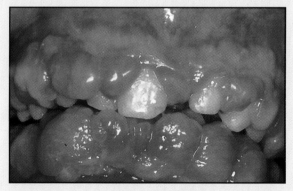

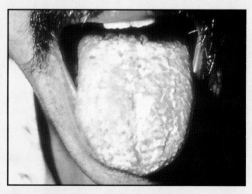

COLOR PLATE 17 Dilantin hyperplasia.

COLOR PLATE 18 Oral candidiasis.

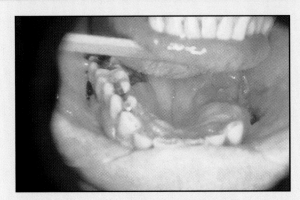

COLOR PLATE 19 Histoplasmosis.
(Courtesy of Daniel J. Barbaro, MD. Infectious Diseases, private practice. Fort Worth, TX.)

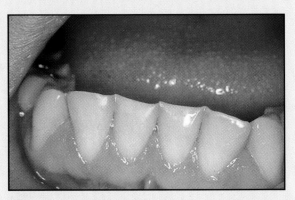

COLOR PLATE 20 Bulimia nervosa.
Erosion occurring on the incisal edges of the mandibular anterior teeth as a result of acid action on the teeth from frequent vomiting.
(Courtesy of Barbara D. Altshuler, BSDH, MS; Clinical Assistant Professor; Caruth School of Dental Hygiene; The Texas A&M University System; Baylor College of Dentistry; Dallas, TX and Larry L. Pace, DDS; private practice, Dallas. TX.)

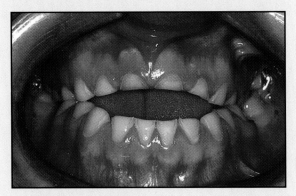

COLOR PLATE 21 Bulimia nervosa.
Generalized enamel erosion as a result of acid action on the teeth from frequent vomiting.
(Courtesy of Barbara D. Altshuler, BSDH, MS; Clinical Assistant Professor; Caruth School of Dental Hygiene; The Texas A&M University System; Baylor College of Dentistry; Dallas, TX and Larry L. Pace, DDS; private practice, Dallas. TX.)

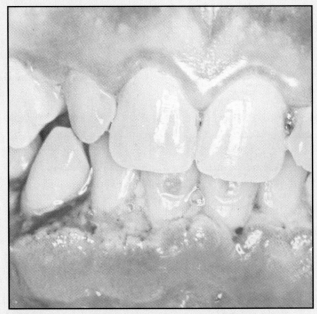

COLOR PLATE 22 Acute necrotizing gingivitis.
(From Pindborg JJ. *Atlas of Diseases of the Oral Mucosa*, 5th ed. Munksgaard: W.B. Saunders, 1992, pg 35.)

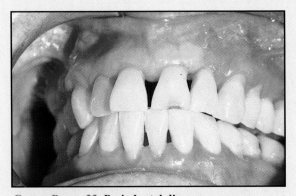

COLOR PLATE 23 Periodontal disease.
(Courtesy of Barbara D. Altshuler, BSDH, MS; Clinical Assistant Professor; Caruth School of Dental Hygiene; The Texas A&M University System; Baylor College of Dentistry; Dallas, TX.)

Section I

ORIENTATION TO BASIC NUTRITION

Chapter 1

Overview of Healthy Eating Habits

The Student Will Be Able To:

- List the general physiologic functions of the six nutrient classifications of foods.
- Identify factors that influence food habits.
- Name the food groups in the Food Guide Pyramid.
- State the number of servings needed from each of the food groups in the Food Guide Pyramid.
- Identify significant nutrient contributions of each food group.
- State the Dietary Guidelines for Americans and their purpose.
- Identify dietary selections in each food group that significantly affect intake of calories, fats, salt, and sugar.
- Assess dietary intake of a client, using the Dietary Guidelines for Americans and the Food Guide Pyramid.
- Explain the different purposes of the RDAs, the Food Guide Pyramid, and the RDIs.
- Apply basic nutritional concepts to help clients with problems related to nutrition.

GLOSSARY OF TERMS

Precursor a substance from which another substance is formed

Recommended Dietary Allowances (RDAs) specific amounts of essential nutrients that adequately meet the known nutrient needs of practically all healthy Americans

Estimated Safe and Adequate Daily Dietary Intakes (ESADDIs) estimated allowances established for nutrients for which data were sufficient to establish a range of requirements but insufficient for a specific RDA

Cruciferous belonging to the botanical family of plants that includes cabbage and mustard

Enrichment the process of restoring nutrients removed from food during processing

Fortification the process of adding nutrients not present in the natural product or to increase the amount above that in the original product

Satiety a feeling of fullness

Reference Daily Intakes (RDIs) a new term for Recommended Dietary Allowances, reflecting nutrient requirements for optimizing health in individuals and groups

Daily Reference Values (DRVs) the desirable levels of nutrients considered important for health: total fat, saturated fatty acids, protein, cholesterol, carbohydrate, fiber, and sodium

Test Your NQ (True/False)

1. Milk is a perfect food for everyone. T/F
2. Only consumption of refined sugar is related to caries formation. T/F
3. Water is the most important nutrient. T/F
4. RDAs are required daily allowances essential for all clients to be healthy. T/F
5. Good nutrition is possible regardless of a patient's cultural habits. T/F
6. Based on the Food Guide Pyramid, two to four servings daily are needed from the fruit and vegetable group. T/F
7. The Dietary Guidelines for Americans were written for healthy people to help reduce their risk of developing chronic diseases. T/F
8. Sugar is the leading cause of chronic health problems. T/F
9. The goal of the Food Guide Pyramid is to convey the importance of variety, moderation, and proportion. T/F
10. The only nutrients that provide energy are carbohydrates, fats, and vitamins. T/F

INTRODUCTION

As the dental hygiene profession continues to grow and rapidly move into the forefront of health care, it is imperative that we be knowledgeable in various aspects of health to be effective practitioners. We are in a unique position in that we generally see our clients more often than other health care professionals. This allows us to observe many physical signs, in particular oral signs, of a nutrient deficiency or medical condition affecting nutritional status before it is diagnosed, thus making the dental hygienist a valuable member of the health care team. Recognition of abnormal conditions and early referral to the appropriate health care professionals can provide very positive outcomes for our clients.

Also, assessment of dietary information obtained from a client can uncover habits detrimental to oral health that may be modified easily or referred to a dietitian or physician.

Finally, we can follow up on the goals established by our clients to evaluate their understanding and compliance. Overall, the dental hygienist is committed to prevention of oral disease and health and wellness promotion. It is important for all health care professionals to work together as a team to enhance the care of our clients.

The purpose of this textbook is to provide the dental hygienist with the nutrition information that can realistically be applied to and practiced with clients.

BASIC NUTRITION

Nutrition is the process by which living things utilize food to obtain *nutrients* for energy, growth and development, and maintenance. Nutrients are

biochemical substances that can only be supplied in adequate amounts from an outside source, normally from food. One aspect of nutrition is the integration of physiologic and biochemical reactions within the body: (1) digesting food to make nutrients available; (2) absorbing and delivering nutrients to the cells, where they are utilized; and (3) eliminating waste products. Psychological and social factors that enter into the frequent decisions concerning food choices are also important aspects of nutrition. Freedom of choice and variety in consumption are important components of an individual's personal and social life; tastes, budget, environment, and cultural attitudes influence food choices. The systemic effects of nutrients, which are determined by these food choices, in turn affect dental health.

PHYSIOLOGIC FUNCTIONS OF NUTRIENTS

Physiologically, foods eaten are used for energy, tissue building and replacement, and obtaining or producing numerous regulatory substances. The six classes of nutrients obtained from foods are (1) water, (2) proteins, (3) carbohydrates, (4) fats, (5) minerals, and (6) vitamins. Nutrients work together, interacting in complex metabolic reactions. Table 1–1 lists the basic functions of the major nutrients.

BASIC CONCEPTS OF NUTRITION

Foods differ in the amount of nutrients they furnish. Any individual food can be compatible with good nutrition but should be evaluated in the context of the client's physiologic needs, the food's nutrient content, and other food choices. The premise of nutritional care is that, in any cultural or environmental circumstance or for any personal taste or preference, good nutrition is possible.

Increasing the variety of foods in the diet reduces the probability of developing isolated nutrient deficiencies, nutrient excesses, and toxicities due to non-nutritive components or contaminants in any particular food. A dietary change to eliminate or increase intake of one specific food component or nutrient usually alters the intake of other nutrients. For instance, since red meats are an excellent source of iron, decreasing cholesterol intake by limiting these meats reduces dietary iron intake.

Essential nutrients are needed throughout life; only the amounts of nutrients needed change. Nutrient requirements change according to the patient's utilization of foods eaten, stage of growth and development, sex, body size, weight, physical activity, and state of health.

Some nutrients can be converted by the body to meet its physiologic needs. Nonessential nu-

TABLE 1–1   *General Functions of Nutrient Classes*

Nutrient	Furnish Energy	Build and Maintain Body Tissues	Regulate Body Processes
Protein	X	X	X
Carbohydrates	X		
Fats	X		
Vitamins		X	X
Minerals		X	X
Water		X	X

From Davis JR, Sherer K. *Applied Nutrition and Diet Therapy for Nurses,* 2nd ed. Philadelphia: W.B. Saunders, 1994.

trients can be utilized by the body but either are not required or can be synthesized from dietary **precursors.** One such example is cholesterol (an essential component of cells present in animal foods); the body can produce all the cholesterol it needs when dietary cholesterol is inadequate.

Water is the most important nutrient. Following water, the nutrients of highest priority are those that provide energy, which must be supplied from foods or can be supplied from quantities stored in the body. Energy is measured in potential calories provided by three of the basic nutrients: carbohydrate, fat, and protein. The human body has adaptive mechanisms that allow toleration of modest ranges in nutrient intakes. For instance, the metabolic rate usually decreases as a result of decreased caloric intake.

Dental Hygiene Considerations

- Because nutrients work interdependently, a lack or excess of one can interfere with or prevent the use of another. Ask the client to record or list food intake for 24 hours so that you can assess nutrient intake. Evaluation of the client's intake of the six classes of nutrients can help determine whether intake is adequate or excessive.

Nutritional Directions

- No single food contains all the essential nutrients in amounts needed for optimum health.
- Nutrition can either improve or adversely affect health.

NUTRITIONAL CONCERNS

The Senate Select Committee on Nutrition and Human Needs originally published *Dietary Goals for the United States* in 1977 to promote healthy food choices. This was followed by *The Surgeon General's Report on Nutrition and Health* in 1988, confirming that 5 of the 10 leading causes of death (coronary heart disease, certain types of cancer, stroke, diabetes mellitus, and atherosclerosis) are associated with diet.

Both of these reports had similar conclusions. The U.S. food supply provides adequate quantities of nutrients to protect healthy Americans from deficiency diseases. In general, nutritional deficiencies that were once prevalent have been replaced by dietary excesses and imbalances. However, groups of isolated or economically deprived people experience undernutrition.

Healthy People 2000 Nutrition Objectives

In 1990, the U.S. Department of Health and Human Services (USDHHS) released *Healthy People 2000,* a report that described the generalized goals of lengthening the healthy lifespan, reducing health disparities, and achieving access to preventative services for all Americans over the next 10 years. To help meet these goals, specific objectives were identified in 21 different priority areas involving nutrition (see *Healthy People 2000:* Nutrition Priority Areas). Many of the Dietary Guidelines for Americans were addressed in these objectives, including the flagship objectives of reduction of overweight and dietary fat intake. Based on a progress review, objectives showing positive results were improved death rate from coronary heart disease and strokes, better control of hypertension, lower blood cholesterol levels, increased numbers of people using nutrition labels to make food choices, decreased fat consumption, and increased numbers of restaurants offering low-fat, low-calorie menu choices. On the other hand, for many of the objectives very little progress had been made: the number of overweight people increased, more food-related illnesses occurred as a result of food contamination, and the number of children with dental caries and elderly adults who are edentulous increased.

Healthy People 2000: Nutrition Priority Areas

- Reduce coronary heart disease deaths to no more than 100 per 100,000 people.
- Reverse the rise in cancer deaths to achieve a rate of no more than 130 per 100,000 people.
- Reduce overweight to a prevalence of no more than 20% among people aged 20 and older and no more than 15% among adolescents aged 12 through 19.
- Reduce growth retardation among low-income children aged 5 and younger to less than 10%.
- Reduce dietary fat intake to an average of 30% of calories or less, and average saturated fat intake to less than 10% of calories among people aged 2 and older.
- Increase complex carbohydrates and fiber-containing foods in the diets of adults to five or more daily servings of vegetables and fruits, and to six or more daily servings of grain products.
- Increase to at least 50% the proportion of overweight people aged 12 and older who have adopted sound dietary practices combined with regular physical activity to attain an appropriate body weight.
- Increase calcium intake so at least 50% of youths aged 12 through 24 and 50% of pregnant and lactating women consume three or more servings daily of foods rich in calcium, and at least 50% of people aged 25 and older consume two or more servings daily.
- Decrease salt and sodium intake so at least 65% of home meal preparers prepare foods without adding salt, at least 80% of people avoid using salt at the table, and at least 40% of adults regularly purchase foods modified or lower in sodium.
- Reduce iron deficiency to less than 3% among children aged 1 through 4 and among women of childbearing age.
- Increase to at least 75% the proportion of mothers who breastfeed their babies in the early postpartum period and to at least 50% the proportion who continue breastfeeding until their babies are 5 to 6 months old.
- Increase to at least 75% the proportion of parents and caregivers who use feeding practices that prevent baby bottle tooth decay.
- Increase to at least 85% the proportion of people aged 18 and older who use food labels to make nutritious food selections.
- Achieve useful and informative labeling for virtually all processed food and at least 40% of fresh meats, poultry, fish, fruits, vegetables, baked goods, and ready-to-eat carry-away foods.
- Increase to at least 5,000 brand names the availability of processed food products that are reduced in fat and saturated fat.
- Increase to at least 90% the proportion of restaurants and institutional food service operations that offer identifiable low-fat, low-calorie food choices, consistent with the *Dietary Guidelines for Americans.*
- Increase to at least 90% the proportion of school lunch and breakfast services and child care food services with menus that are consistent with the nutrition principles in the *Dietary Guidelines for Americans.*
- Increase to at least 80% the receipt of home food services by people aged 65 and older who have difficulty in preparing their own meals or are otherwise in need of home-delivered meals.
- Increase to at least 75% the proportion of the nation's schools that provide nutrition education from preschool through 12th grade.
- Increase to at least 50% the proportion of worksites with 50 or more employees that offer nutrition education and/or weight management programs for employees.
- Increase to at least 75% the proportion of primary care providers who provide nutrition assessment and counseling and/or referral to qualified nutritionists or dietitians.

- Consider cultural influences and personal preferences when assessing intake and planning nutritional interventions.
- A basic understanding of nutrient components in foods is needed for dental hygienists to be able to suggest alternate food choices that provide the needed nutrients for clients who avoid or dislike a particular food. Additionally, this information may help dental hygienists prevent clients from inadvertently deleting needed nutrients.
- If a client has any of the five diseases that are leading causes of death, evaluate food/ nutrient choices by asking the client to list typical intake for 24 hours; or refer the client to a registered dietitian.

- It is the overall balance of the diet that matters, and the best balance incorporates a variety of foods.
- Unrestrained habits, especially overconsumption of certain dietary components, may contribute to the development of many diseases (e.g., saturated fat intake predisposes clients to atherosclerosis).

FOOD GROUPING SYSTEMS

Food grouping systems are tools used to translate technical nutritional needs into practical guidelines for food selections. Since clients eat foods, nutrient requirements and information must be interpreted into the "food" language clients understand. The **Recommended Dietary Allowances (RDAs)** and the recently introduced **Dietary Reference Intakes (DRIs)** attempt to establish required nutrients and amounts suggested for various stages of life. Several guidelines that facilitate appropriate food choices will be discussed, including the new U.S. Department of Agriculture (USDA) Food Guide Pyramid, Dietary Guidelines for Americans, and nutrition labeling.

Recommended Dietary Allowances/Dietary Reference Intakes

The RDAs and DRIs are published by the government but are established by competent scientists and nutritionists who base their recommendations on evidence from different types of studies on the nutrients and their application to individual requirements. RDAs and DRIs are principally used as a measurement by professionals who assess the nutritional status of the American population, establish guidelines for feedings in institutions, and set standards for governmental programs.

The assumption is that nutrients not included in the RDAs, such as water and some trace elements, are supplied in sufficient amounts when a varied diet provides recommended amounts of the nutrients addressed. The RDAs include an **Estimated Safe and Adequate Daily Dietary Intakes (ESADDI)** for two vitamins and five minerals.

The National Academy of Science Food and Nutrition Board is currently updating the RDAs. This revised and expanded information is called the Dietary Reference Intakes (DRIs). **DRIs are based on the observed average or experimentally set intake by individuals that appear to sustain a defined nutritional status, such as growth rate, normal circulating nutrient values, or other functional indicators of health.** They differ from the RDAs in their goal to reduce risks of consuming either excessive or deficient amounts of nutrients. Upper limit (UL) guidelines are indicated to reduce risk of adverse health effects from overconsumption of a nutrient. Adequate intake (AI) indicates a lack of scientific evidence to determine an estimated average requirement. Also, two age groups for the older American population are added.

The first guideline set, covering the nutrients

specific to bone health, was introduced in the fall of 1997. The completion of this planned seven-step overhaul of the outdated RDAs is scheduled for the year 2000. Other nutrient groups include: (1) folate and B vitamins; (2) antioxidants and phytochemicals; (3) macronutrients (protein, carbohydrates, and fat); (4) fiber and trace elements, (iron and zinc); and (5) the electrolytes potassium, sodium, and chloride.

Unfortunately, there are no sure guidelines for establishing at what point diets become inadequate. The government generally considers a diet adequate that provides two thirds of the RDAs, whereas less than 66% is considered poor.

Dental Hygiene Considerations

- Use of RDAs as an assessment guide is for healthy clients only.

Nutritional Directions

- The RDAs are general guidelines for good health rather than specific requirements.

Dietary Guidelines for Americans

Based on recommendations made from goals established in 1977, the U.S. Department of Agriculture (USDA) and the former U.S. Department of Health, Education, and Welfare (USD-HEW) established the Dietary Guidelines for Americans. These guidelines are reviewed every 5 years and were last updated in 1995 (Fig. 1–1). The guidelines provide information about food choices that promote health and decrease the risk of chronic diseases such as family history of obesity, high blood pressure, and elevated cholesterol levels in healthy Americans over the age of 2 (Fig. 1–2). The Dietary Guidelines for Americans is the cornerstone of federal nutrition policy.

EAT A VARIETY OF FOODS   No healthy individual with a broad range of food preferences who regularly eats a wide variety of fruits, vegetables, milk, cereals, and small amounts of animal protein at each meal will be in any danger of developing nutritional deficiencies. Adequate

nutritional status can be achieved by encouraging clients to eat a variety of foods from each of the basic food groups. Recent estimates of nutrients available in the U.S. food supply indicate all nutrient levels are adequate to prevent deficiency diseases (Zizza & Gerrior, 1995).

BALANCE THE FOOD YOU EAT WITH PHYSICAL ACTIVITY TO MAINTAIN OR IMPROVE YOUR WEIGHT   Obesity occurs in clients of all ages and economic groups. The probability of developing hypertension, coronary heart disease, gallbladder disease, diabetes, some cancers, and problems associated with osteoarthritis increases with obesity. Obesity indicates that caloric intake has exceeded output. Preventing weight gain is an achievable goal and is the first step toward reducing the prevalence of obesity and risk for chronic illness.

Physical activity is important for both weight control and health. To stay at the same body weight, the amount of energy in food must be balanced with the amount of energy the body uses. Physical activity is an important way to use up food energy.

Moderation of calorie intake and an increase in calorie output is the key to maintaining ideal weight; it may be the most important dietary goal for clients. All food groups should be included, with more servings of low-calorie foods in each group. When the energy requirement is low, consumption of foods not included in the food groups (i.e., sugar, alcohol, and fats) should especially be reduced because these foods provide calories for energy but few other nutrients. Further discussion of weight control and energy balance may be found in Health Application 1, below, and in chapter 6.

Being underweight also has risks. Numerous health problems are associated with anorexia, and underweight is associated with increased risk of osteoporosis in women.

CHOOSE A DIET WITH PLENTY OF GRAIN PRODUCTS, VEGETABLES, AND FRUITS   Grain products and many vegetables and fruits are especially important because they provide complex

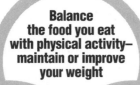

Balance the food you eat with physical activity— maintain or improve your weight

Choose a diet with plenty of grain products, vegetables, and fruits

Choose a diet low in fat, saturated fat, and cholesterol

Eat a variety of foods

Choose a diet moderate in salt and sodium

Choose a diet moderate in sugars

If you drink alcoholic beverages, do so in moderation

FIGURE 1–1 Nutrition and Your Health: Dietary Guidelines for Americans. Seven guidelines that should be used together to choose a healthful and enjoyable diet. (From U.S. Department of Agriculture, U.S. Department of Health and Human Services: *Nutrition and Your Health: Dietary Guidelines for Americans,* 4th ed. Home and Garden Bulletin No. 232. Washington, D.C.: Government Printing Office, 1995.)

carbohydrates (starches) and dietary fiber. Foods rich in complex carbohydrates and fiber are listed in Natural Food Sources of Complex Carbohydrates and Fiber.

Unrefined complex carbohydrates are those that are as close to the form in which they naturally occur as possible (e.g., whole grains or whole legumes as opposed to refined flours, cereals, and meat substitutes). They contain significant amounts of fiber and also vitamins and minerals, especially zinc, vitamin B_6, and folate.

Dietary fiber is important for healthy bowel functioning and can reduce symptoms of chronic constipation, diverticular disease, and hemorrhoids.

To accomplish the goal of increasing intake of grain products requires teaching clients how to modify eating habits. Many have avoided complex carbohydrates because of the misconception that they are fattening. Because of their low fat content, they are relatively low in calories. A diet high in complex carbohydrates may be less fattening than a diet of comparable calories high in fat. Foods containing complex carbohydrates are usually eaten with added fats or sugars, however. For example, sugar is usually added to cereal, and margarine is added to bread or potatoes.

Foods rich in vitamins A and C may help lower

FIGURE 1–2 Comparison of current eating patterns versus recommendations from the Dietary Guidelines for Americans. Data from Raper N. Nutrient content of the U.S. food supply. *Food Rev* 1991; 14(4):13–18; Glinsman WH, et al. Evaluation of health aspects of sugars contained in carbohydrate sweeteners. U.S. Food and Drug Administration, 1986; and Dietary Goals for the United States, 2nd ed. Washington, D.C.: Senate Committee on Nutrition and Human Needs, 1977. (Redrawn from Davis JR, Sherer K. *Applied Nutrition and Diet Therapy for Nurses,* 2nd ed. Philadelphia: W.B. Saunders, 1994.)

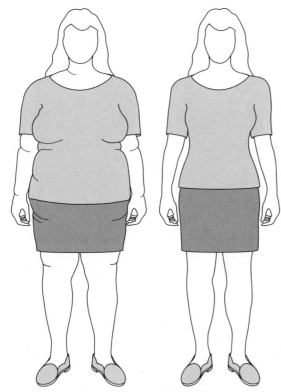

CURRENT DIET
Total carbohydrate: 47%
  (sugars: 10–13%)
Protein: 12%
Fat: 35–45%
  (saturated: 15%;
  monounsaturated: 17%;
  polyunsaturated: 8%)

GOAL DIET
Total carbohydrate: 55–58%
  (sugars: 10–12%)
Protein: 12%
Fat: 30%
  (saturated: 10%;
  monounsaturated and
  polyunsaturated: 20%)

Natural Food Sources of Complex Carbohydrates and Fiber

Good Sources of Complex Carbohydrates

◆ Breads, both whole-grain and enriched

◆ Breakfast cereals, cooked or ready-to-eat (enriched or fortified)

◆ Flours, whole-grain and enriched

◆ Noodles and pasta

◆ Rice, whole-grain or white

◆ Legumes such as dried beans, peas, and lentils

◆ Starchy vegetables such as English peas, potatoes, lima beans, corn

Good Sources of Fiber

◆ Whole-grain breads and other bakery products

◆ Whole-grain cereals, cooked and ready-to-eat

◆ Legumes such as dried beans, peas, and lentils

◆ Fruits, especially with skins (figs, pears, apricots, nectarines, raisins, blueberries) and edible seeds (blackberries, raspberries, strawberries)

◆ Vegetables, especially sweet potatoes, carrots, mushrooms, raw onions, pumpkin, spinach, turnip greens, kale, Brussels sprouts, parsnips, peas, beets, okra, and broccoli

◆ Nuts and seeds

From Davis JR, Sherer K. *Applied Nutrition and Diet Therapy for Nurses,* 2nd ed. Philadelphia: W.B. Saunders, 1994.

the risk for cancers of the larynx, esophagus, and lungs. **Cruciferous** vegetables help reduce cancer susceptibility. Good sources of fiber and vitamins A and C, including cruciferous vegetables, are listed in Table 1–2. One of the B vitamins, folate, is critical in very early pregnancy to reduce the risk of spina bifida and other neural tube defects of the developing fetus. Grains and fresh fruits and vegetables are a good source of folate. Tips for increasing dietary fiber are presented in Implementing the Guideline for Increasing Fiber.

CHOOSE A DIET LOW IN FAT, SATURATED FAT, AND CHOLESTEROL Choosing lower-fat foods from each of the food groups allows one to increase the amount and variety of grain products, fruits, and vegetables without

TABLE 1–2   *Contributions of Selected Fruits and Vegetables to a Healthy Diet*

	Vitamin A	Vitamin C*	Fiber	Cruciferous Vegetable
Acorn squash	X			
Apple			X	
Apricot	X		X	
Avocado	X		X	
Banana			X	
Bell pepper		XX		
Broccoli	X	XX	X	X
Brussel sprouts		XX	X	X
Cabbage		X	X	X
Cantaloupe	X	XX	X	
Carrot	X		X	
Cauliflower		X	X	X
Celery			X	
Collard greens	X	X		
Grapefruit		X	X	
Iceberg lettuce			X	
Kale	X	X		X
Kiwi fruit		X	X	
Kohlrabi				X
Orange		XX	X	
Papaya	X	X	X	
Peach	X		X	
Prune			X	
Spinach	X		X	
Strawberry		XX	X	
Sweet potato	X		X	
Swiss chard	X			X
Tomato		X	X	

*XX, Excellent source of Vitamin C. X, Good source of Vitamin C.

From Davis JR, Sherer K. *Applied Nutrition and Diet Therapy for Nurses,* 2nd ed. Philadelphia: W.B. Saunders, 1994.

exceeding one's caloric needs (see Implementing the Fat and Cholesterol Guideline). The diet should provide no more than 30% of total calories from fat. This guideline applies only to children aged 2 years or older. Children under the age of 2 should have a higher percentage of fat in their diet; after the age of 2, however, the diet should be modified gradually so that by age 5 no more than 30% of the calories are provided by fat.

By decreasing fat intake, caloric intake is likely to be reduced as well. Fats and the different classes of fatty acids and cholesterol affect blood cholesterol levels and the risk of heart disease. Certain cancers have also been linked to fat intake. Fortunately, the type of fats most commonly consumed has changed. A larger percentage of fat intake is from vegetable products, especially margarine, vegetable shortenings, and other consumable oils. The proportion of fat from animal sources markedly declined, from 63% to 52%, between 1970 and

Implementing the Guideline for Increasing Fiber

♦ Include two to four servings of fruits and three to five servings of vegetables daily.

♦ Use breads and cereals if "whole wheat" or "whole grain" is the first listing in the ingredient list.

♦ Choose cereals with at least 2 gm of fiber but no more than 2 gm of fat per serving.

♦ Add a little bran or wheat germ to recipes, even to casseroles, main dishes, pancakes, and cooked cereal.

♦ Prepare raw vegetables to eat with low-fat dip as appetizers.

♦ Serve baked potatoes topped with steamed vegetables (broccoli, cauliflower, carrots).

♦ Add vegetables (mushrooms, peppers, onions, tomatoes) to omelettes or scrambled eggs.

♦ Add leafy greens, tomato, and sprouts to sandwiches.

♦ Add raw vegetables (zucchini, carrots celery sticks) to brown-bag lunches.

♦ Snack on fresh fruits and vegetables or plain popcorn instead of fried chips and cookies.

From Davis JR, Sherer K. *Applied Nutrition and Diet Therapy for Nurses,* 2nd ed. Philadelphia: W.B. Saunders, 1994.

1990 (Zizza & Gerrior, 1995). Americans have reduced their fat consumption from 40% in the late 1970s to 33% in 1994 (Putnam & Duewer, 1995). Fewer people are dying from heart disease.

Food manufacturers have developed fat replacers to help lower the fat content of foods. The potential for fat replacers to decrease fat intake by reducing the amount of calories from fats in dessert and snack foods is promising, but they are not a panacea for obesity, cancer, and heart disease. Fat replacers will not compensate for poor dietary choices or replace the benefits of a diet rich in whole grains, fresh fruits, and vegetables. Further discussion of various fat replacers is found in chapter 5.

CHOOSE A DIET MODERATE IN SUGARS
Scientific studies do not indicate that the amount of sugar eaten by Americans is detrimental to health; nor can it be proven that reduced amounts would improve health. This guideline was not meant to decrease the intake of natural sugars found in fruits, vegetables, and milk; rather, it relates to decreasing intake of refined sugar, a carbohydrate that contains calories but no other nutrients. Dental caries is the only health risk associated with sugar intake; however, many other factors are involved in the formation of caries. Good oral hygiene practices and use of a fluoride dentifrice and/or fluoridated water are also important factors in healthy teeth.

Many forms of sugar can be added to foods by the consumer or manufacturer, including table sugar, brown sugar, raw sugar, glucose (dextrose), fructose, maltose, lactose, honey, syrup, corn sweetener, high-fructose corn syrup, molasses, and fruit juice concentrate. Therefore, teaching clients to read food labels is essential.

Many other sweeteners are now on the market as substitutes for sucrose. Several, including fructose, sorbitol, mannitol, and xylitol, contain the same number of calories as table sugar. "Dietetic" products containing these sweeteners can mislead clients to believe they contain no calories. Based on the prevalence of obesity, it is doubtful whether these products have actually helped curtail either sugar or caloric consumption. These will be discussed further in chapter 3.

USE SALT AND SODIUM ONLY IN MODERATION
The average amount of salt intake in the United States is about 10 gm daily, which is approximately 20 times more than the body's requirement. Most dietary salt and sodium comes from foods to which salt has been added during processing or preparation. The sodium content of many fast foods is significant (a cheeseburger and french fries, for example, may contain more than 1,300 mg). Salt (sodium chloride) intake should be reduced to less than 6 gm/day; this translates into a daily sodium intake of 2,400 mg. Sodium intake is associated with hypertension. It is especially important to identify clients with a family history of hypertension or who are salt-sensitive. Other factors such as weight, potassium intake, physical activity, and alcohol consumption also affect blood pressure. High salt intake may increase calcium

Implementing the Fat and Cholesterol Guideline

Cooking with Fats and Oils

◆ Check labels on foods to determine the amount of fat and saturated fat in a serving.

◆ Choose liquid vegetable oils most often because they are lower in saturated fat. Reduce saturated fats such as butter, lard, and palm and coconut oils.

◆ Limit foods with hidden fats such as chips, doughnuts, cookies, snack crackers, cakes, fried foods, and some processed and convenience foods.

◆ Use fats and oils sparingly in cooking (roast, bake, grill, or broil when possible). Baste meats with broth or stock.

◆ Use nonstick cookware and an aerosol cooking spray.

◆ Use small amounts of salad dressings, gravies, and spreads such as butter, margarine, and mayonnaise.

◆ Use the paste method for making gravy or sauces: add flour or cornstarch to cold liquids slowly and blend well.

◆ Season with herbs, lemon juice, or stock rather than lard, bacon, or ham.

◆ Skim fat from homemade soups or stews by chilling and removing the fat layer that rises to the top.

◆ Use fat-free or low-fat salad dressings.

◆ Use jam, jelly, or marmalade instead of butter or margarine.

◆ Rely on mustard and salad greens to add moisture to sandwiches rather than fat-laden spreads.

◆ Substitute plain low-fat yogurt for mayonnaise or sour cream or use light sour cream (compare fat content on labels).

◆ Limit fruits and vegetables that contain high levels of fat: olives, avocados, and coconuts.

Meat, Poultry, Fish, Dry Beans, and Eggs

◆ Have two or three servings of meat, poultry, or fish, with a daily total of about 6 oz.

◆ Choose a vegetarian entree (dry beans and peas) at least once a week.

◆ Include all types of meat. Consumer demand has resulted in livestock producers breeding animals to produce leaner beef and pork.

◆ Trim visible fat from meat; take skin off poultry before eating.

◆ Choose beef graded "select" because it contains fewer calories as a result of less fat marbling. The fat content of the meat is also dependent on the type of cut; leaner cuts include flank steak, sirloin or tenderloin, loin pork chops, 85% lean ground beef.

◆ Marinate leaner cuts of meat in lemon juice, flavored vinegars, or fruit juices.

◆ Use low-fat ground turkey or extra-lean ground beef in casseroles, spaghetti, and chili.

◆ Moderate the use of egg yolks (maximum of four egg yolks weekly) and organ meats.

◆ Limit organ meats such as liver, brains, and kidney.

◆ Choose tuna packed in water, not in oil (compare fat content on labels).

Milk and Milk Products

◆ Choose skim or low-fat milk and fat-free or low-fat yogurt and cottage cheese most of the time. Look for the words "1% fat," "99% fat-free," or "skimmed."

◆ Choose cheeses with 6 gm or fewer of fat per ounce (90% of the calories in cream cheese are from fat).

From Davis JR, Sherer K. *Applied Nutrition and Diet Therapy for Nurses,* 2nd ed. Philadelphia: W.B. Saunders, 1994.

excretion in the urine, affecting the body's calcium requirement.

The preferred amount of salt is dependent on the level of salt consumption; this preference can be lowered after reducing sodium intake for a while. Implementing the Guideline for Salt Intake presents some suggestions to help lower salt intake. Many food manufacturers have reduced the sodium content of their products or offer a reduced-sodium line.

Implementing the Guideline for Salt Intake

♦ Compare the sodium content of products by reading nutrition labels. Try the lower-sodium versions of canned soups, salad dressings, sauces, and other processed foods.

♦ Minimize intake of foods with a high sodium content due to food processing, such as bacon, cured meats, luncheon meats, sausage, sauerkraut, olives, and pickles.

♦ Learn to enjoy the natural flavors of foods, or try other seasonings such as lemon, garlic, or ginger.

♦ Use little or no salt at the table. Salt gives a sharper taste *on* food than *in* food, so it is better to add salt (in very small amounts) after food is prepared.

♦ Cook with only small amounts of added salt.

From Davis JR, Sherer K. *Applied Nutrition and Diet Therapy for Nurses*, 2nd ed. Philadelphia: W.B. Saunders, 1994.

IF YOU DRINK ALCOHOLIC BEVERAGES, DO SO IN MODERATION   Alcohol is high in calories and contains few if any nutrients. Moderate alcohol consumption is classified as one drink a day for women and no more than two drinks a day for men. An alcoholic beverage is defined as 12 oz of regular beer, 5 oz of wine, or 1½ oz of distilled spirits (80 proof). Alcohol may be retained in the blood for 3 to 5 hours; this poses a risk to clients who engage in activities that require attention or skill, especially driving, after consuming alcoholic drinks. Heavy drinking by pregnant women has been associated with birth defects. Many medications may be adversely affected (decreased benefits or increased toxicity) by alcohol.

SUMMATION OF THE DIETARY GUIDELINES

These goals work in conjunction with the Food Guide Pyramid, described below, to help clarify some points lacking in the food groups relating to optimal health, as shown in Table 1–3. All of these guidelines support healthy eating habits to improve health and quality of life, as shown in the sample menu in Figure 1–3.* Although the initial guidelines were controversial, other health and governmental organizations, such as the National Cancer Institute, American Cancer Society, and American Heart Association, have also issued guidelines regarding nutrition and health advice to reduce the risk of nutrition-related diseases in the United States.

Dental Hygiene Considerations

● These guidelines do not necessarily apply to clients requiring special diets, or with conditions that interfere with normal nutrition, or for children under 2 years of age.

● Assess the client's intake of the food groups, weight, blood pressure, and family history of hypertension, cardiovascular disease (strokes, heart attacks), and cancer.

● Encourage consumption of foods listed in Natural Food Sources of Complex Carbohydrates and Fiber and in Table 1–2.

● Encourage clients to follow suggestions listed in Implementing the Fat and Cholesterol Guideline.

● Evaluate the client's knowledge of foods low and high in fat, saturated fats, and cholesterol. A quick check is to have the client identify one or two foods that are high in these food components followed by one or two foods that can be substituted that are low in fat, saturated fats, and cholesterol. If the client is unable to do this, determine if the client knows where to find this information. If not, provide an educational booklet or information sheet.

* This sample menu will be used throughout this text to identify which foods provide specific nutrients, as appropriate.

TABLE 1–3 *Summary of Foods High in Cholesterol, Fat, Salt, and Sugar*

	Bread/Cereal Group	Fruit/Vegetable Group	Milk/Dairy Group	Meat/Protein Group
High in cholesterol			Butter and cream	Egg yolks, shrimp, organ meats, bacon, salt pork, and animal products
High in salt	Pretzels, salted crackers, highly seasoned rice, and pasta mixtures	Pickled vegetables (pickles and sauerkraut), regular canned vegetables, vegetable juices with added salt	Buttermilk	Canned fish and meats, chipped beef, and textured vegetable protein analogs
High in salt and fat	Salted snacks and chips	Potato chips, frozen vegetables in sauce, and olives	Natural cheeses, especially blue, Camembert, processed cheese, and cheese foods	Canned, dried, salted, cured meats or fish such as bacon, salt pork, ham, corned beef, sausage, frankfurters, luncheon meat, and corned beef
High in fat		French fries, fried vegetables, and avocados	Cream cheese, sour cream, whole milk, butter, cream, and whole milk yogurt	Duck, goose, nuts, brisket, oily fish (mackerel), and fish packed in oil
High in sugar and fat	Commercial granola, doughnuts, and pastries		Sweetened condensed milk; ice cream; malts and shakes; chocolate milk; whole-milk, fruit-flavored yogurt	
High in sugar	Presweetened breakfast cereals	Fruits canned or frozen in heavy syrup, juices with added sugar, and maraschino cherries		
Reduced in fiber; low in salt, fat, and sugar	Refined grains, especially white rice, degerminated cornmeal or flour, and white flour	Fruit juices and peeled fruits and vegetables		

Other foods or accessory foods provide calories and flavor but few nutrients. These foods should not replace foods in the food groups but can be used to enhance a diet. *Use moderation when selecting these foods:*
- Fats: Gravy, mayonnaise, cream and cream sauces, chocolate, coconut, solid shortening, most nondairy creamers
- Condiments (most are high in salt): Barbecue sauce, catsup, horseradish, mustard, olives, pickles, soy sauce, taco sauce

From Davis JR, Sherer K. *Applied Nutrition and Diet Therapy for Nurses,* 2nd ed. Philadelphia: W.B. Saunders, 1994.

Nutritional Directions

◆ Encourage clients to eat a variety of foods, but consume salt, sugar, alcohol, and fat in moderation.

◆ Describe the advantages of a diet high in grains, fruits, and vegetables.

◆ Dietetic and sugar-free foods may not be low in calories; this is dependent on other ingredients in the food.

◆ These guidelines may not be appropriate if the client has been told to follow a special diet or is ill.

◆ A physician or registered dietitian should be consulted before the client radically modifies his/her diet.

FIGURE 1–3 Sample menu based on the Dietary Guidelines for Americans.

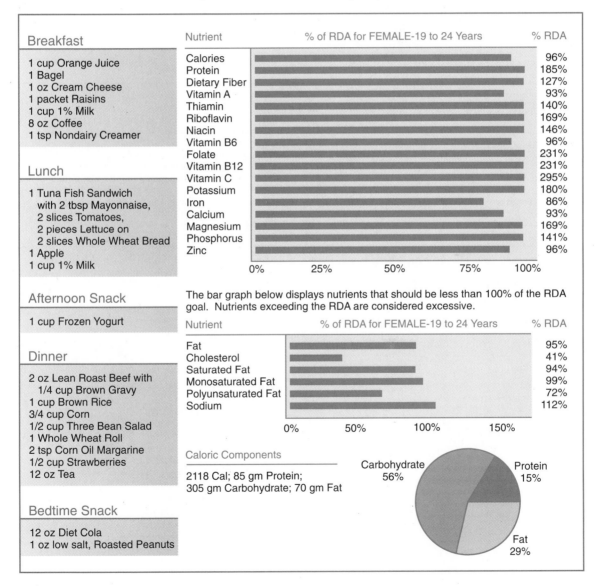

Breakfast

1 cup Orange Juice
1 Bagel
1 oz Cream Cheese
1 packet Raisins
1 cup 1% Milk
8 oz Coffee
1 tsp Nondairy Creamer

Lunch

1 Tuna Fish Sandwich
  with 2 tbsp Mayonnaise,
  2 slices Tomatoes,
  2 pieces Lettuce on
  2 slices Whole Wheat Bread
1 Apple
1 cup 1% Milk

Afternoon Snack

1 cup Frozen Yogurt

Dinner

2 oz Lean Roast Beef with
  1/4 cup Brown Gravy
1 cup Brown Rice
3/4 cup Corn
1/2 cup Three Bean Salad
1 Whole Wheat Roll
2 tsp Corn Oil Margarine
1/2 cup Strawberries
12 oz Tea

Bedtime Snack

12 oz Diet Cola
1 oz low salt, Roasted Peanuts

Nutrient	% of RDA for FEMALE-19 to 24 Years	% RDA
Calories		96%
Protein		185%
Dietary Fiber		127%
Vitamin A		93%
Thiamin		140%
Riboflavin		169%
Niacin		146%
Vitamin B6		96%
Folate		231%
Vitamin B12		231%
Vitamin C		295%
Potassium		180%
Iron		86%
Calcium		93%
Magnesium		169%
Phosphorus		141%
Zinc		96%

The bar graph below displays nutrients that should be less than 100% of the RDA goal. Nutrients exceeding the RDA are considered excessive.

Nutrient	% of RDA for FEMALE-19 to 24 Years	% RDA
Fat		95%
Cholesterol		41%
Saturated Fat		94%
Monosaturated Fat		99%
Polyunsaturated Fat		72%
Sodium		112%

Caloric Components

2118 Cal; 85 gm Protein;
305 gm Carbohydrate; 70 gm Fat

Carbohydrate 56%
Protein 15%
Fat 29%

◆ Explain that 1 tsp salt = 5 gm salt or 2,000 mg (2 gm) sodium.
◆ Instruct women who are pregnant or trying to conceive to abstain from alcohol.

Food Guide Pyramid

The Food Guide Pyramid (see inside cover and Fig. 1–4), which replaced the Basic Four Food Groups, was introduced by the USDA and USDHHS in 1992 as an implementation guide for the Dietary Guidelines for Americans. The Food Guide Pyramid organizes food into six groups, with the amount of space and location allotted to each group reflecting their relative value in the daily diet. Foods providing similar kinds of nutrients are grouped together, and therefore foods in one group cannot replace those in another (Table 1–4). This graphic was chosen to depict the three essential elements of a healthy diet: proportion, variety, and moderation. The five food groups in the lower sections are most important because each of these groups contributes some of the required nutrients. Using the Food Pyramid, the diet can be adapted

FIGURE 1–4 **Serving sizes. (Courtesy of the Education Department of the National Live Stock and Meat Board.)**

What Counts as 1 Serving?	▶ The amount you eat may be more than one serving. For example, a dinner portion of spaghetti would count as 2 or 3 servings.				

Bread, Cereal, Rice, & Pasta Group	Vegetable Group	Fruit Group	Milk, Yogurt, & Cheese Group	Meat, Poultry, Fish, Dry Beans, Eggs, & Nuts Group	Fats & Sweets
1 slice of bread ½ cup of cooked rice or pasta ½ cup of cooked cereal 1 ounce of ready-to-eat cereal	½ cup of chopped raw or cooked vegetables 1 cup of leafy raw vegetables	1 piece of fruit or melon wedge ¾ cup of juice ½ cup of canned fruit ¼ cup of dried fruit	1 cup of milk or yogurt 1½ ounces of natural cheese 2 ounces of process cheese	2½ to 3 ounces of cooked lean meat, poultry, or fish Count ½ cup of cooked beans, or 1 egg, or 2 tablespoons of peanut butter as 1 ounce of lean meat	LIMIT CALORIES FROM THESE especially if you need to lose weight

How Many Servings Do You Need Each Day?

	Women & some older adults	Children, teen girls, active women, most men	Teen boys & active men
Calorie level*	about 1,600	about 2,200	about 2,800
Bread group	6	9	11
Vegetable group	3	4	5
Fruit group	2	3	4
Milk group	2-3**	2-3**	2-3**
Meat group	2 for a total of 5 ounces	2 for a total of 6 ounces	3 for a total of 7 ounces

* These are the calorie levels if you choose lowfat, lean foods from the 5 major food groups and use foods from the fats and sweets group sparingly.

** Women who are pregnant or breastfeeding, teenagers, and young adults to age 24 need 3 servings.

A Closer Look at Fat and Added Sugars

The small tip of the Pyramid shows fats and sweets. These are foods such as salad dressings, cream, butter, margarine, sugars, soft drinks, candies, and sweet desserts. Alcoholic beverages are also part of this group. These foods provide calories but few vitamins and minerals. Most people should go easy on foods from this group.
Some fat or sugar symbols are shown in the other food groups. That's to remind you that some foods in these groups can also be high in fat and added sugars. When choosing foods for a healthful diet, consider the fat and added sugars in your choices from all food groups, not just fats and sweets from the Pyramid tip.

TABLE 1–4   *Principal Nutrient Contributions of Each Food Group*

Nutrients	Vegetable	Fruit	Meat	Milk	Grain
Protein			X	X	X
Vitamin A	X	X			
Vitamin D				X	
Vitamin E	X				
Vitamin C	X	X			
Thiamin			X		X
Riboflavin				X	
Niacin			X		X
Vitamin B_6			X	X	
Folacin	X	X			
Vitamin B_{12}			X	X	
Calcium				X	
Phosphorus			X	X	
Magnesium	X	X		X	
Iron			X		X
Zinc			X		
Fiber	X	X			X

From Davis JR, Sherer K. *Applied Nutrition and Diet Therapy for Nurses,* 2nd ed. Philadelphia: W.B. Saunders, 1994.

and modified imaginatively to meet the needs of clients and families with different levels of income, cultural patterns, and lifestyles.

Figure 1–5 depicts the typical eating practices of Americans today. Every food group except the Meat group and the Fat, Oils, and Sweets group is deficient in the number of servings consumed. Instead of a well-balanced diet, the American diet is top-heavy in high-calorie, low-nutrient value foods and deficient in foods from the groups at the base of the pyramid. Nutrition education is obviously needed to change eating habits and make structural changes to the client's personal food pyramid. When food choices are based on the Dietary Guidelines for Americans, intake of zinc, iron, and vitamin B_6 may be below the RDA (Dollahite et al., 1995).

BREADS, CEREALS, RICE AND PASTA GROUP   Six to 11 servings daily from the bread, cereal, rice, and pasta group are recommended. All whole-grain, refined and enriched, or fortified grain products are included in this group. Enriched

products have had iron, thiamin, riboflavin, folic acid, and niacin replaced approximately to their original levels. **Enrichment** is federally controlled by the U.S. Food and Drug Administration (FDA), which establishes the quantity of nutrients that can be added. Beginning in 1998, folic acid is added to all grain products (enriched bread, flour, cornmeal, pasta, grits, rice, and other grains). Whole-grain products contribute more fiber, magnesium, and folacin than do enriched products (Table 1–5). A variety of grain products should be selected, including wheat, rice, oats, and corn. Most processed breakfast cereals undergo **fortification** to achieve nutrient levels higher than those occurring naturally in the grain.

VEGETABLE AND FRUIT GROUPS   Fruits and vegetables are in two separate groups. Although three to five servings of vegetables and two to four servings of fruits daily are recommended, Americans consume an average of 4.3 servings of fruits and vegetables per day. Only 32% of the population consume the recommended five serv-

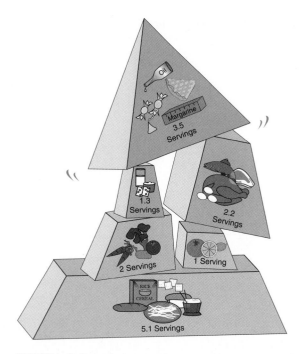

FIGURE 1–5 **Actual consumption pyramid, U.S. total. (From Eating in America Today, 2nd ed. A Dietary Pattern and Intake Report Commissioned by the National Live Stock and Meat Board, 1994.)**

and vitamins C and A, individual fruits and vegetables vary widely in their vitamin C and A content (note that vitamin C occurs naturally only in fruits and vegetables). A good source of vitamin C should be eaten daily; vitamin A-rich foods should be eaten three to four times a week (see Table 1–2). Dark-green vegetables also contribute calcium, iron, magnesium, riboflavin, and folate. Because of their high water and high fiber content, most fruits and vegetables are relatively low in calories.

Consumption of fruits and vegetables has been gradually increasing. Clients now have the opportunity to purchase fruits such as kiwis and papayas and vegetables such as Chinese cabbage and snow peas that were virtually unheard of 10 years ago. Additionally, more clients are choosing fruits as snacks. They are concerned about consuming a well-balanced diet, with fewer calories, and getting their money's worth.

MILK, YOGURT, AND CHEESE The dairy group excludes high-fat products such as butter and cream because they are not high in calcium, riboflavin, and protein. Fortified milk products are important sources of vitamin D; however, many milk substitutes (cheese, yogurt, and ice cream) are not fortified with vitamin D (unless made with fortified milk). Use of low-fat milk products can decrease calorie content significantly. Serving recommendations for this group are based on calcium requirements for various stages of life (see Fig. 1–4).

ings per day, and half the population consume no fruits on any given day. Vegetables and fruits in season (at their peak of production and lowest in price) are the most flavorful and highest in nutrient value in most cases. Although foods in both of these groups are valuable for their contribution of fiber

TABLE 1–5   *Comparison of Nutrient Values of Selected Whole-Grain and Enriched Products*

Types of Bread	Protein (gm)	Total Dietary Fiber (gm)	Thiamin (mg)	Ribo-flavin (mg)	Niacin (mg)	Vitamin B_6 (mg)	Folacin (mcg)	Panto-thenic Acid (mcg)	Iron (mg)	Zinc (mg)	Cal-cium (mg)	Phos-phorus (mg)	Magne-sium (mg)
Whole wheat	2	2.8	0.09	0.05	1	0.05	14	0.18	0.9	0.42	18	65	23
Rye	2	1.6	0.10	0.08	0.8	0.02	10	0.11	0.7	0.32	20	36	6
Enriched white	2	0.4	0.11	0.07	0.9	0.08	8	0.10	0.7	0.14	29	25	5

Nutrient data from Nutritionist IV software, First Data Bank, San Bruno, CA.

From Davis JR, Sherer K. *Applied Nutrition and Diet Therapy for Nurses,* 2nd ed. Philadelphia: W.B. Saunders, 1994.

TABLE 1–6　*Outstanding Contributions of Various Protein Foods*

Protein Food	Nutrient
Lean red meats	Iron
	B vitamins
	Zinc
Pork	Thiamin
Liver and egg yolks	Vitamin A
	Iron
Dry peas and beans, soybeans, and nuts	Magnesium
	Fiber

From Davis JR, Sherer K. *Applied Nutrition and Diet Therapy for Nurses*, 2nd ed. Philadelphia: W.B. Saunders, 1994.

MEATS, POULTRY, FISH, DRY BEANS AND PEAS, EGGS, AND NUTS　The foods in this group are important sources of protein, iron, and essential trace minerals. Choices within this group should include a variety, since each food has distinct nutritional advantages. Various meat choices or high-protein foods are outstanding for their individual contributions (Table 1–6).

OTHER FOODS　Foods at the top of the pyramid might well be called the "icing on the cake"; fats, oils, and sweets provide mainly energy and few other nutrients. These foods contribute to palatability and make some nutritious foods more desirable. For instance, some clients may dislike milk but enjoy pudding or custard. In addition to providing a prolonged feeling of **satiety,** some fats and oils are a good source of vitamin A and E.

In general, the amounts of these foods to include in the diet depend on the energy level needed. When only the specified amounts of foods from the basic food groups are consumed, the caloric intake ranges from about 1,200 to 1,500 calories, far below the energy needs of a teenager or a person with high energy expenditure. But most adults should use these foods sparingly.

Dental Hygiene Considerations

- Assess each client's diet to determine nutrient adequacy or inadequacy. (For example, if a client dislikes fruits and vegetables, vitamin A and C deficiencies may develop; if milk and other milk products are eliminated, calcium deficiencies may develop.)
- Be sure clients are aware of the number and size of servings they should eat from each food group daily to obtain adequate nutrients.

Nutritional Directions

- Within each food group, foods can vary widely in the number of calories furnished; therefore it is important to be knowledgeable about serving sizes.
- Milk products are poor sources of iron and vitamin C, but they are good sources of protein, calcium, and riboflavin.
- Caloric consumption can be decreased by substituting low-fat or skim milk for whole milk.
- Foods in the bread-cereal group are economical as well as nutritious; they may be staple items for those in lower socioeconomic groups. These foods by themselves are not high in calories.
- Cholesterol occurs naturally in all foods of animal origin.
- Foods not classified in the basic food groups (i.e., sugars, fats, and alcohol) are intended to complement, not replace, foods from the other groups.

Nutrition Labeling

In a concerted effort by the USDA and the FDA to improve the health and well-being of the American people by enhancing nutritional knowledge, the U.S. government established in 1994 the Nutrition Facts food label as a graphic tool to inform consumers in the supermarket. Nutrition labels on product packaging help health educators and consumers know what nutrients are in a food and to compare nutritional values of various products.

The new labeling policy requires that 90% of all foods, including some fresh produce, meat, and fish, provide nutritional information based on the nutrients provided in a single serving. For foods that are not packaged, the information must be displayed at the point of purchase (e.g., in a counter card, sign, or booklet). Serving portions are more standardized and are based on the reference amount normally consumed by an average person. The number of servings in a container is expressed to the nearest whole number.

Nutrients provided on the label include total calories, total calories from fats; total fat and saturated fat (gm); cholesterol (gm); total carbohydrates, complex carbohydrates, and sugars (gm); dietary fiber (gm); protein (gm), and sodium (mg); vitamins and minerals (%) are listed as a percentage of Daily Values (DVs) or Reference Values (RVs). Inclusion of the following information is voluntary: calories from saturated and unsaturated fatty acids; kilocalories from total carbohydrate and protein; and amounts (gm) of unsaturated, polyunsaturated, and monounsaturated fatty acids, sugar alcohols, soluble and insoluble fiber, and potassium, and other vitamins (thiamin, riboflavin, niacin).

Two new sets of reference values are used to indicate nutrient content of the product. **Reference Daily Intakes** (RDIs) are the basis for the percentage of the DVs or RVs for protein, vitamins, and minerals. The RDIs are different from the RDAs previously discussed and should not be confused with them. There are actually five sets of RDIs, which are designed for special foods for infants, children under 4, pregnant women, lactating women, adults, and children over 4 years of age (see Appendix B). Following completion of establishing DRIs for all sets of nutrient groups, the DRIs will be this basis for DVs and RVs on nutrition labels.

A product's nutrition profile is based on the percentage of **Daily Reference Values** (DRVs) of the nutrients it contains (Table 1–7). Only DVs are included on the label, which reflects how the food product affects a 2,000-calorie diet. Thus, consumers can use this as a guideline for maintaining appropriate dietary intake. Figure 1–6 depicts a sample of a nutrition label and explains the type information displayed.

A label cannot include an explicit or implied nutrient content claim unless it uses terms that have been defined by the FDA, such as "free," "low,"

TABLE 1–7 *Daily Reference Values**

	% of Calories†	Highest Desirable Amount
Protein	10‡	
Carbohydrate	60	
Fat	30	<65 gm
Satuated fat	10	<20 gm
Cholesterol		<300 mg
Sodium		<2,400 mg
Fiber		11.5 gm per 1,000 calories

*Daily Reference Values (DRVs) do not appear on the nutrient label. The term *Daily Value* which appears on the label for ease of understanding, reflects the DRV and the RDI standards.
†Based on a reference intake of 2000 cal/day.
‡Protein amount is for adults and children over age 4 only. The RDI for protein has been established for certain groups of people: children 1 to 4 years, 16 gm; infants under 1 year, 14 gm; pregnant women, 60 gm; nursing mothers, 65 gm.
From Davis JR, Sherer K. *Applied Nutrition and Diet Therapy for Nurses,* 2nd ed. Philadelphia: W.B. Saunders, 1994.

"more," or "reduced." Table 1–8 and Nutrient Content Descriptors define the established terms and will be helpful as reference tools.

Only health claims that are supported by substantial scientific evidence and authorized by the FDA can be used. Health claims addressed by the FDA include claims dealing with the relationship between sodium and hypertension, calcium and osteoporosis, lipids and cancer, and lipids and cardiovascular disease. Despite an association between consumption of fiber and blood cholesterol levels and some cancers, the FDA has concluded that evidence to support these claims is insufficient to authorize either health claim.

Dental Hygiene Considerations

- The dental hygienist must make sure that the set of RDIs used is appropriate for the client's age or grouping (e.g., when talking to a pregnant client, the RDI for pregnancy should be used).
- To prevent confusion, the acronyms RDI and DRV are not used on labels; however, dental hygienists need to be aware of the basis for the information presented.

The New Food Label at a Glance

The new food label will carry an up-to-date, easier-to-use nutrition information guide, to be required on almost all packaged foods (compared to about 60 percent of products up till now). The guide will serve as a key to help in planning a healthy diet.*

Serving sizes are now more consistent across product lines, stated in both household and metric measures, and reflect the amounts people actually eat.

The list of nutrients covers those most important to the health of today's consumers, most of whom need to worry about getting too much of certain items (fat, for example), rather than too few vitamins or minerals, as in the past.

The label will now tell the number of calories per gram of fat, carbohydrates, and protein.

New title signals that the label contains the newly required information.

Calories from fat are now shown on the label to help consumers meet dietary guidelines that recommend people get no more than 30 percent of their calories from fat.

% Daily Value shows how a food fits into the overall daily diet.

Daily Values are also something new. Some are maximums, as with fat (65 grams or less); others are minimums, as with carbohydrates (300 grams or more). The daily values on the label are based on a daily diet of 2,000 and 2,500 calories. Individuals should adjust the values to fit their own calorie intake.

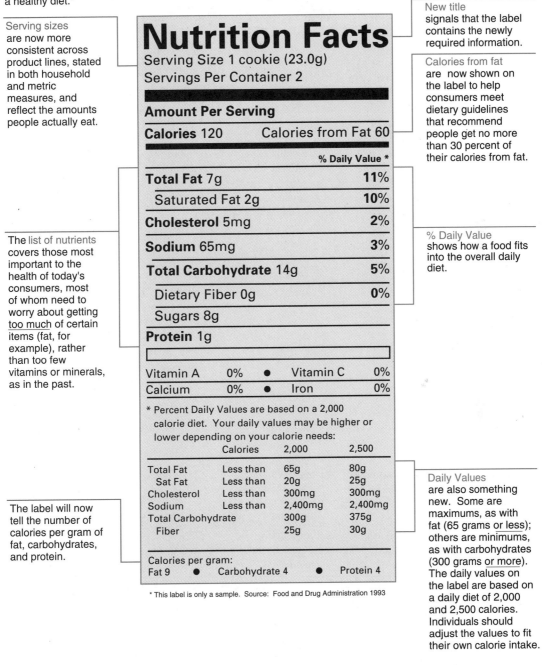

Nutrition Facts

Serving Size 1 cookie (23.0g)
Servings Per Container 2

Amount Per Serving

Calories 120   Calories from Fat 60

	% Daily Value *
Total Fat 7g	**11%**
Saturated Fat 2g	**10%**
Cholesterol 5mg	**2%**
Sodium 65mg	**3%**
Total Carbohydrate 14g	**5%**
Dietary Fiber 0g	**0%**
Sugars 8g	
Protein 1g	

Vitamin A	0%	●	Vitamin C	0%
Calcium	0%	●	Iron	0%

* Percent Daily Values are based on a 2,000 calorie diet. Your daily values may be higher or lower depending on your calorie needs:

	Calories	2,000	2,500
Total Fat	Less than	65g	80g
Sat Fat	Less than	20g	25g
Cholesterol	Less than	300mg	300mg
Sodium	Less than	2,400mg	2,400mg
Total Carbohydrate		300g	375g
Fiber		25g	30g

Calories per gram:
Fat 9   ●   Carbohydrate 4   ●   Protein 4

* This label is only a sample. Source: Food and Drug Administration 1993

FIGURE 1–6 The new food label at a glance. (Adapted from Kurtzweil P. 'Nutrition facts' to help consumers eat smart. *FDA Consumer* 1993; 27(4):22–27.

TABLE 1–8   *Definitions of Nutrition Labeling Terms*

	Free*	Low*	Reduced† or Less‡	Other
Synonyms	No, zero, without, trivial source of, negligible source of, dietarily insignificant source of	Little, few, small amounts of, low source of, low in	Reduced, reduced in, fewer, less, lower, lower in	
Generalized meaning	Contains no or "physiologically inconsequential" amounts of one or more of the following: calories, sugars, fat, saturated fat, cholesterol, or sodium; or no added sugar, salt, or fat	Appropriate for foods that could be eaten frequently without exceeding dietary guidelines for one or more of the following: calories, fat, saturated fat, cholesterol, sodium	Nutritionally altered product that contains ≤25% of a nutrient or of calories than the regular, or reference product	
Calories	≤5 cal/serving	≤40 cal/serving	≥25% fewer calories/serving	"Light": ≥33.3% reduction of cal/serving
Sugars§	≤0.5 gm/serving‖		≥25% less sugar/serving	
Sodium	≤5 mg/serving	≤140 mg/serving	≥25% less sodium/serving	Very low sodium; ≤35 mg/serving Light: ≥50% reduction of sodium/serving
Fat	≤0.5 gm/serving	≤3 gm/serving	≥25% less fat/serving	"Light": ≥50% reduction of fat/serving
Saturated fatty acids¶	≤0.5 gm/serving and ≤1% of total fat from trans fatty acids	≤1 gm/serving and ≤15% of calories from saturated fatty acids	≥25% less saturated fat/serving	
Cholesterol	≤2 mg/serving and ≤2 gm saturated fat	≤20 mg/serving and ≤2 gm of saturated fat	≥25% less cholesterol/serving	

*A claim for a food being "free" or "low" implies that the food differs from other foods of the same type. These foods have been specially processed, altered, formulated, or reformulated to decrease the amount of nutrient in the food.

†The term *reduced* cannot be used if the reference food already meets the requirement for a "low" claim.

‡Whether altered or not, the product contains 25% less than the regular or reference product.

§*Sugars* are defined as the sum of all free monosaccharides and disaccharides (glucose, fructose, lactose, and sucrose).

‖If "sugar-free" or "sugarless" are used, the label must indicate whether the food is "low calorie" or "calorie reduced", or "not a reduced calorie food" or "not for weight control."

¶If claims are made with respect to the level of saturated fat, the level of total fat and cholesterol in the food must be disclosed unless the food contains ≤2 mg of cholesterol/serving and ≤3 gm total fat/serving, in which case the cholesterol or fat content, respectively, can be omitted.

Data from FDA Backgrounder: The New Food Label. Washington, D.C., December, 1992; and *Fed Reg* 1993; 58(3).

From Davis JR, Sherer K. *Applied Nutrition and Diet Therapy for Nurses,* 2nd ed. Philadelphia: W.B. Saunders, 1994.

Nutrient Content Descriptors

Expressed nutrient claim: Any direct statement about the level or range of a nutrient in the food.

Implied nutrient claim: Description of the product in a manner that suggests that a nutrient is absent or present in a certain amount or that the food may be useful in maintaining healthy dietary practices and is made in association with an explicit claim or statement about a nutrient. These misleading claims are prohibited. For example, a product that contains oat fiber must contain enough oat bran to meet the definition of a "good source" of fiber to claim "made with oat bran."

Substitute food: A food that can be used interchangeably with another food that (1) has similar performance characteristics, (2) is not nutritionally inferior to the reference food (unless labeled "imitation"), and (3) complies with compositional requirements set by FDA.

High: Contains 20% or more of the DV per serving for a particular nutrient.

Good source: Contains 10% to 19% of the DV per serving for a particular nutrient.

Relative claim: A statement that compares the level of a nutrient in the product with the level of a nutrient in a reference food. Relative claims include the terms "light," "reduced," "less," "fewer," and "more." Relative claims can be made for a product if the nutrient content of the reference food meets the requirement for "low," "less," "fewer," or "more" or if the product can be compared with a dissimilar food within a product category that can generally be substituted for the product in the diet (e.g., potato chips as reference for pretzels) or a similar food (e.g., potato chips as reference for potato chips). For "light," "reduced," "added," "fortified," and "enriched" claims, the reference food must be a similar food. To bear a relative claim, the amount of the nutrient in that food must be compared with the amount of that nutrient in an appropriate reference food, and the label must do the following: (1) identify the reference food; (2) state as a percentage or fraction the degree to which the reference food has been modified (e.g., "50% fewer calories than _____ "); (3) provide quantitative comparison of the amount of the nutrient in the product with the amount in the reference food; (4) provide information immediately adjacent to the most prominent claim.

More: Natural or added content of a nutrient is at least 10% of the DV more than the reference food; applies to "fortified" and "enriched" foods.

Fresh: Indicates that a food is raw or unprocessed (raw, never been frozen or heated, and contains no preservatives). Low levels of irradiation are allowed. "Fresh frozen," "frozen fresh," and "freshly frozen" can be used for foods that are quickly frozen while still fresh. Blanching is allowed. Exceptions to the use of this term include "fresh" as used in "fresh milk" or "freshly baked bread."

Percent fat free: The product must be a low-fat or a fat-free product. The claim must also reflect the amount of fat in 100 gm of the food.

Lean and Extra lean: Describes fat content of meat and seafood products. "Lean": ≤10 gm fat, ≥4 gm saturated fat, and ≤95 mg cholesterol per serving and per 100 gm. "Extra lean": ≤5 gm fat, ≥2 gm saturated fat, and ≤95 mg cholesterol per serving and per 100 gm.

Meals and main dishes: Must meet same requirements as those for individual foods. "Low calorie": contains <120 calories. "Low sodium": contains <20 mg cholesterol/100 gm and no more than 2 gm saturated fat. "Light": low fat or low calorie, or a low-calorie, low-fat food whose sodium content been decreased by 50%.

Healthy: Describes a food that is low in fat (≤3 gm) and saturated fat (≤1 gm) and contains ≤60 mg cholesterol and ≤480 mg sodium per serving and at least 10% of the RDI or DRV of *one* of the following per reference amount: vitamin A, vitamin C, protein, calcium, iron, or fiber.

Data from FDA Backgrounder: The New Food Label. Washington, D.C., 1992, and *Fed Reg* 1993:58.
From Davis JR, Sherer K. *Applied Nutrition and Diet Therapy for Nurses,* 2nd ed. Philadelphia: W.B. Saunders, 1994.

- From the new label (see Fig. 1–5), the number of teaspoons of sugar in that food product can be determined. Four grams of sugar is equivalent to 1 level teaspoon of sugar. Thus, a product containing 16 gm of sugar has 4 tsp of sugar.
- To determine the percentage of sugar in a serving of a food, (1) multiply the number of grams of sugar in a product by 4 (cal/gm); (2) divide this number by the total number of calories per serving; and (3) multiply by 100 to establish the percentage of calories as sugar. Using the example of the label shown in Figure 1–5:

$$8 \text{ g sugar} \times 4 \text{ Cal/gm} = 32 \text{ Cal from sugar}$$

$$\frac{32 \text{ Cal sugar}}{120 \text{ Cal/serving}} = 0.27 \times 100 = 27\%$$

Nutritional Directions

- Labels should be read carefully. Ingredients are listed in order of quantity (by weight). Choose products that have less fat or oils or in which fats are listed last.
- The RDIs are a useful tool to compare nutrient values of foods and to learn valuable sources of nutrients. Review a label together with the client and/or family.
- Fortified foods and supplements should not be purchased in an attempt to meet 100% of the RDIs because this may result in greater food consumption than is needed, especially for young children. Concerns should be addressed to the physician.
- The DRVs on nutrition labels help in comparing processed foods in terms of their fat, saturated fat, cholesterol, carbohydrate, sodium, and fiber content. Using an actual nutrient label, review the information presented with clients and discuss how the information can be used to compare various products available.
- Because portion sizes between products can vary, remind clients to compare these when comparing products.

- On a label, point out the DVs that indicate calories (carbohydrate, fat, and protein), those that indicate maximum intake (fat, saturated fat, cholesterol, and sodium), and those that reflect minimum recommended amounts (carbohydrate and fiber).
- Unsweetened juices and milk contain significant amounts of sugars because of the natural content of simple carbohydrates. This may be confusing for some clients since both are encouraged in appropriate amounts.
- Soluble fiber is considered in the total carbohydrate calories, but not insoluble fiber.

HEALTH APPLICATION 1

Obesity

According to a 1995 report by the Institute of Medicine, 59% of American adults are clinically obese (Gibbs, 1996); one of the goals of the U.S. Public Health Services' *Healthy People 2000* nutritional objectives is to reduce the prevalence of obesity to less than 20%. Another objective indirectly addresses prevention of obesity: "To increase to at least 30% the proportion of people aged 6 and older who engage regularly, preferably daily, in light to moderate physical activity for at least 30 minutes per day."

The terms "overweight" and "obesity" are used interchangeably, but are technically very different. Desirable body weight (DBW) or ideal body weight (IBW) can be used to denote a weight for height considered to be healthy for a patient. Overweight, defined as excess weight for height, is identified as 10% to 20% above DBW. Obesity, or 20% above DBW, is excess accumulation of body fat. Morbid obesity refers to more than 100 lbs over DBW.

Many people, although normal or below normal in weight, have excess amounts of fat stores. Athletes are usually overweight because of their increased muscle mass, not excess fat. Being overweight is not the same as being fat or obese. Additional muscle tissue aids body functions, but excessive fat interferes with normal body metabolism. A desirable weight for a patient depends on the amount and location of body fat and other weight-related medical problems.

Excess fat in the abdominal area (the "apple-shaped" body), known as android obesity, is characteristic of men. Accumulation of fat in the hips or femoral (thigh) (the "pear-shaped body"), called gynoid obesity, is typical of women. Any amount of upper-body obesity or increased abdominal fat increases health risks. In contrast, lower-body or gynoid obesity is relatively benign. However, clients with this pattern of obesity have more difficulty losing weight and maintaining IBW.

Obesity is the result of consistent caloric overconsumption in excess of energy expenditure. Food intake is controlled by many different mechanisms: hormonal, metabolic, dietary, social, and psychological. Obesity probably has different causes, thereby resulting in different characteristics and warranting differing treatments.

In some cases, understanding physiologic benefits of weight loss can be motivating for some clients. Weight loss is highly desirable in those with certain risk factors and advisable for others. Weight loss is associated with a decrease in serum glucose, cholesterol, systolic blood pressure, and uric acid. Other physical symptoms that can be expected to improve with weight loss include shortness of breath, easy fatigability, fluid retention, gastric disorders, headaches, decreased energy level, decreased sexual interest, joint pains, muscle cramps, elevated pulse rate, restless sleep, urinary infection, and varicose veins.

Treatment of obesity has a high level of noncompliance and failure. Weight loss should be motivated by internal rather than external reasons ("I am doing this for myself" rather than "I will lose weight for my son's wedding"). Any treatment for weight loss should always be a serious undertaking with a high level of motivation and long-term commitment. This ap-

proach increases chances that the plan will be followed until weight is lost, and that weight loss will be maintained.

A pound of fat equals 3,500 calories. Losing weight can be accomplished by eating less, increasing activity, or a combination of both. When 2 lb or more per week are lost, clients are more enthusiastic about the method of loss. To accomplish this goal, food intake must be 500 calories less than needed per day, which will result in a 1-lb loss per week. An additional energy expenditure of 500 calories per day is recommended for the other pound of weight loss. Effective weight loss is a slow process.

Numerous strategies have been used to treat overweight and obesity. No one treatment is best for everyone; each modality varies in effectiveness, risk, and cost. A realistic goal regarding the rate and amount of weight loss must be established for each dieter.

Numerous diets have been devised for weight loss. The mainstay of weight loss is restriction of energy intake. A weight-reduction diet needs to be followed for an extended period of time; therefore, it must be appealing and flexible as well as affordable for the dieter. It can be balanced yet hypocaloric. The diet should include foods from each food group to provide necessary nutrients.

A diet that totally eliminates one category (fat or carbohydrate) or specific group of foods (fruits or meats) is inadvisable because essential nutrients may also be eliminated. Indispensable to any weight loss program is a pre-planned food allotment with specified times for eating throughout the day to lessen feelings of deprivation and to eliminate excessive food intake. The total amount of food should be divided into at least three feedings. Eating only once or twice a day has been associated with increased adipose tissue and serum cholesterol and impulsive snacking. Some "free" foods or beverages may be available for snack periods, but regular mealtimes are important. A diet that requires the least amount of change in usual dietary patterns has better long-term

Evaluating Weight-Loss Diets

Is the program preceded by careful screening to determine the degree of overweight and its contributing causes?

What is the nature of the diet program? (Are special foods, beverages, or vitamins required?)

Are individual differences considered in determining energy needs?

What is the recommended rate of weight loss?

How successful is the program?

Are advertisements and endorsements based on solid facts or testimonials?

How much does the program cost, what do the fees include, and how is payment required? (Are there costs for foods, nutrient supplements, initial membership, or weekly fees?)

What are the side effects and health risks associated with the program?

Is proper medical supervision provided?

Is an exercise and behavior modification component included?

Does the program offer a maintenance plan and, if so, at what cost?

Can you live with the program indefinitely?

From National Dairy Council. Promoting a healthy weight. *Dairy Council Dig* 1991; 62(2):7-12.

success. A 1,200- to 1,500-calorie diet is relatively safe; when accompanied by an exercise program, the rate of weight loss is augmented and muscle mass is maintained.

A weight-reduction diet should satisfy the following criteria: (1) meets all nutrient needs except energy; (2) suits tastes and habits; (3) minimizes hunger and fatigue; (4) is accessible and socially acceptable; (5) encourages a change in eating pattern; and (6) favors improvement in overall health. Evaluating Weight-Loss Diets provides some questions of use in determining the validity of a weight-reduction diet.

Treatment of obesity is improved when increased energy expenditure occurs along with decreased caloric intake. Exercise alone has only a modest effect on weight loss; it affects energy metabolism. Exercise incorporated into a weight-control program offers the advantages of improved cardiovascular fitness, plasma lipoprotein profile, and carbohydrate metabolism, increased energy expenditure, and enhanced psychological well-being. The initiation of an exercise regimen may lead to weight gain in the form of muscle mass.

Behavior Modification

Behavior modification for weight control refers to getting in touch with the reality of which foods are being consumed and in what quantity, and when and why eating occurs. One of the most important components of an effective weight-control program is learning new ways of dealing with old habits (see Behavior Modification Techniques). Comprehensive behavior-modification programs include diet and exercise programs individually tailored for clients. A team approach utilizing a physician,

Behavior-Modification Techniques

1. Eat regularly in the same place.
2. Use smaller plates and containers.
3. Put down the utensils between each bite.
4. Do not watch television or read while eating.
5. Take at least 20 minutes to eat each meal.
6. Store leftover food immediately to avoid returning for second helpings.
7. Buy only appropriate food to have available.
8. Arrange an attractive meal and serve it accordingly.
9. Sit down to eat.
10. Leave a small amount of food on the plate (one or two bites).
11. Do not taste food while preparing: an alternative is to chew sugar-free gum or brush teeth to help resist temptations.

From Davis JR, Sherer K. *Applied Nutrition and Diet Therapy for Nurses,* 2nd ed. Philadelphia: W.B. Saunders, 1994.

psychologist, registered dietitian, and the family is more effective in helping the patient make necessary long-lasting changes in food choices. A food diary for recording amounts and types of food eaten, emotional status, and environmental factors helps to provide new insights to devise strategies for dealing with eating habits. Although behavior-modification approaches to weight control are helpful, maintaining weight loss still remains a problem. Studies indicate that programs need to be approximately 20 to 24 weeks long and more comprehensive, including relapse prevention training and use of social support systems.

CASE APPLICATION FOR THE DENTAL HYGIENIST

A young healthy mother who has a 3-year-old son at home comes to the dental office for a 6-month recall. She expresses concern about foods she should be eating and feeding her husband and son to improve/maintain their nutrition. She has learned a little about new food groups, the Dietary Guidelines for Americans, and labeling changes from the press but does not know how to implement them.

Nutritional Assessment

○ Willingness to seek nutritional information
○ Desire for increased control of nutritional health habits
○ Knowledge of community resources
○ Cultural or religious influences
○ Knowledge regarding the Dietary Guidelines for Americans, food labels, and the Food Guide Pyramid
○ Definition of optimal nutrition

Nutritional Diagnosis

Health-seeking behaviors related to lack of knowledge concerning optimal nutrition and current standards.

Nutritional Goals

Client verbalizes correct information concerning the Dietary Guidelines, food labels, and can name the food groups and the number of servings needed from each group of the Food Guide Pyramid.

Nutritional Implementation

Intervention: Encourage variety of food intake, utilizing the Food Guide Pyramid. Review the number of servings needed and what consists of a serving size.
Rationale: It is the total balance of diet that matters, and the best balance incorporates variety to promote optimal nutrition. Providing the minimal number of servings will prevent nutritional deficiencies in healthy people.

Intervention: (1) Suggest that the mother and her husband have their blood lipid profiles checked if not recently done; (2) emphasize a decreased intake of fats, saturated fats, and cholesterol by trimming excess fat and eating smaller servings of meat (about the size of a fist or a deck of cards).
Rationale: By decreasing fats and saturated fats and cholesterol, one can decrease the risk of heart disease.

Intervention: (1) Stress the importance of eating vegetables, fruits, and grains; (2) explain that complex carbohydrates are not fattening; (3) encourage foods listed in the Natural Food Sources of Complex Carbohydrates and Fiber box; (d) use guidelines in Implementing the Guideline for Increasing Fiber.
Rationale: Dietary fiber is important for healthy bowel functioning and can reduce symptoms of chronic constipation, diverticular disease, and hemorrhoids and decrease the

risk of developing obesity, cancer, and diabetes.

Intervention: (1) Explain how to read labels for sugar. The name of most sugars end in "-ose"; (2) emphasize moderation of sugar intake; (3) explain that "dietetic" and "sugar-free" do not necessarily mean that the product is low in calories; (4) explain the relation between sugar and tooth decay and emphasize the importance of proper oral hygiene after its use.

Rationale: Refined sugar contains calories and no other nutrients but is acceptable when used in items that contain appreciable amounts of other nutrients (e.g., a pudding would provide more nutrients than a congealed dessert or carbonated beverages).

Intervention: (1) Stress using sodium and salt in moderation; (2) follow suggestions in Implementing the Guideline for Salt Intake; (3) emphasize that "no salt added" does not mean that the product is low in sodium.

Rationale: Good habits that do not foster a high level of salt preference are recommended.

Intervention: Emphasize that any alcohol intake should be in moderation (one drink a day for women and two drinks a day for men), if at all.

Rationale: Alcohol is high calorie and contains few if any nutrients.

Intervention: (1) Actually review an entire label with the mother to help her understand how to utilize it; (2) determine a serving size; (3) explain the types of carbohydrates; (4) determine the percentage of fat in a product by multiplying the grams of fat by 9 and compare this number to the total calories; if amount is more than 30%, do not consume that product every day; (5) look at cholesterol levels; (6) emphasize that "no cholesterol" does not necessarily mean that the product contains no saturated fat; (7) identify the product's sodium level and if it is above 400 mg, encourage its use in moderation.

Rationale: Knowledge increases compliance and allows one to make informed choices regarding food selections.

Intervention: Refer the client to county extension agencies or to a registered dietitian.

Rationale: These agencies and nutritional professionals provide practical guidelines via newsletters, workshops, and written materials for healthy clients wanting to improve health.

Evaluation

To determine effectiveness of care, have the client read labels and choose the best buy for the nutrient content; have patient state the seven basic guidelines for nutrition and explain to her that these are not an accurate guide for her son. Additionally, patient should be able to plan a menu utilizing foods recommended and to state how to obtain or actually use community information/support.

Student Readiness

1. A patient asks you the difference between food and nutrition. What would you say?
2. Locate an advertisement in a popular magazine or newspaper for a weight-reduction product and list the merits of the product stated in the ad. Then list information about the product that might have been omitted or should be questioned.
3. Discuss popular weight-reduction diets and how they may have adverse effects.
4. Distinguish between recommendations and requirements.

5. Keep a record of all the foods you eat for 24 hours. Was your intake adequate as evaluated by the Food Guide Pyramid? How does it measure up to the Dietary Guidelines?

6. Collect nutrient labels for three similar products. Compare the nutrient values to determine which is a better source of nutrients. Which is a better buy for the amount of nutrients it contains?

7. List the Dietary Guidelines for Americans. List your favorite food items from each category and the frequency of consumption. Are these moderate amounts? If not, what are some foods that you could substitute for them?

8. Discuss the pros and cons of allowing nutritional claims on products.

9. If a food label indicates that one serving of the product has 23 gm of carbohydrate and 15 gm of sugar with 140 calories (total), how many teaspoons of sugar does the product contain?

References

Dollahite J et al. Problems encountered in meeting the Recommended Dietary Allowances for menus designed according to the Dietary Guidelines for Americans. *J Am Diet Assoc* 1995; 95 (3):341–4, 370.

Gibbs WW. Trends in medicine: gaining on fat. *Sci Amer* 1996; 275(2):88–94.

Leibel RL et al. Changes in energy expenditure resulting from altered body weight. *N Engl J Med* 1995 Mar; 332(10):621–628.

Manson JE et al. Body weight and mortality among women. *N Engl J Med* 1995 Sept; 333(11):677–685.

Putnam JJ, Duewer LA. U.S. per capita food consumption: Record high meat and sugars in 1994. *Food Rev* 1995; 18(2):2–11.

Zizza C, Gerrior S. The US food supply provides more of most nutrients. *Food Rev* 1995; 18(1):40–45.

Chapter 2

The Alimentary Canal: Digestion and Absorption

LEARNING OBJECTIVES

The Student Will Be Able To:

- Discuss factors that influence food intake.
- Describe general functions of each digestive organ.
- Identify chemical secretions necessary for digestion of energy-containing nutrients and in what parts of the gastrointestinal tract they are located.
- Name the nutrients that require digestion and the digested products that can be absorbed.
- Explain the role of gastrointestinal motility in the digestion and absorption process.
- Identify nutritional directions for digestion and absorption.
- Apply digestion and absorption processes that affect nutritional status into dental hygiene practice.

GLOSSARY OF TERMS

Hydrolysis   the splitting of a large molecule into smaller ones that are water-soluble and can be used by cells; the reaction requires water

Enzymes   complex proteins that enable the metabolic reactions to proceed at a faster rate without being exhausted themselves

Peristalsis   the involuntary rhythmic waves of contraction traveling the whole length of the alimentary tract

Valves/sphincter muscles   door-like mechanisms between the digestive segments

Taste buds   the receptors for the sense of taste

Olfactory nerves   the receptors for smell

Anosmia   the loss of smell

Dysgeusia   the persistent, abnormal distortion of taste, including sweet, sour, bitter, salty, or metallic tastes. Dysgeusia without identifiable taste stimuli is called *phantom taste*

Hypogeusia   the loss of taste

Hypergeusia   heightened taste acuity

Anorexia   poor appetite

Xerostomia   dryness of the mouth from inadequate salivary secretion

Masticatory efficiency   how well the client prepares the food for swallowing

Bolus   a mass of food that is swallowed and passed into the stomach

Lower esophageal sphincter   a group of very strong circular muscle fibers located just above the stomach

Bile   an emulsifier that helps in the digestion of fats

Emulsify   to break up fats into smaller particles by lowering the surface tension

Osmosis   the passage of water through a semi-permeable membrane to equalize osmotic pressure exerted by ions in solutions

Residue   the total amount of fecal solids, including undigested or unabsorbed food, and metabolic (bile pigments) and bacterial products

Test Your NQ (True/False)

1. The alimentary tract is about 30 feet long. T/F
2. The hydrolysis of carbohydrate yields fatty acid and glycerol. T/F
3. Most absorption occurs in the stomach. T/F
4. Fat-soluble nutrients always enter the portal circulation. T/F
5. Taste disorders are often the result of problems in smell rather than taste. T/F
6. Lactose is the name of an enzyme. T/F
7. The digestive process begins in the oral cavity. T/F
8. Villi are located in the large intestine. T/F
9. Missing, decayed, or poorly restored teeth can affect food intake. T/F
10. Saliva aids in the oral clearance of food. T/F

Foods are composed of large chemical molecules that cannot be utilized unless they are broken down to an absorbable form. The digestive system is designed to (1) ingest foods, (2) digest or break down complex molecules into simple, soluble materials that can be absorbed, and (3) eliminate unused residues. Only the three energy-providing nutrients (carbohydrate, protein, fat) must be digested for absorption. Most vitamins, minerals, and water can be absorbed as eaten.

The gastrointestinal tract may be used to deliver oral medications, which are also complex chemical substances. Medications can frequently affect or be affected by foods, thereby modifying absorption, metabolism, or excretion of either the food or the drug. They may also affect nutritional status as a result of changes in taste or salivary flow; both of these conditions influence the amount and types of foods consumed. Dental hygienists need to become familiar with normal gastrointestinal processes because disturbances in the gastrointestinal tract may affect the nutritional status of clients.

PHYSIOLOGY OF THE GASTROINTESTINAL TRACT

The digestive system includes the *alimentary canal* and several accessory organs (Fig. 2–1). The alimentary canal comprises all the body parts through which food passes, extending from the mouth to the anus. The alimentary canal is a tubular structure, with a length of about 30 feet (five times the height of an average man). It includes the oral cavity, pharynx, esophagus, stomach, *small intestine,* and *large intestine.* The small intestine includes the duodenum, jejunum, and ileum; the large intestine includes the cecum, colon, and rectum. *Accessory organs* include the salivary glands, liver, gallbladder, and pancreas. Accessory organs provide secretions essential for the digestive process.

Digestion involves two basic types of action on food: (1) *Mechanical* activities and (2) *chemical* activities. Mechanical actions include chewing and

ALIMENTARY TRACT

ACCESSORY ORGANS

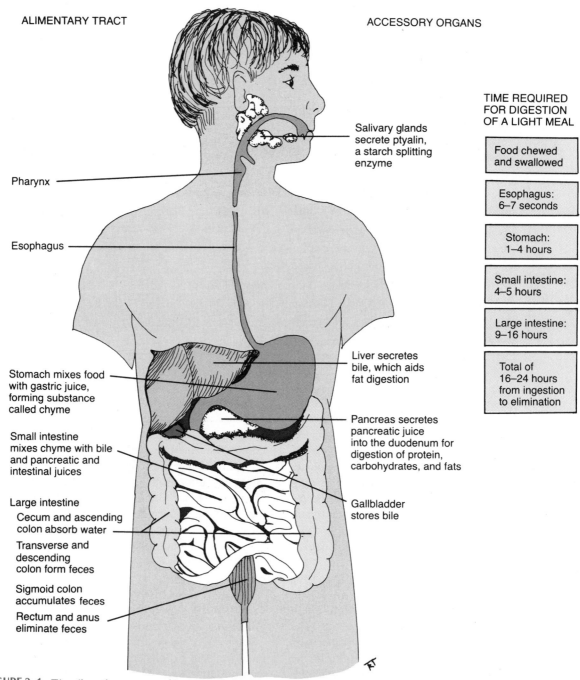

Salivary glands
secrete ptyalin,
a starch splitting
enzyme

Pharynx

Esophagus

Stomach mixes food
with gastric juice,
forming substance
called chyme

Small intestine
mixes chyme with bile
and pancreatic and
intestinal juices

Large intestine

Cecum and ascending
colon absorb water

Transverse and
descending
colon form feces

Sigmoid colon
accumulates feces

Rectum and anus
eliminate feces

Liver secretes
bile, which aids
fat digestion

Pancreas secretes
pancreatic juice
into the duodenum for
digestion of protein,
carbohydrates, and fats

Gallbladder
stores bile

TIME REQUIRED
FOR DIGESTION
OF A LIGHT MEAL

Food chewed
and swallowed

Esophagus:
6–7 seconds

Stomach:
1–4 hours

Small intestine:
4–5 hours

Large intestine:
9–16 hours

Total of
16–24 hours
from ingestion
to elimination

**FIGURE 2–1   The digestive process. (From Davis JR, Sherer K. *Applied Nutrition and Diet Therapy for Nurses,*
2nd ed. Philadelphia: W.B. Saunders, 1994.)**

peristalsis, which break up and mix foods, permitting better blending with the chemicals; chemical actions involve salivary enzymes and digestive juices that reduce foodstuffs to absorbable molecules.

Chemical Action

The process of digesting energy nutrients involves **hydrolysis.** The following are basic hydrolysis reactions in food digestion:

$$Protein + H_2O \rightarrow amino\ acids$$
$$Fat + H_2O \rightarrow fatty\ acids + glycerol$$
$$Carbohydrate + H_2O \rightarrow monosaccharides$$

These reactions are dependent on **enzymes.** In protein hydrolysis, the substrate for the enzyme is protein, and amino acids are the product. The enzyme forms a temporary chemical compound with the substrate. When the reaction is completed, the complex separates, releasing new chemical compounds and the enzyme.

Because the enzyme is reused, only small amounts are needed. Enzymes function somewhat like keys in that they are very specific and will function on only one substrate, similar to a key fitting a particular lock (Fig. 2–2). The name for some enzymes is derived from the name of the substrate, with the suffix "-ase" (e.g., lactase is the enzyme produced to catalyze the breakdown of lactose).

Mechanical Action

The wall of the gastrointestinal tract is similar from the esophagus to the rectum (Fig. 2–3). A circular layer of muscles encircles the tube, allowing the diameter of the tube to expand and contract. Food particles are broken up and mixed by the churning action. The outer fibers of the muscular coat (longitudinal muscle) run lengthwise and are responsible for **peristalsis.**

Valves, or **sphincter muscles,** are designed to (1) retain food in each segment until the work of the mechanical actions and digestive juices has been completed, (2) allow measured amounts of food to pass into the next segment, and (3) prevent food from "backing up" into the preceding area. The regulation of these valves is complex, involving muscular function and different pressures on each side of the valve.

Dental Hygiene Considerations

- Gurgling sounds, caused by air and fluid in the normal abdomen, indicate peristalsis is occurring.
- If the alimentary tract is not functioning properly, adequate amounts of nutrients may not be provided to the body as a result of alterations in digestion and absorption. The client may be prone to nu-

---

FIGURE 2–2 **Lock-and-key mechanism of enzyme action. Like keys, substrates fit into the active sites of the enzyme. Following the reaction, the products separate and the unchanged enzyme is available to catalyze production of additional products. (Redrawn from Davis JR, Sherer K. *Applied Nutrition and Diet Therapy for Nurses,* 2nd ed. Philadelphia: W.B. Saunders, 1994.)**

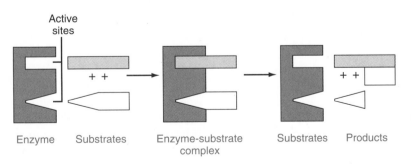

Active sites

Enzyme   Substrates   Enzyme-substrate complex   Substrates   Products

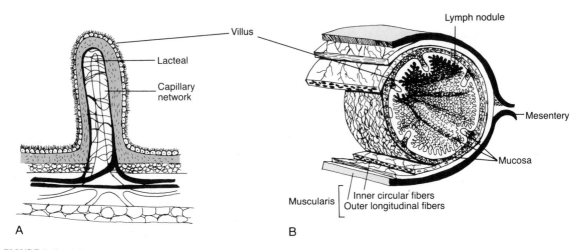

FIGURE 2–3   (A) A villus, the absorptive organ of the small intestine. (B) Layers composing the intestinal wall. (From Davis JR, Sherer K. *Applied Nutrition and Diet Therapy for Nurses*, 2nd ed. Philadelphia: W.B. Saunders, 1994.)

trient deficiencies, poor healing, or fecal impactions.

● Loss of motility in the stomach and small intestine results in impaired gastric and intestinal emptying. This allows excessive growth of bacteria, which may injure the surface of the intestine, cause diarrhea, and interfere with nutrient absorption. Clients who are immobile (due to injury, trauma, or debilitating illness) are more prone to these disorders.

℞ Food-drug interactions have the potential to cause nutritional problems or erratic drug responses. Therefore, knowledge of the drugs taken and how they interact with food is necessary. For example, giving milk with tetracycline decreases the amount of tetracycline and calcium available to the body.

Nutritional Directions

◆ Taking over-the-counter enzyme tablets may not be beneficial because the enzymes are digested before they can be utilized. Prescription pancreatic enzymes are effective because of a special enteric coating that prevents the enzyme from exposure to gastric juices. Lactase, a nonprescription enzyme, is also effective because it is either added to or taken with lactose-containing foods, allowing the conversion of lactose into glucose and galactose before the gastric juices can affect the enzyme (lactase).

◆ Digestion involves two types of action: mechanical and chemical. Proper functioning of the gastrointestinal tract facilitates the digestive process.

ORAL CAVITY

Taste and Smell

Generally, food choices are influenced by the three sensory perceptions: sight, smell, and taste. Gustatory (taste) sensations evoke pronounced feelings of pleasure or aversion; in the United States, taste is the primary determinant of food choices. The presentation of food, its color and aroma, may be the basis for acceptance or rejection. Food flavors are prompted from characteristics of substances ingested, including taste, aroma, texture, temperature, and irritating properties. Approximately 75% of flavor is derived from odors (Mott et al., 1993).

The mouth, or oral cavity, plays an important role in the digestive system, not only because it is the "port of entry," but also because of the presence of **taste buds.** A taste bud consists of approximately 50 cells. These cells replace themselves every 10 days and can be affected by disease, drugs,

nutritional status, radiation, and age. Food stimulates taste buds, and aromas stimulate **olfactory nerves.** The average lifespan of an olfactory nerve cell is 30 days. Satisfaction derived from food determines its acceptability. The basic gustatory sensations, which are limited to sweet, sour, salty, and bitter, are located on different parts of the tongue (Fig. 2–4). These four basic tastes reflect

FIGURE 2–4 **(A) Regions of taste on the tongue. (From Davis JR, Sherer K.** *Applied Nutrition and Diet Therapy for Nurses,* **2nd ed. Philadelphia: W.B. Saunders, 1994.) (B) The human oropharyngeal cavity showing the regions that contain taste buds. (From Miller IJ, Bartoshuk LM. Taste perception, taste bud distribution and spatial relationships. In Getchell TV, Doty RL, Bartoshuk LM, et al. (eds).** *Smell and Taste in Health and Disease.* **New York: Raven Press, 1991, 205–234.)**

specific constituents of food. Taste buds also are found on the soft palate, epiglottis, glossopalatine arch, larynx, and posterior wall of the pharynx. In general, taste and smell are essential for maintaining intake to meet physiologic needs.

In contrast to gustatory sensations, an almost unlimited number of unique odors can be detected. There is no tactile sensation to indicate the origin of odor sensations. Hence, food-related aromas may be confused with taste sensations, and taste disorders are often the result of problems in smell rather than taste. Taste is stable with aging but up to 50% of elderly persons have some loss of olfactory perception (Duffy 1996). This is usually the reason an elderly client will state that food "just doesn't taste good."

Upper respiratory infections, nasal and/or sinus problems, neurologic disorders, endocrine abnormalities, aging, or head trauma may cause **anosmia.** The rate of the continuous renewal process undergone by olfactory receptor cells is depressed in malnutrition and by some antibiotics. These disorders are self limited. Chemosensory losses from infections and aging are irreversible.

Anosmia results in a limited capacity to detect the flavor of food and beverages. One's ability to smell food being prepared and eaten influences food selection. Foods are sometimes judged to be harmful or spoiled because of their odors, so the sense of smell is also a protective mechanism. Persons with a cold usually lose their appetite because of a decreased sense of smell, which affects the ability to "taste" and enjoy food.

Gustatory disorders, or **dysgeusia,** may be caused by a previous viral upper respiratory infection, head trauma, neurologic or psychiatric disorder, systemic condition, decreased salivation, severe nutritional deficiencies, and some oral or dental disorders (Table 2–1), or it may have an iatrogenic causation (medications, irradiation, surgery). These conditions may also cause **hypogeusia** and **hypergeusia.** Dysgeusia may also result from breathing through the mouth. The dental hygienist is frequently the first health care provider who detects a client's taste disorder. Hyperkeratinization of the epithelium may be observed during an oral exam; blockage of taste buds may affect intake.

Gustatory and olfactory disorders, whether caused by disease states or drugs, are not mere inconveniences or neurotic symptoms. They affect food choices and dietary habits. Drug-induced loss of taste acuity may result in **anorexia** (Table 2–1). Taste stimulants affect salivary and pancreatic secretions, gastric contractions, and intestinal motility; therefore, gustatory disorders can also affect digestion.

Because gustatory and olfactory disorders can result in deterioration of a client's general condition or nutritional status, these abnormalities must always be considered in dental and nutritional care. Potentially adverse compensatory habits may develop (e.g., decreased sweetness or saltiness perceptions may result in excessive usage of sweets or salts, which may be potentially harmful, especially for clients with diabetes or hypertension, respectively). Also, the addition of sugar can lead to higher incidence of caries. Persistent taste distortions can lead to inadequate caloric intake with resultant weight loss or malnutrition.

Saliva

Adequate saliva flow is essential for oral health and maintenance of soft tissues in the oral cavity, including the taste buds. Saliva, secreted by the salivary glands, is essential in taste sensations, functioning (1) as a solvent, (2) to transport tastants to the receptors, (3) to provide ions for taste transduction, and (4) to provide secretory proteins. This complex fluid also helps maintain the integrity of the teeth against physical, chemical, and microbial insults. Saliva is supersaturated with calcium phosphates that allow demineralized areas of the hydroxyapatite in enamel to be remineralized.

Acidic or bitter tastes stimulate saliva flow. Saliva production is also increased when tasty foods are consumed. This increases the oral clearance rate, decreasing risk of caries formation. Saliva blended with food particles moistens foods so they are more easily manipulated and prepared for swallowing.

Some chemical action or hydrolysis of nutrients

TABLE 2–1   *Some Factors Affecting Taste and Smell**

Factor	Gustatory Effect	Olfactory Effect
Disorders		
Damage to chorda tympani	Absent/diminished	
Familial dysautonomia	Absent/diminished	
Head trauma	Absent/diminished	Absent/diminished
Cancer	Absent/diminished (sweet); heightened (bitter)	
Head and neck radiation therapy	Absent/diminished/distorted	
Chronic renal failure	Absent/diminished/distorted (sweet, salt, sour)	Absent/diminished
Cirrhosis	Absent/diminished	Absent/diminished
Thermal burn	Absent/diminished/distorted	
Niacin deficiency	Absent/diminished/distorted	
Vitamin B_{12} deficiency		Absent/diminished
Zinc deficiency	Absent/diminished	
Adrenal cortical insufficiency	Increased detection but decreased recognition	
Multiple sclerosis	Absent/diminished/distorted	Absent/diminished
Cushing syndrome	Absent/diminished	Absent/diminished
Hypothyroidism	Absent/diminished/distorted	Absent/diminished/distorted
Diabetes mellitus	Absent/diminished (sweet)	Absent/diminished
Allergic rhinitis, nasal polyposis, sinusitis, bronchial asthma		Absent/diminished
Cystic fibrosis	Individual variation, frequently increased	Individual variation, frequently increased
Hypertension	Absent/diminished (salt)	
Drugs		
Dimercaprol, fluorouracil, lincomycin, griseofulvin, sulfasalazine, amphotericin B, phenindione, carbamazepine, cholestyramine, azathioprine, levodopa, nifedipine, chlorhexidine, hexitidine, sodium lauryl sulfate, phenytoin	Altered/distorted	
Phenformin, lithium, metronidazole, disulfiram, methotrexate, sulfonylureas, streptomycin, procaine, penicillin, tetracycline, ethambutol, allopurinol, auranofin, enalapril	Metallic taste	
Cephalosporin, chloral hydrate, metaproterenol, potassium supplements	Bad taste	
Amphetamines	Increased sensitivity (bitter)	
Enalapril, furosemide	Peculiar sweet taste	

Table continued on following page

TABLE 2–1   *Some Factors Affecting Taste and Smell* (Continued)*

Factor	Gustatory Effect	Olfactory Effect
Drugs		
Penicillamine, clofibrate, amrinone, methylthiouracil, methimazole, phenylbutazone, bleomycin, cisplatin, methotrexate, baclofen, carbamizole, thiamazole, diltiazem, enalapril, nitroglycerin, spironolactone, chlorhexidine	Diminished	
Acetazolamide, bretylium, bromide-containing medications	Salty, bitter taste	
Amiloride, chlorhexidine	Decreased salt taste	
Dextroamphetamine	Diminished sweet taste	

*Data from Pronsky ZM. *Food-Medication Interactions,* 8th ed. Pottstown, PA: Food-Medication Interactions, 1993; Mandel ID. The role of saliva in maintaining oral homeostasis. *J Am Diet Asoc* 1989; 119(8):298-303; and Schiffman S. Taste and smell in disease. *N Engl J Med* 1983; 308(21):1275. From Davis JR, Sherer K. *Applied Nutrition and Diet Therapy for Nurses,* 2nd ed. Philadelphia: W.B. Saunders, 1994.

begins in the mouth. The functions of the different constituents in saliva are shown in Table 2–2. Because food is normally in the mouth briefly, ptyalin, or salivary amylase, just initiates starch digestion. If a carbohydrate food, such as a cracker, is chewed and held in the mouth for a few seconds, it will begin to taste sweet, denoting the fact that some starch is being hydrolyzed to dextrin and maltose.

TABLE 2–2   *Digestive Functions of Saliva*

Saliva Component	Classification	Function
Mucin	Glycoprotein	Lubricates food for easier passage
Amylase	Enzyme	Begins hydrolysis of starch to maltose
Lysozyme	Enzyme	Kills some ingested bacteria
Lingual lipase	Enzyme	Begins digestion of fats

From Davis JR, Sherer K. *Applied Nutrition and Diet Therapy for Nurses,* 2nd ed. Philadelphia: W.B. Saunders, 1994.

Xerostomia leads to diminished gustatory function. Xerostomia may result in frequent oral ulcerations and increased sensitivity of the tongue to spices and flavors as well as an increased risk of dental caries. Diuretics, which are frequently prescribed to help the body eliminate fluids, will also cause a decrease in salivary flow. Increasing fluid intake to 8 to 10 cups daily is important to compensate for these losses.

Teeth

Another important role of the mouth in food digestion is the mechanical action of teeth. Unlike bone, neither the tooth enamel nor dentin can be repaired or replaced by any natural process other than simple remineralization of small areas and deposition of secondary dentin around the pulp chamber (Fig. 2–5). Mineral deposition and resorption influence the supporting bone structure. Alveolar bone is principally trabecular bone. Thus, the maxilla and mandible are dependent on the presence of teeth and occlusal forces associated with chewing to maintain calcium balance. Chewing firm foods helps maintain proper balance between alveolar bone resorption and new bone formation. Teeth and supporting bone structures are affected by intake of adequate nutrients, adequate digestive function, and hormonal balance.

Chewing reduces food particle size. Inability to masticate food adequately may result in larger chunks of food being swallowed. The loss of even one permanent molar may decrease **masticatory efficiency.** Even after clients become fully adjusted to well-fitted dentures, masticatory efficiency is 27% that of clients with their natural teeth.

Swallowing larger pieces increases the potential for food obstruction in the airway. Food asphyxiation, which may result in sudden death, occurs in a large number of people with defective, incomplete, or poorly fitting dentures.

Digestion of food is facilitated by increasing its surface area. Whether or not particle size affects its digestibility is uncertain, but when elderly clients have digestive problems, masticatory capability is usually a factor. Frequently when masticatory efficiency declines, foods that require less chewing are chosen or special techniques may be taken to change the resistance of food, such as stewing meats, steaming vegetables, or dunking cookies or toast. In many circumstances, hypersensitive, poorly restored, decayed or abscessed, or periodontally involved teeth will affect food choices and limit the variety of foods consumed.

Dental Hygiene Considerations

- Assessment of nutritional status is indicated because nutritional status may have a bearing on chemosensory function and changes in dietary habits, and poor nutritional status may result from chemosensory dysfunction.

- An evaluation of the dietary history of clients with dysgeusia may reveal limited total caloric intake or avoidance of specific foods.

- Clients commonly complain about the ''taste'' or ''flavor'' of food when in fact olfactory as well as gustatory sensations are impaired.

- Assess clients for possible dietary deficiencies (niacin, vitamins B_{12} and A, zinc, copper, nickel) because these can cause gustatory abnormalities.

- Assess clients with gustatory or olfactory disorders for appetite, increased use of spices (especially salt and sugar), and development of food cravings and/or dislikes.

- Toddlers have the largest number of taste buds (and a higher degree of taste sensitivity), resulting in an aversion for highly seasoned foods. Thus, bland-tasting foods are more appealing to youngsters, and a variety of foods are encouraged.

- Xerostomia may result in impairment in the preparation of food for mastication, deglutition, digestion, and enjoyment in addition to an increased risk of both the hard and soft tissues to a variety of destructive processes.

- Xerostomia may compound nutritional intake problems related to taste loss, as clients with dry mouth experience difficulty chewing and swallowing food.

- Clients who have difficulty chewing are likely to develop decreased taste acuity; therefore, monitor food intake.

FIGURE 2–5 Diagram of a tooth.

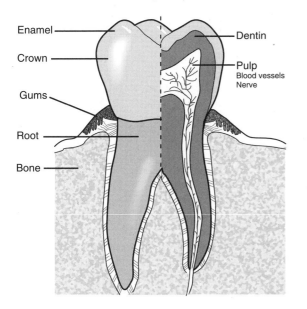

Enamel
Crown
Gums
Root
Bone
Dentin
Pulp
Blood vessels
Nerve

- Edentulous clients or those with ill-fitting dentures should be monitored because both quality and quantity of food intake may be compromised.
- Subjective alterations in taste perception in denture wearers theoretically could be due to altered masticatory ability or shielding of palatal taste buds by the prosthesis. Clients with complete dentures exhibit poorer taste and texture tolerance compared with those with partial dentures or with compromised natural dentition (Cauncey et al., 1984).
- Food intake often decreases when clients receive a set of dentures. However, after an initial adjustment period, food intake usually increases with improved ability to chew.
- Carefully evaluate anecdotal reports or studies involving limited numbers of clients supporting a beneficial effect of vitamins or minerals on dysgeusia.
- Refer clients with persistent gustatory, masticatory, or swallowing difficulties to a physician or registered dietitian to determine types of foods needed to obtain adequate nutrients.

Nutritional Directions

- Natural teeth are more efficient for chewing and biting than any prosthesis.
- Tooth losses are not inevitable; most people can maintain their natural dentition throughout life if preventive dental measures are practiced routinely.
- If salivary flow is diminished, fluid intake with meals should be increased to assist in oral clearance. Nutrient-dense foods in a liquid or semiliquid form are beneficial.
- There is no proven intervention to either enhance taste acuity or abolish dysgeusia; encourage experimentation with texture, spiciness, temperature, and enhanced visual presentation of food.
- To improve nutrient intake when mastication is less efficient, special cooking techniques (such as stewing meats), chewing longer, and choosing soft foods is preferable to pureeing foods. For example, cream-style corn can replace corn on the cob, and applesauce can replace raw apples.
- Artificial salivas may be used between meals to improve oral comfort and hydration. Fluid intake with meals facilitates chewing and swallowing foods.
- Particularly for new denture wearers, herbs and spices and contrasting food taste combinations (e.g., sweet and sour) can be used to enhance taste perception.

ESOPHAGUS

The swallowing reflex moves a **bolus** into the esophagus, where it is transported to the stomach by peristalsis and gravity. The esophagus, a continuous tube about 10 inches long connecting the mouth with the stomach, penetrates the diaphragm through an opening called the esophageal hiatus. The **lower esophageal sphincter** (LES) relaxes to permit food entrance into the stomach, but contracts tightly to prevent the regurgitation or "backwashing" of the stomach contents.

GASTRIC DIGESTION

A bolus entering the stomach is mixed with gastric secretions by peristaltic contractions, producing chyme, a semifluid paste. Gastric secretions include mucus, hydrochloric acid (HCl), enzymes, and a component called intrinsic factor.

The low pH of the stomach contents (about 1.5 to 3.0) is beneficial for several reasons: (1) it kills or inhibits the growth of most food bacteria, (2) it denatures proteins and makes them more easily hydrolyzed to amino acids, (3) it activates gastric enzymes, (4) it hydrolyzes some of the sugars, and (5) it increases solubility and absorption of calcium and iron.

Two major enzymes are found in gastric juice: pepsin and lipase. Pepsin is capable of hydrolyzing large protein molecules to smaller fragments. Gastric lipase is involved in digestion of short- and medium-chain triglycerides (such as those found in butterfat). Mucus forms an alkaline coating on the lining of the stomach for protection against digestion of the stomach by pepsin. Intrinsic factor secreted in the stomach is essential for absorption of vitamin B_{12} in the small intestine.

Normal gastric secretion is regulated by nerve and hormonal stimuli. Visual, olfactory, and gustatory senses stimulate gastric secretions. Gastric secretions are affected by emotions. Fear, sadness, pain, and depression are generally accompanied by decreased secretions; anger, stress, and hostility, by increased secretions.

The adult stomach functions as a reservoir to hold an average meal from 3 to 4½ hours. The stomach empties at different rates depending on its size and the composition of the chyme. The rate of passage through the stomach (fastest to slowest) is liquids, carbohydrates, proteins, fats. However, when a mixture of foods is presented, this pattern is not as well defined. The smaller the stomach capacity, the more rapidly it will empty. (This is exemplified in the infant or person with a partial gastrectomy who must be fed frequently until the stomach size expands.) Fats remain in the stomach longer, increasing feelings of fullness for a longer time than proteins or carbohydrates. Chyme is released from the stomach through the pyloric sphincter in small amounts to allow for adequate digestion and absorption in the small intestine.

Very little absorption takes place in the stomach because few foods are completely hydrolyzed to nutrients the body can use at this stage. Nutrients that can be absorbed from the stomach include some water, alcohol, and a few water-soluble substances (amino acids and glucose).

Dental Hygiene Considerations

- Peptic ulcers are usually due to the digestive action of pepsin; when the HCl somehow overwhelms the mucous protective coating of the stomach, the stomach lining becomes vulnerable to the digestive action of pepsin.

- Dietary constituents that increase HCl and pepsin secretions are proteins, calcium, caffeine, coffee, and alcohol. These may need to be limited in clients with ulcers or certain gastrointestinal tract disorders.

- Since gravity facilitates the movement of food down the esophagus, clients who are in a horizontal position may have some difficulty swallowing and may have reflux of gastric contents, especially after eating.

Nutritional Directions

- Vomiting is one of the methods the body has of eliminating toxins from contaminated foods. Vomiting can also be stimulated by rapid changes in body motion or by drugs.

- Heartburn is a result of regurgitation of the stomach contents back into the esophagus. Acidic gastric secretions produce discomfort or pain, which may be relieved if the client remains in the upright position after eating.

- Eating in a relaxing atmosphere will help reduce gastric secretions.

- Chronic problems with vomiting or reflux can result in sensitive teeth and superficial or deep tooth erosion, especially on lingual surfaces.

SMALL INTESTINE

Within the small intestine, most of the energy-providing nutrients are completely hydrolyzed and absorbed. Most vitamins and minerals are also absorbed in the small intestine. The small intestine is specially designed to perform these tasks with juices secreted by the accessory organs and its complex luminal wall (Table 2–3). The small intestine is approximately 15 feet long, and foods are retained therein for 3 to 10 hours.

Digestion

Throughout the walls of the small intestine are villi, finger-like projections rising out of the mucosa into the intestinal lumen (see Fig. 2–3). These villi increase the surface area of the alimentary tract to about 3,000 square feet. Each villus is also covered with a layer of epithelial cells containing microvilli that collectively form the brush border cells. This further increases the surface area. The pH change and motility in the small intestine inhibit bacterial growth.

Acidic chyme entering the intestine stimulates hormones to release pancreatic juices into the duodenum. Cholecystokinin, released in response to the presence of fat in chyme, stimulates the gallbladder to contract and release **bile.**

Pancreatic enzymes enter the duodenum through the pancreatic duct and function best in the neutralized chyme. Pancreatic enzymes hydrolyze carbohydrates, protein, and fats. The *proteolytic enzymes* are produced and stored in the pancreas in inactive form. Proteolytic enzymes function to hydrolyze proteins.

Bile is secreted by the liver and is stored in the gallbladder, where reabsorption of water concentrates the bile. Bile salts **emulsify** fats, allowing greater exposure to intestinal and pancreatic lipases. This allows insoluble molecules to be divided into smaller particles. Peristalsis facilitates the mixing and emulsification process by bile.

Specific digestive enzymes located within the microvilli are responsible for completing the hydrolysis of carbohydrates, proteins and fats. Not everything in foods can be completely digested; for example, the human body does not have enzymes to digest cellulose, a carbohydrate found in plants.

Other factors affecting digestion and absorption are as important to nutritional status as adequate intake: (1) the amount of the nutrient consumed; (2) the physiologic need; (3) the condition of the digestive tract, such as the amount of secretions, motility, and absorptive surface; (4) the level of circulating hormones; (5) the presence of other nutrients or drugs ingested at the same time that enhance or interfere with absorption; and (6) the presence of adequate amounts of digestive enzymes.

Absorption of Nutrients

The small intestine is the principal site for nutrient absorption (Fig. 2–6). Only after the nutrient is absorbed into the intestinal mucosa is it considered to be "in" the body. As a general rule, absorption of nutrients occurs by passive diffusion or active transport mechanisms. Passive diffusion is the passage of a permeable substance from more concentrated solution to an area of lower concentration. Active transport occurs when absorption is from a region of low concentration to one of a higher concentration and requires a carrier and cellular energy. Approximately 80% to 90% of fluid intake is absorbed in the small intestine by **osmosis.** Actually, water moves freely in both directions across the intestinal mucosa.

Absorbable nutrients pass through the microvilli and enter the portal circulation if they are water soluble and the lymphatic circulation if they are fat soluble.

ABSORPTION INTO PORTAL CIRCULATION

Monosaccharides, amino acids, glycerol, water-soluble vitamins, minerals, and short-chain and medium-chain fatty acids are absorbed from the small intestine through the mucosa into the portal circulation. They are transported through the portal vein directly to the liver, where metabolism begins.

ABSORPTION OF FAT-SOLUBLE NUTRIENTS

The absorption process for long-chain fatty acids is complex because the molecules are large and insoluble. Long-chain fatty acids are broken apart to allow passage through the intestinal wall into the lymphatic system, which transports them to the left subclavian and internal jugular veins. Absorption of the four fat-soluble vita-

TABLE 2–3   *Digestion in the Gastrointestinal Tract*

Location	Secretion/Enzyme	Function	Nutrient Action
Mouth	Salivary amylase (ptyalin)		Hydrolyzes starch into disaccharides
Stomach	Hydrochloric acid	Antibacterial Activates pepsinogen, which is then called pepsin	Converts Fe^{3+} to Fe^{2+}
	Pepsin		Hydrolyzes proteins into polypeptides
	Gastric lipase		Hydrolyzes emulsified fats (butterfat) into glycerol and fatty acids
	Intrinsic factor	Combines with vitamin B_{12}	
	Mucin	Protects mucosa	
Small intestine			
Pancreatic juices	Trypsin		Hydrolyzes proteins and polypeptides into dipeptides
	Chymotrypsin		Hydrolyzes proteins and polypeptides into dipeptides
	Carboxypeptidase		Hydrolyzes polypeptides and dipeptides into amino acids
	Pancreatic lipase (requires bile salts)		Hydrolyzes fats into glycerol, monoglycerides, diglycerides, and fatty acids
	Pancreatic amylase		Hydrolyzes starch into maltose
Intestinal juices (in microvilli)	Aminopeptidase		Hydrolyzes polypeptides and dipeptides into amino acids
	Dipeptidases		Hydrolyzes dipeptides into amino acids
	Intestinal lipase		Hydrolyzes fats into glycerol, glycerides, and fatty acids
	Sucrase		Hydrolyzes sucrose into glucose and fructose
	Maltase		Hydrolyzes maltose into glucose
	Lactase		Hydrolyzes lactose into glucose and galactose
	Lecithinase		Hydrolyzes lecithin into fatty acids, glycerol, and phosphoric acid
	Bile	Accelerates action of pancreatic lipase Emulsifies fats Neutralizes chyme Stabilizes emulsions	
Large intestine	Mucus	Protects mucosa	

From Davis JR, Sherer K. *Applied Nutrition and Diet Therapy for Nurses,* 2nd ed. Philadelphia: W.B. Saunders, 1994.

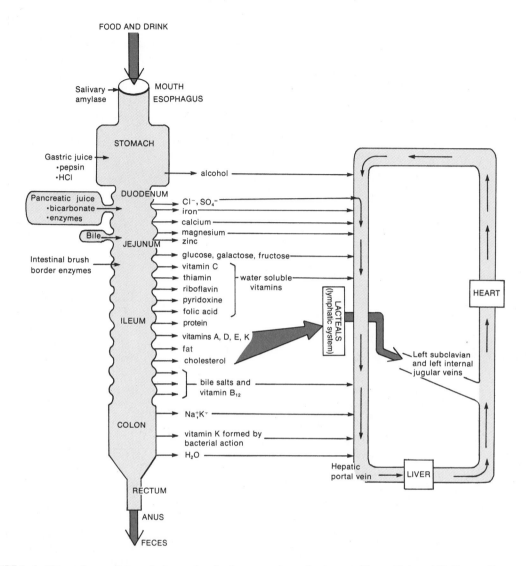

FOOD AND DRINK

Salivary amylase → MOUTH / ESOPHAGUS

STOMACH

Gastric juice →
• pepsin
• HCl

alcohol →

Pancreatic juice
• bicarbonate →
• enzymes

DUODENUM

Cl^-, $SO_4^=$ →
iron →
calcium →
magnesium →
zinc →

Bile →

JEJUNUM

glucose, galactose, fructose →
vitamin C →
thiamin →
riboflavin →
pyridoxine →
folic acid →

water soluble vitamins

Intestinal brush border enzymes →

protein →
vitamins A, D, E, K →
fat →
cholesterol →

LACTEALS (lymphatic system)

ILEUM

Left subclavian and left internal jugular veins

bile salts and vitamin B_{12} →

HEART

$Na^+_+K^-$ →

COLON

vitamin K formed by bacterial action →
H_2O →

Hepatic portal vein → LIVER

RECTUM

ANUS

FECES

FIGURE 2–6   **Sites of secretion and absorption in the gastrointestinal tract. (From Mahan LK, Escott-Stumps.** *Krause's Food, Nutrition, and Diet Therapy,* **9th ed. Philadelphia: W.B. Saunders, 1996.)**

mins—A, D, E, and K—is not as complex. Bile salts and lipases increase their water solubility so that these vitamins are absorbed along with other fats in the lymphatic system.

Dental Hygiene Considerations

- An enzymatic deficiency in the gastrointestinal tract will result in some nutrients not

being digested; therefore, they cannot be absorbed. The most prevalent enzyme deficiency is lactase deficiency, which is prevalent in Asians, native Americans, African Americans, and Hispanics.

- Unless preventive care is taken, clients having had large portions of the gastrointestinal tract removed may develop nutritional deficiency symptoms because digestive secretions or absorptive areas are removed (see Fig. 2–6).

- If motility is increased, such as in diarrhea, nutrients are not exposed to digestive secretions and absorptive surfaces long enough for maximum absorption. Severe or prolonged diarrhea may result in numerous deficiencies, the most rapid being a fluid deficit or dehydration.

Nutritional Directions

- The rate of digestion is affected by how well the food is broken apart. If food is not chewed well, the food passes through the gastrointestinal tract at a slower rate.
- Dietary fat should not be eliminated entirely because it is necessary for absorption of fat-soluble vitamins.
- Most nutrients are absorbed in the small intestine.
- Routine use of mineral oil as a laxative is not advisable because it reduces absorption of fat-soluble vitamins.

LARGE INTESTINE

Chyme remaining in the ileum is released through the ileocecal valve into the cecum in small amounts. Only about 1/20 of the ingested foods and digestive secretions arrives in the large intestine. For most adults, it takes between 16 to 24 hours for foodstuffs to travel the full length of the gut.

Functions

The large intestine, so named because of its large diameter, has little or no digestive function. Its main functions are to reabsorb water and electrolytes (mainly sodium and potassium) and to form and store the residue (feces) until defecation. Chyme entering the large intestine with 500 to 1,000 ml water is excreted as feces containing only 100 to 200 ml fluid. Essentially, all absorption occurs in the proximal half of the colon.

The inner lining of the large intestine is relatively smooth, lacking the numerous villi found in the small intestine. The only important secretion is mucus, which protects the intestinal wall, aids in holding particles of fecal matter together, and helps to control the pH of the large intestine.

Undigested Residues

Fiber, obtained from fruits and vegetables and whole-grain products, results in increased **residue** and has a water-holding capacity, contributing to bulkier feces. Residue has a beneficial side effect of stimulating peristalsis, resulting in better muscle tone. Dietary fiber is undigestible and works as a laxative, but foods may contain other substances that increase fecal output. One example is prune juice, which yields no residue on chemical digestion but is classified as a high-residue food because it contains a laxative that indirectly increases the volume of the stool. Conversely, milk is fiber free and medium residue.

Microflora

Due to decreased peristalsis and the neutral pH, microflora thrive in the colon. Some microflora can break down substances that human enzymes are unable to digest; others synthesize vitamins needed by humans. Vitamin K, vitamin B_{12}, biotin, thiamin, and riboflavin are produced in this manner. This source for obtaining vitamin K is especially important because the food supply normally contains amounts insufficient for adequate blood coagulation. The types of food and medications ingested influence the activity and relative numbers of bacteria. Bacterial activity produces various gases that contribute to flatus in the colon. Fecal odor is a result of the compounds produced by these bacteria.

Peristalsis

After chyme enters the large intestine, it takes about 18 hours to reach the distal colon. The purpose of peristalsis in the large intestine is to force the feces into the rectum. These large waves occur only two to three times daily.

Dental Hygiene Considerations

- Bowel habits, stress, exercise, and diet (especially the amount of fiber and fluid intake) affect the gastrointestinal transit rate.
- Retention of feces in the large intestine for too long allows more reabsorption of water, causing the feces to become hard and dry, leading to constipation.
- ℞ Antibiotic therapy normally kills the bacteria in the colon and inhibits bacterial production of vitamins. Thus, clients on long-term antibiotic therapy may develop vitamin K, vitamin B_{12}, and biotin deficiencies.

Nutritional Directions

- Constipation can be treated by increasing fluid intake and/or by gradually increasing nondigestible materials in the diet. Activity also affects gastrointestinal mobility. Active clients who routinely choose high-fiber foods and drink adequate amounts of liquids are less likely to become constipated than their sedentary counterparts.
- The frequency of bowel movements is an individual matter, and patterns can vary from after each meal to once every 2 days.

HEALTH APPLICATION 2

Lactose Intolerance

Some clients are unable to digest specific carbohydrates because of insufficient amounts of disaccharide enzymes. When those carbohydrates are eaten, the disaccharide is fermented by intestinal bacteria rather than being broken down into simple sugars. This results in malabsorption of the disaccharide, accompanied by diarrhea, abdominal cramps, and flatulence.

Suggestions for Lactose-Intolerant Clients

Milk and milk products provide the most readily available source of calcium to the body; efforts are needed to provide adequate amounts of calcium when these products are avoided. Milk/milk products are also good sources of protein, riboflavin, potassium, and magnesium. Because of different tolerance levels, each client needs to experiment to determine which method is most effective for providing necessary nutrients without discomfort.

- Consume small amounts of whole milk (4 to 6 oz) with meals several times a day.
- Consume fermented dairy products: yogurt,* buttermilk, aged cheese (Swiss, Colby, Longhorn), soft cheese (cream cheese, Neufchatel, cottage cheese, farmer's, ricotta).
- Use over-the-counter lactase enzymes available in tablet/liquid form to hydrolyze the lactose in milk products or lactose-hydrolyzed commercially available milk.
- Increase consumption of other calcium-containing foods: salmon and sardines canned with bones, spinach, kale, broccoli, turnip and beet greens, molasses, tofu, almonds, orange, eggs, shrimp.
- Consider commercially available nutrition supplements such as Ensure (Ross), Resource (Sandoz), Sustacal (Mead Johnson).
- If the above suggestions are not feasible to maintain an adequate intake of at least 600 mg calcium, consult a physician/dietitian for calcium supplements that are well absorbed. These supplements may also need to include vitamin D.

*Unflavored yogurt is usually the best tolerated.

From Davis JR, Sherer K. *Applied Nutrition and Diet Therapy for Nurses,* 2nd ed. Philadelphia: W.B. Saunders, 1994.

Based on the results of a double-blind cross-over study, it was thought that some people who believe they are lactose intolerant may mistakenly attribute gastric distress to milk or dairy products when other foods are the culprit (Suarez et al., 1995).

Lactase, an intestinal enzyme responsible for lactose digestion, is the only disaccharidase whose activity is reduced in a significant proportion of older children and adults. Lactose intolerance occurs in about 92% of Asians, 79% of native Americans, 75% of African Americans, 51% of Hispanics, and 21% of Caucasians. Lactase deficiency may be (1) present at birth because of an inborn error of metabolism, (2) an inherited problem with gradual decreases in lactase activity throughout the lifespan, or (3) a temporary condition caused by gastrointestinal diseases or intestinal mucosa damage.

Nutritional Care

Treatment of lactase deficiency is simple: reduce lactose-containing foods. Because milk provides significant amounts of calcium, phosphorus, riboflavin, vitamins, and sometimes protein, elimination is not advisable. The ability to digest lactose is not an all-or-nothing phenomenon; most clients with lactose intolerance can tolerate up to 6 gm of lactose per serving (Hertzler et al., 1996). Therefore, the amount of dairy products is reduced to a client's tolerance level (see the Suggestions for Lactose-Intolerant Clients). Milk is tolerated better when taken with a meal and limited to 8 oz at a time. Whole milk is tolerated better than skim milk.

Fermented dairy products—especially yogurt but also buttermilk, aged cheese, and sour cream—are often better tolerated by lactase-deficient individuals. Yogurt made with the organisms *Lactobacillus bulgaricus* or *Streptococcus thermophiles* is better tolerated than nonfermented dairy products because it contains active lactase and less lactose. Yogurt buffers stomach acid, preventing lactase-producing bacteria from being killed. Most commercially available yogurt can be beneficial to lactose-intolerant clients, but unflavored yogurt generally has a higher level of lactase activity. Many commercially available frozen yogurts are pasteurized to increase their shelf life. This process decreases lactase activity and kills lactose-producing bacteria, so most frozen yogurts are not well-tolerated by lactose-intolerant clients.

Studies indicate an increased frequency of lactose intolerance in clients with osteoporosis (Gudmand-Hoyer, 1994). Clients should be taught about the approximate calcium composition of the milk products they tolerate (see Table 8–3) so they can increase their calcium intake.

Commercially available lactase in tablet or liquid form can be beneficial. Lactose tablets, taken with a lactase-containing food, are effective in the stomach's acidic environment for approximately 45 minutes. Liquid lactase is effective in a neutral pH; lactose in milk is hydrolyzed prior to ingestion. Specialized lactose-reduced products are also commercially available.

CASE APPLICATION FOR THE DENTAL HYGIENIST

Mr. A. complains that he can hardly talk because his mouth is dry and sticky. Sores in his mouth make his dentures very uncomfortable. He states he does not leave his home often because he is unable to readily find liquids to prevent his tongue from sticking to the sides and the roof of his mouth. He also complains that eating is difficult. A diuretic has been prescribed by his physician because of his hypertension.

Nutritional Assessment

○ Current and normal weight
○ Dietary intake
○ Preferred fluids, frequency of intake
○ Food preparation techniques
○ Medications taken
○ Oral examination to determine the condition of the underlying tissues
○ Fit of dentures
○ Willingness to learn and to change habits

Nutritional Diagnosis

Knowledge deficit of the effects of diuretics on hydration of the body related to lack of information and understanding.

Nutritional Goals

The client will continue taking diuretic; his nutrient intake will improve to prevent further weight loss; and his fluid intake will increase to 8 to 10 glasses fluid a day.

Nutritional Implementation

Intervention: Discuss the importance of adequate salivary flow for maintenance of soft tissues, taste functions, and teeth. If indicated and desired, suggest use of an artificial saliva product to provide temporary comfort as needed.
Rationale: Xerostomia has severe deleterious effects not only on a client's ability to talk, but also on the integrity of the oral tissues.

Intervention: Review the importance of meticulous oral hygiene and removal of dentures for periods of time.
Rationale: Xerostomia promotes plaque formation, which can lead to further gingival irritations and caries. Removal of dentures will allow the underlying tissue to become healthy again.

Intervention: Discuss that although diuretics may cause this condition, the diuretic is important for his health.
Rationale: To prevent other health problems, it is important for Mr. A. to continue the medication as prescribed by the physician.

Intervention: Discuss ways he can increase his fluid intake to 8 to 10 glasses daily: (1) drink more fluid with meals; (2) carry fluids with him in a large covered thermal container.
Rationale: To replace fluids excreted because of the diuretic, adequate fluid intake is essential.

Intervention: Encourage increased intake of nutrient-dense liquid or semiliquid foods, such as milkshakes, cream soups, gravies, and sauces.
Rationale: These foods contain larger proportions of nutrients, which will help Mr. A. to consume adequate amounts and will prevent weight loss.

Intervention: Recommend tips to relieve the dryness in his mouth, such as sugar-free mints and gum or ice chips.
Rationale: The client's comfort will be enhanced if his mouth is moist; oral complications associated with xerostomia will be minimized.

Evaluation

If the client continues to take the prescribed diuretic, consumes a well-balanced diet, increases fluid intake, uses correct oral hygiene practices, maintains body weight, and can state why he was having all these problems, dental hygiene care was effective.

Student Readiness

1. Make a chart or diagram showing the gastrointestinal secretions, where they are produced, and their digestive actions on the nutrients present in milk. Homogenized milk contains the following: lactose (a disaccharide), proteins, emulsified fats, calcium, riboflavin, and vitamins A and D. Where would the end products be absorbed?

2. Define alimentary canal, hydrolysis, enzyme, fiber, and residue.

3. A client has problems secreting too much HCl. What foods would you tell a client to avoid?

4. If caloric intake were equal, which of the following breakfasts would probably delay the feeling of hunger the longest? Explain your reason.

    (A) Dry cereal with skim milk, toast with jelly, and coffee with sugar.
    (B) Egg with ham, toast with butter, and coffee with cream.

5. What are the absorbable products resulting from digestion of carbohydrates, proteins, and fats?

6. Within what section of the alimentary canal does most of the digestion and absorption take place?

7. Discuss the fallacy of diets that claim only one type of food (such as fruits) should be eaten at a given time.

8. Could constipation be called a nutrient deficiency? Defend your answer.

9. What types of problems might be encountered when a client does not chew his/her food well?

10. Your client has had radiation to the mouth and salivary gland area, resulting in diminished salivary secretions. List some advice you should give to the client. Determine suitable salivary substitute liquids that would begin the process of hydrolysis. Evaluate the frequency and volume needed at each time and approximate daily cost.

CASE STUDY

A 22-year-old Asian female client reports a history of lactose intolerance. She is concerned about her calcium intake since she has eliminated all dairy products from her diet.

1. What should be included in the dietary recommendations made by the dental hygienist?

2. Can this client consume dairy products?

3. Which dairy products are best tolerated by lactose-deficient individuals?

4. When should lactase tablets be taken?

5. What symptoms may the client report that are associated with lactose intake?

References

Chauncey H et al. The effect of the loss of teeth on diet and nutrition. *Int Dent J* 1984; 34(2):98–104.

Duffy VB. The flavor of food—It's all in your head! *J Am Diet Assoc* 1996; 96(7):655–656.

Gudmand-Hoyer E. The clinical significance of disaccharide maldigestion. *Am J Clin Nutr* 1994; 59 (Suppl 3S):735S–741S.

Hertzler SR et al. How much lactose is low lactose? *Am J Diet Assoc* 1996; 96(3):243–246.

Mott AE et al. Diagnosis and management of taste disorders and burning mouth syndrome. *Dent Clin North Am* 1993; 37(1):33–71.

Suarez FL et al. A comparison of symptoms after the consumption of milk or lactose-hydralized milk by people with self-reported severe lactose intolerance. *N Engl J Med* 1995; 333(1):1–4.

Chapter 3

Carbohydrate: The Efficient Fuel

LEARNING OBJECTIVES

The Student Will Be Able To:
- Identify major carbohydrates in foods and in the body.
- List ways glucose can be used by the body.
- State the functions of dietary carbohydrate.
- State why carbohydrates should be included in the diet.
- Identify dietary sources of lactose, other sugars, and starches.
- State the role and sources of dietary fiber.
- State the number of calories provided per gram of carbohydrate.
- Describe the role of carbohydrate in the caries process.
- Make recommendations concerning carbohydrate consumption when counseling clients about preventing dental caries.

GLOSSARY OF TERMS

Monosaccharides   simple sugars containing two to six carbon atoms

Disaccharides   double sugars (two simple sugars joined together) containing 12 carbon atoms

Polysaccharides (complex carbohydrates)   sugars containing over 12 carbon atoms

Dextrins   intermediate products of the digestive enzymes on the starch molecules; they are long glucose chains split into shorter ones

Glycogen   the carbohydrate storage form of energy in humans

Structural polysaccharides (dietary fiber)   a mixture of several different types of polysaccharides and lignin; these are undigestible and arrive intact in the large intestine

Lipogenesis   the process of converting glucose to fats

Hyperglycemia   elevated blood sugar (above 126 mg/dl)

Hypoglycemia   low blood sugar (below 60 mg/dl)

Phenylketonuria   a genetic disorder characterized by an inability to metabolize the amino acid phenylalanine

Test Your NQ (True/False)

1. Raw sugar is nutritionally superior to white sugar. T/F
2. Fructose is the principal carbohydrate in honey. T/F
3. All caloric sugars can be metabolized by bacterial plaque. T/F
4. The desire for sweetness in the diet is an acquired taste. T/F
5. Fiber tends to regulate the rate of foods passing through the gastrointestinal tract. T/F
6. Carbohydrates are absorbed as monosaccharides. T/F
7. Excessive consumption of carbohydrates is the main cause of obesity. T/F
8. Glucose is the same as table sugar. T/F
9. Eliminating sucrose from the diet prevents the development of dental caries. T/F
10. Natural sugars in foods can be just as cariogenic as added sugars. T/F

INTRODUCTION

Carbohydrates have been the major source of energy for people since the dawn of history. Worldwide, carbohydrates are the most important source of energy, furnishing up to 90% of the calories for many African nations. There is no basis for the popular belief that carbohydrates are "fattening." They add variety and palatability to the diet and are the most economical form of energy.

Carbohydrates are made by all plants from carbon, hydrogen, and oxygen. In the process of *photosynthesis,* the carbon is combined with a molecule of water, as in $C-H_2O$:

$$6\ CO_2 + 6\ H_2O \rightarrow C_6H_{12}O_6 + 6\ O_2$$
(air)   (water)   (glucose) (oxygen)

It has been stated that a hydrated carbon is a carbohydrate.

During the 1950s, carbohydrates acquired a bad reputation in the United States. Statements have been made in best-selling books to the effect that we are the victims of "carbohydrate poisoning." Naturally, these unscientific statements affected food consumption patterns. Since the government began advising Americans in late 1977 that their risk of various chronic diseases could be reduced by eating foods containing more complex carbohydrates (fruits, vegetables, grains, legumes, and cereal products), dietary patterns have been changing. Between the 1980s and 1994, vegetable and fruit consumption increased 14% and the intake of rice, pasta, and breakfast cereals increased significantly (Putnam & Duewer, 1995). Americans are still consuming less dietary carbohydrate than is recommended (49% versus 58%) although sugar consumption is higher than recommended (Zizza & Gerrior, 1995), only 10% to 15% of the total calorie intake should be from added sugars.

Other misconceptions surrounding the intake of sugars are that (1) sugar rots the teeth, (2) food with a high sugar concentration is more dangerous to the teeth, and (3) avoidance of sticky sweets will prevent tooth decay. The incidence of caries has decreased and the number of totally caries-free children has increased dramatically in the last 20 years; during this time there were no parallel changes in the eating habits or types of food consumed (Moss, 1992) (however, fluoride usage has increased). Since 90% of all snack foods contain some form of *fermentable carbohydrate* (i.e., those that can be metabolized by bacteria in plaque, including all sugars as well as cooked or processed starches). Therefore, dental hygienists need to be knowledgeable about carbohydrates' effect on soft and hard tissues in the oral cavity as well as chronic health problems caused by low-carbohydrate, high-fat intake. Dental hygienists need to be able to counsel patients about ways to modify carbohydrate consumption that are consistent with overall physiologic health.

CLASSIFICATION

Generally, the chemical components of carbohydrate are in these proportions: $C_n(H_2O)_n$. Hence, empiric formulas such as $C_6H_{12}O_6$ or $C_{12}H_{22}O_{11}$ could readily be identified as carbohydrates. The number of carbon atoms in the molecule is used to classify carbohydrates as **monosaccharides** (two to six carbon atoms), **disaccharides** (12 carbon atoms), or **polysaccharides** (more than 12 carbon atoms).

Monosaccharides and disaccharides contribute to the palatability of a food because of their sweetness. Temperature, pH, and the presence of other substances influence the sweetness of a food. Relative sweetness of sugars is measured by subjective sensory tasting; sucrose is used as the standard of comparison (Table 3–1).

Monosaccharides

The simplest carbohydrates, monosaccharides, are absorbed without further digestion. The monosaccharides of greatest significance in foods and body metabolism are glucose, fructose, and galactose. Figure 3–1 identifies slight differences between three of the six-carbon sugars, as compared with glucose. They are less likely to be cariogenic than other sweeteners.

GLUCOSE

Also called dextrose or corn sugar, glucose is naturally abundant in many fruits, such as grapes, oranges, and dates, and in some vegetables, including fresh corn and carrots. It is prepared commercially as corn syrup or by special processing of starch. Glucose is the principal product formed by the digestion of disaccharides and polysaccharides. It provides energy for cells via the bloodstream.

FRUCTOSE

This sugar, also known as levulose, is found naturally in honey and fruits. It is the sweetest of the monosaccharides and is a product of the digestion of sucrose. Fructose can be manufactured from glucose.

GALACTOSE

Another six-carbon sugar is galactose, which is a product of lactose digestion (milk sugar). Although the primary source of galactose is milk, legumes also contain some galactose. Physiologically, it is a constituent of nerve tissue and is produced from glucose during lactation in the synthesis of lactose.

TABLE 3–1 *Relative Sweetness and Cariogenicity of Sugars and Sweeteners*

Sugar or Sweetener	Relative Sweetness*	Relative Cariogenicity*
Sugars/Natural Sweeteners		
Fructose	173	80 to 100
Honey (fructose and glucose)	130	100
Sucrose	100	100
Molasses (sucrose and invert sugar)	100	100
Brown sugar (sugar and molasses)	100	100
Dextrose/glucose (corn syrup)	74	**
Galactose	60	**
Maltose	50	**
Lactose	16	40 to 60
Sugar Alcohols		
Xylitol	90	0
Sorbitol	60	10 to 30
Mannitol	50	0
High-Intensity, Low-Calorie Sweeteners		
Alitame†	2000	**
Sucralose†	600	**
Saccharin	300	0
Acesulfame K	200	**
Aspartame	180	0

*Relative to sucrose (=100).
**Information not available.
†Pending FDA approval.

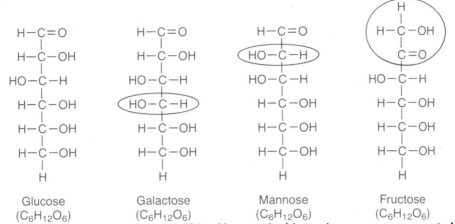

FIGURE 3–1 **The chemical structure of monosaccharides. Monosaccharides, or hexoses, are represented as straight chains called stick formulas. The chemical formula is the same, but the atoms are arranged differently, as shown by the encircled grouping. (From Davis JR, Sherer K. *Applied Nutrition and Diet Therapy for Nurses*, 2nd ed. Philadelphia: W.B. Saunders, 1994.)**

SUGAR ALCOHOLS

Sugar alcohols, such as sorbitol, may appear naturally in foods or be added by a manufacturer. Sugar alcohols, also called polyols, are formed from or converted to sugar. Polyols most frequently used or found naturally in the body include sorbitol, xylitol, and mannitol.

For a given quantity, a sugar alcohol adds about the same amount of sweetness as glucose; it also furnishes the same amount of calories. Poor absorption of all the sugar alcohols causes a laxative effect. Their advantage is that they probably do not contribute to tooth decay.

The benefit of sorbitol is that it is absorbed and metabolized more slowly than sucrose. Mannose is a six-carbon sugar derived from some legumes. Mannitol, derived from mannose, is found in foods. Xylitol is a sweetener with approximately the same perceived sweetness and caloric value as sugar. It is found in fruits and vegetables (lettuce, carrots, and strawberries).

PENTOSES

Five-carbon sugars, called pentoses, include ribose, xylose, and arabinose. Ingested pentoses are not absorbed but eliminated in the urine and feces. The body synthesizes pentose sugars from other carbohydrates as needed by the cell. Physiologically, ribose is important as a constituent of the B vitamin, riboflavin, and ribonucleic acid (RNA) and deoxyribonucleic acid (DNA), which are important in cell synthesis.

OTHER SUGARS

Raffinose, a trisaccharide, and stachyose, a tetrasaccharide, cannot be hydrolyzed by humans. Their presence in dry beans may cause flatulence.

Disaccharides

Disaccharides are not important in human metabolism because they contribute to body function only after they have been digested. All are hydrolyzed during digestion to their constituent monosaccharides for absorption as shown:

Sucrose = glucose + fructose
Maltose = glucose + glucose
Lactose = glucose + galactose

SUCROSE

Granulated table sugar is the most common form of sucrose. Commercially, sucrose is produced from sugar cane or sugar beets (not to be confused with red beets). It is also found in molasses, maple syrup, and maple sugar. Some fruits and vegetables (apricots, peaches, plums, raspberries, honeydew, cantaloupe, beets, carrots, parsnips, winter squash, peas, corn, and sweet potatoes) naturally contain large amounts of sucrose.

LACTOSE

The sugar found in milk is lactose. Lactose is unique to mammalian milk. In the fermentation of milk, some of the lactose is converted to lactic acid, giving buttermilk and yogurt their characteristic flavors.

MALTOSE

Also called malt sugar, maltose does not occur naturally. It is created in bread making and brewing and is present in beer, some processed cereals, and baby foods. It is also combined with dextrins in infant formulas.

Dental Hygiene Considerations

- Assess clients with an increased risk of dental caries for frequency of sugar intake, including sources of natural and added monosaccharides and disaccharides.
- The desire for sweetness is not considered an acquired taste because newborn infants exhibit a preference for it.
- Judgment or criticism by the dental hygienist is not beneficial in decreasing a client's use of sugar, so be nonjudgmental.

Nutritional Directions

- All caloric sugars, whether they are naturally occurring in foods or added to foods, have some cariogenic effect.
- All disaccharides contain the same caloric and nutrient content. The body cannot distinguish between natural honey or refined table sugar; both are absorbed and metabolized in the same manner.

- Encourage use of hard candies and chewing gum containing sugar alcohols (mannitol, sorbitol) to prevent caries, but alert clients to the fact that more than three to four pieces of sugar alcohol-containing items a day may cause gastric cramping and diarrhea.

Polysaccharides or Complex Carbohydrates

Some **polysaccharides** have a role in energy storage and are digestible; the second group, largely indigestible by human intestinal enzymes, is called dietary fiber (Table 3–2). Complex carbohydrates, also called polysaccharides, are composed of many (1,500 or more) monosaccharides. The chains have different structures and can be branched or straight.

STARCH

Most complex carbohydrates in the diet are in the form of starch from cereal grains, roots, vegetables, and legumes. The amount of starch present in a vegetable increases with its maturity. For example, corn tastes much sweeter immediately after it is picked than it does several days after it has been picked because its simple sugars have not developed into starch. In contrast, the amount of starch in fruit decreases as it ripens, that is, complex carbohydrates are broken down in the ripening process into simple sugars.

The presence of the cell wall, or cellulose, surrounding the starch granule is the reason starches are insoluble in cold water. Cooking facilitates the digestive process by causing the granules to swell, rupturing the cell wall so that digestive enzymes have access to the starch inside the cell. In cooking, this swelling is referred to as thickening, as occurs in making gravy. Industrially, food starch is modified by chemicals to produce a better thickening agent.

GLUCOSE POLYMERS

Industrially produced carbohydrate supplements are composed of glucose, maltose, and **dextrins.**

TABLE 3–2   *Synopsis of Fiber*

Type of Fiber	Major Food Sources	Physiologic Mechanism	Clinical Implication
Insoluble fiber			
Noncarbohydrate			
Lignin	Fruits and mature vegetables; whole grains	Decreases free radicals in GI tract	Possibly anticarcinogen
Carbohydrate			
Cellulose	Whole-wheat flour, bran, cabbage family, peas/beans, apples, root vegetables	Increases fecal bulk: Lowers GI transit time Lowers intraluminal pressure	May prevent: Constipation Hemorrhoids Diverticulosis Colon cancer
Hemicellulose	Bran, cereals, whole grains	Lowers GI exposure time to cancer-causing toxins Decreases mineral absorption	Potential for mineral deficiency
Soluble fiber			
Gums and mucilages	Oat products, dried beans, and legumes	Decreases rate for stomach emptying, delaying absorption of sugar Increases mouth to cecum transit time	Increased satiety Improved glycemic control Decreased serum lipids Cholelithiasis
Pectin	Apples, citrus fruits, strawberries	Binds with bile acids, increasing their excretion	

From Davis JR, Sherer K. *Applied Nutrition and Diet Therapy for Nurses,* 2nd ed. Philadelphia: W.B. Saunders, 1994.

Carbohydrate supplements include Polycose (Ross) and Moducal (Mead Johnson). They are used to increase caloric intake when requirements are increased and/or inadequate amounts of calories are consumed from regular foods. They are well-suited for clear-liquid diets and fat-restricted diets, or when appetite is poor. These products can be mixed easily with most foods and beverages without making them excessively sweet. Glucose polymers are absorbed as rapidly as glucose. The glucose provides 4 cal/gm, similar to other carbohydrate products.

GLYCOGEN

Stored in the muscle and liver, **glycogen** is readily available as a source of glucose and energy. Carbohydrates are frequently consumed in excess of immediate energy needs. Excess glucose is converted to glycogen until the limited glycogen storage capacity is filled; simultaneously, glucose is also converted into fats and stored as adipose tissue. The total amount of glycogen stores is actually

FIGURE 3–2   **The structure of glycogen. (From Davis JR, Sherer K. *Applied Nutrition and Diet Therapy for Nurses,* 2nd ed. Philadelphia: W.B. Saunders, 1994.)**

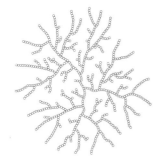

relatively small, only enough to meet energy demands for less than a day.

STRUCTURAL POLYSACCHARIDES

Dietary constituents that contribute to **dietary fiber** cannot be digested by human gastrointestinal enzymes. A large percentage, however, are digested in the large intestine by microflora, which produce fatty acids and flatus. Each type has different physiologic roles (Table 3–2), which are discussed later in the chapter.

Of concern to clients is the measure of dietary fiber, not crude fiber, which consists mainly of cellulose and lignin. For every gram of crude fiber, the food probably contains 2 or 3 gm of dietary fiber per serving. The amount of dietary fiber varies from plant to plant, and with its location within the plant (outer layers, stalk, leaf) and the age of the plant. Most plant foods contain both soluble and insoluble dietary fiber.

INSOLUBLE FIBER

Insoluble fiber does not dissolve in water and is nonfermentable in the colon. The most plentiful insoluble polysaccharide found in plants is cellulose. Although it is not digested by human digestive enzymes, it serves as a substrate for microbial fermentation and is hydrophilic (i.e., it has the ability to attract water), promoting efficient intestinal function.

Another important food fiber, hemicellulose, absorbs and retains water in the gut but has little effect on stool size. Gastrointestinal bacteria can digest much of the hemicellulose.

Lignin is a woody substance closely associated with cellulose in plants. Although it is the only noncarbohydrate fiber, it is grouped with the polysaccharides. Lignified fiber is less digestible by gut bacteria than other polysaccharides. Lignin combines with bile acids to prevent their absorption.

SOLUBLE FIBER

Pectins are nondigestible polysaccharides that form a gel with water. They are used in the preparation of fruit jams and jellies.

Gums, mucilages, and algal polysaccharides are water-soluble components of dietary fiber. These products are frequently used as additives, especially in milk products such as ice cream.

PHYSIOLOGIC ROLES

Energy

The principal role of absorbed sugars is to provide a source of energy for the body and heat to maintain body temperature. Glucose is the preferred source of energy for the brain and central nervous system, red blood cells, and the lens of the eye. Although many organs can use fats for energy, glucose is the preferred fuel. Carbohydrate, whether it was originally from a sugar or a starch, provides 4 Cal/gm. Glycogen stores are a readily available source of glucose for the tissues.

Lipogenesis

Blood sugars ensure replenishing of glycogen stores; however, excessive intake results in less fat being oxidized and in **lipogenesis.** When carbohydrates are eaten in excess of needs, lipogenesis results in increased fat stores.

Conversion to Other Carbohydrates

Monosaccharides are important constituents of many compounds that regulate metabolism. Examples include heparin, which prevents blood clotting; galactolipins, which are constituents of nervous tissue; and dermatan sulfate, which is present in tissues rich in collagen (especially the skin).

Conversion to Amino Acids

The liver can utilize part of the carbon framework from the sugar molecule and part of the protein molecule contributed by the breakdown of an amino acid to produce *nonessential amino acids,* which are essential to the body but are not required in the diet.

Normal Fat Metabolism

Oxidation of fats requires the presence of some carbohydrates. When carbohydrate intake is low, the body relies on energy from fat intake or stores. Fats are metabolized faster than the body can oxidize them; the resulting intermediate products are called *ketone* bodies. Ketones are normal products of lipid metabolism in the liver; they can only be used by muscles for energy if adequate amounts of glucose are available. An accumulation of ketones, or incompletely oxidized fatty products, results in ketosis.

Protein-Sparers

Carbohydrates, by furnishing energy in the diet, are said to be protein-sparing. Energy is an essential physiologic requirement. With insufficient carbohydrate intake, the body burns protein for fuel. If carbohydrate intake is adequate, protein can be used to build and repair tissue.

Intestinal Bacteria

Lactose and dietary fiber remain in the gastrointestinal tract longer than other nutrients. This encourages the growth of bacteria that synthesize certain vitamins (B complex and vitamin K).

Gastrointestinal Motility

The presence of fiber in the gastrointestinal tract has several functions (see Table 3–2). Insoluble fiber *accelerates* the transit rate (the time it takes for waste products to move through the intestine) in those with a slow transit time (constipation), and soluble fiber *decreases* it in those with rapid transit time (diarrhea). Fiber's ability to bind water in the intestine and increase bulk from nondigestible substances decreases the length of time waste products are in the alimentary tract. An *increased transit time* causes tissues to be exposed to cancer-causing nitrogenous waste products for longer periods of time. An added benefit of fiber is its stool softening ability, which helps prevent constipation.

Water-insoluble fiber affects the large bowel. Lignin, cellulose, and hemicellulose serve as substrates for microbial fermentation, producing fatty acids that can be used by colonic bacteria for growth. These fibers increase stool bulk, exercising the digestive tract muscles by increasing the radius of the colon and preventing the muscle from being chronically contracted. As muscle tone is maintained and colonic pressure is diminished the gut is able to resist bulging out into the pouches known as diverticuli. Insoluble fiber accelerates intestinal transit rate, slows starch hydrolysis, and delays glucose absorption.

Water-soluble fibers such as pectins, gums, psyllium, mucilages, and algal polysaccharides influence the physiology of the upper gastrointestinal tract. They are physiologically important for their gel-forming ability. Pectin increases the viscosity of chyme in the gut, thereby delaying gastric emptying and glucose absorption. These can also bind bile acids and decrease serum cholesterol levels. Another benefit is that because fiber-rich foods are not calorie-dense, they may cause one to feel full on a fewer number of calories. Whether or not it plays a significant role in weight management has yet to be determined. Guidelines for assisting clients in increasing dietary fiber are given in Table 3–3.

Other Nutrients

Carbohydrates are normally accompanied by other nutrients. Starchy foods are especially important for their contribution of protein, minerals, and B vitamins. Whole-grain products are superior be-

TABLE 3–3 *High-Fiber Diet*

Principles*	Guidelines*
1. Assess current dietary fiber intake before initiating a fiber increase. The optimal level is 35 gm of dietary fiber daily.	Fiber normalizes bowel movements to one to two a day. Cooking, freezing, and other preservation methods only slightly decrease fiber content, but grinding of foods before cooking and by the teeth may have pronounced effects on fiber action.
2. Eating food rather than fiber supplements is the best way to increase both soluble and insoluble dietary fiber.	Supplementation with concentrated or purified dietary fiber lacks the nutritional balance provided by a diet containing a variety of fruits, vegetables, whole-grain products, and legumes.
	Avoid large amounts of purified fiber such as lignin and bran because many minerals, especially calcium, iron, and zinc, may be bound by the fiber and excreted.
3. Fiber absorbs water in the intestines, so adequate fluids are important to keep the intestinal contents moving.	Ensure intake of 10 to 12 cups of water a day.
4. Increase the consumption of high-fiber foods gradually. Begin with 5- to 10-gm increments to avoid adverse side effects. A period of at least 6 to 8 weeks should be allowed for adaptation and preventing flatulence, abdominal cramping, and diarrhea/constipation.	Insoluble fiber comes principally from whole-grain products; brown color is no guarantee of whole-grain content.
	Substitute whole-wheat flour for some of the white flour in baked goods.
	Add bran, bran flakes, or oatmeal to mixed meat dishes, muffins, and pancake batter.
	Enjoy fresh fruits and vegetables in season, preferably unpeeled.
	Use whole-grain crackers and unbuttered popcorn. Incorporate beans into soups and casseroles.
	Use bran flakes for a crispy coating on meats or fish.
5. Increase intake of oat bran, beans, barley, and psyllium to help lower cholesterol levels.	Rice bran and corn bran may be just as effective in lowering serum cholesterol levels as oat bran.
	Substitute dried beans and peas occasionally for animal proteins.
	The cholesterol-lowering properties of soluble dietary fiber are more effective when the diet is also low in fat.
	Increase intake of oat bran, beans, barley, and psyllium to help lower serum cholesterol levels.

*Data from Earll L, et al. Feasibility and metabolic effects of a purified corn fiber food supplement. *J Am Diet Assoc* 1988; 88(9):950–952; Flock MH, et al. Practical aspects of implementing increased dietary fiber intake. *Am J Gastroenterol* 1986; 81(10):936–939; Hegsted M, et al. Stabilized rice bran and oat bran lower cholesterol in humans. *FASEB J* 1990; 4(3):A368; Eastwood MA. The physiological effect of dietary fiber: An update. *Annu Rev Nutr* 1992; 12; 19–35.

From Davis JR, Sherer K. *Applied Nutrition and Diet Therapy for Nurses,* 2nd ed. Philadelphia: W.B. Saunders, 1994.

cause they contain fiber plus other nutrients (see Table 1–4); enriched products should always be used in preference to those processed but not enriched.

Dental Hygiene Considerations

- Utilization of carbohydrate requires an adequate supply of B vitamins and two minerals, phosphorus and magnesium. Usually adequate amounts of these nutrients accompany the increased carbohydrate intake. However, this may not be true if refined sugars and breads are the predominant choices because adequate amounts of B vitamins and minerals may not be provided.

- Ketosis frequently occurs in persons with uncontrolled diabetes mellitus or in those who are not eating (due to illness or dieting) because they are burning fat rather than carbohydrate. Therefore, question clients with fruity smelling breath about their recent dietary intake.

Nutritional Directions

- Carbohydrates are not fattening.
- Fiber tends to regulate the rate of foods in the gastrointestinal tract; the best source of dietary fiber to relieve constipation is bran.
- Enthusiastic patients who eat excessive amounts of bran (50 to 60 gm) gain no benefit from the surplus and expose themselves unnecessarily to known hazards, such as decreased mineral and vitamin absorption.
- Some vegetables and fruits (bananas, white potatoes, and apples) are high in pectins, which bind water. They are frequently used to control diarrhea but can also help relieve constipation by softening the stool.
- Even when dieting, it is important to consume carbohydrates, especially vegetables, fruits, whole-grain breads and cereals, to provide vital nutrients.
- Carbohydrates supply 4 Cal/gm and are a less concentrated source of energy than fats (9 Cal/gm).

REQUIREMENTS

Since amino acids and a portion of fats consumed can be converted to glucose, a specific requirement for carbohydrate has not been established by the National Research Council. A reasonable proportion of the caloric intake should consist of carbohydrates (minimum of 50 to 100 gm digestible carbohydrate) to avoid ketosis, excessive breakdown of protein, loss of electrolytes, and involuntary dehydration. The importance of complex carbohydrate rather than sugar intake is emphasized.

Although dietary fiber is important, a specific RDA has not been made. Approximately 20 to 35 gm of dietary fiber daily is suggested as an appropriate fiber intake. This can be provided by incorporating adequate whole grains, fruits, and vegetables into the diet (Table 3–4). The average daily intake of dietary fiber in the United States is about 12 gm (Smallwood & Blaylock, 1994).

SOURCES

Presently, the American diet furnishes about 45% of the calories from carbohydrates, or almost 400 gm carbohydrate daily. Carbohydrates are furnished by the following food groups: milk, grain, fruits, and vegetables. The average sugar intake is about 11% to 13% of daily caloric intake.

The only animal foods supplying significant quantities of carbohydrate are milk and milk products, which furnish the disaccharide lactose. In cheese making, the lactose remains in the whey, which is removed as a byproduct. Consequently, most cheeses contain only trace amounts of lactose.

TABLE 3–4   *Sources of Fiber*

	Insoluble Fiber	Soluble Fiber
Wheat bran	X	
Whole-wheat products	X	
Corn bran	X	
Oat bran	X	X
Whole-grain oats	X	X
Barley	X	X
Rice bran	X	
Brown rice	X	
Nuts	X	
Lentils	X	X
Navy beans	X	X
Soy beans	X	X
Kidney beans	X	X
Bananas	X	X
Apples	X	X
Cauliflower	X	
Potatoes	X	X
Citrus fruits		X
Green beans and peas	X	
Broccoli	X	X
Carrots	X	X
Psyllium		X
Pectin		X
Carrageenan		X
Guar gum		X
Flax seed		X

From Davis JR, Sherer K. *Applied Nutrition and Diet Therapy for Nurses,* 2nd ed. Philadelphia: W.B. Saunders, 1994.

Other sugars are furnished by table sugar, syrups, jellies, jams, and honey. Sugars are incorporated into many popular foods (e.g., candy, beverages, cakes and desserts, chewing gum, and ice cream). Only about 25% of the sugar we consume is added to foods in the home and by institutions and restaurants; the remainder is added to foods during processing and in canning and freezing; breakfast cereals; condiments and salad dressings; soft drinks; cookies, crackers, and can-dies; flavored extracts and syrups; flour and bread products; and milk and milk products.

Approximately 18% of the caloric intake is from natural sugars that occur in fruits and vegetables. (This amount does not include sugar in milk.) Sugars, mainly glucose and fructose, are furnished in fruits and vegetables in varying amounts depending on their maturity (ripe bananas contain more simple sugars than green bananas) and their water content (spinach contains less carbohydrate than potatoes) (Table 3–5).

The dietary guideline, "choose a diet moderate in sugar," is rather vague for most professionals and consumers because of the many different ways sugar is incorporated into foods. In the Food Guide Pyramid, sugars are grouped with fats at the small

TABLE 3–5   *Free Sugars in Selected Fruits and Vegetables**

	Glucose	Fructose	Sucrose
Apricots	1.73	1.28	5.84
Beets	0.85	0.85	4.24
Blackberries	2.48	2.15	0.59
Blueberries	3.76	3.82	0.19
Carrots	0.85	0.85	4.24
Corn	0.34	0.31	3.03
Currants	3.33	3.68	0.95
Grapes	6.86	7.84	2.25
Honeydew melon	0.18	0.16	6.11
Lettuce	0.25	0.46	0.10
Parsnips	0.18	0.24	2.98
Peaches	0.91	1.18	6.92
Pears	0.95	6.77	1.61
Plums	3.49	1.53	4.94
Raspberries, red	2.4	1.58	3.68
Strawberries	2.09	2.40	1.03
Sweet Potato	0.33	0.30	3.37
Winter Squash	0.96	1.16	1.61

*Percentage of Fresh/Raw Edible Portion

From Shallenberger RS. Occurrence of various sugars in foods. *In* Sipple HL, McNutt KW. *Sugars in Nutrition.* New York: Academic Press, 1974; 67–80.

TABLE 3–6   *Dietary Fiber Content of Sample Menu**

Sample Menu	Dietary Fiber Content (gm)
Breakfast	
Orange juice (1 cup)	0.5
Bagel (1) with	1.2
cream cheese (1 oz)	0
Raisins (1 packet)	0.7
1% Milk (1 cup)	0
Coffee	0
Creamer (1 tsp)	0
Lunch	
Sandwich: Tuna (1 oz)	0
Mayonnaise (2 Tbsp)	0
Tomato (2 slices)	0.5
Lettuce slices	0.4
Whole-wheat bread (2 slices)	5.6
Apple (1)	3.0
1% Milk (1 cup)	0
Afternoon Snack	
Frozen yogurt (1 cup)	0
Dinner	
Lean roast beef (2 oz)	0
Gravy (¼ cup)	0
Brown rice (1 cup)	3.3
Corn (½ cup)	1.7
Three-bean salad (½ cup)	5.3
Whole-wheat roll (1)	1.8
Margarine (1 Tbsp)	0
Strawberries (½ cup)	1.6
Iced tea	0
Evening Snack	
Diet cola (12 oz)	0
Dry roasted nuts (1 oz)	2.3
Totals	28.1

*This menu could easily be further increased by changing from orange juice to 1 whole orange (3.1 gm of fiber), increasing to 1 cup strawberries (additional 1.6 gm of fiber), and/or increasing the amount of three-bean salad.

Nutrient data from *Nutritionist IV* software. The Hearst Corporation, San Bruno, CA. From Davis JR, Sherer K. *Applied Nutrition and Diet Therapy for Nurses,* 2nd ed. Philadelphia: W.B. Saunders, 1994.

tip of the Pyramid as well as being found in other food groups (a sugar sign appears next to these foods to remind people that some foods in all food groups can be high in sugar).

People's consumption of these products varies, with some finding it easier to change their soft drink consumption than to give up their candy bars, and others preferring to give up their breakfast roll or donut to changing their choice of sugar-containing beverage. Eating sugar in *moderation* implies that appropriate balance among foods or nutrients is the overriding consideration in food selection.

Complex carbohydrates or starches are furnished by grain products (wheat, corn, rice, oats, rye, barley, buckwheat, and millet). Some vegetables, especially root and seed varieties (potatoes, sweet potatoes, beets, carrots, peas, and winter squashes), also contain considerable amounts of starch. Dried beans and peas are excellent sources of complex carbohydrates.

Dietary fiber, especially hemicellulose and cellulose, is furnished by whole-grain breads and cereals. Cellulose is found principally in the stems, roots, leaves, and seed coverings of plants; unpeeled fruits and leafy vegetables are good sources. Legumes are also a good source of dietary fiber. The pectin contributed by fruits and vegetables is an important source of fiber. Table 3–4 shows specific foods containing large amounts of soluble and/or insoluble fiber, and Table 3–6 indicates the fiber-containing foods provided in a sample menu.

Dental Hygiene Considerations

- Assess not only total sugar intake, but also the frequency, form, and time of day of carbohydrate intake.
- Encourage patients to increase fiber intake. Fiber helps reduce constipation and diverticulosis, and may help reduce some colon cancers.
- Encourage patients to consume a diet high in carbohydrate to maintain glycogen reserves, whereas a diet high in fat and low in carbohydrate and protein results in poor glycogen reserves. Because glycogen

stores in the heart are critical for continuous functioning of heart muscles, the importance of carbohydrates should be emphasized.

Nutritional Directions

◆ Encourage clients to consume more complex carbohydrates and less refined sugar.

◆ A tablespoon of honey has more calories than a tablespoon of sugar and only trace amounts of other nutrients. (Honey is not appropriate for children under 2 years of age because of the risk of botulism it poses.) Because of its retentive nature, honey is also more cariogenic than refined sugar.

◆ Inform clients on weight-reduction diets that food labels must indicate the total amount of carbohydrate (starch, sugar, and fiber) in a serving. Because fiber is not absorbed, it

does not contribute any calories. Hence a product with 25 gm of carbohydrate may have only 80 calories if at least 5 gm of the carbohydrate are from fiber.

◆ The U.S. FDA has labeled raw sugar as "unfit for direct use as food or as a food ingredient because of the impurities it ordinarily contains."

◆ Clients should be aware that sugar may be identified as any of the following on food labels: sucrose, fructose, corn sweetener, cane sugar, honey, molasses, high-fructose corn syrup, raw sugar, and maple syrup. Patients trying to reduce concentrated sweets should avoid foods if the first ingredient is any of the aforementioned.

◆ Only about one-third of the sugars in some corn syrups are identified as "sugar" on laboratory analysis of foods. Products containing corn syrup may appear to be lower in sugar than they actually are.

HYPER- AND HYPO- STATES

The role of sugar on nutritional health and behavior continues to be misrepresented by the press and many professionals. Many stories have been published in the media linking sugar to practically every modern-day illness, including malnutrition, hypoglycemia, diabetes mellitus, blood lipid abnormalities, cardiovascular disease, hyperactivity, criminal behavior, obesity, malabsorption syndrome, allergies, gallstones, and cancer. Thus, the public's perception of sugar consumption continues to be at odds with scientific facts.

In 1986 the Sugars Task Force of the U.S. FDA, after an extensive review of the scientific literature, concluded that sugar consumption at typical American levels does not directly contribute to any chronic health or behavioral problems. Normal physiologic conditions and disease states affect carbohydrate metabolism, which is reflected in serum glucose levels (**hyperglycemia** or **hypoglycemia**). Other factors concerning too much or too little carbohydrate are discussed below.

Carbohydrate Excess

Sugars contain no other nutrients (vitamins and minerals), and, when consumed as soft drinks and hard candies, provide nothing other than pleasure and energy. Soft drinks are increasingly being substituted for milk and coffee. Annual soft drink consumption reached approximately 45 gallons per person in 1992, an increase of about 60% since 1977–78 (Tippett & Goldman, 1994). A diet high in sugar from too many pastries, candies, and soft drinks is less likely to be adequate in other nutrients.

On the other hand, sugar increases palatability and may induce ingestion of certain foods otherwise disliked. Combining sugar with other nutritious foods, as in milk used for pudding, may increase the variety of foods consumed and enjoyed.

Carbohydrate Deficiency

Frequently, complex carbohydrates are eliminated in the belief that they are fattening. This can result in an insufficient intake of B vitamins, iron, and fiber.

There is no evidence that sugar can cancel the nutritive value of a food or an otherwise adequate diet. Vitamins and minerals are necessary for the body to utilize sugar, but it is not essential for these nutrients to be present in the same foods. Only when sugar consumption interferes with or replaces a well-balanced intake does the diet become inadequate, and only then does sugar deserve the designation of "empty calorie," which indicates that it is inadequate in vitamins, minerals, and trace elements. There is no evidence to prove that sugar consumption actually contributes to micronutrient deficiencies in people who consume adequate calories.

Dental Caries

For many years, sucrose has been considered the "arch-criminal" in dental caries formation. Not only does sucrose have unusual biochemical properties that promote bacterial growth, but it is also the most frequently consumed form of sugar. The presence of sucrose in the mouth increases the volume and rate of plaque formation. High sucrose concentrations promote the production of polysaccharides (glucans) by *Streptococcus mutans* which permit bacterial colonies to adhere to the tooth. Sucrose can lower the pH of dental plaque, hastening the dissolution of the hydroxyapatite crystals of the enamel. Glucose available from sucrose can be used by oral bacteria in the dental plaque.

Many health professionals and consumers believe that removing sucrose from the diet would largely eliminate dental caries. However, only a small amount of sugar is needed for maximum acid formation and demineralization of the teeth. Despite differences in the sugar content of carbonated beverages, fruit drinks and juices (about 10%), and sport drinks (about 4.4% sugar), all appear to have similar cariogenic potential.

Other monosaccharides and disaccharides, such as glucose, fructose, maltose, and lactose, are also readily metabolized by oral microorganisms, with resultant demineralization of tooth enamel. These sugars diffuse rapidly into dental plaque to become available for bacteria. In laboratory tests, fructose and glucose rapidly lower plaque pH similar to sucrose; thus they are considered as cariogenic as sucrose. Substituting glucose or fructose for sucrose would not be significantly effective in lowering caries rates (Rugg-Gunn, 1990). On the other hand, a 2-year study in humans found significantly fewer dental caries in the fructose group than in the sucrose group (Scheinin & Mäkinen, 1975). Lactose is less cariogenic than other sugars.

Although the picture is not completely clear, it appears that sucrose is the most cariogenic of sugars, but it is not the only cariogenic sugar. The kind of sugar is not significant; neither is the concentration of sugar in a foodstuff critical to its cariogenic potential.

Most studies of large populations have correlated caries rates with total sugar consumption (Navia, 1994). Conversely, no clear-cut relationship has been shown between total carbohydrate consumption of individuals and caries. Starches can cause accumulation of plaque acid when consumed as part of a mixed diet containing fermentable carbohydrates. Some foods, such as potato chips, that have a high-carbohydrate, low-sugar content can be active participants in the caries process (IADR, 1986).

The starch molecule is large and cannot penetrate into dental plaque. Cooked and refined cereal grains are more readily hydrolyzed by salivary and plaque amylases to produce maltose, which can lower the pH and demineralize enamel (Mundorff et al., 1990). Some foods high in sugar are removed quicker and do not lower the pH of plaque as much as starchy foods with less sugar. Starches, such as breads and pasta, are considered less cariogenic than sugars but may tend to prolong the caries attack once it has been initiated, especially when sugar is added, as in sweet breads and cookies.

The total amount of fermentable dietary carbohydrate appears to be of less importance than the form in which it is eaten and the frequency of consumption. This may be related to variables that influence the length of time carbohydrate is in contact with the teeth and its potential for promoting growth of caries-forming, acid-producing bacteria.

Because of the belief that sucrose restriction would curtail dental caries, attempts have been made to replace sucrose in popular snack products with sweeteners that are less cariogenic. Sugar alcohols may decrease the risk of dental caries through any one of the following mechanisms: (1) inhibiting the growth of *S. mutans*, (2) not promoting the synthesis of dental plaque, or (3) not lowering plaque pH.

Sorbitol causes only a slight pH decrease in dental plaque. Plaque bacteria are able to ferment sorbitol and mannitol, but only at a very slow rate over several weeks. After a period of adaptation, however, acid production increases.

Xylitol is anticariogenic because oral bacteria lack the enzymes to ferment it; therefore plaque pH does not drop. Xylitol stimulates secretion of saliva, which contains a larger number of bicarbonate ions that help to neutralize plaque acid. Xylitol may inhibit growth of *S. mutans*. Certain mixtures of sorbitol and xylitol may be more protective against dental caries than sorbitol alone.

Lactitol has not been approved for use in the United States by the FDA; however, it is used in other countries. Lactitol cannot be metabolized by plaque bacteria and may even provide a protective effect for teeth. However, it is only about one-third as sweet as sucrose.

Saccharin inhibits tooth decay in rats. Aspartame does not support the growth of *S. mutans*, acid production, or plaque formation.

Dental Hygiene Considerations

- Counsel clients that they can maintain healthy teeth and still include sweet-tasting foods without increasing the risk of caries.
- Approximately 90% of commonly consumed snack foods contain fermentable carbohydrates (sugars and/or cooked starch).
- Snacks contribute significantly to the nutri-

tional intake of young children and teenagers, who need larger amounts of calories for growth.
- Clients unable to tolerate adequate amounts at meals require snacks to promote healing and avoid loss of lean tissue.
- Although sucrose is a major factor in caries risk, provide factual information that does not overblame or overclaim sugar's role in caries formation.
- Some foods, such as milk and aged cheese, actually protect the teeth by raising the pH of the mouth and inhibiting acid production. If snacks are needed when oral hygiene cannot be performed, suggest snacks consisting of milk or aged cheese or follow snacks with these items.
- Be aware of adaptive changes by microorganisms that may occur when sugar sources are changed.
- Total elimination of sweets permanently is unrealistic. The best advice is to use sugar in moderation and limit the frequency of sugar exposure.

Nutritional Directions

- All sugars and cooked starches are potentially cariogenic.
- Natural sugars, primarily fructose and glucose, in unprocessed foods, such as bananas and apples, are potentially as cariogenic as sucrose.
- Vegetables such as lettuce, celery, and broccoli that do not contain sugars do not cause acid production or demineralization of enamel in humans (DePaula et al., 1994).
- Sugar alcohols do not promote caries; xylitol may even prevent caries formation.
- The most important cause of dental caries is the frequency of intake of fermentable carbohydrates, which supply substrate to the caries-producing oral bacteria.
- The potential for caries exists every time a food is eaten because most foods will promote acid formation if no procedures are

taken to remove food debris or plaque, or to interfere with acid production.

♦ Replacing potentially cariogenic snacks with foods such as fresh fruits and vegetables; low-fat cottage cheese, cheese, and yogurt; peanuts, or low-fat popcorn can decrease caries and promote other health-conscious nutritional habits.

♦ To prevent dental caries (1) always brush after eating, and (2) eat sweets as part of a meal rather than as snacks.

♦ Using a straw with beverages such as carbonated drinks may lessen contact with the teeth and lessen the risk of caries.

♦ The amount of sugar in a food is unrelated to its caries-forming potential; all carbohydrate foods are potentially cariogenic.

♦ High-carbohydrate foods, especially complex unrefined carbohydrates, are high in fiber and other nutrients.

Obesity

Many people continue to believe that sugar is uniquely fattening. Because the taste of sugar is so pleasant, some rationalize that sugar becomes irresistible to the point of overconsumption. However, most people have a limit as to how sweet they like their foods and how much sweetness they can eat at a time.

There is no evidence that carbohydrates or sugars are a cause of obesity. Excessive caloric intake leads to obesity, whether from carbohydrates, proteins, fats, or alcohol. Although excessive calories from sugar intake could lead to obesity, epidemiologic studies and several individual studies have shown that obese patients actually consume less sugar than thin patients. Many sweet foods contain large amounts of fat. Too much carbohydrate is likely to be consumed as fat consumption is limited but overall food intake is not restricted to some degree.

Dental Hygiene Considerations

● Scientific studies do not support the claim that sugars interfere with bioavailability of vitamins, minerals, or trace nutrients or the notion that dietary imbalances are preferentially caused by increased sugar consumption. Thus, do not assume that just because a client is obese, increased sugar intake is the culprit.

Nutritional Directions

♦ A well-balanced diet that contains adequate nutrients with larger amounts of fruits and vegetables is advisable.

♦ Several organs are dependent on glucose to function. A change to a low-carbohydrate, high-fat diet usually results in an increase in food intake without an increase in glucose; however, an increase in calories from carbohydrate foods with a concurrent decrease in fats has strong scientific support because it provides increased glucose for organ function.

SUGAR SUBSTITUTES

The practice of flavoring foods without additional calories is one of many approaches to the problems of excess calorie intake and a sedentary life. The use of sugar substitutes also has beneficial ramifications for dental hygiene. The desire to decrease sugar consumption is being met through the widespread and increasing use of numerous sugar substitutes (Fig. 3–3). In the 1980s, consumption of low-calorie sweeteners increased faster than that of caloric sweeteners. Total use of caloric sweeteners rose from 123 lbs per capita in 1970 to 148 lbs in 1994 (17% increase); low-calorie sweetener use increased from 5.8 to 24.3 lbs per capita (319% increase) during the same time period.

These products are used principally for their sweetening power, but they also make some foods more palatable. The large variety of sweeteners is desirable because each has certain advantages and

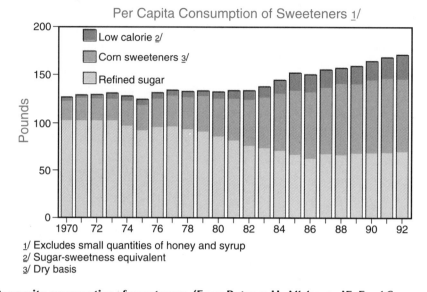

Per Capita Consumption of Sweeteners 1/

1/ Excludes small quantities of honey and syrup
2/ Sugar-sweetness equivalent
3/ Dry basis

FIGURE 3–3   **Per capita consumption of sweeteners. (From Putnam JJ, Allshouse JE. Food Consumption, Prices, and Expenditures, 1970–92. USDA, Economic Research Service, Statistical Bulletin No. 867. Washington, D.C., 1993.)**

limitations. Because each sweetener has different properties, the availability of various products helps satisfy various flavor and texture requirements in foods and beverages. Sweeteners are combined because of their *synergistic* effect, that is, when combined sweeteners yield a sweeter taste than that provided by each sweetener alone.

Although taste buds may be fooled by their sweetness, artificial sweeteners do not produce a prolonged feeling of satiety. On the other hand, numerous studies indicate that low-calorie sweeteners do not increase the appetite. Use of these artificial sweeteners may or may not decrease the total caloric intake, depending on other food choices. Compensatory food choices such as drinking a diet carbonated beverage to permit a piece of cheesecake will be ineffective in weight control, whereas using a low-calorie food to replace a high-calorie food, watching other food intake, and engaging in some form of exercise may be beneficial.

Many patients question the safety of these products. All the products on the market have been extensively researched and are safe for most people if consumed in moderation (except for aspartame,

which should be avoided by patients with **phenylketonuria**). Information regarding sugar substitutes is summarized in Table 3–7.

Dental Hygiene Considerations

- Sugar substitutes can reduce the caloric content and decrease cariogenicity of a product. Used in moderation, sugar substitutes are beneficial for many people, especially those with diabetes.

- Because aspartame contains phenylalanine, aspartame-containing products are labeled to warn persons with phenylketonuria to avoid their use.

- The use of sugar substitutes is especially advocated for between-meal snacks to decrease frequency of exposure of the teeth to sugar. For those who do not need to decrease caloric intake, sugar alcohols may be recommended.

- Sugar substitutes are nonfermentable and therefore do not promote caries formation; antimicrobial activity has not been observed.

TABLE 3–7   *Low-Calorie Sweeteners*

	Saccharin	Aspartame	Cyclamate	Acesulfame K
Description	Noncaloric sweetener	Nutritive noncaloric sweetener made from two amino acids: phenylalanine and aspartic acid	Noncaloric sweetener; used widely during the 1960s in low-calorie foods and beverages	Noncaloric sweetener; odorless, crystalline sweetener
Assets	Stable shelf life; combines well with other sweeteners; synergistic effect when combined with other low-calorie sweeteners	Sugar-like taste; enhances some flavors; synergistic effect when combined with other low-calorie sweeteners; appropriate for many applications	Stable in heat and cold, good shelf life; soluble in liquids; has synergistic effect when combined with other low-calorie sweeteners	Sweet taste is quickly perceptible; good shelf life; high degree of stability
Limitations	Slight aftertaste, which can be lessened when blended with another low-calorie sweetener	Unstable at prolonged high heat; not suitable for cooking or in products exposed to high temperatures; can be added to heated recipes after cooking; loses sweetness gradually depending on temperature and acidity; restrict intake for patients with phenylketonuria	Least "sweetening power" of the commercially acceptable intense sweeteners	Some aftertaste noted at levels required to achieve adequate sweetness when used alone; when blended with other low-calorie sweeteners, provides improved taste; economic and stable
Applications	Primarily in soft drinks, tabletop sweeteners, and other beverages and foods, as well as cosmetics and pharmaceuticals	Wide variety of products, including tabletop sweeteners, soft drinks, other beverages, puddings, fillings, milk beverages, frozen desserts and novelties, candies, baked goods and mixes	Before 1970, widely used as tabletop sweetener, in sugar-free beverages and other low-calorie foods, particularly with saccharin	Potentially useful for almost all applications, including soft drinks and baked goods

Table continued on following page

TABLE 3–7   *Low-Calorie Sweeteners* (Continued)

	Saccharin	Aspartame	Cyclamate	Acesulfame K
Safety	Nearly a century of safe human use; 30 human studies found no association between saccharin and bladder cancer; NCI concluded that there was "no evidence of increased risk with long-term use of artificial sweeteners in any form or with use that began decades ago"; FDA now has less concern about saccharin than in 1977. "The actual risk, if any, of saccharin to humans still appears to be slight." Research now demonstrates that saccharin is unlikely to cause cancer in humans; differences in rat urine and the type of saccharin used in rat studies cause the differences observed	Extensive animal and human studies provide strong evidence that aspartame is no more hazardous than normal dietary protein consumption; in 1984, the CDC found that the complaints "do not provide evidence of the existence of serious widespread, adverse health consequences; the majority of frequently reported symptoms were mild and uncommon in the general populace. In July, 1985, AMA's Council on Scientific Affairs concluded that consumption of aspartame is safe and "is not associated with serious adverse health effects"	Banned in the US in 1970; current petition for reapproval in the US	Tested in approximately 90 studies; on approval, FDA said it "found that the safety studies did not show any toxic effects that could be attributed to the sweetener"

TABLE 3–7 *Low-Calorie Sweeteners (Continued)*

	Saccharin	Aspartame	Cyclamate	Acesulfame K
Status	A 1977 proposed ban on saccharin in the United States was stayed by Congress pending further research; congressional moratorium on saccharin ban was extended five times; current moratorium is in effect; in 1991, the FDA formally withdrew its 1977 proposal to ban saccharin use; it is used in more than 90 countries	Approved for use in more than 95 countries and is available in more than 5,000 products worldwide	In June, 1985, NAS concluded, "the totality of the evidence from studies in animals does not indicate that cyclamate or its metabolites is carcinogenic by itself"; petitioned for reapproval pending; approved for use in more than 50 countries	Approved by FDA in July 1988 for use in dry beverage mixes, instant coffee and tea, chewing gum, gelatins, puddings, dairy product analogues, and tabletop sweetener; approved for use in more than 40 countries

NCI, National Cancer Institute; NAS, National Academy of Sciences; CDC, Centers for Disease Control.

Adapted from Sweetener Fact Sheets: Saccharin, May 1992; Aspartame, September 1992; Cyclamate, September 1992; Acesulfame K, September 1992. Calorie Control Council, 5775 Peachtree-Dunwoody Road, Ste 500-G. Atlanta, GA 30342.

● Saccharin and aspartame exhibit microbial inhibition and caries suppression.

Nutritional Directions

◆ Noncaloric sweeteners do nothing to appease the appetite, but they do provide the pleasure of sweetness. They enable clients to choose a wide variety of foods while managing their caloric intake.

◆ Clients who need to rely on sugar substitutes to help with blood glucose control should use multiple types so that only small amounts of any one sweetener are consumed.

◆ When deciding whether a young child should be given artificially sweetened foods, consider the child's body weight and limit the sweetener to below recommended levels (500 mg/day for saccharin, 50 mg/kg body weight for aspartame, and 15 mg/kg body weight for Acesulfame-K). One packet of Sweet & Low (Cumberland Packing Corp.) contains 40 mg of saccharin; one packet Sweet One (Stadt Corp.), 50 mg of acesulfame; 1 packet of Equal (Nutrasweet Co.), 35 mg of aspartame. Remember, children need calories for growth and development.

◆ Combinations of sweeteners can produce a sweet taste more similar to that of sugar than can a single high-intensity sweetener.

◆ During pregnancy, aspartame (limited amounts) is the preferred sweetener because it is metabolized like other amino acids, whereas saccharin is known to cross the placenta. Refer the client to her obstetrician for counseling about use of nonnutritive sweeteners.

HEALTH APPLICATION 3

The Effects of Sugar on Behavior

Many parents and teachers believe that sugar causes hyperactivity in children. Attention deficit hyperactivity disorder (ADHD) is the latest term for hyperkinetic behavior syndrome, hyperactivity, learning disabilities, or minimal brain dysfunction. It is characterized by chronic age-inappropriate behaviors, with inattention, impulsiveness, hyperactivity, or restlessness. For a diagnosis of ADHD, the child must exhibit specific symptoms before age 7. Many theories have been proposed on the causes of hyperactivity, but none has been proven conclusively.

In the 1970s, the late Dr. Benjamin Feingold suggested a diet for ADHD free of all foods containing artificial colorings, flavorings, and naturally occurring salicylates. Sugar per se was not restricted, but the overall acceptable sugar intake was lowered because of its close association with colorings and flavorings in processed foods. However, numerous controlled studies failed to reproduce the dramatic behavioral improvement Feingold reported. While a minority of children may be helped by this diet, benefits may be associated with increased family involvement, increased individual attention, and expectations rather than the diet per se.

Meta-analysis of 16 scientific studies (double-blind, placebo-controlled) indicates that sugar does not affect behavior or cognitive performance of children (Wolraich et al., 1995). Whether sugar intake is a symptom or a cause of this behavior disorder is unknown. While a few studies testing the effect of sugar on hyperactive behavior have found a positive correlation, most have found no association or observed a calming effect.

In a study by Wender and Solanto (1992), neither sugar nor aspartame-sweetened placebos caused aggressive behavior of normal or ADHD-affected children, but inattentiveness of ADHD children increased only after sugar intake. Since some studies have noted an improvement in vigilance and motor behavior of hyperactive children with sugar intake, Conners (1991) has hypothesized that an elevated brain serotonin level might be beneficial to these hyperactive children. Studies suggest hyperactive children may have chronically elevated blood sugar levels and exaggerated responses to sucrose challenges related to abnormal neuroendocrine or catecholamine regulation. It is possible that children with ADHD may inadvertently choose a diet with a high sugar content to increase energy intake.

The belief that high sugar intake causes ADHD is in direct opposition to the results of many research studies. Sugar intake of normal boys and boys with ADHD was similar in one study, averaging 15% of the caloric intake (Wolraich et al, 1986). External clues, such as parties or celebrations, possibly associated with sugar intake will cause hyperactivity. The National Institute of Health has concluded that dietary changes other than a well-balanced diet cannot be recommended until clinical significances have been documented.

Evidence of an association between diet and behavior is considered weak, and health professionals need to be critical of scientific claims regarding diet and behavior. Inappropriate dietary treatment without scientific backing could (1) detract from efforts to identify effective treatment and prevention of delinquent behavior, (2) lead to nutritional deficiencies or excesses, and (3) provide offenders with a dietary excuse for their behavior rather than assuming responsibility for their own behavior.

CASE APPLICATION FOR THE DENTAL HYGIENIST

A healthy client needs information on how to eat less refined sugar and more complex carbohydrate. He knows this regimen is being encouraged but is not sure about all the health reasons. Fiber intake is also important to him, but he is not knowledgeable about the types of food needed or the benefits.

Nutritional Assessment

○ Willingness/motivation to learn
○ Usual dietary habits; focus especially on carbohydrate
○ Basic knowledge of carbohydrate and carbohydrate principles
○ Usual food/nutrient intake
○ Financial status, employment status and place
○ Support persons, married, divorced, single
○ Use of community resources
○ Food shopping practices

Nutritional Diagnosis

Health-seeking behavior related to lack of knowledge concerning carbohydrate and carbohydrate principles for optimal nutrition.

Nutritional Goals

Client will consume a high-fiber food and complex carbohydrate foods daily and state three principles concerning carbohydrate.

Nutritional Implementation

Intervention: Explain (1) that the main function of carbohydrate is to provide energy for the body; (2) that excessive amounts of carbohydrate in conjunction with excessive calories are converted to triglycerides and stored as fat but that carbohydrates themselves do not cause obesity; and (3) roles of carbohydrate.
Rationale: Knowledge corrects misinformation.

Intervention: (1) Follow suggestions in Table 3–4. (2) Explain the importance of fiber. Recommend 20 to 35 gm of fiber daily, and help the client plan a diet that will provide this amount, incorporating his food preferences. Stress the importance of adequate fluid intake.

Rationale: These will increase fiber in the diet. Fiber increases stool bulk, exercising digestive tract muscles and thus preventing them from being chronically contracted. Therefore, muscle tone is maintained, colonic pressure is diminished, and the gut is able to resist bulging out into pouches. Additionally, fiber slows starch hydrolysis and delays glucose absorption.

Intervention: Explain sources of complex carbohydrates and fiber sources and provide the client with a list of these foods.
Rationale: These measures will help the client consume more complex carbohydrate and fiber by increasing knowledge and providing concrete information.

Intervention: (1) Recommend substituting artificial sweeteners for sugar, especially at snacktime. (2) Actually read a label with the client to determine how to recognize sugars (they usually end in "-ose"). (3) Recommend substituting fresh fruit for juices. (4) Instruct him to avoid products like cookies and pastries that contain complex carbohydrates and sugar.
Rationale: He wanted to reduce refined sugar intake, and these measures will help meet this personal goal.

Intervention: Refer him to a registered dietitian and county extension agencies.
Rationale: These will provide expert knowledge and community resources for continued compliance.

Intervention: Review labeling: (1) a high-fiber food has been defined as containing 5 gm or more per serving; (2) "no sugar added" means sugar was not added, although the product may naturally contain sugar; (3) "sugar-free" means the product contains no added sucrose but may have other sugars added such as sorbitol; (4) incorporate foods with 3 gm or more of fiber per serving.

Rationale: If a client does not know how to read labels, unhealthy food choices may be selected inadvertently.

Evaluation

The client consumes a bran muffin, beans, or other high-fiber foods daily and verbalizes that carbohydrates provide energy and fiber, carbohydrate has several roles in maintaining gut functioning, and most sugars end in "-ose." Other indicators of success include reading a label correctly, reducing intake of refined sugars, and using the community resources.

Student Readiness

1. Differentiate between the three classes of carbohydrates.

2. Identify sources of complex carbohydrates in the diet.

3. What are the main sources of fiber in the American diet? What are the main sources of starch? List three of your favorite foods high in sugar. What realistic modifications can you make to your diet with respect to these high-sugar foods?

4. Explain the functions of sugars and fiber in the diet in terms a client can understand.

5. From cereal boxes at the local grocery store, identify some of the products that claim to be high in fiber. (a) Evaluate the source of fiber on the ingredient label to determine if those are soluble or insoluble fibers. (b) Rank the cereals according to the amount of dietary fiber they contain. Which would you recommend?

6. Discuss why a diet with limited amounts of carbohydrate is neither healthy nor wise.

7. How would you advise a mother who has been told she should never give her infant anything that contains sugar because the infant will develop a sweet tooth?

8. Match the carbohydrates on the left with the appropriate answer in the right column.

Dextrose	Cannot be used by the body
Glycogen	Milk
Fructose	Sweetest sugar
Lactose	Glucose
Cellular	Storage form of carbohydrate in the body

CASE STUDY

A 22-year-old African American male presents with four carious lesions acquired since his last dental hygiene recall appointment. Questioning the client reveals that he frequently skips meals and relies heavily on snacks to get him through the day.

1. What further information about his dietary intake do you need?

2. Could the client's snacking habits be related to his increase in dental caries?

3. Which types of foods should be suggested as snack foods and why?

4. What other precautions could the client practice that might be helpful in preventing further caries problems?

References

Connors CK. Sugars and hyperactivity. *In* Kretchmer N, Hollenbeck CB (eds). *Sugars and Sweeteners.* Boca Raton, FL: CRC Press, 1991.

DePaula DP et al. Nutrition in relation to dental medicine. *In* Shils ME, Young VR (eds). *Modern Nutrition in Health and Disease.* 8th ed, Philadelphia: Lea & Febiger, 1994; 1007–1028.

International Association of Dental Research (IADR). Proceedings of the Scientific Consensus Conference on Methods for the Assessment of the Cariogenic Potential of Foods, 1986.

Moss SJ. The relationship of diet and dental caries. Presented at the 75th Annual Meeting of The American Dietetic Association. Washington, D.C., October, 1992.

Mundorff SA et al. Cariogenic potential of foods. *Caries Res* 1990; 24(5):344–355.

Navia JM. Carbohydrates and dental health. *Am J Clin Nutr* 1994; 59 (Suppl 3S):519S–527S.

Putnam JJ, Duewer LA. U.S. per capita food consumption: Record-high meat and sugars in 1994. *Food Rev* 1995; 18(2):2–11.

Rugg-Gunn AJ. Diet and dental caries. *Dental Update* 1990; 5:198–201.

Scheinin A, Mäkinen KK. Turku studies V. Final report on the effect of sucrose, fructose, and xylitol diets on the caries incidence in man. *Acta Odontol Scand* 1975; 34(4):179–216.

Smallwood DM, Blaylock JR. Fiber: Not enough of a good thing? *Food Rev* 1994; 17(1):23–29.

Tippett KS, Goldman JD. Diets more healthful, but still fall short of dietary guidelines. *Food Rev* 1994; 17(1):8–14.

Wender EH, Solanto MV. Effects of sugar on aggressive and inattentive behavior in children with attention deficit disorder with hyperactivity and normal children. *Pediatrics* 1992; 89(1):960–966.

Wolraich ML et al. The effects of sugar on behavior or cognition in children. *JAMA* 1995; 274(20):1617–1621.

Wolraich ML et al. Dietary characteristics of hyperactive and control boys. *J Am Diet Assoc* 1986; 86(4):500–504.

Zizza C, Gerrior S. The U.S. food supply provides more of most nutrients. *Food Review* 1995; 18(1):40–45.

Chapter 4

Protein: The Cellular Foundation

LEARNING OBJECTIVES

The Student Will Be Able To:

- List the possible fates of amino acids.
- Classify foods as sources of high-quality or lower-quality proteins.
- Explain how protein foods can be used to complement one another.
- Plan menus to include the recommended protein level for a meat-containing diet and a vegetarian diet.
- Explain why various physiologic states require different amounts of protein.
- State the problems associated with protein deficiency or excess.
- Assess a client's protein consumption in terms of deficiency or excess.
- Incorporate nutrition principles regarding food intake to prevent protein deficiency and protein excess into client counseling.

GLOSSARY OF TERMS

Amino acids   basic building blocks for proteins

Radical   a group of atoms that forms a fundamental constituent of a molecule

Interstitial fluid   fluid located between cells and in body cavities, including the joints, pleura, and gastrointestinal tract

Bioavailability   the amount of nutrient available to the body following absorption

Incaparina   a food powder made from corn, cottonseed, and sorghum with mineral and vitamin supplements

Test Your NQ (True/False)

1. A protein deficiency during childhood may lead to increased caries susceptibility related to alterations in tooth development and diminished salivary flow. T/F
2. Brown-shelled eggs are more nutritious than white-shelled eggs. T/F
3. Gelatin is a good source of high-quality protein. T/F
4. Elderly clients require less protein than younger clients. T/F
5. High protein intake strengthens the enamel of the tooth. T/F
6. An increase in protein intake may lead to an increase in fat rather than muscle. T/F

7. Amino acids are the building blocks of proteins. T/F
8. Marasmus is a protein-deficiency disorder. T/F
9. Lactovegetarians eat eggs and plant foods. T/F
10. A biological value of 3.5 indicates a lower-quality protein. T/F

Until the middle of the 19th century, many scientists thought that all life was composed of a single basic chemical: protein. Protein is present in each living cell, making up almost half of the dry weight of a cell. Second to water, protein is the most plentiful substance in the body. Americans are a nation of meat eaters, more so now than ever. Most Americans are unable or unwilling to plan a balanced meal without a meat entree. Customers clamor for half-pound hamburgers and "value-priced" buckets of fried chicken. Between 1970 and 1990, protein consumption increased 6% (Zizza & Gerrior, 1995). The greater variety of low-fat and reduced-fat meat choices now available probably has contributed to this increased meat consumption.

AMINO ACIDS

Proteins are very large molecular structures containing the elements carbon, hydrogen, oxygen, nitrogen, and sometimes sulfur and phosphorus. The billions of proteins associated with life are all made from combinations of 22 different **amino acids.** Amino acids can be compared to letters of the alphabet used in different sequences and combinations to make billions of words. An amino acid contains a basic, or amino, grouping ($-NH_2$) and an acidic, or carboxyl, grouping ($-COOH$). The general design of an amino acid is

$$NH_2 \quad \text{(amino group)}$$
$$\text{Radical group} - - - C - - - COOH \quad \text{(acid group)}$$
$$H$$

The distinguishing feature of amino acids is the amine group, which is the body's source of nitrogen. The **radical** group shown is the part of the structure that varies to form 22 different amino acids.

Amino acids combine with each other to make long chains. Two amino acids together form a dipeptide, as shown:

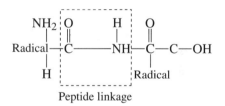

Peptide linkage

Several amino acids form a polypeptide. Food and body proteins contain polypeptides. The number of amino acids in proteins varies greatly (from 100 to 300), but each protein has a specific number.

CLASSIFICATION

A very important classification of amino acids is whether they are *essential* or *nonessential*. Essential amino acids (EAAs) are required in the diet. Nonessential amino acids (NEAAs) are essential for the body, but since they can be made from EAAs they are not required in the diet. The nine EAAs are listed in Table 4–1. If any one of the EAAs is not present when the cell needs it for protein synthesis, the protein cannot be produced. The body is able to make adequate amounts of NEAAs if a sufficient amount of protein is available to furnish the nitrogen needed and

TABLE 4–1   *Classification of Amino Acids*

Essential Amino Acids	Nonessential Amino Acids
Threonine	Glycine
Valine	Alanine
Leucine	Serine
Isoleucine	Tyrosine*
Phenylalanine	Proline
Tryptophan	Cysteine (cystine)*
Histidine	Methionine
Lysine	Arginine*
	Hydroxylysine
	Aspartic acid (asparagine)
	Glutamic acid (glutamine)*

*Semiessential or conditionally essential amino acids.

From Davis JR, Sherer K. *Applied Nutrition and Diet Therapy for Nurses,* 2nd ed. Philadelphia: W.B. Saunders, 1994.

enough calories are present to spare the catabolism of amino acids.

Other amino acids are *conditionally essential* in certain nutritional or disease states or in certain stages of development; these are arginine, cysteine, tyrosine, and glutamine.

The amount of EAAs furnished by a food determines its ability to support growth, maintenance, and repair. Several methods of classification are used to evaluate a food's protein quality or its ability to support these functions. Foods that supply amounts of the nine EAAs adequate to maintain *nitrogen balance* (Table 4–2) and permit growth are known as *high-quality proteins* or proteins of high *biological value. Nitrogen balance* refers to the balance of reactions in which protein substances are broken down or destroyed and rebuilt. High-quality proteins are well-balanced in their EAA content. Biological value is a measure of how well proteins from a food can be converted into body proteins. Biological values range from 1 to 100, with a higher score for proteins of higher quality. Foods of high

biological value containing high-quality proteins are derived from animal sources: egg, dairy products, meat, fish, and poultry. One exception is gelatin, which contains no tryptophan.

Most protein-containing foods have all the EAAs present. Although in some foods the quantity of one or more of the EAAs may be insufficient for optimum protein synthesis, these foods are still sources of *lower-quality* proteins. Lower-quality proteins, if fed as the only protein source, support life but not normal growth and are intermediate in biological value. These include proteins found in legumes, nuts, and grains. The amino acid in short supply relative to need is referred to as the "limiting amino acid" (Table 4–3).

Proteins that do not contain EAAs in adequate amounts to support life have a low biological value. Vegetable and some grain proteins fall into this category; they contain all the EAAs, but because one or more EAAs are present in a very low ratio, the protein they furnish has a low biological value.

Dental Hygiene Considerations

- Inquire about the client's use of amino acid supplements because toxicity and amino acid imbalance syndromes may occur when an excess of one amino acid is ingested. For example, when large doses of tryptophan are taken, toxic metabolites build up, causing an unusual syndrome called tryptophan-induced eosinophiliamyalgia syndrome.

Nutritional Directions

- The biological value indicates how well the body utilizes a particular protein. The higher the number, the higher the protein quality.
- Animal foods (except for gelatin) and fish are high-quality proteins but are not essential to an adequate diet.

PHYSIOLOGIC ROLES

Proteins perform many important physiologic roles, but it is inaccurate to say that protein is more important than any other required nutrient because

other nutrients are essential for the body to fully use available protein. Proteins are the principal source of nitrogen for the body and are fundamental

TABLE 4–2   *Nitrogen Balance**

N balance: body protein constant
N intake = N excretion
Positive N balance: increase in body protein
N intake > N excretion
Negative N balance: decrease in body protein
N excretion > N intake

Positive N Balance	Negative N Balance
Growth	Inadequate intake or protein (fasting, GI tract diseases)
Pregnancy	Inadequate kilocalorie intake
Convalescent periods	Illnesses, such as fevers, trauma, infections, or wasting diseases
Athletic training	Injury or immobilization
	Deficiency of EAAs
	Accelerated protein loss (albuminuria, protein-losing gastroenteropathy)
	Burns
	Increased secretion of thyroxine and glucocorticoids

*Because nitrogen is a unique component of protein metabolism, measurements of nitrogen and nitrogenous constituents in the blood and urine assess protein equilibrium in the body. Although "nitrogen balance" means that the output is equal to input, the amount of excreted nitrogen atoms is usually not the same as that ingested. For nitrogen equilibrium, not only must the diet contain the required amounts of protein, but also caloric intake must also be adequate, or else protein will be used for energy.
From Davis JR, Sherer K. *Applied Nutrition and Diet Therapy for Nurses,* 2nd ed. Philadelphia: W.B. Saunders, 1994.

TABLE 4–3   *Amino Acid Content of Selected Foods*

Food	Limiting Amino Acids	High Amounts of Amino Acids
Corn	Lysine, threonine, tryptophan	
Cereal	Cystine, lysine, threonine	Methionine
Legumes	Cystine, methionine, tryptophan	Lysine, threonine
Whole grains	Threonine	Methionine, lysine
Nuts and soybeans	Methionine	Lysine, threonine
Sesame and sunflower seeds	Lysine	Cystine, methionine, tryptophan
Peanuts	Methionine, lysine, threonine	
Green leafy vegetables	Methionine	
Gelatin	Methionine, lysine, tryptophan	
Yeast	Phenylalanine	Methionine, threonine

From Davis JR, Sherer K. *Applied Nutrition and Diet Therapy for Nurses,* 2nd ed. Philadelphia: W.B. Saunders, 1994.

components of all body cells. Proteins are necessary for many bodily functions, which can be classified into the seven categories described below. Some of the more familiar functions are included in Table 4–4.

1. *Generation of new body tissues.* Because protein is a constituent of all cells, it is necessary for growth. During periods of increased growth (infancy, childhood, adolescence, and pregnancy) as well as in periods of wound healing or recovery (illness, surgery, burns, or fever), the need for protein to build new tissues is increased.
2. *Repair of body tissues.* Body proteins are continuously being broken down, necessitating their replacement. Therefore, assessment of both recent and usual protein intake is important.
3. *Production of essential compounds.* Amino acids and proteins are constituents of regulatory enzymes, hormones, and other body secretions. The structural compound collagen is a protein that provides a framework for bones and teeth. A low protein intake may affect all of these functions.
4. *Regulation of fluid balance.* Protein dissolved in water forms a colloidal solution; in other words, it attracts water. Blood albumin (a protein) draws water from **interstitial fluid** or cells to maintain blood volume. During protein deficiency, a decreased amount of protein in the blood causes a loss of osmotic balance, resulting in an accumulation interstitial fluid (edema).
5. Resistance to disease. Antibodies, or immunoglobulins, the body's main protection from disease, are proteins. Thus, low protein levels may result in an inability to fight bacteria and other harmful organisms.
6. Transport mechanisms. Proteins enable insoluble fats to be transported through the blood.
7. Energy. When the nitrogen grouping is removed, the remaining carbon skeleton can be used for energy, furnishing 4 Cal/gm. Although this is not one of its main functions, protein is utilized in this manner when (1) caloric intake from carbohydrate and fat is inadequate, (2) protein intake exceeds requirements, and (3) EAAs are not available for synthesis of proteins.

REQUIREMENTS

Protein requirements for health are based on body size and rate of growth. (The body needs more protein during growth periods or for maintenance and repair of a larger body mass.) To a certain extent, the better the quality of protein, the lesser the quantity is required. Protein requirements are based on the assumption that EAAs and calories are provided in adequate amounts.

The Recommended Dietary Allowances (RDAs) for protein are proportionately higher for different ages and stages of life to adjust for growth rates. The National Research Council has determined that the daily minimum requirement of protein for adults is about 0.6 gm/kg. Using 0.6 gm/kg, a client weighing 120 lbs (54.5 kg) would require 33 gm of protein. Because RDAs provide a margin of safety, the National Research Council has established 0.8 gm/kg daily as the RDA for all adults. With this standard, a client weighing 120 lbs (54.5 kg) would require 44 gm of protein. The amount of protein in

the RDAs for various stages of life are listed in Table 4–5.

When any condition of health or disease causes a significant protein loss, an increased protein intake (above the RDAs) prevents excessive loss of tissue and plasma proteins. Although these states increase protein requirements, RDAs have not been established for these conditions. Supplementation with high-quality proteins can help prevent protein malnutrition and shorten recovery periods.

Americans commonly ingest significantly more protein than is recommended. Ordinarily, dietary protein is only restricted in some physiologic disease states affecting the liver and kidney because these organs are heavily involved in protein utilization and excretion of protein waste products. If they are diseased, excessive amounts of protein cannot be properly handled.

TABLE 4–4 *Classification of Protein by Function*

Classification	Body Location	Example	Function
Structural proteins	Skin, cartilage, bone	Collagen	Principal substance in connective tissue
Contractile proteins	Skeletal muscle	Actin myosin	Muscle contraction
Antibodies	Blood plasma, spleen, lymphatic cells	Alpha globulins	Disease protection
Blood proteins	Blood plasma	Albumins	Control osmotic pressure of blood
			Maintain the buffering capacity of blood pH
	Blood	Fibrinogen	Blood clotting
	Blood	Hemoglobin	Transports oxygen from lungs to all parts of the body
Hormones	Endocrine or ductless glands (thyroid, pancreas, parathyroid, adrenals, pituitary)	Insulin	Regulates carbohydrate metabolism
		Growth hormone	Stimulates overall protein synthesis and growth
Enzymes	Throughout body—nearly 2,000 different enzymes known; each highly specific in function		Biological catalysts: proteins that allow chemical reactions to proceed at their proper rate
	Stomach	Pepsin	Protein digestion
	Pancreas	Trypsin and chymotrypsin	Protein digestion
Nutrient proteins		Meat, fish, chicken, milk, cheese, eggs, peanut butter, nuts, soybeans, tofu, dried peas and beans	Sources of amino acids required by humans and other animals
Viruses	Microscopic infective agents	Smallpox, measles	Cause disease
Nucleoproteins	Cell nucleus	DNA	Determines and transmits hereditary characteristics: carries genetic (hereditary) code

From Howard RB, Herbold NH. *Nutrition in Clinical Care,* 2nd ed. New York: McGraw-Hill, 1982.

SOURCES

Foods with a high protein content are readily available in the United States. The average protein content of some foods is shown in Table 4–6. Most of the protein is furnished by the meat and milk food groups. As Americans increase their intake of cereal products, this food group will contribute

TABLE 4–5 *Recommended Dietary Allowances for Protein*

Life Stage/Gender	Age (Years)	Protein (GM)*
Infants	0–.5	13
	0.5–1	14
Children	1–3	16
	4–6	24
	7–10	28
Males	11–14	45
	15–18	59
	19–24	58
	25–50	63
	51+	63
Females	11–14	46
	15–18	44
	19–24	46
	25–50	50
	51+	50
Pregnant		60
Lactating	First 6 months	65
	Second 6 months	62

*Additional protein is needed with physiologic stresses (e.g., postsurgery, dental procedures such as periodontal surgery) for healing.

Data from National Research Council Subcommittee on the Tenth Edition of the RDAs. *Recommended Dietary Allowances,* 10th ed. Washington, D.C.: National Academy Press, 1989.

significantly more to the protein intake. The protein content of items from the sample menu displayed in Figure 1–3 is shown in Figure 4–1.

In most cases, digestibility and nutritional value are not unfavorably affected by cooking procedures. Proper cooking sometimes facilitates digestion and utilization. For example, cooking makes egg albumin more readily digestible, and cooking soybeans increases amino acid **bioavailability.** On the other hand, processing affects proteins in cereal by binding lysine (an amino acid), making it unusable by the body.

Dental Hygiene Considerations

- Most Americans consume almost twice as much protein as recommended in the RDAs.

When assessment indicates a normal consumption of 1.5 gm/kg or more above the RDA for protein, this is considered a high-protein diet. Further increases would probably not be beneficial and may contribute to increased fat stores.

- The protein requirement of the elderly is equal to or more than that of the young adult, so monitor protein intake accordingly. Decreased protein intake is common as a result of ill-fitting dentures or loss of teeth, poverty, or poor access to the grocery store.
- A decreased protein intake could affect any or all of protein's physiologic functions of the

TABLE 4–6 *Protein Content of Selected Foods*

Food	Quantity	Protein (gm)
Beef, cooked, lean cuts	2 oz	17
Chicken breast, cooked	2 oz	16
Pork chop, lean, cooked	2 oz	16
Cottage cheese	½ cup	16
Navy beans, cooked	1 cup	15
Cheddar cheese	2 oz	14
Thick milkshake	12 oz	13
Cod fish, cooked	2 oz	13
Egg, hard cooked	2	13
Milk, protein fortified	1 cup	10
American processed cheese	2 oz	9
Whole milk	1 cup	8
Peanut butter	2 tbsp	8
Macaroni, cooked	1 cup	7
Oatmeal, cooked	1 cup	6
Nonfat dried skim milk powder	¼ cup	6
Rice, cooked	1 cup	5
Ice cream, 10% fat	1 cup	5
Corn muffin	1	3
Enriched white bread	1 slice	2
Vegetables	½ cup	1–2
Fruits	½ cup	0.1–1

Nutrient data from Nutritionist IV software, The Hearst Corporation, San Bruno, CA.

From Davis JR, Sherer K. *Applied Nutrition and Diet Therapy for Nurses,* 2nd ed. Philadelphia: W.B. Saunders, 1994.

Sample Menu	Protein Content	Vegetarian Menu*	Protein Content
Breakfast			
Orange juice (1 cup)	1.7		1.7
Bagel (1)	6.0		6.0
Cream cheese (1 oz)	2.2		2.2
Raisins (1 packet)	0.5		0.5
1% Milk (1 cup)	8.0		8.0
Coffee	0		0
Creamer (1 tsp)	1.0		1.0
Lunch			
Tuna sandwich (1 oz)	7.6	Peanut butter (2 tbsp)	7.9
Mayonnaise (2 tbsp)	0.4	Jam (2 tbsp)	0
Tomato (2 slices)	0.6	Omit	
Lettuce slices	0.4	Omit	
Whole wheat bread (2 slices)	5.4		5.4
Apple (1)	0.3		0.3
1% Milk (1 cup)	8.0		8.0
Dinner			
Lean roast beef (2 oz)	15.5	Cheese-brown rice-broccoli	
Gravy (1/4 cup)	0.5	casserole (1 1/4 cup with	
Brown rice (1/2 cup)	2.8	2 oz cheese)	19.7
Corn (1/2 cup)	2.5		2.5
Three bean salad (1/2 cup)	2.8	Three bean salad (3/4 cup)	4.3
Whole wheat roll (2)	7.0		7.0
Margarine (1 tbsp)	0		0
Strawberries (1/2 cup)	0.5	Strawberries (1 cup)	1.0
Iced tea	0		
Evening Snack			
Diet cola (12 oz)	0.4		0.4
Dry roasted nuts (1 oz)	7.5		7.5
Totals	81.6		83.4

* Only items changed are listed; all others are the same.

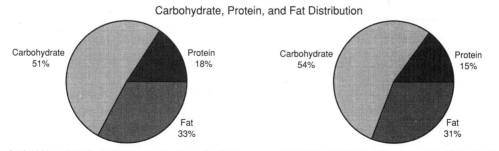

Carbohydrate, Protein, and Fat Distribution

Carbohydrate 51%   Protein 18%   Fat 33%

kcal, 1969; carbohydrate, 264 gm; protein, 82 gm; fat, 75 gm

Carbohydrate 54%   Protein 15%   Fat 31%

kcal, 2179; carbohydrate, 311 gm; protein, 83 gm; fat, 79 gm

FIGURE 4–1   **Protein content of Sample Menu and Modifications for Ovolactovegetarian Diet. Nutrient data from Nutritionist IV software, First Data Bank, San Bruno, CA. (From Davis JR, Sherer K. *Applied Nutrition and Diet Therapy for Nurses,* 2nd ed. Philadelphia: W.B. Saunders, 1994.)**

body. If dietary intake appears inadequate, evaluate the client's status in the areas described under Physiologic Roles, above.

- One rule of thumb is that protein should never exceed 15% to 20% of caloric intake. If protein intake appears excessive, determine caloric and protein intake. The adequacy of intake can be established using either of two methods. As an example, for a client consuming 2,000 calories and 115 gm protein, the *recommended amount of protein based on total energy intake* is calculated as follows:

2,000 calories × 0.20 (% of total calories) =
    400 calories from protein or less
400 calories ÷ 4 (Cal/gm protein) =
    100 gm protein recommended

Thus, the intake of 115 gm of protein is more than the recommended amount. The *actual intake based on the actual protein intake* is figured as follows:

115 (gm protein) × 4 (Cal/gm protein) =
    460 calories from protein
460 (calories from protein) ÷ 2,000 (total calorie intake) × 100 (%) =
    23% of total calories from protein

Because 20% is the upper limit, this client is consuming 3% more protein than is recommended.

- Do not overemphasize animal sources of protein to clients on restricted incomes (elderly, homeless, impoverished). Too much emphasis on high-protein foods may result in inadequate amounts of other nutrients in the diet, especially when the food budget is low. Complementary sources of protein (de-

scribed later in this chapter), which are less expensive, can provide adequate protein.

- Healthy clients will be in nitrogen balance appropriate for their stage of life if their diet contains adequate calories with the recommended number of servings from all the Food Guide Pyramid groups. Evaluate food intake by gathering data from the client and comparing it with the Food Guide Pyramid, stage of growth, and RDAs for calories and protein needed.

Nutritional Directions

- Increased muscular activity does not appear to elevate the protein requirement except for the small increase needed for muscle development during conditioning.

- Protein requirements should be met by foods from several sources (even animal protein foods) because of other nutrients that accompany the protein. For example, pork is an excellent source of thiamin; red meats furnish a significant amount of iron. In contrast, too many egg yolks in the diet contribute excessive cholesterol.

- Animal sources of protein are generally the most expensive. When clients have limited resources, counsel them to (1) eat protein in adequate but not excessive amounts, (2) use a variety of proteins of lower quality (which are less expensive), and (3) purchase less expensive kinds of protein foods (see chapter 14).

- The color of the eggshell is not related to its nutritional value. The breed of the hen determines the color.

- Reinforce the need to avoid amino acid supplements.

UNDERCONSUMPTION AND HEALTH-RELATED PROBLEMS

Although protein supplies in the United States are plentiful and drastic protein deficiency is uncommon, several groups are susceptible to insufficient intakes: (1) the elderly who are unable to prepare nutritious meals or are uninspired to eat, (2) low-income groups, (3) strict vegetarians, (4) those with a lack of education or who are unwilling to shop wisely, and (5) the chronically ill and hospitalized (e.g., AIDS, anorexia nervosa, or cancer patients). Certain physiologic conditions and impaired digestion or absorption cause excessive protein losses and may also precipitate *protein-energy malnutrition* (PEM). Although PEM is uncommon in the United States, given the above mentioned conditions, malnutrition is frequently unrecognized.

In other areas of the world, where quantities of high-quality protein and calories are insufficient, PEM is commonly seen. Kwashiorkor develops when young children receive adequate calories, but not enough high-quality protein (Fig. 4–2). It usually appears after the child has been weaned from breast milk. Marasmus occurs in infants when both protein and calories are deficient in the diet.

PEM is usually accompanied by other nutritional deficiencies. Separating out the effects of different nutrient deficiencies on the observation of clinical symptoms is often difficult. PEM affects the whole body, including every component of the orofacial complex.

The occurrence of PEM during critical developmental stages, including the prenatal and postnatal periods, may affect any developing tissue and can lead to irreversible changes affecting oral tissues. During tooth development in animal studies, mild to moderate protein deficiency results in smaller molars, significantly delayed eruption, and retardation during development of the mandible in the offspring. Smaller salivary glands result in diminished salivary flow; this saliva is different in its protein composition and amylase and aminopeptidase activity.

Poor nutrition results in delayed eruption and exfoliation of deciduous teeth. In addition to the increased rate of caries in malnourished children, the peak caries experience is delayed by approximately 2 years. The increased caries rate may simply be related to the length of time a tooth is in

FIGURE 4–2 One child in this picture is healthy; the other three, all from the same community and of about the same age, are victims of the deficiency disease kwashiorkor. Note that the faces and abdomens of the two on the left look quite full, because of the accumulation of water as edema. The fact that the children are in reality pitifully thin is apparent from looking at their arms. (Courtesy of World Health Organization, photo by H. Omen.)

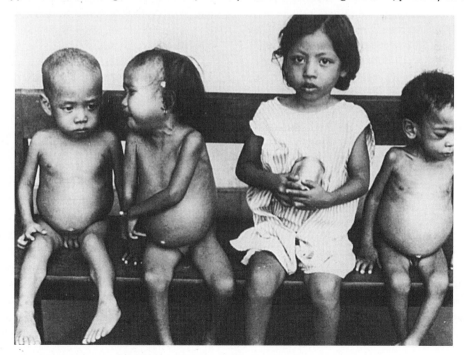

the oral cavity; if the delay in exfoliation is greater than the delay in eruption, the tooth is in the mouth a longer period of time, and it is exposed to caries-producing bacteria longer.

Increased caries susceptibility may be related to alterations in structure of tooth crowns and diminished salivary flow. An increase in acid solubility associated with chemical alterations of the exposed enamel surface may contribute to increased caries susceptibility.

Children in developing countries suffering from malnutrition have different dietary habits overall and oral environments that were not conducive to dental caries in some studies. However, when fermentable carbohydrates are available, the teeth in these populations are highly susceptible to dental caries.

An insufficient intake of protein calories causes a negative nitrogen balance. Tissues are depleted of reserves, blood protein levels are lowered, and resistance to infections is lowered. Also, the ability to withstand the stress of injury or surgery is lowered and recovery periods are longer.

In malnourished children, *secretory immunoglobulin A* (sIgA) levels are depressed. SIgA is the predominant immunoglobulin, or antibody, in oral, nasal, intestinal, and other mucosal secretions and provides the first line of defense in the oral cavity. Low sIgA levels in malnourished children probably play a role in their increased susceptibility to mucosal infections.

PEM may be a major reason for the increased incidence of *noma* and *acute necrotizing ulcerative gingivitis* (ANUG) (see color plate 1), which are clearly associated with depressed immune responses caused by nutritional deficiencies, stress, and infection. Noma is a severe gangrenous process usually presenting as a small ulcer on the gingiva that becomes necrotic and spreads to produce extensive destruction of the lips, cheek, and tissues covering the jaw. ANUG is characterized by erythema and necrosis of the interdental papillae. This painful gingivitis is generally accompanied by a metallic taste and foul oral odor. Cratered papillae often remain after treatment of the disease.

While occasionally observed in severely debilitated or immunocompromised individuals in developed countries, ANUG is relatively common in children between the ages of 2 and 6 who are malnourished and have recently experienced a stressful event such as a viral disease in socioeconomically deprived countries.

The development of this disease in the late teens to early adult years is often associated with psychological stress. It is possibly precipitated by emotionally stressful situations that affect eating patterns, leading to acute deficiencies, and lowering the host's response to bacteria normally found in most oral cavities. Decreased host resistance to infection may permit gingival lesions to spread rapidly into adjacent tissues, producing extensive necrosis and destruction of orofacial tissues, whereas in a healthy person, the lesion is limited to the gingivae alone. Wound healing is also delayed.

Kwashiorkor and marasmus are very serious health problems that have received much attention by the United Nations and the World Health Organization. Supplementation has been made in the form of skim-milk powder, **Incaparina,** and the addition of lysine to cereal products. However, most of these efforts to improve the status of nutrition worldwide have not been well accepted for various reasons, and the protein-energy problems of the world still exist.

Dental Hygiene Considerations

- When assessing for marasmus or kwashiorkor, remember that the main difference between the two conditions is that edema is present in kwashiorkor, especially in the feet and legs, but is absent in marasmus.

- Assess the client's financial status because poverty is a major cause of PEM.

- To assess for inadequate protein intake, look for or identify frequent or extended periods of fasting, medications that cause anorexia, abnormal food intake, nausea and vomiting, and problems with hair (dull, dry, brittle, breaks easily) or skin (flaky and dry).

- Treatment of malnutrition will require referral to a physician and/or a dietitian.

- Malnourished clients take longer to heal and regain strength and are at risk for frequent infections. Adequate infection control procedures are particularly important for these clients.
- Elderly people are frequently not motivated to eat because of low income level, transportation problems, depression and loneliness, edentulous status, and gustatory changes. Assess elderly clients closely for possible malnutrition.
- In the United States, noma-like lesions may occur in clients with cancer whose immune systems have been severely impaired by chemotherapy.

Nutritional Directions

- Suggest Meals on Wheels for elderly clients and refer them to a social worker.
- The protein content of the diet can be supplemented by adding skim-milk powder to milk, soups, or mashed potatoes and by adding cheese to foods, provided the client is not lactose intolerant.

OVERCONSUMPTION AND HEALTH-RELATED PROBLEMS

An upper limit for safe levels of protein intake has not been determined. Most clients believe there is no such thing as too much protein in the diet. Frequently, Americans eat 150% to 200% of the RDA for protein. Excessive protein intake can contribute to obesity since protein in excess of physiologic needs is converted to fat and stored.

One concern regarding high-protein intake is its effect on calcium balance. RDAs in the United States for calcium are approximately double those established in most other nations. Studies indicate that high-protein foods with a high phosphorus content do not cause calcium loss in clients.

When protein intake is excessive, fluid imbalances may occur in all age groups, but especially in infants. Metabolism of 100 calories of protein requires 350 gm of water, compared with 50 gm of water for a similar amount of carbohydrates or fats. Therefore, water requirements are increased as well as the end-products of protein metabolism in the blood stream.

Dental Hygiene Considerations

- Too much protein can result in additional fat stores and obesity.

Nutritional Directions

- Extremely high intake of protein is especially undesirable in infants.

- Since proteins must be metabolized by the liver and filtered by the kidneys, excessive amounts (over 200% of the RDA) result in additional work by or stress on these organs.

HEALTH APPLICATION 4

Vegetarianism

Despite the fact that protein is not limited in the food supply, some people choose plant sources of protein for health reasons or because of their philosophical, ecological, or religious convictions. The large numbers of newly published vegetarian cookbooks and meatless vegetable burgers and sausage-style products would lead one to believe that vegetarianism is a growing consumer movement. Yet, surveys indicate that only 5% of the population, the same amount as 16 years ago, are true vegetarians (Putnam & Duewer, 1995).

EAAs can be provided by plants but larger amounts of these plant products must be consumed to match the protein obtained from animal sources. EAAs that are present in low levels in grains are abundant in other plants, such as legumes. As can be seen in Table 4–3, beans are low in methionine and tryptophan, and corn is low in lysine and threonine. When both are eaten together, as in pinto beans and cornbread, they are said to be *complementary* to each other and less volume is required.

When a combination of plant proteins are eaten throughout the day, the amino acids provided by each complement each other; that is, the deficiencies of one are offset by the adequacies of another. Additionally, small amounts of high-quality proteins can be combined with plant foods, as in macaroni and cheese or cereal and milk, to provide adequate amounts of EAAs.

Protein from a single source is seldom consumed alone. Foods are usually eaten without awareness that they are complementary to each other (e.g., beans are usually combined with rice, bread or crackers [wheat], or tortillas or cornbread [corn]. Thus, the variety of protein-containing foods commonly eaten throughout the day will provide enough EAAs; therefore it is unnecessary that foods providing complementary amino acids are eaten at the same time (ADA, 1993).

With some basic nutrition knowledge, a vegetarian diet can be created that is healthy and nutritionally balanced. Nutrient needs of a vegetarian are the same as those for any other person. The major difference is the protein source. The Food Guide Pyramid can still be used for planning well-balanced menus, using combinations of foods allowed. As shown in Table 4–7 and Tips for Planning Vegetarian Diets, the only food group changed is the meat and/or dairy group. The four types of vegetarian diets differ in the types of foods included.

The *vegan* (or strict vegetarian) diet contains only food from plants, including vegetables, fruits, and grains. No foods of animal origin are allowed (meat, milk, cheese, eggs, butter) This is the strictest type of diet and requires cautious planning to achieve combinations that provide necessary amounts of amino acids and other nutrients, such as vitamins B_{12} and D and the mineral iron. The use of complementary proteins can provide proper quantities of EAAs. By utilizing a variety of principally unrefined foods, and enough calories to promote good health, protein quality and quantity and nutrients can be adequate

for most individuals. Because of the difficulty of consuming adequate volumes of food to meet caloric requirements, the vegan diet is not recommended for infants, children, or pregnant women.

In a *lactovegetarian* diet, dairy products are consumed in addition to plant foods ("lacto-" comes from the Latin word for milk, *lactis*). Meat, poultry, fish, and eggs are excluded. Milk and cheese products, which complement plant foods and enhance the amino acid content, are included.

The *ovolactovegetarian* diet is supplemented with milk, cheese, and eggs ("ovo-" comes from the Latin word for egg, *ovum*). Only meat, poultry, and fish are excluded. If adequate quantities of eggs, milk, and milk products are consumed, all nutrients are likely to be provided in sufficient quantities (Table 4–7). Strict supervision is not warranted unless serum cholesterol levels require dietary fat restrictions.

The ovovegetarian diet consists of foods from plants with the addition of eggs. Meat, poultry, fish, and dairy products are excluded.

Much can be said of the healthy aspects of vegetarian diets. Indeed, the latest version of the Dietary Guidelines for Americans acknowledges that vegetarian diets can meet the RDAs as long as the variety and amounts of foods are adequate. That vegetarian diets and lifestyles appear to be conducive to good health is borne out by the fact that vegetarians exhibit better weight control, improved gastrointestinal function, fewer breast and colon cancers, better glycemic control, a lower incidence of gallstones, lower blood pressure, and a decreased rate of coronary heart disease. When working with a vegetarian, keep lines of communication open by respecting the client's decision, unless eating habits are clearly potentially harmful. Clients who have an interest in pursuing a vegetarian diet should be encouraged to do so; all clients should be encouraged to have more meatless meals and to consume more plant foods.

TABLE 4–7 *Vegetarian Food Guide*

Food Group	Standard Serving Size	Number of Servings Daily (by Age)			
		1–2 Yrs	3–6 Yrs	7–10 Yrs	Adolescents & Adults
Bread, cereal, rice, and pasta¶	1 slice bread; 1 small roll; ½ cup cooked rice, pasta, or cooked cereal; 1 oz dry cereal	4	4–5	9–11	6–11
Protein foods, total daily*					
a. Legumes, lentils, peas, limas; tofu; soy products; meat analogues	½ cup	2–3	2–3	2–3	2–4‡,§
b. Nuts and seeds; peanut or almond butter; tahini	2–3 oz 1 oz or ¼–⅓ cup 2 Tbsp				
c. Eggs	½ (<3 egg yolks/week)				
Vegetables, total daily*	½ cup cooked; 1 cup raw; ¾ c juice	2–3	2–3	4–5	3–5
Fruits, total daily	¾ cup juice; ½ cup cooked or canned fruit; ¼ cup dried fruit; 1 medium upfresh fruit	1–2	1–2	3–4	2–4
Milk and milk products*	1 cup lowfat or nonfat milk or yogurt; 1–2 oz lowfat cheese; 1 cup soy milk (fortified with calcium, vitamins D and B_{12}); 1 cup tofu	2–3**	2–3	2–3	2–3†
Fats, oil	1 tsp oil, margarine, mayonnaise; 2 tsp salad dressing; ⅛ avocado				
Sugar	1 tsp sugar, jam, jelly, honey, syrup, etc.				

*Vegans must include at least two servings of calcium-rich foods daily, such as 1 cup milk alternative fortified with calcium, vitamins D and B_{12}; 1 cup firm tofu, 1 cup cooked broccoli or greens (collards, dandelion, kale, mustard).

**Low-fat products are not recommended for children under 2 years of age.

†Pregnant or breastfeeding women, teenagers, and young adults to age 24 need three servings.

‡To help meet the adult requirement for iron, include 2 cups of legumes.

§Include 1 cup dark greens to help meet the adult female iron requirement.

¶Include at least half of the servings from whole-grain breads and cereals.

Adapted from Haddad EH. Development of a vegetarian food guide. *Am J Clin Nutr* 1994; 59(5 Suppl): 1130S–5S.

Tips for Planning Vegetarian and Vegan Diets

Tips for a Vegetarian Diet

- Follow the vegetarian food guide (Table 4–7).
- Use unrefined foods as much as possible; based on their caloric contribution, they provide a greater variety of nutrients. Substantially reduce high-calorie, low-nutrient-density foods.
- Replace meat with plant proteins from legumes, seeds, and nuts.
- Ensure that all the EAAs are present in adequate amounts. Suggestions are provided below for combining complementary proteins in appropriate combinations. (If a diet contains variety, combining the foods at the same meal is not essential.)

  —*Grains and legumes:* rice and beans, wheat-soy bread, corn-soy bread, cornbread and black-eyed peas, corn tortillas and beans, lentil soup and rye crackers, baked beans with brown bread, beans in a tostada, or brown rice and peas.

  —*Legumes and nuts/seeds:* roasted soybean snacks with bean dip, raw peanuts and sunflower seeds, stir-fried tofu with slivered almonds and broccoli, seed bread with split-pea soup.

  —*Grains and nuts/seeds:* rice and sesame seeds, wheat germ and peanuts, rice and cashews, peanut butter on wheat bread, or noodles and cashews.

  —*Vegetables and legumes, grains or corn, or potatoes:* dark green leafy vegetables with pinto beans, stir-fried vegetables with kidney beans, steamed broccoli and corn over brown rice, fresh lima beans and corn, corn and potato casserole, spinach-potato salad, or gumbo with okra, corn, and lima beans.

  —*Grains and milk products:* cottage-cheese salad with sesame seeds and garbanzo beans, milk in legume soup, cheese sauce for beans, or vegetable quiche with peanut-butter muffins.
- Commercially prepared plant protein products are not essential for adequate protein intake but may be used to replace the traditional entree.
- If milk/milk products are used, utilize low-fat or nonfat milk/milk products (low-fat cheese, ice cream, and yogurt).
- Increase whole-grain breads and cereals to meet energy requirements.
- Use a variety of fruits and vegetables. Include a vitamin C-rich food at each meal.
- Use fortified or enriched products.
- Limit egg yolks to three to four per week.

Tips for a Vegan Diet

- Obtain adequate energy intake using whole-grain breads and cereals, legumes, nuts, and seeds.
- Use a variety of legumes and whole-grain products with some seeds and for nuts.
- Since milk/milk products are eliminated, foods need to replace the nutrients contained in milk:
  —Use a fortified soybean milk drink.
  —Incorporate a modest amount of nutritional yeast.
  —Increase the use of green leafy vegetables.
  —Increase the use of legumes, nuts, and dried fruits.
- Obtain vitamin D by daily exposure to sunshine (20–30 minutes).
- Use foods fortified with vitamin B_{12} or obtain the vitamin by taking a supplement.

From Davis JR, Sherer K. *Applied Nutrition and Diet Therapy for Nurses,* 2nd ed. Philadelphia: W.B. Saunders, 1994.

Some groups, especially Seventh-Day Adventists, supplement protein intake with many textured vegetable protein (TVP) products. These are meat analogues produced from vegetable proteins, usually soybeans. The protein in TVP products is of good quality, but they may have a high sodium content.

CASE APPLICATION FOR THE DENTAL HYGIENIST

A male client brags to you that he is principally eating protein foods to build muscle. He is a college student and participates in intramural sports on weekends but usually does not work out on weekdays. He believes that protein foods are the best and that the others are of "no value."

Based on his diet diary, his caloric intake is 1,800 calories and his protein intake is 150 gm. He does not understand why you are so concerned about his intake; he is just making sure enough protein is available for body building.

Nutritional Assessment

○ Willingness to learn
○ Knowledge base of protein, carbohydrate, and fat principles of optimal nutrition
○ Cultural beliefs
○ Recent percentage of calories from protein (33%)
○ Types of protein intake and total nutrient intake
○ Kidney functioning and fluid intake
○ Carbonated beverage intake
○ Source of information

Nutritional Diagnosis

○ Altered health maintenance related to insufficient knowledge of protein and optimal nutrition.

Nutritional Goals

The client will verbalize three principles concerning protein as well as the benefits from other nutrients. Client will consume 15% to 20% of total calories from protein.

Nutritional Implementation

Intervention: Teach (1) the seven functions or roles of protein; (2) the difference between EAAs and NEAAs; (3) the difference between high-quality and lower-quality protein; and (4) the interaction among carbohydrate, fats, and protein and the recommended percentages of each.
Rationale: Knowledge corrects inaccurate information.

Intervention: Explain that protein may be fattening. High protein intake does not necessarily increase muscle tissue.
Rationale: Excess protein is stored as fat.

Intervention: Encourage adequate fluid intake (minimum of 8 cups daily).
Rationale: Metabolism of 100 calories of protein requires 350 gm of water, compared with 50 gm of water for similar amounts of carbohydrate or fats.

Intervention: Exercise through the week is effective for building muscle.
Rationale: After 3 days, muscle not being used will break down, after which an individual begins to retrain.

Evaluation

The client should understand that some of his concepts about protein were inaccurate. To determine this, have the client repeat three of the principles he remembers from your teaching. He should say that 12% to 20% of the total calories should come from protein, and that excessive protein can be harmful and does not necessarily turn into muscle but may increase fat deposits. The client should also state that he uses complementary proteins to provide adequate amounts of amino acids, which will also provide other nutrients that are of "value" and will limit his fat intake.

Student Readiness

1. Define amino acid, essential amino acid, nitrogen balance, high-quality protein, and complementary proteins for a client.

2. Name the functions of proteins.

3. Using your desirable body weight, how many grams of protein should you consume?

4. Given a client weighing 150 lbs who has a caloric intake of 2,500 calories, if the diet averages 15% protein, how many calories are provided by protein? How many grams of protein is this? How does this compare with the RDA for this client?

5. What would you tell strict vegetarian parents about feeding their infant?

6. What are the effects of too much protein in the diet? Too little?

7. Explain the relationship between calories and protein.

8. What are two methods of obtaining the EAAs from vegetarian foods? List two food combinations for each type of vegetarian diet that would provide adequate amounts of EAAs.

9. If a client eats more protein than his or her body needs, what happens to the excess protein?

10. Using Table 4–7, what suggestions would you offer to reduce a client's protein intake? Would this significantly affect intake of other nutrients?

References

American Dietetic Association. Position of the American Dietetic Association: Vegetarian diets—technical support paper. *J Am Diet Assoc* 1993; 93(11):1317–1319.

Putnam JJ, Duewer LA. U.S. per capita food consumption: Record-high meat and sugars in 1994. *Food Rev* 1995; 18(2):2–11.

Sanders TAB, Reddy S. Vegetarian diets and children. *Am J Clin Nutr* 1994; 59 (5 Suppl):1176S-1181S.

Zizza C, Gerrior S. The U.S. food supply provides more of most nutrients. *Food Rev* 1995; 18(2):2–110.

Chapter 5

Lipids: The Condensed Energy

LEARNING OBJECTIVES

The Student Will Be Able To:

- Identify the basic structural units of dietary lipids.
- Describe how fatty acids affect the properties of fat.
- Name the essential fatty acid and some of its functions.
- List the functions of fats in the body.
- List dietary sources for saturated, monounsaturated, and polyunsaturated fatty acids, and cholesterol.
- Distinguish between chylomicrons and other lipoproteins.
- State the number of calories provided per gram of fat.
- Consider appropriate interventions when dietary modification of fat intake has been recommended to a client.
- Identify nutritional directions for clients concerning fats.

GLOSSARY OF TERMS

Fatty acid   a structural component of fats

Melting point   temperature at which a product becomes a liquid

Eicosanoids   hormone-like compounds of prostaglandins derived from arachidonic acid

Adipose tissue   body fat

Hyperlipidemia   elevated concentrations of any or all of the serum lipids, especially triglycerides and/or cholesterol

Test Your NQ (True/False)

1. No food that contains more than 30% of its calories from fat can be considered healthy. T/F
2. Americans are being poisoned by manufacturers adding tropical oils to foods. T/F
3. Products containing more unsaturated fatty acids than saturated fatty acids are healthier food choices than products containing a higher proportion of saturated fatty acids. T/F
4. Dietary fat intake should be less than 30% of total calories. T/F

   5. Bananas and avocados contain a lot of cholesterol. T/F

   6. Oils are less fattening than solid fats. T/F

   7. Fat intake has been linked more frequently to cancer than any other dietary factor. T/F

   8. Nuts and cheeses are nutritious foods that should be recommended to all patients for snacks because they reduce caries rate. T/F

   9. Fats contain 9 Cal/gm. T/F

   10. Omega-3 fatty acids are polyunsaturated fatty acids. T/F

INTRODUCTION

Unsweetened coconut, mayonnaise, blue cheese salad dressing, almonds, pecans, olives, avocados, and sausages—what do all these foods have in common? More than one-half of the calories in each of these food items comes from fat, a vital constituent in our diet.

Examination of food supply trends in the United States indicates a slight increase in total fat intake with a greater portion of the fat coming from vegetable products, whereas saturated fat and cholesterol intake has decreased. Consumer concerns about healthy food choices explain these changes. Food manufacturers, producers, and grocers have responded by (1) trimming fat from meats, (2) providing leaner cuts of beef and pork, (3) replacing tropical oils in processed foods, and (4) manufacturing foods containing less fat. Even though prices for seafood and chicken rose faster than those for beef and pork, consumers have increased their consumption of fish and poultry and substituted lower-fat milk for whole milk (Putnam, 1993). The fat content of very lean beef and pork cuts currently compares favorably to a skinless chicken breast.

CLASSIFICATION

Fats in the diet should actually be called *lipids.* Lipids contain the same three elements as carbohydrates: carbon, hydrogen, and oxygen. Lipids contain less oxygen in proportion to hydrogen and carbon than carbohydrates. Because of their structure, they provide more energy per gram than either carbohydrates or protein.

The two classes of water-insoluble substances are (1) *simple lipids,* or *triglycerides,* which occur both in foods and in the body, and (2) *structural lipids,* which are produced by the body for specific functions. Triglycerides with at least one of the fatty acids replaced with carbohydrate, phosphate, and/or nitrogenous compounds are called *compound lipids.* Dietary lipids utilizable by the body include triglycerides, fatty acids, phospholipids, and cholesterol. Lipoproteins are found solely in the body.

CHEMICAL STRUCTURE

Triglycerides are composed of *fatty acids* and glycerol, as shown:

monoglycerides = glycerol + one fatty acid

diglycerides = glycerol + two fatty acids

triglycerides = glycerol + three fatty acids

A fatty acid is a chain of carbon atoms attached to hydrogen atoms with an acid grouping on one end. Glycerol is the alcohol portion of a triglyceride to which the fatty acids attach. Triglycerides (also called triacylglycerols) are the most common fat present in animal or protein foods (Fig. 5–1). Monoglycerides and diglycerides are found in the small intestine and result from hydrolysis of triglycerides during digestion.

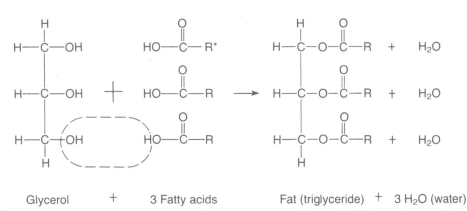

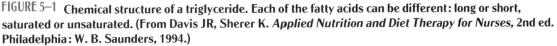

Glycerol   +   3 Fatty acids   Fat (triglyceride) + 3 H₂O (water)

FIGURE 5–1 **Chemical structure of a triglyceride. Each of the fatty acids can be different: long or short, saturated or unsaturated. (From Davis JR, Sherer K. *Applied Nutrition and Diet Therapy for Nurses*, 2nd ed. Philadelphia: W. B. Saunders, 1994.)**

Each of the three fatty acids in a triglyceride can be long, medium or short, and saturated or unsaturated. *Medium-chain* and *short-chain fatty acids* are readily digested and absorbed, but most fats in foods (especially vegetable fats) contain predominantly *long-chain fatty acids*. Short-chain fatty acids contain 4 to 6 carbon atoms; medium-chain fatty acids, 8 to 12 carbon atoms; and long-chain fatty acids, more than 12 carbon atoms.

Saturated Fatty Acids

Fatty acids are classified according to their degree of *saturation*. Saturation of a fatty acid depends on the number of hydrogen atoms attached to the carbon. Saturated fatty acids contain only single bonds, with each carbon atom having two hydrogen atoms attached to it. If each carbon atom has two hydrogen atoms attached, the fat is saturated (Fig. 5–2). Palmitic and stearic

FIGURE 5–2 **Structure of a fatty acid. Saturated fatty acid: stearic acid, an 18-carbon fatty acid (18:0). These numbers indicate the number of carbon atoms and how many double bonds are present. Thus stearic acid, a saturated fatty acid containing 18 carbon atoms and no double bonds, is labeled 18:0. (A) Detailed structure. (B) Simplified structure. Each of the C's at the corners of the zigzag lines represents a carbon atom with two atoms of hydrogen attached. The structure can rotate around single bonds and is constantly twisting and bending. A flat space with an extra line indicates a double bond, as will be seen in future examples. (From Davis JR, Sherer K. *Applied Nutrition and Diet Therapy for Nurses*, 2nd ed. Philadelphia: W.B. Saunders, 1994.)**

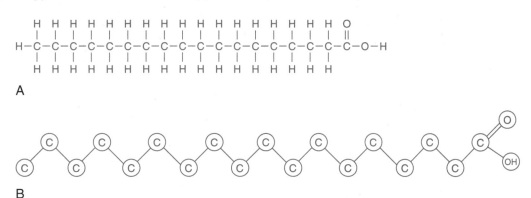

acids, the most prevalent saturated fatty acids, are found in animal fats, butter, coconut oil, and chocolate (Fig. 5–3). These two saturated fatty acids are structural components of tooth enamel and dentin.

Monounsaturated Fatty Acids

When adjacent carbon atoms are joined by a double bond because two hydrogen atoms are lacking, the fatty acid is *monounsaturated.* Monounsaturated fats contain only one double bond (Fig. 5–4). The most abundant monounsaturated fatty acid is oleic acid, which is found in olive, peanut, and canola oils (Fig. 5–3). Oleic acid is also a structural component of the tooth.

Polyunsaturated Fatty Acids

When numerous carbons in a fatty acid are connected by double bonds, the fatty acid is *polyunsaturated.* A polyunsaturated fatty acid (PUFA) has more than two double bonds (Fig. 5–5). Linoleic, linolenic, and arachidonic acids are polyunsaturated. *Linoleic acid* is the only fatty acid that must be provided in the diet. It is the most prevalent PUFA and is the predominant fatty acid in safflower, sunflower, corn, soybean, and cottonseed oils (Fig. 5–3). These PUFAs are *omega-6* fatty acids, having their first double bond on the sixth carbon from the omega (terminal) end.

Omega-3 fatty acids make up another class of PUFAs. These fatty acids are unique in that the first double bond is located three carbon atoms from the omega end of the molecule; hence they are called omega-3s or n-3s.* Omega-3 fatty acids include eicosapentaenoic acid (EPA) which has 20 carbon atoms and five double bonds, and docosahexaenoic acid (DHA), which has 22 carbon atoms and six double bonds) (Fig. 5–6). It appears to have many health benefits, including reduction of cholesterol and triglyceride levels and the risk of blood clots. Fish oils contain omega-3 fatty acids and are also low in saturated fat. The use of omega-3 fatty acid supplements are not recommended because their long-term benefits have not been clearly defined (Report of the Nutrition Committee, 1993).

*Fatty acids are more clearly identified by numbers to indicate the position of any double bonds. The double bond can be designated in two ways. If the structure is numbered from the carboxyl group (C-OH), the symbol "Δ" is used. In the alternate system, carbon atoms are numbered from the omega end, which is indicated by "n-" or "ω" (Omega, or "ω," is the final letter in the Greek alphabet.)

CHARACTERISTICS OF FATTY ACIDS

The carbon chain length and the degree of saturation determine various properties of fats, including their flavor and **melting point** or hardness. Most saturated fatty acids are solid at room temperature; therefore most animal fats, which are predominately saturated fats, are solid at room temperature. Short-chain fatty acids (12 carbon atoms or less), monounsaturated fatty acids, and PUFAs that are liquid at room temperature are called *oils.* Milk fat contains a large amount of short-chain saturated fatty acids.

The proportion of saturated fatty acids can be increased. Polyunsaturated vegetable oil can be converted to a solid margarine or shortening by a commercial process called *hydrogenation* in which hydrogen is added to the oil. Hydrogenation can be controlled so that "tub" or "soft" margarine is "partially hydrogenated," or not completely saturated.

During hydrogenation, the shape of the fatty acid is altered. PUFAs naturally occur in what is called the "cis" configuration (i.e., the carbon chain bends so that hydrogens stick out on the same side of the molecule). During hydrogenation, the groups may rotate so they are on opposite sides of the bond, in the "trans" position (Fig. 5–7). Based on the results of metabolic and epidemiologic studies, high levels of trans fatty acids may slightly lower high-density lipoprotein (HDL) levels (the "good" cholesterol) and may

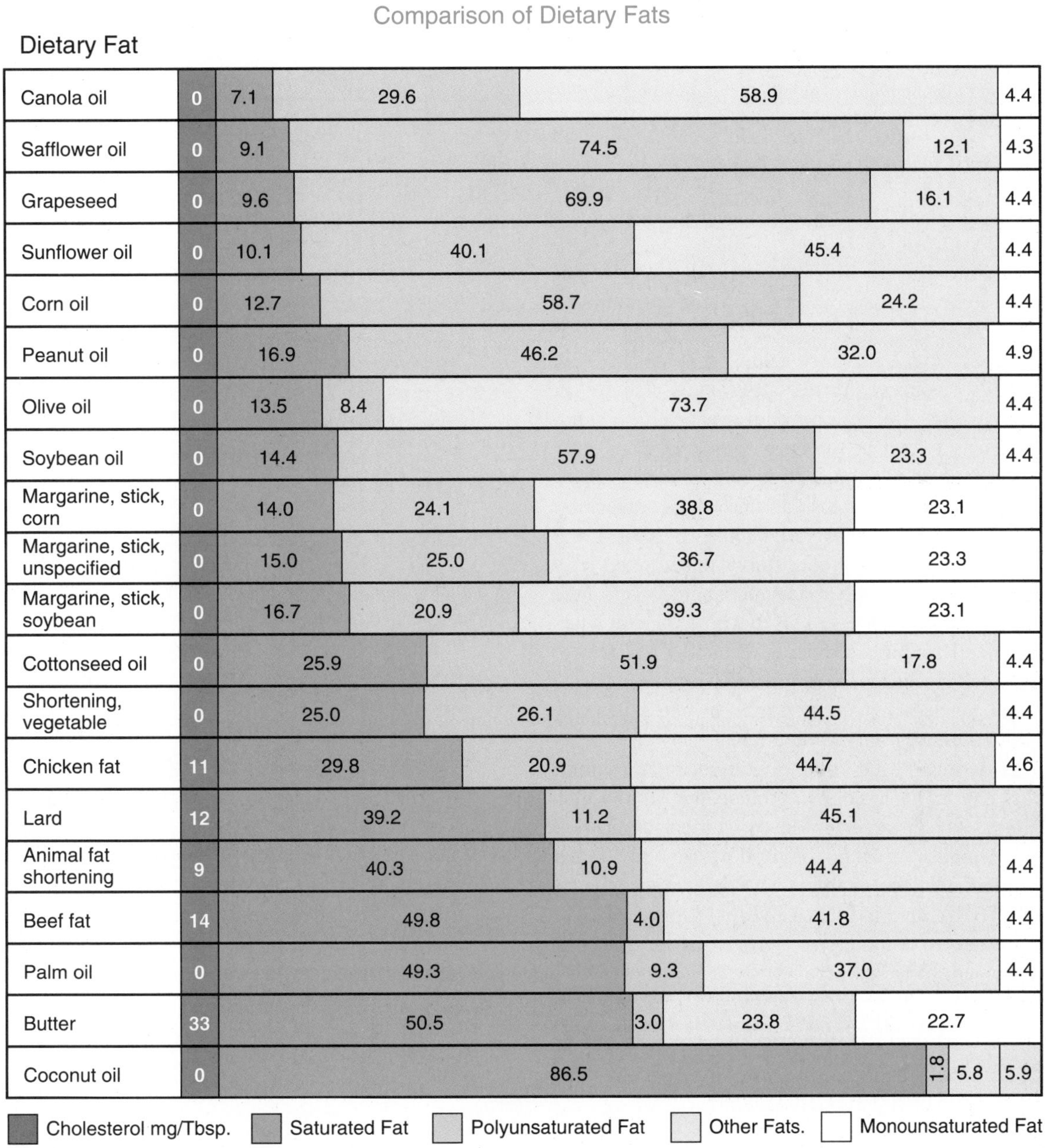

Comparison of Dietary Fats

Dietary Fat	Cholesterol mg/Tbsp.	Saturated Fat	Polyunsaturated Fat	Other Fats	Monounsaturated Fat
Canola oil	0	7.1	29.6	58.9	4.4
Safflower oil	0	9.1	74.5	12.1	4.3
Grapeseed	0	9.6	69.9	16.1	4.4
Sunflower oil	0	10.1	40.1	45.4	4.4
Corn oil	0	12.7	58.7	24.2	4.4
Peanut oil	0	16.9	46.2	32.0	4.9
Olive oil	0	13.5	8.4	73.7	4.4
Soybean oil	0	14.4	57.9	23.3	4.4
Margarine, stick, corn	0	14.0	24.1	38.8	23.1
Margarine, stick, unspecified	0	15.0	25.0	36.7	23.3
Margarine, stick, soybean	0	16.7	20.9	39.3	23.1
Cottonseed oil	0	25.9	51.9	17.8	4.4
Shortening, vegetable	0	25.0	26.1	44.5	4.4
Chicken fat	11	29.8	20.9	44.7	4.6
Lard	12	39.2	11.2	45.1	
Animal fat shortening	9	40.3	10.9	44.4	4.4
Beef fat	14	49.8	4.0	41.8	4.4
Palm oil	0	49.3	9.3	37.0	4.4
Butter	33	50.5	3.0	23.8	22.7
Coconut oil	0	86.5	1.8	5.8	5.9

Legend: Cholesterol mg/Tbsp. · Saturated Fat · Polyunsaturated Fat · Other Fats. · Monounsaturated Fat

FIGURE 5–3 **Comparison of dietary fats. The values shown for saturated and polyunsaturated fats are based on Federal Regulations, Title 21, Section 101.25(c)(2)(ii)(a&b). These state that: (a) saturated fat is the sum of lauric, myristic, palmitic, and stearic acids, and (b) polyunsaturated fat is cis, cis-methylene-interrupted polyunsaturated fatty acids. "Other fats" include saturated and polyunsaturated fatty acids that are outside of these definitions. (Data from USDA Handbook 8-, Fats and Oils. Washington, D.C.: U.S. Government Printing Office.)**

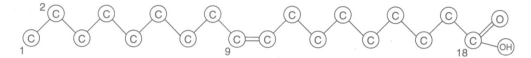

FIGURE 5-4   **Structure of oleic acid, a monounsaturated fatty acid. (From Davis JR, Sherer K. *Applied Nutrition and Diet Therapy for Nurses,* 2nd ed. Philadelphia: W.B. Saunders, 1994.)**

raise low-density lipoprotein (LDL) levels (the "bad" cholesterol), but not as much as saturated fatty acids do. Currently 2% to 4% of energy is supplied from trans fatty acids, compared to 12% to 14% from saturated fatty acids (Hunter & Applewhite, 1991). The consensus of most nutritionists is that at the current rate of trans fatty acid consumption the need to reduce consumption of saturated fatty acids far outweighs any cause for alarm about trans fatty acids in food.

Fats with a high proportion of unsaturated fatty acids may deteriorate or become rancid, resulting in off flavors and odors. Fats become rancid when subjected to high temperatures and exposure to light, which causes oxidation and decomposition of fats. The decomposition results in peroxides that may be toxic in large amounts.

Vitamin E, a fat-soluble vitamin, is an antioxidant and, to some degree, protects the oil to which it is added; however, in doing so the vitamin E is inactivated so it cannot be used by the body. Other antioxidants, for example, butylated hydroxyanisole (BHA) and butylated hydroxytoluene (BHT), are added to commercially processed fats and oils to prevent their spoilage.

Dental Hygiene Considerations

- Lipids are an integral part of many foods and are important physiologically.

- Lipids provide an excellent source of energy: 9 Cal/gm.
- Fish consumption may have a favorable effect on blood platelets and other blood-clotting mechanisms, reducing the risk of clot formation.
- The primary form of fat in the body is triglyceride, not cholesterol.

Nutritional Directions

- Foods that contain hydrogenated fats include stick margarine, vegetable shortening, peanut butter, cookies, biscuits, cake, and white bread. The use of products containing hydrogenated or partially hydrogenated fats should be limited.
- Frying foods at low temperatures causes the food to absorb excessive amounts of fats, whereas frying at very high temperatures results in decomposition of some fats, which can be irritating to the intestine and cause gastrointestinal discomfort after meals containing fried foods.
- BHA and BHT are added to processed foods to retard or prevent spoilage.

FIGURE 5-5   **Structure of linoleic acid, a polyunsaturated fatty acid. (From Davis JR, Sherer K. *Applied Nutrition and Diet Therapy for Nurses,* 2nd ed. Philadelphia: W.B. Saunders, 1994.)**

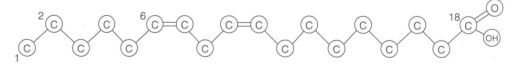

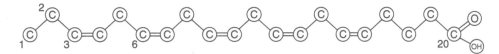

FIGURE 5–6 Structure of eicosapentaenoic acid (EPA), an omega-3 fatty acid. (From Davis JR, Sherer K. *Applied Nutrition and Diet Therapy for Nurses,* 2nd ed. Philadelphia: W.B. Saunders, 1994.)

COMPOUND LIPIDS
Phospholipids

Fats from both plant and animal foods contain *phospholipids,* but they are not necessary in the diet because the body produces all the phospholipids it needs. Phospholipids contain phosphorus and a nitrogenous base in addition to fatty acids and glycerol. These substances cannot be absorbed intact; they are broken down into their chemical components before absorption. As a structural component of cell membranes, tooth enamel, and dentin, they are the second most prevalent form of fat in the body. As such, these substances are not utilized for energy, even in a state of severe starvation. Although the mechanism is not fully understood, phospholipids are involved in the initiation of calcification and mineralization in teeth and bones and are present in higher amounts in the enamel matrix of teeth than in dentin (Kabara, 1986).

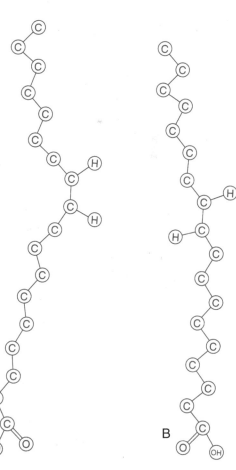

FIGURE 5–7 Note structural differences of *trans-* and *cis-* fatty acids. (From Davis JR, Sherer K. *Applied Nutrition and Diet Therapy for Nurses,* 2nd ed. Philadelphia: W.B. Saunders, 1994.)

Phospholipids can mix with either fat- or water-soluble ingredients and transport these products across membrane barriers. Phospholipids are important in fat absorption and transport of fats in the blood.

Phospholipids include lecithin, cephalin, and sphingomyelins. Lecithin, the most widely distributed phospholipid, is present in all cells. Lecithin supplements have been marketed as reducing the risk of atherosclerosis, however, its value in this role is questionable as lecithin is digested before it is absorbed. Cephalin is present in thromboplastin, necessary for blood clotting. Sphingomyelins are important constituents of brain tissue and of the myelin sheath around nerve fibers. Phospholipids, especially lecithin, are used as additives in commercial products to prevent fat and water components from separating.

Lipoproteins

Lipoproteins are found in foods and are produced by the body. Lipoproteins are compound lipids composed of triglycerides, phospholipids, and cholesterol combined with protein. The liver and intestinal mucosa produce lipoproteins, which transport insoluble fats in the body. Four different types of lipoproteins are present in the blood: high-density lipoproteins (HDLs), low-density lipoproteins (LDLs), very low-density lipoproteins (VLDLs), and chylomicrons.

The ratio of lipid to protein in lipoproteins varies widely; these variations affect their density. Density increases as lipids decrease and the protein increases (i.e., HDLs which are protective, contain larger amounts of protein and less lipid). Lipoproteins can be classified according to their density and composition, as shown in Figure 5–8. Phospholipids in lipoproteins are present in approximately the same proportions in all individuals. Serum HDL, LDL, and VLDL are important predictors of heart disease; their role in heart disease is discussed in Health Application 5.

CHOLESTEROL

Cholesterol is a fat-like waxy substance classified as a sterol (lipid). Cholesterol has a complex ring structure (Fig. 5–9). Because the body can produce all the cholesterol it needs, cholesterol intake is not essential.

Cholesterol has important functions as a con-

FIGURE 5–8 **Characteristics of lipoproteins.**

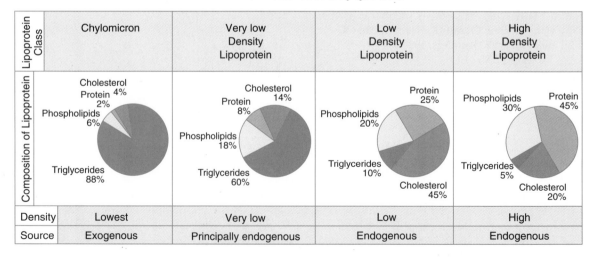

Lipoprotein Class	Chylomicron	Very low Density Lipoprotein	Low Density Lipoprotein	High Density Lipoprotein
Composition of Lipoprotein	Cholesterol 4% Protein 2% Phospholipids 6% Triglycerides 88%	Cholesterol 14% Protein 8% Phospholipids 18% Triglycerides 60%	Protein 25% Phospholipids 20% Triglycerides 10% Cholesterol 45%	Phospholipids 30% Protein 45% Triglycerides 5% Cholesterol 20%
Density	Lowest	Very low	Low	High
Source	Exogenous	Principally endogenous	Endogenous	Endogenous

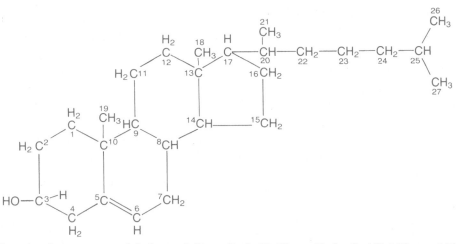

FIGURE 5–9   **Complex ring structure of cholesterol. (From Davis JR, Sherer K. *Applied Nutrition and Diet Therapy for Nurses,* 2nd ed. Philadelphia: W.B. Saunders, 1994.)**

stituent of brain and nervous tissue, a precursor of vitamin D and steroid hormones, a constituent of bile salts, and a structural component of cell membranes and teeth. It is transported in the blood via lipoproteins.

PHYSIOLOGIC ROLES

Concentrated Energy

Dietary fats are a concentrated source of energy, furnishing 9 Cal/gm. Foods high in fats are generally referred to as *calorie dense,* which has its merits in some cases. Calorie-dense foods are usually high in fats (or fat and sugar) and low in other nutrients. The advantage of calorie-dense foods is that less volume of food is needed to furnish energy requirements.

Protein Sparers

As an energy source, fats are also referred to as *protein sparing* because they allow protein to be used for important functions such as building and repairing tissues. Fats are also vitamin sparing when they are used for energy, as opposed to carbohydrates, which require thiamin and other B vitamins.

Satiety Value

Dietary fats are important for their **satiety** value. Fats contribute to a feeling of fullness for a longer period of time than carbohydrates or protein because digestion of high-fat meals is slower than of other energy-containing nutrients. This has given rise to such descriptions as "sticks to the ribs" in reference to rich meals. The higher the fat content of a meal, the longer the food remains in the stomach. Nevertheless, about 95% of the ingested fats is absorbed. Soft fats that are liquids at body temperature (like margarine) are digested more quickly than hard fats (such as meat fats).

Palatability

Fats contribute to palatability and flavor of foods. Their use in cooking improves texture. Preference for high-fat foods develops at an early age and persists through adulthood.

Complementary Relationships

Fat-soluble vitamins and linoleic acid are generally found in foods containing fat. Linoleic acid is necessary for the production of phospholipids and the **eicosanoids.** The absorption of fat-soluble vitamins is facilitated by the presence of fats in the gastrointestinal tract.

Linoleic acid, an omega-6 fatty acid with 18 carbon atoms and two double bonds, cannot be synthesized by the body and must be supplied from dietary sources. If linoleic acid is not furnished in the diet, deficiency symptoms will result. For this reason linoleic acid is an *essential fatty acid.* Arachidonic (an 18-carbon chain with four double bonds) and linolenic (18-carbon chain with three double bonds) acids are also considered essential fatty acids, but healthy children and adults can produce them from sufficient quantities of linoleic acid). Linoleic acid is required for proper growth and healthy skin. It is also incorporated into the phospholipids of dentin (Gilder & Boskey, 1990).

Eicosapentaenoic acid and arachidonic acid, both omega-3 fatty acids, can be used to produce eicosanoids. Eicosanoids are important physiologically in regulation of blood pressure, blood clotting, immune responses, gastrointestinal secretions, cardiovascular function, and inflammatory reactions. The presence of omega-3 fatty acids in the diet has been linked to reduction or amelioration of several chronic diseases, including atherosclerosis, rheumatoid arthritis, psoriasis, and inflammatory and immune disorders. The mechanism by which these polyunsaturated fatty acids reduce the risk of heart disease is unknown.

As a result of consumer awareness of the early studies indicating beneficial effects of omega-3 fatty acids, fish oil preparations are increasingly being promoted as a cure-all for a variety of diseases. However, some fish oil preparations are made from fish livers, which can be high in pesticides, heavy metals, and other environmental contaminants. They may contain potentially toxic amounts of the fat-soluble vitamins A and D and appreciable quantities of cholesterol. Fish oil capsules are expensive, and there are no controls on their manufacture. Because of these concerns regarding the effectiveness and safety of fish oil preparations, consumption of fish two to three times a week is recommended rather than fish oils.

Fat Storage

Adipose tissue has several roles: (1) it provides a concentrated energy source, (2) protects internal organs, and (3) maintains body temperature.

ENERGY

Excess carbohydrates and protein are converted to fat and stored in adipose tissue. Fatty acids can be utilized as an energy source by all cells except red blood cells and those of the central nervous system. People have been known to survive total starvation for 30 to 40 days with only water to drink.

PROTECTION OF ORGANS

Fatty tissue surrounds vital organs and provides a cushion, thereby protecting them from traumatic injury and shock.

INSULATION

The subcutaneous layer of fat functions as an insulator that preserves body heat and maintains body temperature. Excessive layers of fat can also deter heat loss during warm weather.

DIETARY FATS AND DENTAL HEALTH

Obviously, dietary fats are essential for oral health because they are incorporated into the tooth structure. There is some evidence from epidemiologic and laboratory studies that fats may have an anticariogenic effect. Eskimos, whose diet contains 70% to 80% fat from animal and seafood sources, have a very low incidence of dental caries. Another factor that may affect caries rate in these people is that carbohydrate in these diets is low.

Dietary fats probably have local rather than systemic influence since fats added to foods protect the teeth more than foods naturally high in fat (Kabara, 1986). Precisely how fats reduce the caries rate is unknown; several hypotheses have been explored:

1. Some fatty acids, specifically oleic acid, are growth factors for lactic acid bacteria whereas streptococcal organisms are inhibited by lauric acid (Lauricidin) (Kabara, 1986).
2. Long-chain fatty acids may reduce dissolution of hydroxyapatite by acids.
3. Oral food retention is reduced by increasing fat intake.
4. Fats may lubricate the tooth surface and prevent penetration of acid to the enamel (i.e., the "greased" tooth is impervious to acid, protecting caries susceptible areas).
5. Fats may produce a film on the food particles and prevent digestion of food particles.
6. Dietary fat delays gastric emptying, enhancing fluoride absorption and increasing tissue fluoride concentration.

Dental Hygiene Considerations

- Although fat intake may have a positive effect on dental health, the medical history of the client needs to be considered when providing nutritional counseling.
- Interview the client to evaluate total fat intake. Everyone needs adequate amounts of fat to allow protein to perform its function (to build and repair). If total energy intake is inadequate, healing is slower. Also, inadequate fat intake could lead to secondary deficiencies of the fat-soluble vitamins.
- Foods such as nuts and certain cheeses

(cheddar, Monterrey Jack, Swiss, etc.) may protect teeth against acid attack, especially when consumed after fermentable carbohydrates. Even though they are generally considered nutritious foods, for most Americans, their use should be limited because of their high fat content.

- Because omega-3 fatty acids may be beneficial to health, determine the client's frequency of fish consumption.
- Do not advocate indiscriminate use of omega-3 fatty acids. Fish oils may have a negative effect on blood glucose levels in clients with diabetes mellitus.
- ℞ If the client is taking anticoagulants or aspirin, evaluate use of omega-3 fatty acids. These clients may be prone to bleeding problems or poor wound healing.

Nutritional Directions

- Although the digestion of fried foods takes longer, their digestion is as complete as that of other foods in most persons if fried at the proper temperature.
- Fats act as a lubricant in the intestines, thereby decreasing constipation.
- There are currently no regulations or controls for manufacturing omega-3 supplements.
- Omega-3 fatty acid supplements should not be taken unless ordered by a physician.
- Counsel clients to read labels of omega-3 fatty acid supplements. Those made from livers should be avoided because high levels of pesticides or heavy metals may be present. Fish should be eaten instead.

DIETARY REQUIREMENTS

The essential fatty acid linoleic acid is the only specified dietary requirement for fat. The adult requirement for essential fatty acid intake is about 3 to 6 gm/day, or approximately 1 Tbsp polyunsaturated vegetable oil daily (NRC, 1989a). When

dietary intake is high, linoleic acid is stored in the tissues.

Human requirements for omega-3 fatty acids have long been disputed. Research by scientists at the U.S. Department of Agriculture Research

Service has determined that linolenic acid in soybean oil can rapidly be converted into omega-3 fatty acids. The conversion of linolenic acid to EPA and linoleic acid to arachidonic acid causes competition for the same enzyme. If intake of linoleic acid is substantially higher than intake of linolenic acid, the result is that less EPA becomes available. Omega-3 fatty acids may prove to be essential as further studies examine their many and varied effects.

Some fat is essential in the diet; however, approximately 40% of the calories in the typical American diet is from fat (Zizza & Gerrior, 1995). As discussed in chapter 1, numerous health organizations recommend total fat intake be limited to 30% of total calories. A minimum of 15 to 25 gm of fat is recommended to provide adequate amounts of fat-soluble vitamins and essential fatty acid. The method of calculating the appropriate amount of dietary fat is shown in Table 5–l.

TABLE 5–1   *Total Daily Fat Recommendations for Specific Caloric Levels* *

Calorie Level	Grams of Fat/Day
1,200	<40
1,500	<50
1,800	<60
2,000	<66
2,200	<73
2,400	<80

*Total fat intake limited to less than 30% of the total daily calories.

To calculate dietary fat:

1. Determine caloric level of the diet (RDA tables can be used) (e.g., client needs 2,000 cal).
2. Multiply the calories by 0.30 to determine the number of calories of fat the diet can contain (e.g., 2,000 cal × 0.30 [% of total cal] = 600 cal from fat).
3. Divide the answer by 9 to determine the grams of fat allowed daily (e.g., 600 cal from fat ÷ 9 Cal/gm of fat = 66.6 gm of fat).

SOURCES

Foods containing saturated, monounsaturated, and polyunsaturated fatty acids are itemized in Table 5–2. Animal products contribute the largest proportion of fat, although their share declined from 63% to 52% between 1970 and 1990 (Zizza & Gerrior, 1995). The most important sources of saturated fats are the meat and milk groups; for monounsaturated fatty acids, the meat and grain groups; and for PUFAs, the grain group and additional fats and oils. Linoleic acid is highest in safflower, sunflower, and corn oils, with lesser amounts present in soybean and canola oils. Linolenic acid is present in linseed oil (not available in the United States), canola oil, and soybean oil and in small amounts in green leafy vegetables, seaweed or plankton, and meat fats (see Fig. 5–3). High sources of omega-3 fatty acids include mackerel, Atlantic salmon, herring, lake trout, and tuna (presented in order of highest to lowest).

Only animal products contain cholesterol (Table 5–2); it is not found in egg whites or plant foods (i.e., vegetables oils). It is highest in egg yolks, liver, and other organ meats.

Food Choices

The percentage of fat by weight is widely used on food labels and advertising. Although this information is correct, it is misleading to the American public. The recommendation that fat intake should be limited to 30% refers to the percentage of fat based on the total calories of the product. As shown in Table 5–3, the percentage of fat in whole milk by calories is 49%, not 3.3% as the label normally indicates.

Wide publicity about the benefits of a lower-fat diet has resulted in some Americans changing their food habits without the benefit of adequate information regarding the fat content of foods and changes in food composition by the food industry. For most people, a decrease in red meat consumption is probably desirable, but the decision to completely eliminate it from the diet is not advisable. In recent years, through improvements in breeding and feeding livestock, these products are lower in fat, calories, and cholesterol, as shown in Figure 5–10. Other important

TABLE 5–2   *Fatty Acid and Cholesterol Content of Selected Foods*

Food	Portion	Total Fat (gm)	SFA* (gm)	MUFA† (gm)	PUFA‡ (gm)	Cholesterol (mg)
Milk and Milk Products						
Cheddar cheese	1 oz	9.4	6.0	2.7	0.27	30
Monterey Jack cheese	1 oz	8.6	5.4	2.5	0.26	25
2% Cottage cheese	½ c	2.2	1.4	0.6	0.07	10
Cream cheese	1 oz	10.0	6.3	2.8	0.36	31
1% milk	1 c	2.6	1.6	0.8	0.10	10
2% milk	1 c	4.7	3.0	1.4	0.17	18
Whole milk	1 c	8.1	5.1	2.4	0.30	33
Ice cream, 10% fat	1 c	14.3	8.9	3.6	0.32	59
Meats, Fish, and Eggs						
Lean beef tenderloin	3 oz	9.5	3.6	3.6	0.36	71
Beef liver	3 oz	4.2	1.6	0.6	0.91	331
Skinless chicken breast	3 oz	3.0	0.9	1.1	0.65	72
Chicken breast (with skin)	3 oz	10.6	0.6	4.5	1.7	42
Skinless chicken thigh	3 oz	9.3	2.6	3.5	2.11	80
Lean pork chop	3 oz	13.0	4.5	5.8	1.59	81
Lean veal loin	3 oz	5.9	2.2	2.1	.05	90
Canned salmon	3 oz	4.7	1.3	1.6	1.29	33
Cod fish	3 oz	0.7	0.1	0.1	0.25	47
Shrimp	3 oz	0.9	0.3	0.2	0.37	166
Whole egg	1	5.0	1.5	1.9	0.67	212
Egg white	1	0	0	0	0	0
Egg yolk	1	5.1	1.6	2.0	0.70	213
Fats and Oils						
Butter	1 Tbsp	11.4	7.1	3.3	0.42	31
Half and half cream	¼ c	7.0	4.3	2.0	0.26	22
Corn oil margarine, hard	1 Tbsp	11.4	1.8	6.6	2.4	0
Corn oil margarine, soft	1 Tbsp	11.4	2.1	4.5	4.5	0
Corn oil	1 Tbsp	13.6	1.7	3.3	8.0	0
Vegetable shortening	1 Tbsp	12.8	3.2	5.6	3.3	0
Mayonnaise type salad dressing	1 Tbsp	4.9	0.7	1.3	2.6	4

*Saturated fatty acids.
†Monounsaturated fatty acids.
‡Polyunsaturated fatty acids.
Nutrient data from Nutritionist IV software; First Data Bank, San Bruno, CA. From Davis JR, Sherer K. *Applied Nutrition and Diet Therapy for Nurses,* 2nd ed. Philadelphia: W. B. Saunders, 1994.

TABLE 5–3   *Analysis of Fat Content of Milk*

	Calories (1 Cup)	Total Fat (gm)	Percent of Fat by Weight	Percent of Fat by Calories
Whole milk	150	8.1	3.3	49
Low-fat milk (2%)	120	4.7	2	35
Low-fat milk (1%)	102	2.6	1	23
Skim milk	86	0.4	<1	4

From Davis JR, Sherer K. *Applied Nutrition and Diet Therapy for Nurses,* 2nd ed. Philadelphia: W.B. Saunders, 1994.

nutrients are present in beef, pork, and lamb; moderate use of these products is encouraged for everyone. Loin (sirloin, tenderloin, or center loin) and round cuts (top, bottom, eye, or tip) and lean or extra lean ground beef contain the least amount of fat. After consideration of total fat content of a product, the next priority is its saturated fat content.

Dental Hygiene Considerations

- Use Table 5–1 when assessing fat recommendations.
- Clients frequently consume more fat than they realize because of the "invisible" fats in milk (including cheese) and meat products. Therefore, interview clients to assess their intake of these foods.
- Foods having a higher fat content are more calorie-dense. For example, ¼ cup of peanuts and seven whole carrots have the same number of calories (210). Carrots have only a trace of fat; peanuts contain 18 gm of fat per ¼ cup. Therefore, knowledge of fat content of foods is necessary to assess for fat intake.
- Have clients actually read a nutrition label to determine whether the product is a good buy as well as a healthy choice with regard to fat. A rule of thumb to remember is that if the fat content is greater than 3 gm/100 calories, the fat content is too high.

Nutritional Directions

- Butter contains more saturated fats than most margarines; it also contains cholesterol, whereas most margarines do not.

- Tropical oils, including palm oil, palm kernel oil, and coconut oil, are saturated fats; thus their consumption should be limited.
- Purchase processed foods that contain more polyunsaturated and monounsaturated fatty acids than saturated fatty acids. If the food label contains only the required information (total fat and saturated fat content), subtract the number of grams of saturated fat from the total fat. For example, if the product contains 8 gm of fat and 3 gm of saturated fat, the 5 gm of monounsaturated and polyunsaturated fatty acids is more than the 3 gm from saturated fat. This product is acceptable, but if there is another similar product that contains less than 3 gm of saturated fat, that product would be a wiser choice.
- A few fruits and vegetables contain a small amount of fat. For example, bananas contain a trace of fat (0.55 gm or 0.5% fat by weight and 6% of the calories); avocados contain 31 gm of fat (15% by weight and 86% of the calories). Both are good sources of several vitamins and minerals.
- Teach clients to read labels and to understand that the percentage of fat should be determined based on the total calories, not the weight, of the food. To determine fat content use either of the following formulas:

grams of fat × 9 = calories provided by fat, or
calories of fat ÷ the total calories of the
   product × 100 = % fat content of the product

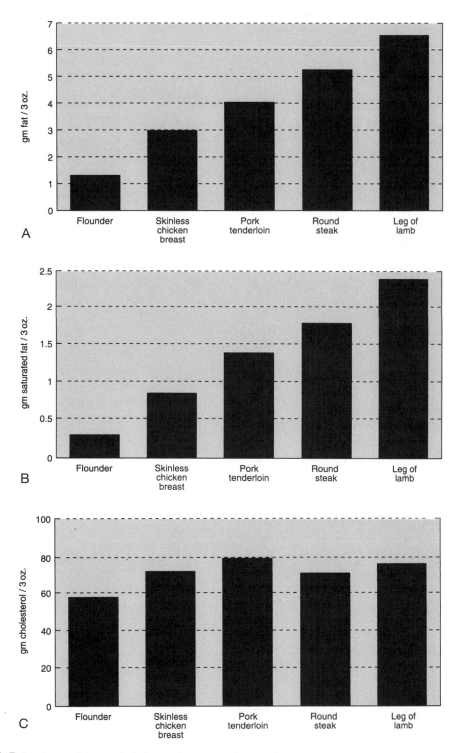

FIGURE 5–10 Fat, saturated fat, and cholesterol content of meats (3 oz cooked [baked /roasted] and trimmed). (A) Fat content comparison. (B) Saturated fat content comparison. (C) Cholesterol content comparison. (From Davis JR, Sherer K. *Applied Nutrition and Diet Therapy for Nurses,* 2nd ed. Philadelphia: W.B. Saunders, 1994.)

If the food contains less than 30% fat, it is generally a wise choice. Fats and oils that are 100% fat are necessary to provide adequate PUFAs and fat-soluble vitamins; therefore, food items are averaged together to determine if an item exceeding 30% fat would cause the day's or week's intake to exceed the overall 30% desired fat level.

◆ Children under the age of 2 are growing rapidly; fat restriction is potentially unsafe for this age group because of uncertainties about the amounts of energy, cholesterol, and essential fatty acid required for growth. After 2 years of age, the Dietary Guidelines for Americans are applicable.

OVERCONSUMPTION AND HEALTH-RELATED PROBLEMS

Some conditions related to fat will be observed in dental hygiene practice. The following conditions suggest alteration of the amount and/or type of fat in the diet: obesity, diabetes mellitus, hyperlipidemia, fatty infiltration of the liver, and certain types of cancer.

Obesity

Excessive fat stores are a common disorder in the United States. Although the cause is usually overconsumption of all energy nutrients, calories from fat are so concentrated that relatively small quantities may rapidly increase caloric intake. Kendall and colleagues (1991) found that weight loss can occur by reducing dietary fat without any other food restrictions. Men who normally consume a larger percentage of fat have more body fat stores and consume more calories than men with a low fat intake.

Blood Lipid Levels

Elevated blood lipids are related to diet. **Hyperlipidemia** is associated with heart disease. While many factors can affect blood lipid levels, the strongest dietary determinant of the blood cholesterol level is the saturated fat content of the diet. In contrast, stearic acid, found in beef and cocoa butter, has no detrimental effect on serum cholesterol. Cholesterol and total fat content also affect serum lipid levels, but to a lesser extent. Reduction of the total dietary fat content to less than 30% of the intake helps lower saturated fat content of the

diet. Factors and dietary modifications that affect serum lipid levels are discussed in more detail in Health Application 5.

Cancer

Thirty to 40% of all cancers in men and 60% of all cancers in women have been attributed to diet; fat has been linked more frequently to cancer than any other dietary factor. Epidemiologic studies of human populations indicate a correlation of total fat intake and breast, colon and, to some extent, prostate cancer. Evidence linking dietary fat and particular fatty acids with risk of cancer has elicited considerable interest and debate because of the diversity of findings. Different mechanisms may be involved in tumor development at different sites and stages of the cancer.

The incidence of colon cancer is strongly correlated with per capita consumption of red meat and animal fat in various countries (Willett et al., 1990). Despite many uncertainties about a relationship between dietary fat and cancer risk, the consensus of opinion is to limit total fat intake by increasing fish and lean chicken consumption while concurrently decreasing high-fat meats.

Dental Hygiene Considerations

● To distinguish obesity from edema, when the skin of an obese subject is palpated, it will have a flabby consistency, unlike the mushy or spongy consistency found in edematous skin.

- A high serum HDL level is desirable to prevent heart disease.
- Ask adult clients if they know their blood lipid levels. If they are high and mainly animal products are consumed, their risk for cardiovascular disease may be increased because of high saturated fat intake.
- Ask adult clients about a family history of cardiovascular disease.

Nutritional Directions

- Diets high in fat may lead to obesity, coronary heart disease, and possibly breast and colon cancer and strokes.
- Advise clients that 10% of the total caloric intake should come from saturated fats, with the remaining 20% from mono- and polyunsaturated fatty acids. Serum cholesterol can be lowered by diets low in total fat and higher in monounsaturated fatty acids and PUFAs (see Table 5–2).
- Because of inadequate information regarding long-term consequences of high PUFA intake, the Committee on Diet and Health of the Food and Nutrition Board recommends that PUFAs not exceed 10% of intake (NRC, 1989b).
- Reduce dietary cholesterol intake to less than 300 mg daily by limiting meats, whole milk and cheese, and eggs.
- "Low cholesterol" in relation to a food or diet can be misleading. A cholesterol-free product can still be high in saturated fat, which will elevate blood cholesterol. Dietary saturated fat has a greater effect on serum cholesterol than dietary cholesterol.
- The consumption of soluble fibers may decrease serum cholesterol.

UNDERCONSUMPTION AND HEALTH-RELATED PROBLEMS

Obviously overconsumption of fat is a primary concern in health care, whereas underconsumption of fats is virtually nonexistent in the United States. However, clinical symptoms of fat deficiency may occur, especially in clients with malabsorption syndromes such as cystic fibrosis or those in later stages of AIDS. Because medications used to lower blood lipid levels interfere with fat absorption, clients taking these medications should be assessed for fat-soluble vitamin and essential fatty acid deficiencies.

When client's whose overall intake including fats is poor, they lose weight, and the subcutaneous fat stores needed to maintain body temperature are depleted. Patients with anorexia nervosa are especially of concern. Severely inadequate fat intake may have a more pronounced influence on dentin lipids than on enamel lipids.

Dental Hygiene Considerations

- Fat deficiency results in poor growth, dermatitis (Fig. 5–11), lowered resistance to infection, and poor reproductive capacity.

- If a client has a poor reserve of subcutaneous fat, monitor temperature closely. These clients are not able to regulate temperature as effectively as those who have subcutaneous fat reserves.
- A client with inadequate fat intake will be thin, will have dry skin and dull hair, and will be sensitive to cold temperatures. If these signs and symptoms are noted, suggest examination by a physician.

Nutritional Directions

- Although much is heard about the problems of fat consumption, fats have important physiologic functions and a certain amount must be provided in the diet.

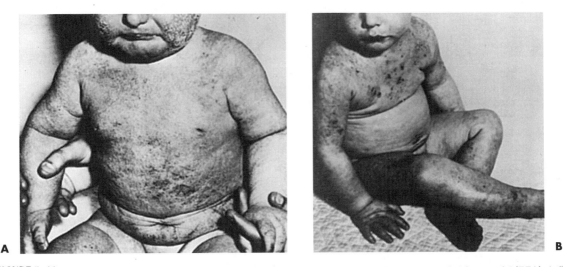

FIGURE 5–11 The first indications of disease identified specifically as being due to essential fatty acid (EFA) deficiency were skin lesions in rats. Similar lesions were then seen in infants given formulas devoid of EFAs. This research was carried out before the critical nature of EFAs was known. Ethical considerations would prohibit such research today. (A) Six-month-old infant with very resistant eczema appearing at 2½ months of age. (B) The same child 6 months later after a source of linoleic acid had been included in the diet. (Courtesy of the late Dr. A. E. Hansen.) (From Davis JR, Sherer K. *Applied Nutrition and Diet Therapy for Nurses,* 2nd ed. Philadelphia: W.B. Saunders, 1994.)

FAT REPLACERS

As a result of growing concern over dietary fats, numerous foods are being manufactured containing less fat. Because of the possible connection between excessive fat intake and chronic diseases, fat replacers may be helpful in reducing fat consumption. Most of the formulations to replace fat are carbohydrate and protein based. Lipid-based materials have been formulated; some are not on the market, pending FDA approval. Each of these fat replacers possesses diverse sensory, functional, and physiologic properties that affect their incorporation into various types of products (Table 5–4). Low-calorie salad dressing, low-fat yogurt, and imitation margarine are all made by using modified starches and gums to reduce the oil or fat in the product.

Simplesse® is a fat substitute made from egg white and milk protein. Simplesse® mimics fat by producing a creamy smooth feeling in the mouth like fats, but it coagulates and loses this creaminess at high temperatures. Thus, this product is limited to use in dairy products (such as ice cream and cream cheese) and in oil-based products (such as salad dressings and margarine) that do not require heat in processing. A more versatile version of Simplesse® has been introduced on the market that is a whey-protein concentrate. It can be used in all food categories, including baked goods, cheese for hamburgers and pizza, soups and sauces. Trailblazer® is another protein-based fat substitute similar to Simplesse®.

Sucrose polyester (Olestra) is a synthetic fat that resembles conventional dietary fats and can be substituted in many foods. Its recent FDA approval has caused a stir in the scientific community because of its association with decreased absorption of vitamins A, D, E, and K, and common effects of intestinal cramps and lose stools. Olestra has been extensively researched through 100 studies with five animal species and 25 clinical studies involving more than 2,500 people. The industry has agreed to supplement Olestra-containing products

TABLE 5–4 *Fat Replacers*

Generic Name	Trade Name	Appropriate Uses	Calories/gm
Carbohydrate-Based Fat Replacers			
Cellulose	Avicel®	Can replace part or all of the fat in dairy-type products, sauces, frozen desserts, and salad dressings	0
Gums		Reduced-calorie, fat-free salad dressings and to reduce fat content in other formulated foods, including processed meats	0
Dextrins	N-Oil®, Oatrim®	Salad dressings, puddings, spreads, dairy-type products, and frozen desserts	4
Maltodextrins	Lycadex®, Maltrin®, Paselli SA2®, STAR-DRI®	Baked goods, dairy products, salad dressings, spreads, sauces, frostings, fillings, processed meat, and frozen desserts	4
Modified food starch	STA-SLIM®	Used with emulsifiers, proteins, gums, and other modified food starches in processed meats, salad dressings, baked goods, fillings and frostings, sauces, condiments, frozen desserts, and dairy products	4
Polydextrose	Litesse®	Approved for use in baked goods, chewing gums, confections, salad dressings, frozen dairy desserts, gelatins, and puddings	1
Protein-Based Fat Replacers			
Microparticulated protein*	Simplesse®	Dairy-type products, salad dressing, margarin, and mayonnaise-type products	1–2
Other protein blends	Trailblazer®, ULTRA-BAKE®, ULTRA-FREEZE®	Frozen desserts and baked goods	1–2
Fat-Based Fat Replacers			
Emulsifiers	Dur-Lo®, Veri-Lo®	Can replace all or part of the shortening in cake mixes, cookies, icings, and vegetable dairy products	9
Dialkyl dihexadecylmalonate (DDM)†		Mayonnaise and margarine-type products as well as high-temperature applications	0
Esterified propoxylated glycerol (EPG)†		Formulated products, baking and frying	
Sucrose polyesters	Olestra®	Home cooking oils and shortenings and in commercial frying and snack foods	0
Trialkoxytricarballylate (TATCA)		Under development for use in margarine and mayonnaise-type products	0

*Currently not available for use.
†Requires FDA approval.
Data from Calorie Control Council: *Fat Replacers.* Atlanta GA: Calorie Control Council, 1992; and Fat Substitute Update. *Food Technol* 1990; 44(3):92–97.

with the poorly absorbed vitamins to compensate for decreased absorption and to replace the amounts of the vitamins normally found in vegetable oils.

Because Olestra is not digested or absorbed, it contributes no calories. It provides the taste, texture, and oral feeling of conventional fats. Olestra has been approved for use in replacing the fats in savory snacks. Caprenin® is a reduced-calorie fat that resembles cocoa butter but contains only 5 cal/gm. It has been approved for use in soft candy and confectionery coatings.

In the near future, countless other fat replacers will be available. By substituting fat replacers for fats, total fat intake can be reduced and some weight loss may be achieved. However, an overall weight loss program is still needed to effect weight loss. Those who consume large portions of lower-fat products potentially negate the caloric and fat savings of the replacement foods. Fat substitutes appear to pose little risk to health, but data are sparse regarding possible benefits under conditions of normal consumer use.

Dental Hygiene Considerations

- Assess use of fat replacers.
- Evaluate overall dietary habits because a client may think using fat replacers will make a desirable change in health without considering other aspects of the diet.

Nutritional Directions

- Simplesse® cannot be used for frying or baking and contains 1 to 2 Cal/gm. Other proposed fat replacers may be used for frying.
- Patients allergic to eggs or cow milk could be at risk for an allergic reaction to Simplesse®.
- Intake of fat replacers needs to be balanced with variety and moderation in food choices to achieve an overall healthy, nutritious diet.

HEALTH APPLICATION 5

Hyperlipidemia

Cardiovascular disease is still the leading cause of death in the United States. Cardiovascular disorders include coronary heart disease (CHD), hypertension, peripheral vascular disease, congestive heart failure, and congenital heart disease. Nearly one-fourth of all persons who die from cardiovascular disease are under age 65.

Hyperlipidemia, or increased plasma cholesterol and LDL levels, appears to be a major risk factor in CHD. In 1993, the *Second Report of the Expert Panel on Detection, Evaluation, and Treatment of High Blood Cholesterol in Adults* updated earlier guidelines for detection and treatment of hyperlipidemia (NCEP, 1993). The Panel encourages that everyone tested for serum cholesterol be assessed for other risk factors (Table 5–5) and provided appropriate treatment. Heredity is a risk factor that cannot be controlled; however, individuals from families in which heart disease is common can follow a preventive diet. Diet can be manipulated to alter two risk factors: hyperlipidemia and hypertension. Lifestyle changes such as increased exercise, cessation of smoking, and moderation in alcohol intake can also alter risk factors.

Average cholesterol intake in the United States is 415 mg/day. The body synthesizes approximately two to four times more cholesterol than it obtains from exogenous sources. Of all the dietary changes recommended, cholesterol intake probably has the least effect on plasma cholesterol concentrations in most individuals because of less endogenous cholesterol production in response to cholesterol absorption.

The National Cholesterol Education Program has recommended a reduction of dietary cholesterol to less than 300 mg/day. Those who initially have a total plasma cholesterol level closer to normal are expected to have a lesser effect from cholesterol restriction.

Currently the American diet contains approximately 35% of the total calories as fat, with 13% of the fat from saturated fats (animal origin, palm oil, coconut oil, cocoa butter, hydrogenated margarine) (Tippett & Goldman, 1994). The remainder of ingested fat is derived from monounsaturated sources, such as olive,

TABLE 5-5 *Treatment Recommendations Based on Serum Lipids*

Risk Category	Cholesterol (mg/dL)			Recommendations*		
	Total	HDL	LDL	Diagnosis	Diet	Drugs
Desirable						
	<200	≥35	<130	Remeasure in 5 years	Educate on general population eating pattern	
	<200	<35		Reevaluate in 1–2 years	Provide information on dietary modification	
Borderline						
Without CHD *or* fewer than two risk factors†	200–239	≥35		Reevaluate in 1–2 years	Provide information on dietary modification	
Without CHD *or* fewer than two risk factors†	200–239	<35	139–159	Lipoprotein analysis and evaluate annually	Initiate Step-1 diet‡ if LDL >160	
With CHD *or* two or more risk factors†	200–239	<35	139–159	Lipoprotein analysis	Initiate Step-1 diet‡ if LDL >130 or if LDL >100 with CHD	May initiate drug treatment
High						
Without CHD *or* fewer than two risk factors†	>240		>160	Lipoprotein analysis	Initiate Step-1 diet‡	Initiate if LDL ≥190
With CHD *or* two or more risk factors†			≥160	Lipoprotein analysis	Initiate Step-1 diet‡	Initiate if LDL >160 or ≥130 with CHD

HDL, high-density lipoprotein; LDL, low-density lipoprotein; CHD, coronary heart disease.

*Patients are also counseled about physical activity and risk factor reduction.

†*Positive risk factors* are (1) age (male ≥45, female ≥55 or premature menopause without estrogen replacement therapy); (2) family history of premature CHD (definite myocardial infarction or sudden death before 55 years of age in father or other male first-degree relative, or before 65 years of age in mother or other female first-degree relative); (3) current cigarette smoking; (4) hypertension (blood pressure ≥140/90 mmHg, confirmed by measurements on several occasions or taking antihypertensive medication); (5) low HDL cholesterol (<35 mg/dL, confirmed by measurements on several occasions; and (6) diabetes mellitus. A *negative risk factor* is a high HDL cholesterol (≥60 mg/dL).

‡Step-1 diet is initiated first; blood lipid levels are measured and dietary compliance is assessed at 4 to 6 weeks and at 3 months. If goals for serum lipids are met, no change is made. If the goals for serum lipids have not been achieved, the client is referred to a registered dietician for implementation of the Step-2 diet, which is followed by another reassessment after 4 to 6 weeks and 3 months.

Adapted from the *Second Report of the Expert Panel on Detection, Evaluation, and Treatment of High Blood Cholesterol in Adults* (Adult Treatment Panel II). Bethesda, MD: National Institutes of Health (NHLBI). NIH Publications No. 93-3095. Sept. 1993.

canola, and peanut oils, which may be significant in lowering cholesterol. Monounsaturated fats can effectively lower plasma LDL concentrations (the "bad" cholesterol) without reducing HDL cholesterol levels (the "good" cholesterol).

Most studies have found that reductions in total dietary fat lower serum cholesterol. Because fat consumption generally coincides with decreased saturated fat intake, changes in blood lipids may be related more to type of fat consumed rather than to total fat. A diet limiting fat to 30% of its calories with 10% from PUFAs and 10% from saturated fats reduces total and LDL cholesterol concentrations in most hyperlipidemic persons. By

replacing some of the saturated fatty acids with monounsaturated fatty acids and some PUFA, and decreasing total fat, LDL is lowered without decreasing HDL concentrations. These changes result in a more palatable diet that is better received by Americans.

Some plant fibers, especially soluble carbohydrates (pectin, guar gum, carrageenan, or oat bran) found in apples, citrus fruit, legumes, oats, and barley, can have significant hypocholesterolemic effects, with a reduction in plasma LDL concentration and a rise or no change in plasma HDL. Mechanisms involved are not clearly established. In studies using insoluble fibers (alfalfa, wheat bran, or cellulose), no hypocholesterolemic effect is seen.

CASE APPLICATION FOR THE DENTAL HYGIENIST

A 50-year-old patient complains to his dental hygienist that he has recently been having chest pain. He states a recent testing at his grocery store indicated his blood cholesterol level was elevated. A physician told him several years ago that his cholesterol was elevated, and that he probably should lower his cholesterol intake. No formal diet education was ordered, and no follow-up work has been done.

He continues to eat anything he wants. He realizes that some foods are high in fat and should be avoided, but he is unable to identify these foods nor is he willing to eliminate them from his diet. When questioned about fat requirements and different types of fat, he says that he does not understand all of those big medical terms. He also indicates that his parents ate what they wanted without all these problems and concerns.

Nutritional Assessment

- Readiness/willingness to learn
- Knowledge level concerning fat principles and how these relate to his diagnosis
- Total amount of fat intake

- Typical foods eaten
- Type of dietary habits: who purchases and prepares the food, where he lives, where most meals are eaten
- Weight and height, ideal body weight, blood pressure
- Serum lipids, if known
- Family medical history (parents still living, cause of death)

Nutritional Diagnosis

Altered health maintenance related to lack of knowledge of fat principles; diet and how it relates to the condition.

Nutritional Goals

Client will adhere to a low-fat, low-cholesterol diet, list foods high and low in fat, and state how disease may improve or deteriorate with diet.

Nutritional Implementation

Intervention: Emphasize the importance of having a thorough examination by a physician and a confirmation of laboratory work.

Rationale: Dietary changes as well as lifestyle changes are probably indicated; however, the best person to diagnose and prescribe treatment is a physician.

Intervention: Explain how diet affects his condition:

1. saturated fat increases rate of fatty deposits in the arteries;
2. high cholesterol intake adversely affects this process;
3. roles of fat.

Rationale: Knowledge increases compliance.

Intervention: Explain the difference between PUFAs and saturated fats:

1. use actual food labels;
2. provide a list of foods high and low in these two types of fat;
3. keep fat intake to less than 30% of total calories;
4. 10% from saturated fats and 20% from monounsaturated and PUFAs;
5. assist the client in learning to calculate these numbers.

Rationale: If the client knows the difference between the two types of fat, he can make informed choices to help decrease progression of heart disease.

Intervention: Explain the difference between types of lipids and cholesterol:

1. provide a list of foods high and low in cholesterol;
2. limit daily cholesterol intake to 300 mg or less;
3. explain that "cholesterol-free" does not necessarily mean "fat-free."

Rationale: Serum cholesterol lowering may help slow effects of heart disease.

Intervention: Monitor lipid levels by inquiring at each visit if the client has had his cholesterol checked recently (cholesterol less than 200 gm/dL, HDLs >30 mg/dL, LDLs <130 mg/dL). Use these as motivators to stay on healthy diet.
Rationale: These values can provide concrete evidence for motivation and compliance.

Intervention: Maintain records on the client's reported weight.
Rationale: Ideal body weight can help minimize adverse effects of heart disease.

Intervention: Teach the client how to read nutrition labels (use an actual food label for teaching) and calculate grams and or calories of fat; use a margarine brand that lists the first ingredient as either liquid oil or water. Explain the difference claims on labels, "fat-free," "low-fat," "reduced-fat," etc. (refer to Table 1–8).
Rationale: Labels can be confusing. Accurate information can promote healthy food choices and lower the incidence of heart disease.

Intervention: Teach the client how to decrease the amount of fat and saturated fats in his diet: advise him to

1. eat smaller servings of meat;
2. trim visible fat from meats;
3. use more poultry and fish;
4. avoid fried foods.

Rationale: These are all ways to decrease intake of fat, thereby decreasing progression of atherosclerosis. The use of more fish will increase intake of omega-3 fatty acids.

Evaluation

If the client lists foods higher and lower in fat; can choose a low-fat, low-cholesterol meal from a restaurant menu; and consumes a low-fat, low-cholesterol diet, dental hygiene care was effective. In addition, if the client can choose the healthiest low-fat, low-cholesterol choices from three food labels; state how fat and cholesterol can lead to further deterioration of his disease; and verbalize that fat speeds up the progression of fatty deposits, dental hygiene care was successful. Other factors to evaluate include whether blood lipid levels decrease to within levels listed in the care plan, and whether the client can plan a diet that is low in fat and cholesterol.

Student Readiness

1. Define the terms *lipid, hydrogenation, triglyceride,* and *lipoprotein* to a client.

2. A client wants to know foods to consume to (1) increase polyunsaturated fats and (2) decrease saturated fats. Name three sources of each.

3. In observing physical properties of fats, how could you make an intelligent guess about the polyunsaturated and saturated fat content of a food?

4. What unsaturated fatty acid is essential in the diet? What are the functions of unsaturated fatty acids in the body?

5. Compare the labels of three brands of stick margarine, three brands of tub margarine, and two brands of diet margarine. How do they differ in their polyunsaturated/saturated fat ratio?

6. List the functions of fat in the diet.

7. Evaluate one day of your intake for types of foods consumed and amounts of cholesterol and saturated fat. If that day represented your average cholesterol and saturated fat intake over a period of some time, determine whether the cholesterol or saturated fat content of intake should be reduced. List some simple suggestions for decreasing their intake.

8. Describe the role of cholesterol in the body.

9. Calculate the caloric value of the following items:
   2 slices bacon (8 gm of fat, 4 gm of protein)
   1 Tbsp margarine (12 gm of fat)
   1 Tbsp whipped margarine (8 gm of fat)
   1 Tbsp mayonnaise (6 gm of fat)
   1 Tbsp lard (13 gm of fat)

10. A client asks if it is possible to lose or gain 1 lb of body fat per day. What would you say?

11. Calculate the grams of fat a client could consume on (1) a 1,500-calorie diet; and (2) a 2,000-calorie diet to meet the Dietary Guidelines.

12. List five points you think a client should know about fats in general.

References

Gilder H, Boskey AL. Dietary lipids and the calcifying tissues. *In* Simmons DJ (ed): *Nutrition and Bone Development.* New York: Oxford University Press, 1990, 244–265.

Hunter JE, Applewhite TH. Reassessment of trans fatty acid availability in the US diet. *Am J Clin Nutr* 1991; 54(2):363–369.

Kabara J. Dietary lipids as anticariogenic agents. *J Environ Pathol Toxicol Oncol* 1986; 6(3–4):87–113.

Kendall A et al. Weight loss on a low-fat diet: Consequences of the imprecision of the control of food intake in humans. *Am J Clin Nutr* 1991; 53(5):1124–1129.

National Cholesterol Education Program (NCEP). *Second Report of the Expert Panel on Detection, Evaluation, and Treatment of High Blood Cholesterol in Adults.* Bethesda, MD: National Institutes of Health, 1993.

National Research Council (NRC). *Recommended Dietary Allowances.* 10th ed. Washington, D.C.: National Academy Press, 1989a.

National Research Council (NRC). *Diet and Health: Implications for Reducing Chronic Disease Risk.* Report of the Committee on Diet and Health, Food and Nutrition Board. Washington, D.C.: National Academy Press, 1989b.

Report of the Nutrition Committee. Rationale of the diet-heart statement of the American Heart Association. *Circulation* 1993; 88(6):3008–3029.

Tippett KS, Goldman JD. Diets more healthful, but still fall short of dietary guidelines. *Food Rev* 1994; 17(1):8–14.

Willett WC et al. Relation of meat, fat and fiber intake to the risk of colon cancer in a prospective study among women. *N Engl J Med* 1990; 323(24):1664–1670.

Zizza C, Gerrior S. The US food supply provides more of most nutrients. *Food Rev* 1995; 18(1):40–45.

Chapter 6

Utilization of the Energy Nutrients: Metabolism and Balance

OBJECTIVES

The Student Will Be Able To:

- Calculate energy needs according to the client's weight and activities.
- Explain physiologic sources of energy.
- Identify factors affecting the basal metabolic rate.
- Assess factors affecting energy balance.
- Describe the effects of inadequate energy intake.
- Explain the principles for regulating energy balance to a client.

GLOSSARY OF TERMS

Metabolism   the continuous processes whereby living organisms and cells convert nutrients into energy, body structure, and waste

Catabolism   the breaking down of complex substances into simpler substances

Anabolism   the use of absorbed nutrients to build or synthesize more complex compounds

Coenzyme   molecule needed to activate an enzyme

Glycogenesis   the process by which sugars, including fructose, galactose, sorbitol, and xylitol, are stored as glycogen

Insulin   a hormone that lowers blood sugar levels

Gluconeogenesis   the synthesis of glucose from noncarbohydrate sources

Lipogenesis   fat synthesis

Lipolysis   fat breakdown

Oxidation   the process of hydrolyzing triglycerides into two-carbon entities to enter the Krebs cycle for energy production

Ketone bodies   acidic metabolic products of normal lipid catabolism

Ketosis   the accumulation of ketone bodies in the blood

Energy   the ability or power to do work

Calorimeter   a device used to measure calories

Basal metabolic rate   the energy required for involuntary physiological functions to maintain life, including respiration, circulation, and maintenance of muscle tone and body temperature

Postabsorptive state   when digestive and absorptive processes are minimal

Basal energy expenditure   a person's total caloric requirement

Hunger   the physiologic drive to eat

Test Your NQ (True/False)

1. Insulin is a hormone that increases blood glucose levels. T/F
2. Even during sleep, the body requires energy. T/F
3. BMR stands for blood malnutrition reaction. T/F
4. A malnourished client will have a low BMR. T/F
5. The hypothalamus controls hunger and satiety. T/F
6. Hunger is the same as appetite. T/F
7. Fats are a good source of quick energy. T/F
8. The kidneys play an important role in maintaining nutrient balance within the body. T/F
9. Ketosis can occur as a result of strict dieting. T/F
10. Vitamins are a source of energy. T/F

INTRODUCTION

After foods are chewed and digested, the *energy-providing nutrients* carbohydrate, protein, fat, and alcohol, which supply physiologic energy for the body, are converted to glucose, fatty acids, and amino acids. These basic nutrient units are delivered to cells where, at the direction of specific enzymes, they can be utilized.

As you may recall from your study of earlier chapters no single nutrient can be isolated from the others because nutrients are concurrently distributed in foods and share many points of interaction in digestion and absorption. Their **metabolism** is also interrelated.

METABOLISM

In metabolic activity, the two major chemical reactions are **catabolism** and **anabolism.** Anabolism and catabolism are continuous reactions in the body. Cells in the epithelial lining of the oral and gastrointestinal mucosa are replaced about every 3 to 7 days. In spite of this rapid turnover, the rate of catabolism is usually equal to that of anabolism in an adult. During certain stages of life, such as growth periods or pregnancy, more anabolism is occurring than catabolism. Conversely, when illness or stress occurs, excessive catabolism is evident.

Other phases of metabolism include delivery of nutrients to the cells where they are needed, and delivery of wastes to sites where they can be excreted. After energy-yielding nutrients are absorbed, glucose, fatty acids, and amino acids can be utilized via a common pathway within the mitochondria of cells to yield energy (Fig. 6–1). The catabolic end-products of carbohydrates, proteins, and fats are carbon dioxide, water, and energy. Nitrogen is an additional end-product of protein.

The Krebs cycle converts glucose, fatty acids, and amino acids to a utilizable form of energy, and requires many enzymes in this process. For the

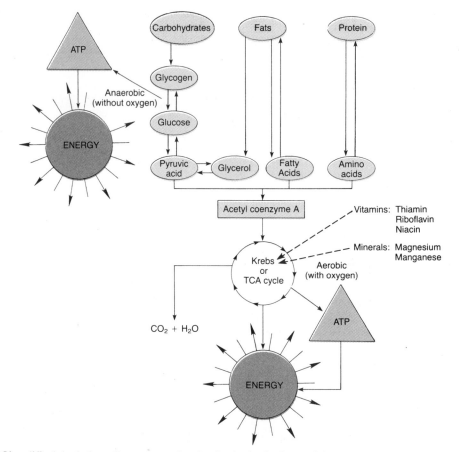

FIGURE 6–1 Simplified depiction of energy production in the body. Potential energy from the storage of glycogen is dependent on the increased intake of carbohydrates. Because this pathway is anaerobic (without oxygen), it can be used without delay. The major pathway of energy production is the Krebs cycle, which is dependent on adequate coenzymes of certain vitamins and minerals plus oxygen (aerobic). ATP, adenosine triphosphate; TCA, tricarboxylic acid. (From Davis JR, Sherer K. *Applied Nutrition and Diet Therapy for Nurses,* 2nd ed. Philadelphia: W.B. Saunders, 1994.)

activity of some of these enzymes, vitamins and/or minerals must be available. Some B vitamins function as **coenzymes** in the Krebs cycle. An enzyme may also require a *cofactor.* A coenzyme usually contains a vitamin; a cofactor usually contains a mineral or electrolyte.

Anabolic processes require energy. Examples of anabolism are the building of new muscle tissue or bone, and the secretion of cellular products such as *hormones.* Hormones are "messengers" produced by a group of cells that stimulate or retard the functions of other cells. Hormones principally control different metabolic functions that affect growth and secretions. Anabolism involves the utilization of glucose, amino acids, fatty acids, and glycerol to build various substances that make up the body itself and the other substances necessary for the body to function. All nutrients are intertwined in this process. For instance, nonessential amino acids are ordinarily used to build proteins; but glucose can be the basis for anabolism of amino acids and fatty acids.

The Role of the Liver

The liver plays a major regulatory role by controlling the kinds and quantities of nutrients in the blood stream. In the liver all monosaccharides are converted to glucose, the major energy supply for cells. The polysaccharide glycogen can also be broken down to glucose and released into the circulating blood as needed. Other end-products of digestion may be either oxidized to provide energy; converted to glucose, protein, fat, or other substances; or released to circulate at prescribed levels in the blood to be used by cells throughout the body.

The Role of the Kidneys

The kidneys perform the important metabolic task of removing waste products from the blood, and along with the liver, control the amount of many nutrients in the blood. Metabolic end-products from cells, unnecessary substances absorbed from the gastrointestinal tract, potentially harmful compounds that have been detoxified by the liver, and drugs are all removed from the blood by the kidneys.

The kidneys accomplish this by a process of filtration and reabsorption. Glucose, amino acids, vitamins, water, and various minerals are reabsorbed or excreted by the kidneys, depending on the body's need. Excess nitrogen from protein catabolism is also excreted by the kidneys. Thus, kidneys help maintain nutrient balance within the body.

Other routes of excretion of waste products are through the bowel; the skin, which excretes water and electrolytes; and the lungs, which remove carbon dioxide and water.

Dental Hygiene Considerations

- Elevated or depressed blood glucose levels may cause numerous complications, such as poor wound healing and loss of consciousness.
- A dental hygiene goal of nutrition is to promote anabolism for growth or healing.
- Assess a client's ability to promote anabolism by monitoring weight and evaluating adequacy of dietary intake.
- The kidneys' ability to reabsorb nutrients may be altered by certain medications, especially diuretics, or a kidney disorder. Function is dependent on fluid balance.

Nutritional Directions

- The liver is a vital organ for metabolism of food and drugs.
- The kidneys help rid the body of waste products and drugs. Adequate fluid intake (8 to 10 cups/day) facilitates this process.
- If the kidneys are not working properly, drugs and nutrients may either be retained or lost. Both are undesirable.

CARBOHYDRATE METABOLISM

Monosaccharides are transported through the portal vein to the liver for **glycogenesis.** Glucose is the most common circulating sugar in the blood; it is the main energy source for cells. The level of circulating glucose is closely monitored by the liver, and is constantly maintained at a level between 70 and 110 mg/dl in normal individuals. After a meal, blood glucose levels will peak in 30 to 60 minutes and return to normal within 3 hours in normal individuals with normal **insulin** secretion. This consistent blood glucose level is significant,

indicating the necessity of a certain amount of sugar in the blood for normal functioning of body tissues. *Hyperglycemia* (elevated blood glucose) and *hypoglycemia* (decreased blood glucose) are very serious conditions and their precipitating cause should be identified. Many clients exhibit symptoms of hypoglycemia if they have not eaten within a 4- to 5-hour time span.

In the past, it was assumed that all monosaccharides or disaccharides (sugars) produced a higher blood glucose response than starches. However, the blood glucose response to different foods and different combinations of food cannot be accurately predicted from the amount of simple sugars or complex carbohydrates ingested (Jenkins et al, 1988). Sucrose has a glycemic effect similar to that of bread, potatoes, and rice.

A complex hormonal system maintains a constant blood glucose level (Table 6–1). When hyperglycemia occurs, insulin is secreted to lower blood glucose levels. Conversely, hypoglycemia elicits the secretion of several hormones (thyroid hormone, epinephrine, glucagon, and growth hor-

mone) to increase blood glucose levels. Blood glucose levels can be increased by converting amino acids and glycerol (from fats) to glucose by a process called **gluconeogenesis** and by breaking down glycogen to glucose.

Dietary carbohydrates ensure optimal glycogen stores and are digested faster than other energy nutrients. The amount of calories available from glycogen stores is generally less than a day's energy expenditure, or about 1,200 to 1,800 calories. Brain cells, red blood cells, and cells of the renal medulla require glucose as their energy source.

PROTEIN METABOLISM

Amino acids are transported through the portal vein into the liver. The liver is an "aminostat," monitoring the intake and breakdown of most of the amino acids. Individual amino acids are released by the liver to enter the general circulation at specific levels; so each amino acid is available as needed by the cells to synthesize each individual protein. Amino acids transported in the blood are rapidly removed for use by cells. If individual amino acids rise above the prescribed level in the blood, they are removed and oxidized for energy.

Protein metabolism is always in a constant dynamic state, with catabolism and anabolism occurring continuously to replace worn-out proteins. Even during anabolic periods such as growth, muscle catabolism is elevated as the cell remodels itself. Anabolic and catabolic processes are controlled not only by the liver but also by hormones (Table 6–1).

A small reservoir of amino acids called the "amino acid metabolic pool" is available for anabolism and to maintain the dynamic state of equilibrium. This metabolic pool, containing about 70 gm of amino acids, is less than most Americans consume in a day and could hardly be classified as a large storage of protein. Increasing muscle size is considered an increase in body mass, not protein storage. Thus, high-protein diets are neither safe nor effective as a means to increase muscle mass in athletes. To maintain a satisfactory protein status, a daily supply of essential amino acids is necessary.

Anabolism

Anabolism is dependent on the presence of all essential amino acids simultaneously. It is not a stepwise process, in which a protein can be started and completed when the needed amino acid appears.

Protein synthesis is also affected by caloric intake. If caloric intake is inadequate, tissue proteins are used for energy, resulting in increased nitrogen excretion. This process requires the B vitamin pyridoxine.

Catabolism

Amino acids are catabolized principally in the liver, but metabolism also occurs to some extent in kidney and muscle. The removal of the nitrogen grouping from amino acids, a process that requires the B vitamins pyridoxine and riboflavin, yields carbon skeletons and ammonia. The carbon skeletons then can be used to (1) make nonessential amino acids, (2) produce energy via the Krebs cycle, or (3) be converted to fats and stored as fatty tissue. Thus, not all ingested protein is used to build muscle.

When amino acids are not needed for protein anabolism and energy is not needed, they are converted to fat and stored in the body. If caloric intake is inadequate, proteins are used for energy rather than to build or repair lean body mass or produce essential protein-based compounds.

TABLE 6–1 *Hormonal Effects on Glucose, Fat, and Protein Metabolism*

Hormone	Glucose	Fat	Protein
Insulin	↑ glycogen stores ↑ glucose utilization	↑ fat synthesis ↓ fat utilization and uptake	↑ protein synthesis
Thyroxine	↑ glucose absorption ↑ glycogen breakdown ↑ glucose synthesis from amino acids or fats	↑ fat mobilization	↑ protein synthesis
Epinephrine	↑ glycogen breakdown ↓ insulin release	↑ fat mobilization	
Glucagon	↑ glycogen breakdown ↑ glucose synthesis from amino acids or fats ↑ insulin release	↑ production of ketones	
Growth hormone	Antagonistic effect on insulin ↓ glucose uptake of cells	↑ fat mobilization	↑ protein synthesis and amino acid uptake during infancy and childhood
Glucocorticoid	↑ glucose production from fat and amino acids ↓ glucose utilization	↑ fat mobilization	↑ glucose production from protein
Adrenocorticoids			↑ nitrogen excretion

123

Urea is the major waste product of protein catabolism. Ammonia, a toxic substance, is transformed to urea in the liver and excreted by the kidneys. The levels of urea and ammonia vary directly with dietary protein levels.

LIPID METABOLISM

Hormones involved in carbohydrate metabolism also control fat metabolism (Table 6–1). The liver is the principal regulator of fat metabolism and lipoprotein synthesis. Fatty acids can be hydrolyzed or modified by shortening, lengthening, or adding double bonds before their release from the liver into the circulation. Cholesterol is produced, removed from the blood, and used to make bile acids by the liver.

Metabolism of chylomicrons in the liver results in triglycerides being transported to the tissues for energy or other uses or carried to adipose tissue to be stored. Serum triglycerides are the result of not only absorption from foods, but also the conversion of carbohydrates and proteins into fats. Triglycerides can be synthesized in the intestinal mucosa, adipose tissue, and liver. **Lipogenesis** and **lipolysis** are continual processes, which are in equilibrium when energy needs are balanced.

The **oxidation** of 1 lb of fat results in the release of 3,500 Cal for energy. (This is more than most clients use in a 24-hour period.) When excessive amounts of fats are oxidized for energy, the liver is overwhelmed, and **ketone** bodies are formed. Ketone bodies are not oxidized in the liver but are carried to the skeletal and cardiac muscles, where they are rapidly metabolized under normal circumstances.

When the glucose supply is reduced, the capacity of the tissues to use ketone bodies may be exceeded, causing **ketosis.** Ketosis can be a dangerous condition for several reasons. These strong acids must be neutralized by bases to maintain acid-base balance in the blood. Thus, they are generally excreted in the urine with sodium (a condition known as *ketonuria*). If the amount of base available is inadequate, acidosis may result. In addition to the loss of sodium ions, large amounts of water are lost, which can lead to dehydration (or rapid weight loss for the dieter). When blood glucose levels remain low for several days, brain and nerve cells adapt to utilize ketones for some of their fuel requirements.

Carbohydrate plays a dominant role in heavy exercise when the muscle's oxygen supply is limited, but triglycerides provide about half the energy with continued exercise. Although fats can be stored in body depots in virtually inexhaustible amounts, their slower rate of metabolism makes them a less efficient source of quick energy. The amount of energy available is highly variable in individuals, but usually at least 160,000 Cal are available from body fat stores.

ALCOHOL METABOLISM

Although alcohol is considered a drug or toxin, the calories it provides can be utilized by the body for energy, providing approximately 7 Cal/gm. Caloric content of alcoholic beverages can be calculated by using Table 6–2. Alcoholic beverages contain negligible nutrients.

Alcohol is metabolized primarily by the liver. Alcohol provides an alternate fuel that is oxidized instead of fat; this may result in accumulation of lipids in the liver. There is little information on how much alcohol can be consumed without risk of liver damage. Habitual consumption of ethanol in excess of energy needs probably favors lipid storage and weight gain when consumed in excess of normal energy needs (Sonko et al., 1994). The Dietary Guidelines for Americans advise moderation in alcohol consumption: one drink a day for women and no more than two drinks a day for men. (An alcoholic beverage is defined as 12 oz of regular beer, 5 oz of wine, or 1½ oz of 80 proof distilled spirits). In addition to causing liver damage, alcohol can interfere with the transport, activation, catabolism, and storage of almost every nutrient.

METABOLIC INTERRELATIONSHIPS

To put it mildly, the body is a very complex system. Whether excessive food intake is in the form of protein, carbohydrate, alcohol, and/or fat, most of the excessive energy intake is stored as adipose tissue. (Glycogen is another storage form of energy; however, normal glycogen stores are limited.) Protein from the metabolic pool of amino acids and in lean muscle mass is generally not considered a good source of calories, but it can be used for energy if caloric intake is below caloric expenditure.

Lipids do not contribute significantly to the synthesis of amino acids, but glycerol from triglycerides can be used for synthesis of carbohydrates. Even though fat is a good source of energy, carbohydrate is the preferred fuel. However, the body cannot metabolize excessive quantities of fat without some side effects, namely ketosis, hyperlipemia, and accumulation of fat in the liver. Carbohydrates can be used in forming nonessential amino acids. Fatty acids and some amino acids can be converted to glucose. Proteins contribute to synthesis of some lipids (e.g., lipoproteins).

Catabolism of all classes of foodstuffs involves oxidation through the Krebs cycle to produce energy. The quantity of calories in the diet from carbohydrate or lipids influences protein metabolism. In some situations, one nutrient can be substituted for another because of their interrelationship. For example, a decrease in carbohydrate intake increases lipolysis; a protein excess can be used for energy.

Not only are energy-providing nutrients necessary; vitamins and minerals are essential for their digestion, absorption, and metabolism of carbohydrate, protein, and fat. Although they are not required in large quantities, as are the energy nutrients, their presence is just as important. When a deficiency occurs, reactions do not proceed normally. For example, even though protein may be consumed alone (as in liquid protein supplements), many other nutrients, including vitamins and minerals, must be present for the protein to be utilized by cells. Each nutrient has its specific function; all the nutrients must be present simultaneously for optimal benefits.

A detailed discussion of metabolic interrelationships is beyond the scope of this text. These interrelationships are important, and for optimal utilization of nutrients, food sources of all the nutrients should be incorporated into every diet. The easiest way to obtain optimal nutrition is to include a variety of foods from all the food groups.

TABLE 6–2 *Caloric Value of Alcoholic Beverages*

For Gin, Rum, Vodka, and Whiskey

To estimate the calories, multiply the number of ounces by the proof and then again by the factor 0.8.

Example: 2 oz × 86 proof × 0.8 Cal/proof/oz = 137.6 Cal

For Beer and Wines

To estimate the calories, multiply the ounces by the percentage of alcohol and then by the factor 1.6.

Example: 6 oz × 9% (0.09) × 1.6 Cal/%/oz = 86 Cal

From Davis JR, Sherer K. *Applied Nutrition and Diet Therapy for Nurses,* 2nd ed. Philadelphia: W.B. Saunders, 1994.

Dental Hygiene Considerations

- Glycogen stores are depleted with a carbohydrate-poor diet even when high levels of fat and protein are eaten. A client who ingests a carbohydrate-poor diet will have decreased energy reserves and be prone to prolonged healing periods and fatigue.

- Blood glucose concentrations are increased only slightly when fructose, sorbitol, or xylitol is given because these sugars are absorbed more slowly; less insulin is required for their metabolism. Encourage clients with diabetes to limit foods containing these sugars so that total caloric intake will not be adversely affected (with weight gain) and to avoid diarrhea.

- Clients with compromised liver or renal function may postpone progression of their condition by avoiding excessive amounts of protein.
- Ketosis does not result from the rapid breakdown of adipose tissue alone; severe curtailment of carbohydrate intake must occur simultaneously. Thus, be sure clients are consuming an adequate amount of carbohydrate.
- Ketosis frequently occurs in those with uncontrolled diabetes mellitus or who are not eating (as a result of illness or dieting) because they are burning fat rather than carbohydrate. Therefore, question clients with fruity-smelling breath about recent food and fluid intake, weight loss, and conditions such as diabetes mellitus.
- Evaluate the client's weight and use of diets because high ketone levels may be associated with starvation or high-protein, low-carbohydrate, low-calorie diets. These result in decreased appetite and occasionally nausea, which can worsen the condition.
- Symptoms of hypoglycemia include weakness or light headedness, confusion, pale color, sweating, and rapid, shallow breathing.

Nutritional Directions

- ◆ A diet high in protein may be fattening because excess protein is stored as fat.
- ◆ Increasing protein intake does not necessarily increase muscle tissue and may lead to dehydration.
- ◆ High-protein, low-carbohydrate diets have been promoted as an effective way of excreting calories to lose weight through ketonuria. However, at most, about 20 gm/day of ketones may be excreted in the urine, or less than 100 Cal/day. This is an insignificant amount and not worth the risk involved.

METABOLIC ENERGY

Without energy from chemical reactions, people could not bat an eye, wiggle a toe, or think a thought. **Energy** from food is converted into forms the body can use: electrical for the brain and nerves, mechanical for muscles, thermal for body heat, and chemical for synthesis of new compounds.

The potential energy value of foods and energy exchanges within the body are expressed in terms of the *kilocalorie*. A kilocalorie (kcal or Cal) is the amount of heat required to raise the temperature of 1 kg of water 1° C. A kilocalorie is 1,000 times larger than the small calorie. While *kilocalorie* is the proper terminology, it is commonly used interchangeably with *calorie* or *large Calorie* (abbreviated Cal).

Carbohydrate, fat, protein, and even alcohol are chemical sources of energy for humans. (Vitamins and minerals are not energy sources but are necessary for energy-producing reactions.) Physiologic energy values commonly used are: 4 Cal/gm carbohydrate, 9 Cal/gm fat, 4 Cal/gm protein, and 7 Cal/gm alcohol.

Measurement of Potential Energy

The amount of energy, or calories, available in a food may be precisely calculated by placing a weighed amount of food inside a **calorimeter.** As it is burned, an increase in water temperature indicates the heat given off or potential (free) energy of that food.

Energy Production

The metabolism of basic nutrients results in production of cellular energy, which is stored as *adenosine triphosphate* (ATP). ATP is an instant source of cellular energy for mechanical work, transport of nutrients and waste products, and synthesis of chemical compounds generated from the Krebs cycle. ATP units, also called *high-*

energy phosphate compounds, are the currency or "money" the body uses for energy. Since ATP can be metabolized without oxygen, the reaction is classified as anaerobic. The body must always have a supply of ATP, and several systems within the body ensure a constant supply.

Increasing calorie intake from carbohydrates and fats will not produce optimum energy without adequate protein intake. Energy utilization is remarkably sensitive to both the quantity and quality of dietary protein.

BASAL METABOLIC RATE

Even during sleep, the body requires energy for the obvious minimum tasks of respiration and circulation as well as many intricate activities within each cell. A client's **basal metabolic rate** (BMR) is lowest while lying down, awake, rested, and relaxed in a comfortable environment, not having eaten for 12 to 15 hours. Since digestion and absorption require energy, the BMR is the amount of energy required when the body is in a **post-absorptive state.**

Factors Affecting the Basal Metabolic Rate

Various factors can increase or decrease the BMR, which determines caloric needs.

SLEEP: THE EBB OF LIFE After a few hours of sleep, metabolic rate is lowest be-cause muscles are more relaxed. About 10% less energy is needed for the BMR during this relaxed state.

AGE From birth through age 2, growth results in the highest BMR, which decreases until the puberty growth spurt, and is followed by a gradual decline for the rest of the life cycle (Fig. 6–2).

PREGNANCY AND LACTATION During the last trimester of pregnancy, the BMR increases about 15% to 30%. The amount of energy necessary to produce milk for lactation increases the BMR as much as 40%.

SURFACE AREA The more surface area, the greater the BMR. Because of greater surface area, a tall, thin person would require more energy than a short, heavy one of similar weight.

FIGURE 6–2 **Normal basal metabolic rates at different ages for each sex. (From Guyton AC, Hall JE. *Textbook of Medical Physiology,* 9th ed. Philadelphia: W.B. Saunders, 1996.)**

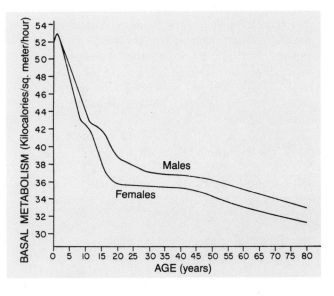

STATE OF HEALTH   Certain illnesses and diseases may increase or decrease the BMR. Those recovering from a wasting illness require extra energy to build new tissue. Additionally, the activity level may be influenced by such conditions as lack of sleep or exhaustion, tenseness, fatigue, or depression.

BODY COMPOSITION AND GENDER   In adulthood, lean body mass is the best single predictor of the BMR. Because cells in muscles and glands are more active than those in bone and fat, body composition influences the BMR. The amount of lean body tissue versus fat tissue in adults is a distinguishing factor; normally, women have more fat tissue and use fewer calories. Therefore, differences in the BMR may be primarily related to typical variations in body composition rather then directly related to gender.

Muscle tone is an important factor in metabolism; thus, the state of tension or relaxation also has an effect. An athlete, who has better muscle tone than sedentary people, requires more calories than a nonathletic person of similar size and shape.

ENDOCRINE GLANDS: CHEMICAL MESSENGERS   Thyroxine, the iodine-containing hormone from the thyroid gland, has a greater influence on the rate of metabolic processes than secretions from any other gland. However, thyroid problems as the cause of obesity are rare.

Adrenal glands affect metabolism to a lesser degree. Stimulations by fright, excitement, or even joy can cause a temporary rise in the BMR by releasing catecholamines, particularly epinephrine. The pituitary gland accounts for about 15% to 20% increase in the BMR during growth of children and adolescents.

TEMPERATURE   The BMR can be affected by body temperature or climate. The BMR will be slightly higher in cooler climates to maintain normal body temperature. The BMR increases when fever is present.

FASTING AND STARVATION   Clients who are undernourished or fasting for long periods of time have a lower than normal BMR. This is a result of decreased muscle mass as well as an adaptive body process to conserve energy. Several studies indicate that the body responds to dieting the way it does to famine, by decreasing the BMR.

TOTAL ENERGY REQUIREMENTS

Basal energy expenditure (BEE) includes calories necessary to maintain BMR, plus additional calories needed for *thermogenic effect,* voluntary activities, and any increased needs from catabolic (disease states, fever) or anabolic (growth, pregnancy) processes. The thermogenic effect (formerly called *specific dynamic action*) of food refers to increased heat production resulting from the metabolism of food.

There are several methods of estimating the BMR. For most clients, the BMR accounts for 65% to 70% of the body's total energy requirement. Determining a client's precise BMR is still inexact, but many general guidelines have been formulated. One quick guideline for adults is:

10–11 × ideal weight (lb) =
                     calories needed for BMR daily

Voluntary Work and Play

The most variable factor affecting total energy needs is muscle activity, which is influenced by the physical activity level (Table 6–3). Mental activity uses almost no extra energy (about 3 to 4 Cal/hr). Activity level normally accounts for 20% to 30% of the daily energy requirement.

3 × ideal weight (lb) =
            calories for inactive, bedfast, or obese persons

5 × ideal weight (lb) =
            calories for sedentary or persons over 55

10 × ideal weight (lb) =
            calories for thin or very active persons

TABLE 6–3 Caloric Expenditure for Various Activities

Kcal/Hr for 150-lb Body Weight	Cal/Hr for 150-lb Body Weight
100–200 Cal/hr	**400–450 Cal/hr**
Billiards	Disco dancing
Golf	Square dancing
Music Playing	Hunting (carry load)
200–250 Cal/hr	Lawn mowing (hand)
	Bicycling (11 mph)
Jazzercise, light	Wood chopping, sawing
Walking (20–26 min/mile)	Jogging (14 min/mile)
Aerobics, light	**450–500 Cal/hr**
Shuffleboard	
Gardening	Tennis, singles
Canoeing (2.5 mph)	Jogging (13 min/mile)
Archery	Water skiing
Sailing	**500–550 Cal/hr**
Fishing	
Bicycling (6 mph)	Hiking, mountain
Golf (pull cart)	Fencing
Lawn mowing (power)	Bicycling (12 mph)
250–300 Cal/hr	Football, touch
	Canoeing (5 mph)
Bowling	Swimming, slow
Jogging (17 min/mile)	Aerobics, heavy
Roller skating	Calisthenics, heavy
Housework	Jazzercise, heavy
Calisthenics, light	Skiing, downhill
Weight lifting, light	**550–600 Cal/hr**
Badminton, doubles	
Row boating (2.5 mph)	Boxing, sparring
300–350 Cal/hr	Bicycling (13 mph)
	Jogging (12 min/mile)
Jazzercise, medium	Racquetball, social
Aerobics, medium	Tennis, vigorous
Carpentry	**600–650 Cal/hr**
Golf (carry clubs)	
Tennis, doubles	Weight lifting, heavy
Jogging (15 min/mile)	Backpacking
Volleyball	Swimming, fast
Badminton, singles	Basketball, nonvigorous
Horseback trotting	**650–700 Cal/hr**
Roller skating	
350–400 Cal/hr	Ice hockey, vigorous
	Climbing, mountain
Table tennis	Racquetball, vigorous
Fishing (wading)	Jogging (10 min/mile)
Hiking (cross-country)	Handball, vigorous
Bicycling (10 mph)	Skiing, cross–country
Ditch digging (hand)	**700–800 Cal/hr**
Ice skating (10 mph)	
	Jogging (9 min/mile)
	Basketball, vigorous
	Over 800 Cal/hr
	Running (5-8 min/mile)
	Rowing (11 mph)
	Boxing, competition
	Swimming, competition

Data from FIT III software, The Hearst Corp, San Bruno, CA.

From Davis JR, Sherer K. *Applied Nutrition and Diet Therapy for Nurses,* 2nd ed. Philadelphia: W.B. Saunders, 1994.

Thermogenic Effect

Food digestion requires energy. The thermogenic effect of a mixed diet is estimated to be about 10% of the energy required for BMR. Many times this factor is omitted in calculations to determine total energy expenditure.

In the 1989 RDAs, the National Research Council recommended energy allowances for reference adults with light to moderate activity levels (Table 6–4). These recommended allowances can be adjusted for increased physical activity and body size.

To calculate total energy expenditure for a client based on his/her ideal body weight, (1) calculate the basal metabolism based on ideal body weight, and (2) add the energy costs of voluntary activities, as shown in Table 6–5.

Dental Hygiene Considerations

- Determine a client's energy requirements and encourage intake of adequate amounts of both protein and energy so protein can be used for growth or healing, as needed. If energy is insufficient, healing is prolonged.

- Low-carbohydrate diets are not as effective in supporting high activity levels as a high intake of complex carbohydrates. Thus, in athletic clients, advise increased intake of complex carbohydrates.

- For healthy men, the BMR usually ranges from about 1,500 to 1,800 calories daily, whereas approximately 1,200 to 1,350 calories is needed for women. If energy intake is inadequate, physical status may deteriorate. A dietary consult or supplemental feedings may be needed to maintain this level.

- Increased thyroxine activity (hyperthyroidism) may double the BMR and can cause vitamin deficiencies because the quantity of many of the different enzymes is increased (vitamins are essential parts of some of these coenzymes).

- A naturally higher BMR is a reason why children and pregnant females do not feel as cold as adults under the same weather

TABLE 6-4 *Median Heights and Weights and Recommended Energy Intake*

Category	Age (years) or Condition	Weight (kg)	(lb)	Height (cm)	(in)	REE* (Cal/day)	Average Energy Allowance (Cal)† Multiples of REE	Per kg	Per day‡
Infants	0.0–0.5	6	13	60	24	320		108	650
	0.5–1.0	9	20	71	28	500		98	850
Children	1–3	13	29	90	35	740		102	1,300
	4–6	20	44	112	44	950		90	1,800
	7–10	28	62	132	52	1,130		70	2,000
Males	11–14	45	99	157	62	1,440	1.70	55	2,500
	15–18	66	145	176	69	1,760	1.67	45	3,000
	19–24	72	160	177	70	1,780	1.67	40	2,900
	25–50	79	174	176	70	1,800	1.60	37	2,900
	51+	77	170	173	68	1,530	1.50	30	2,300
Females	11–14	46	101	157	62	1,310	1.67	47	2,200
	15–18	55	120	163	64	1,370	1.60	40	2,200
	19–24	58	128	164	65	1,350	1.60	38	2,200
	25–50	63	138	163	64	1,380	1.55	36	2,200
	51+	65	143	160	63	1,280	1.50	30	1,900
Pregnant	1st trimester								+0
	2nd trimester								+300
	3rd trimester								+300
Lactating	1st 6 months								+500
	2nd 6 months								+500

*Calculation based on FAO equations, then rounded. (FAO, Food and Agriculture Organization; REE, Resting energy expenditure.)

†In the range of light to moderate activity, the coefficient of variation is ±20%.

‡Figure is rounded.

Reprinted with permission from *Recommended Dietary Allowances*, 10th ed. Copyright 1989 by the National Academy of Sciences, published by the National Academy Press, Washington, D.C.

conditions. Do not over- or underdress children based on an adult's perception.

- Unless physical activity is above average, the BMR represents the largest proportion of a client's energy requirement. Determination of the BMR can be used to evaluate adequacy of caloric intake.

Nutritional Directions

- ◆ Teach clients how to figure the calorie content of foods. For example, if a food contains 10 gm of fat (fat supplies 9 Cal/gm), multiply 10 gm by 9 Cal/gm = 90 calories. The same principle applies to calculating the amount of calories from carbohydrate or protein, using 4 Cal/gm.
- ◆ The BMR may be elevated or depressed. A high BMR requires more calories; fewer calories are needed for a low BMR.
- ◆ Since the BMR decreases about 2% every 10 years after age 25, many clients gain weight because previous eating habits are maintained without increasing activity.

TABLE 6–5   *Calculation of Total Energy Needs*

1. Determine IBW; see Appendix C.
2. Calculate basal metabolic needs:
   10–11 Cal × IBW = calories for BMR
   Example: IBW 180 lb
   10 Cal/lb × 180 = 1,800 calories for BMR
3. Add a factor for calories needed for voluntary activities
   Sedentary: 30%
   Light: 50%
   Moderate: 75%
   Very active: 100%
   Example: Patient's activity level light
1,800 calories for BMR × 0.50 calories for light activity = 900 calories for light activity
1,800 calories for BMR + 900 calories for light activity = 2,700 total caloric daily requirement

IBW, ideal body weight; BMR, basal metabolic weight.

Sedentary, sedentary job or bedrest.

Light, sedentary job such as sitting or working with hands with routine workouts three times a week.

Moderate, work performed principally in a standing position with several sports or workout activities a week.

Very active, engages in manual labor or participates in vigorous play or heavy exercise regimen five or more times a week.

From Davis JR, Sherer K. *Applied Nutrition and Diet Therapy for Nurses,* 2nd ed. Philadelphia: W.B. Saunders, 1994.

ENERGY BALANCE

The proper energy balance for stable weight is maintained when the caloric intake equals the amount of energy needed for body processes and physical activities (Fig. 6–3). "Energy balance is maintained when the calorie intake equals the amount of energy needed for body processes and physical activities." This statement sounds innocent and simple. Very few Americans are able to maintain energy balance at an appropriate body weight. Based on findings from *Healthy People 2000,* increasing numbers of Americans are overweight; caloric consumption increased by 400 calories a day between 1970 and 1990 (Zizza & Gerrior, 1995). Dental hygienists need to have an awareness of the complexities of maintaining energy balance to be more understanding of clients who have problems with their weight.

Many healthy clients are able to control energy intake to balance energy output with little effort; their *appetite* controls food intake to balance energy expenditure. Appetite, or the desire to eat, is related to the pleasurable sensations of eating.

When more calories are consumed than the body needs, the excess is stored as fat, resulting in weight gain. One pound of body fat is equivalent to 3,500 Cal. Overweight clients have a very difficult time losing extra pounds and maintaining their energy balance to keep off unwanted pounds. Weight control can be approached by either decreasing the number of calories consumed or increasing physical activities. Generally, a combination of both is most effective.

Many factors enter into this unbalanced equation; since it is a complex system, there are no easy

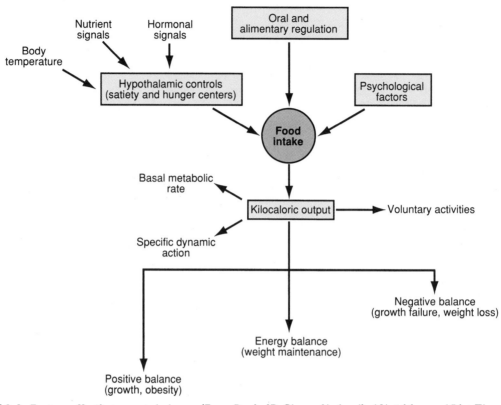

FIGURE 6–3 **Factors affecting energy balance. (From Davis JR, Sherer K. *Applied Nutrition and Diet Therapy for Nurses,* 2nd ed. Philadelphia: W.B. Saunders, 1994.)**

answers. **Hunger** is regulated by a complex network of factors (Fig. 6–3). The opposite of hunger is satiety. "Appetite" is frequently used in the same sense as "hunger," but it usually implies desire for specific types of food. Hunger and appetite greatly affect weight balance.

Intake has generally been regarded as the key to weight regulation. Most clients' weight tends to remain stable for long periods. Even small daily deviations from balance could result in gradual significant fluctuations in fat stores (100 additional calories daily would result in a 10-lb weight gain over a year's time and a 100-lb increase over 10 years). Most clients are unaware of changing their intake or physical activity level to maintain stable weight. Klesgas and colleagues (1992) deter-

mined in a longitudinal study that high fat intake and increases in total energy intake were related to higher weight gain in women; but in men, dietary fat intake alone was related to weight gain.

Physiologic Factors

The hypothalamus, located in the middle of the brain, is especially important in controlling hunger. Within the hypothalamus, both a satiety center and a hunger or feeding center are present.

Stimulation of the hunger center causes insatiable hunger (hyperphagia); damage to this area results in no desire for food. Stimulation of the satiety center will result in complete satiety. If the satiety center of the hypothalamus is destroyed, the appetite becomes voracious, resulting in obesity. The feeding center stimulates the drive to eat while the satiety center inhibits the feeding center.

Metabolic factors control the feeding center. The knowledge that hypoglycemia causes hunger has led to the glucostatic theory of hunger and feeding regulation. An increase in blood glucose activates the satiety center and deactivates neurons in the hunger center.

Several mechanisms affect the amount eaten at a particular meal. Distention of the stomach results in inhibitory signals that suppress the feeding center, reducing the desire to eat. The release of cholecystokinin in response to fat in the duodenum has a strong direct effect on the feeding center, causing the person to cease eating. Food in the stomach and duodenum causes the secretion of glucagon and insulin, both of which suppress the feeding center.

Additionally, the hypothalamus is responsive to body temperature. Cold temperatures result in increased food intake, resulting in a higher metabolic rate and more fat stores for insulation.

The relationship between exercise and food intake is unclear. Exercise has been reported to increase, decrease, or have no effect on appetite. As a general rule, acute exercise decreases food intake following the exercise, but regular exercise promotes increased caloric intake.

Nutrient and hormonal signals affect the brain and liver to stimulate satiety and feeding centers in the brain (Table 6–6). Numerous studies have shown that physiologic control of energy intake is unreliable. Therefore, energy balance must be adjusted through some other mechanism.

Psychological Factors

Appetite is affected by the fact that eating is rewarding or pleasurable and makes us feel good. The eating behavior of obese individuals is thought to be influenced more by external cues, including time, taste, smell, and sight of food, than persons of normal weight. Greater weight usually means the person is responding to feelings and emotions

TABLE 6–6 *Stimuli Affecting Food Intake*

Signal	Food Intake Increased	Decreased
Food odors	Pleasant	Repulsive
Taste	Desirable	Offensive
Climate (temperature)	Cold	Hot
Gastrointestinal	Hunger pains	Distention Cholecystokinin Glucagon
Glucose level	Low	High
Lipoprotein	High	Low
Nutrient stores	Decreased	Increased

From Davis JR, Sherer K. *Applied Nutrition and Diet Therapy for Nurses,* 2nd ed. Philadelphia: W.B. Saunders, 1994.

rather than actual hunger. Boredom and stress are frequent factors affecting eating habits of obese persons.

Energy Expenditure

Contrary to popular opinion, obese females have a similar or higher metabolic rate than thinner women. The effect of this is less weight gain for a given increase in caloric intake. Genetics may also play a role in the BMR. Some families have low metabolic rates but not all persons with a low BMR are obese (Ravussin et al., 1988). Infants of overweight mothers had a lower BMR by 3 months of age; these infants later became obese (Roberts et al., 1988).

Exercise tolerance of obese individuals is less than normal, but any activity utilizes more calories because of the amount of additional mass that has to be moved. Not all inactive clients are obese, so activity level does not appear to be a principal determinant in the development of obesity. The BMR as a result of body composition affects energy expenditure for activities.

In summation, weight loss resulting from a specific caloric deficit is invariably smaller than expected. Conversely, overconsumption fails to produce weight gains anticipated. Adjustments in energy expenditure appear to be adaptive.

Inadequate Energy Intake

Inadequate amounts of energy may result in a depressed rate of growth in children and weight loss in adults. Intentional weight loss may be helpful or harmful, depending on the methods used for losing weight. Decreased fat stores are normally the goal, but loss of muscle may be an undesirable side effect.

Inadequate energy intake may result in malnutrition and become a serious problem in the face of a physiologically stressful situation. Inadequate intake may be intentional, as in the case of anorexia nervosa, a psychological disorder in which one's undernourishment is not perceived. Inadequate intake causes a vicious downward spiral in which metabolic imbalances decrease hunger and may become life-threatening without proper treatment.

Dental Hygiene Considerations

- Assess emotional factors. Depression and other emotional factors result in overeating and decreased activity in some clients.

- A positive energy balance is desirable during periods of growth; therefore, a proportionately larger amount of energy is needed by pregnant women and children.

- When nutrient stores decrease, the feeding center of the hypothalamus becomes active and the client becomes hungry; when nutrient stores are abundant, the client feels satiated and loses the desire to eat. If the hypothalamus is injured in any way (as in a head injury or stroke), hunger and satiety may be altered.

- If calories are underestimated, the body must utilize stored energy (fat and protein), making the client at risk for malnutrition. If excessive calories are given, the body converts excess calories to fat. Evaluation of energy requirement is needed to prevent malnutrition or obesity.

Nutritional Directions

- ◆ Exercise may enhance the BMR by increasing the amount of lean body mass, which utilizes more calories.
- ◆ To gain 1 lb of fat, a client must consume 3,500 Cal more than are used.
- ◆ To lose 1 lb of weight, energy intake must be 3,500 Cal less than the number of calories used.
- ◆ Boredom or stress may trigger the desire to eat in some clients.
- ◆ A decrease from prior activity level or additional caloric intake may result in weight gain.

HEALTH APPLICATION 6

Diabetes Mellitus

Diabetes mellitus is a heterogenous group of endocrine diseases in which carbohydrates are ineffectively metabolized, leading to disturbances in lipid and protein metabolism, and fluid and electrolyte imbalances (Fig. 6–4). This condition is specifically related to hormonal pancreatic secretions but also involves the entire endocrine system.

Diabetes mellitus is presently one of the most common diseases, affecting 6% of the U.S. population in 1990. African Americans, Hispanic Americans, and Native Americans have the highest incidence of diabetes mellitus of all population groups. In addition to metabolic complications secondary to diabetes mellitus, life expectancy is about 70% to 80% that of the general population.

Classifications

The two prevalent types of diabetes mellitus are characterized by different metabolic defects and can appear to be very different conditions (Table 6–7). Insulin-dependent diabetes mellitus (IDDM) is distinguished by little or no endogenous insulin production. This condition most commonly manifests itself in young

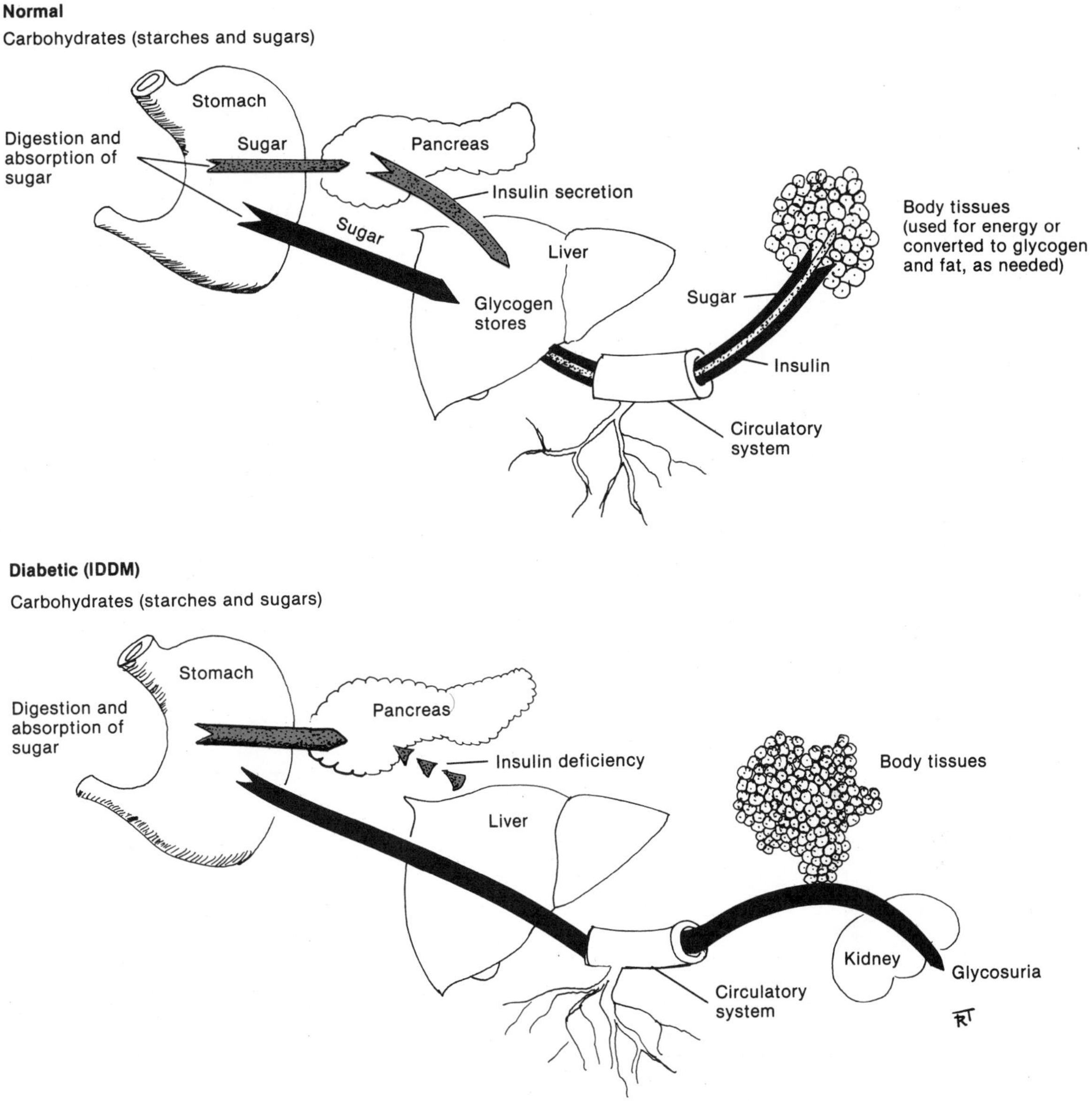

Normal

Carbohydrates (starches and sugars)

Diabetic (IDDM)

Carbohydrates (starches and sugars)

FIGURE 6–4 **Comparison of carbohydrate utilization of the nondiabetic and diabetic client. (Adapted from What Is Diabetes? Indianapolis, IN: Eli Lilly & Co, 1973.)**

people but can occur at any age. Onset is sudden with all the clinical symptoms associated with this condition. Clients are ketosis prone and must receive exogenous insulin for life.

More than 16 million persons in the United States have diabetes mellitus; half of the total number of persons with diabetes do not know they have it. Approximately 95% of the diabetes is non-insulin-dependent diabetes mel-

TABLE 6–7   *Comparison of Type I and Type II Diabetes*

	NIDDM	IDDM
Age at onset	Frequently over 35	Most frequently during childhood or puberty
Type of onset	Usually gradual	Sudden
Family history of diabetes	Usually positive	Frequently positive
Nutritional status at time of onset	Usually obese	Frequently undernourished
Symptoms	Frequently none	Polydipsia, polyphagia, polyuria
Stability	Blood sugar fluctuations are less marked	Blood sugar fluctuates widely in response to changes in insulin, dose, exercise, and infection
Control of diabetes	Easy, expecially if a diet is followed	Difficult
Ketosis	Uncommon except in the presence of unusual stress or moderate-to-severe sepsis	Frequent
Plasma insulin	Plasma insulin may be low, but not absent, or high	Negligible to zero
Vascular complications and degenerative changes	Frequent	Occurs after diabetes has been present for about 5 years
Diet	Diet therapy may eliminate the need for hypoglycemic agents	Required
Insulin	Used by a few clients	Necessary for all clients
Oral agents	Effective	Not suitable

Adapted from *Diabetes Mellitus,* 8th ed. Indianapolis, IN: Eli Lilly & Co, 1980.

litus (NIDDM). NIDDM is diagnosed most frequently in overweight individuals over 40 years of age. In most cases, clients with NIDDM are insulin resistant, that is, insulin is secreted in adequate or higher-than-normal amounts but glucose uptake by body cells (except for the brain) is decreased. Obesity and weight gain are associated with insulin resistance.

In diabetes mellitus, insulin is absent, deficient, or ineffective; glucagon is present in excessive amounts. These problems then precipitate clinical manifestations (Fig. 6–4). Insulin deficiency results in hyperglycemia, the main manifestation of diabetes mellitus. Symptoms of hyperglycemia include thirst, frequent urination, hunger, blurry vision, fatigue, frequent infections, and dry, itchy skin.

Chronic complications develop slowly over long periods of time as body tissues are adversely exposed to hyperglycemia and hypoglycemia. Treatment should be implemented as soon as possible after diagnosis to prevent complications of metabolic alterations secondary to diabetes mellitus. Most diabetic authorities believe that early, tight control of diabetes can postpone and minimize many of these severe complications.

Diabetic clients experience slow wound healing, frequent abscesses, periodontal disease, skin irritations, pruritus, numbness and tingling of the extremities, and visual disturbances. These are generally associated with vascular problems. Hyperlipidemia and hypertension are common. Changes in capillary membranes result in renal complications (leading to renal failure), obstruction of circulation in the extremities (leading to gangrene), and progressive blood vessel damage in the retina of the eye (leading to blindness). Neuropathy, or deterioration of nervous tissue, is also frequently seen in diabetes mellitus. Abnormalities of the gastrointestinal tract causing nausea, early satiety, and frequent vomiting interfere with food intake and absorption.

Diabetes mellitus is a chronic, life-long disease. Consensus supports dietary therapy as the cornerstone for preventing hyperglycemia and hypoglycemia as well as decreasing chronic complications. No single dietary plan can be appropriate for all people with different personalities and lifestyles. The objective of the diet is to enable clients to maintain good control of their diabetes or to promote near-normal blood glucose and lipid levels. Additionally, the diet should promote overall health by providing optimum nutrition; achieve and/or maintain an ideal body weight; and prevent and/or delay development or progression of cardiovascular, renal, retinal, neurologic, and other complications associated with diabetes, insofar as these are related to metabolic control.

The American Diabetes Association, The American Dietetic Association, and the U.S.

Public Health Service compiled the Exchange System to allow flexibility of the diet in addition to achieving a reasonable constancy of carbohydrate, protein, fat, and energy intake. These exchange lists divide foods into six groups; within each group, all food items are approximately equal in calories and in carbohydrate, protein, and fat content. Serving sizes vary so foods in each list are calorically equivalent. Therefore, foods within any group can be traded, or exchanged, with other foods in the same group. Because of increased awareness of nutrient metabolism in diabetes, the "diabetic diet" has been liberalized in favor of modifying the client's usual eating habits to be more consistent with the Dietary Guidelines for Americans and the Food Guide Pyramid. When calorie content is controlled, all foods containing carbohydrate, protein, fat, and alcohol are restricted to some degree because these sources of energy are potential sources of glucose.

Carbohydrate counting focuses on total carbohydrate consumption. Since carbohydrate is the major factor in glucose fluctuations, the given amount of carbohydrate affects insulin requirements more than the protein and fat content. Carbohydrate counting provides greater precision in estimating carbohydrate intake than the Diabetic Food Exchange Lists.

CASE APPLICATION FOR THE DENTAL HYGIENIST

On a routine recall, Mrs. White reports that she has been on a semistarvation diet because her physician told her she needed gall bladder surgery, but because of the risks involved, recommended the surgery be postponed until she lost about 50 lbs. You note that she has a fruity-smelling breath. With further questioning you learn she has been eating only meats and salads, once or twice a day.

Nutritional Assessment

○ Height, weight, IBW, age
○ Previous methods used to lose weight
   Motivation level
   Food/nutrient/calorie intake
   Eating habits
   Support from family, significant others

Nutritional Diagnosis

Altered nutrition: Body requirements more than calorie intake in relation to energy expenditure.

Nutritional Goals

Client will lose 1 lb/week until desirable weight is reached.

Nutritional Implementation

Intervention: Provide Mrs. White with the name of a registered dietitian who can provide necessary nutritional counseling.
Rationale: A well-balanced reduction diet is needed to maintain her health while she is losing weight. A dietitian's knowledge of nutrition and expertise in counseling is recommended to safely and effectively reduce weight.

Intervention: Explain that her current method of losing weight is not safe and may cause further health problems.
Rationale: By consuming inadequate amounts of carbohydrates, the body cannot properly metabolize the fats that are being catabolized for energy, thus causing ketosis or the fruity-smelling breath. This can be harmful. The protein she is eating is not necessarily used to prevent muscle loss. Additionally, a diet made up principally of meat products may be high in saturated fats, which may contribute to elevated serum cholesterol levels.

Intervention: Explain that carbohydrates, protein, and fats all provide calories, but that fats are the most concentrated source of energy.
Rationale: To lose weight, it is necessary to consume 3,500 Cal less than the body is using to lose 1 lb. Since fats contain 9 Cal/gm and carbohydrates and proteins, 4 Cal/gm, a calorie deficit is more easily achieved by curtailing fat intake.

Intervention: Stress the importance of consuming some complex carbohydrate and fiber, and reducing intake of fat and calories.
Rationale: Complex carbohydrate and fiber intake is effective in a weight-loss program by increasing satiety and discouraging binge eating. Fat reduction enhances weight loss because caloric intake is closely associated with the amount of total caloric intake.

Intervention: Discuss other benefits of weight loss.
Rationale: Understanding physiologic benefits of weight loss can be motivating for some clients and may help her to maintain the lower weight after the surgery.

Intervention: Discuss the importance of a plan incorporating diet, exercise, and behavior modification.
Rationale: This combination of therapies has proven more effective for long-term weight control.

Intervention: (1) Encourage client to maintain a food diary. (2) Explain the difference between hunger and appetite.
Rationale: (1) A food diary helps the client to become aware of eating patterns and antecedents that precede eating, and to determine why she is eating. (2) Hunger is the physiologic drive to eat or the body's need for food. Appetite, or the desire to eat, is related to the pleasurable sensations of eating.

Intervention: Suggest simple exercises such as walking.
Rationale: Treatment of obesity is improved when energy expenditure is increased along with decreased caloric intake. Additionally, this will help maintain muscle mass and prevent it from being used for energy.

Evaluation

Client consulted with the dietitian and was able to have the surgery in 6 months (weight was lost at a rate of about 2 lb/week).

Student Readiness

1. Define the following: *calorimetry, energy, thermogenic effect, basal metabolism, basal energy expenditure.*

2. Figure your total caloric needs for 1 day (BMR plus estimated voluntary energy expenditures plus thermogenic effect).

3. Assuming height and weight are the same, is the BMR higher or lower in:
   a. Men or women?
   b. An athlete or a sedentary person?
   c. A person 40 years old or one who is 20 years old?
   d. A woman who is not pregnant or one who is pregnant?

4. How many calories of protein, fat, and carbohydrate are in 1 cup of homogenized milk that contains 8.5 gm of protein, 8.5 gm of fat, and 12.0 gm of carbohydrate?

5. A boxer achieved a dramatic weight loss of about 18 kg (39.6 lb) in about 60 days. A strict diet, heavy exercise, thyroid supplements, and a diuretic drug produced his large weight loss. His defeat in a boxing match shocked some of his fans. What happened to his physical condition?

CASE STUDY

Jay G. is a 16-year-old high school athlete on the football and baseball teams. He has recently had three dental caries. His classmates have encouraged him to eat a high-protein, low-carbohydrate diet. His mother is concerned about this and talks to her best friend who is a dental hygienist.

1. What points do you think the dental hygienist should mention to this mother?

2. For increased energy expenditure, what should be the primary source of nutrients?

3. Would decreasing the carbohydrate content of the diet have a positive effect on the rate of dental caries?

4. What is the effect of a high protein intake?

5. On a high-protein, low-carbohydrate diet (approximately 120 gm of protein, 80 gm of carbohydrate, 2,800 calories), where would most of his calories come from? Is this good or bad?

6. Which vitamins are important in the production of energy?

7. Is the diet varied? Does the diet provide recommended amounts of fruits, vegetables, grains, and other nutrients?

References

Diabetes Control and Complications, Trial Research Group (DCCTRG). The effort of intensive treatment of diabetes on the development and progression of long-term complications in insulin-dependent diabetes mellitus. *N Engl J Med* 1993; 329(14):977–986.

Nutrition recommendations and principles for people with diabetes mellitus. *J Am Diet Assoc* 1994; 94(5): 504–506.

Ravussin E et al. Reduced rate of energy expenditure as a risk factor for body weight gain. *N Engl J Med* 1988; 318(8):467–472.

Roberts SM et al. Energy expenditure and intake in infants born to lean and overweight mothers. *N Engl J Med* 1988; 318(8):461–466.

Sonko BJ et al. Effect of alcohol on postmeal fat storage. *Am J Clin Nutr* 1994; 59(3):619–625.

Surveys show socioeconomic trends in diabetes. *Hospitals* 1991; 65(4):14.

Zizza C, Gerrior S. The U.S. food supply provides more of most nutrients. *Food Rev* 1995; 18(1):40–45.

Chapter 7

Vitamins Required for Calcified Structures

OBJECTIVES

The Student Will Be Able To:

- Name and define the fat-soluble vitamins.
- Compare the characteristics of water-soluble vitamins with those of fat-soluble vitamins.
- Identify functions, deficiencies, surpluses and toxicities, and oral symptoms for vitamins A, D, E, K, and C.
- Select food sources for vitamins A, D, E, K, and C.
- Identify dental hygiene considerations for vitamins A, D, E, K, and C.
- Discuss nutritional directions for patients regarding vitamins A, D, E, K, and C.

GLOSSARY OF TERMS

Vitamins   general term for a number of related organic, noncaloric substances present in foods in small amounts

Rhodopsin   light-sensitive pigment that allows the eye to adjust to changes in light

Night blindness   an inability to adapt to bright lights when the eyes are adapted to darkness

Ameloblasts   tall columnar epithelial cells in the inner layer of the enamel

Odontoblasts   tissue cells that deposit dentin and form the outer surface of dental pulp adjacent to the dentin

Lysosomes   intracellular bodies that contain hydrolytic enzymes that promote the breakdown of materials taken into the cells

Alopecia   hair loss

Xerophthalmia   abnormally dry and thickened surface of the conjunctiva and cornea as a result of vitamin A deficiency

Xeroderma   dry, rough, scaly skin

Keratinization   production of hardened eruptions around hair follicles by the epithelial tissues

Hormone   substance produced by cells of the body, and transported in the blood stream to another site, where it has a specific regulatory effect

Hematopoiesis   formation of red blood cells

Epiphyses   growing points

Osteomalacia   the adult form of rickets

Calciotraumatic line   line of disturbed calcification of dentin

Prostaglandins   hormone-like compounds derived from unsaturated fatty acids

Collagen   the basic protein substance of connective tissue that helps support body structures such as skin, bones, teeth, and tendons

Fibroblasts collagen-forming cells

Petechiae small pinpoint round red spots caused by submucous hemorrhage

Scorbutic similar to scurvy

Hyperemetic engorged and dilated with increased blood

Test Your NQ (True/False)

1. Fat-soluble vitamins are stored in the body. T/F
2. A daily intake of water-soluble vitamins is necessary. T/F
3. Vitamin E is found in vegetable oils and green leafy vegetables. T/F
4. Fat-soluble vitamins include K, A, D, and E. T/F
5. Animal foods are the principal dietary source of beta carotene. T/F
6. Xerophthalmia occurs with a deficiency of vitamin A. T/F
7. Vitamin D is called the sunshine vitamin. T/F
8. An excess of vitamin D causes rickets. T/F
9. Vitamin K is essential for regulation of blood calcium and phosphorus levels. T/F
10. Vitamin C is needed for wound healing. T/F

OVERVIEW OF VITAMINS

Nutrients never work single-handedly but in partnership with each other. **Vitamins** are catalysts for all metabolic reactions using proteins, fats, and carbohydrates for energy, growth, and cell maintenance. Because only small amounts of these chemical substances obtained from food facilitate millions of processes, they may be regarded as "miracle workers."

Eating fats, carbohydrates, and proteins without enough vitamins means the energy from these nutrients cannot be utilized. The opposite is also true. These vitamins do not provide energy, and they cannot be used without an adequate supply of fats, carbohydrates, proteins, and even minerals. Most vitamins come in several forms; each form may perform a different task. Vitamins are easily destroyed by heat, oxidation, and chemical processes used in their extraction. In this text, water-soluble vitamins, fat-soluble vitamins, and minerals are presented based on their function in calcified structures (teeth and periodontium) or on their role in oral soft tissues (oral mucous membranes and salivary glands) to familiarize you with which nutrients might be involved when oral changes are

observed. Most dental hygiene students are well aware of the role of several minerals in calcified structures in the oral cavity, but vitamins presented in this chapter are also important for healthy teeth and the periodontium (Table 7–1).

Most nutrients have various functions; thus, some are involved in both calcified and soft oral tissues. Oral physiologic roles for these nutrients will be presented in appropriate chapters, but duplication of information, such as requirements and food sources, will only be found when the vitamin is first discussed. Fat-soluble and water-soluble vitamins are different in many ways; a basic

TABLE 7–1 *Vitamins Required for Calcified Structures*

Fat-Soluble Vitamins	Water-Soluble Vitamins
Vitamin A	Vitamin C
Vitamin D	
Vitamin E	
Vitamin K	

understanding of their fundamental similarities can facilitate learning.

Requirements

Although vitamins are vital to life, they are required in minute amounts. Vitamins are like hormones because of their potent effects, but they must come from an outside source because they cannot be produced by the body. Each vitamin is essential even though the amount may vary from 2 to 4 mcg for vitamin B_{12} to as much as 45 to 60 mg/day for vitamin C, a 10,000-fold difference.

Even though the RDAs list the amounts of vitamins for different ages and sexes, many factors, such as smoking, use of alcohol, caffeine, or drugs, and stress, modify one's requirements. Periods of unusually rapid growth, pregnancy or lactation, fever, and recovery from accidents, disease, surgery, or burns are all considered stressful. Requirements for most vitamins, especially the water-soluble ones, are increased during periods of stress because of elevated metabolic activity. Dietary energy components affect some vitamin requirements; for example, a protein-rich diet or a high-calorie diet increases vitamin requirements.

Deficiencies

If adequate amounts of the nutrient are not available to sustain biochemical functions, a *nutritional deficiency* occurs. A nutritional deficiency as a result of decreased intake is called a *primary* deficiency. A vitamin deficiency caused by inadequate absorption or utilization, increased requirements, excretion, or destruction is called a *secondary* deficiency. Nutrients are codependent; a deficiency of one may cause deficiency symptoms of another because it relies on a metabolic product from the initial vitamin deficit.

Although specific vitamin deficiency syndromes are relatively rare in the United States, several groups are at risk: the elderly, those who consume minimal amounts of food, alcoholics, and those with a chronic debilitating condition, such as cancer or AIDS. Because vitamin levels in the blood are often nondiagnostic, a nutritional deficiency is identified on the basis of clinical signs and symptoms and response to vitamin supplementation. One of the peculiarities of vitamins is that the symptoms of a deficiency frequently resemble those caused by an overdose.

Characteristics of Fat-Soluble Vitamins

Although the four fat-soluble vitamins (A, D, E, and K) differ in function, utilization, and sources, they have several similar characteristics in common: (1) they are soluble in fat or fat solvents; (2) they are fairly stable to heat, as in cooking; (3) they do not contain nitrogen; (4) they are absorbed in the intestine along with fats and lipids in foods; and (5) they require bile for absorption.

Fat-soluble vitamins are different from water-soluble vitamins mainly because larger amounts can be stored in the body. Vitamins A and D are stored for long periods of time; hence minor shortages may not be identified until drastic depletion has occurred. For example, vitamin A can be stored in the liver to meet basic needs for at least a year; *dietary deficiencies* may occur for some time before the shortage is obvious. Dietary deficiencies occur when foods consumed do not provide recommended amounts for that nutrient.

Several forms of each of the fat-soluble vitamins can be used by the body; therefore, in the past, vitamins A, D, and E were measured by their biologic activity based on the growth of animals. International units (IUs) reflect biologic activity in animal studies and do not always represent absorption rates in humans. Because various forms of vitamins A and E have varying activity levels, the RDAs for these vitamins were determined based on the biologic effectiveness of each. Following measurement of all active forms of the vitamins, they are converted to micrograms or milligrams and totaled to indicate the amount of the vitamin in that food. Thus, retinol equivalents (RE) reflect vitamin A activity of foods, and tocopherol equivalents (TE) reflect vitamin E activity. Although many food tables still list IUs, conversions are being made to the more accurate weight measurements in micrograms or milligrams. A summary of all the vitamins is provided in Appendix B.

Characteristics of Water-Soluble Vitamins

Vitamins B complex and C are all water soluble. In contrast to vitamin C and fat-soluble vitamins, B vitamins contain nitrogen. Water-soluble vitamins have vital roles as coenzymes necessary for almost every cellular reaction in the body (Fig. 7–1). Vitamin C is discussed in this chapter, along with the fat-soluble vitamins because of its vital role as a structural component of the tooth; it is also important in oral soft tissues. The B complex vitamins will be discussed in chapter 10.

Most water-soluble vitamins are readily absorbed in the jejunum. As a rule, high concentrations of these vitamins result in decreased absorption efficiency. The body stores very small amounts of each of these vitamins, therefore few water-soluble vitamins produce toxic symptoms.

Due to their limited storage, daily intake is important.

Dental Hygiene Considerations

- Assessment is crucial to determine requirements for vitamins. Assess for the following: smoking, alcohol use, excessive caffeine use, medications, physiologic stress, or surgery. If any of the mentioned are present, vitamin requirements may be elevated.
- Dietary and physical assessments are more diagnostic for vitamin deficiencies than laboratory values.
- Evaluate nutrient intake of groups at high risk for developing nutritional deficiencies by questioning elderly clients, impoverished/low-income clients, and those with chronic diseases. If indicated, refer the client to a registered dietitian.

Nutritional Directions

- No vitamin contains calories, but some vitamins, especially the B vitamins, are essential to the production of energy.

VITAMIN A (RETINOL, CAROTENE)

Retinol is the dietary source of vitamin A from animal sources, and beta-carotene is the principal carotenoid present in plant pigments. Retinoic acid is the most biologically active form of vitamin A.

Physiologic Roles

Vitamin A has many hormone-like roles in the body. It is also required for normal bone growth and development and for facilitating the transcription of DNA into RNA.

VISION

Retinal combines with opsin, a protein in the eye, to form **rhodopsin.** Retinol is converted to retinal in the eye. **Night blindness** may be the result of inadequate vitamin A to permit rhodopsin produc-

tion. This condition takes years to develop in adults, but occurs much sooner in children because they have less body stores.

GROWTH

Vitamin A is necessary for growth of both soft tissues and bones. In skeletal tissue, vitamin A is necessary for resorption of old bone and synthesis of bone. Vitamin A also has an important role in the development of teeth, especially in the formation of **ameloblasts** and **odontoblasts.** Vitamin A deficiency during pre-eruptive stages of tooth development leads to enamel hypoplasia and defective dentin formation in experimental animals (Sweeney & Shaw, 1988). Enamel hypoplasia in vitamin A-deficient humans is controversial. Vitamin A is also involved with normal teeth spacing

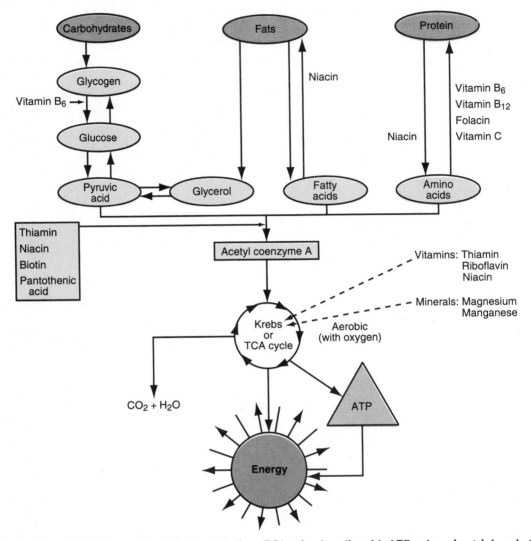

FIGURE 7–1 The role of vitamins in nutrient metabolism. TCA, tricarboxylic acid; ATP, adenosine triphosphate. (From Davis JR, Sherer K. *Applied Nutrition and Diet Therapy for Nurses,* 2nd ed. Philadelphia: W.B. Saunders, 1994.)

and promotes osteoblast function of the alveolar bone. The main functions relating to health and integrity of the body openings and their linings are discussed in chapter 10.

CANCER

Vitamin A and carotene have consistently been associated with cancer prevention because of their importance to the development and integrity of cells. The *antioxidant* role of vitamin A is discussed in Health Application 7. Antioxidants prevent cell membrane damage by free radicals that are produced by cells and tissues using free oxygen. These free radicals have unpaired electrons seeking to combine with whatever is available. They attack cell membranes or DNA, producing a chain reaction with the formation of more free radicals.

is enamel hypoplasia contributes to increased susceptibility to caries.

Dental Hygiene Considerations

Assess for signs of vitamin A deficiencies (loss of night vision, keratomalacia, corneal ulceration, Bitot's spots), especially in young and elderly clients. When in doubt, refer to a physician and/or dietitian.

Unlike vitamin A, beta-carotene is not toxic even in megadoses, but large amounts can cause a temporary change in skin color. Hypercarotenemia may be distinguished from jaundice by the fact that the sclera retains its normal white color in hypercarotenemia.

Jaundice or any disorder that affects fat absorption also affects fat-soluble vitamin absorption, making these individuals prone to vitamin A deficiency.

The alcoholic or alcoholic-cirrhotic client may be deficient in vitamin A because of the effects of ethanol and impaired liver function.

Vitamin A toxicity can be masked, especially when protein-energy malnutrition is present.

- Excessive intake of vitamin E or C may decrease absorption of vitamin A. Do not encourage use of vitamin E and C supplements or vitamin E- or C-rich foods if the client is at risk of vitamin A deficiency.

Nutritional Directions

- Vitamin A from animal sources is better used by the body.
- Vitamin prescriptions should be followed explicitly; severe life-threatening liver damage can result from increasing the amounts.
- Discourage clients from taking more than the RDA in over-the-counter vitamin preparations unless specifically advised to do so by a physician or registered dietitian.
- Recommend storing vitamins in a cool, dark place to prevent deterioration.
- The use of mineral oil as a laxative can interfere with the absorption of vitamin A.
- Women of childbearing age need to limit intake of preformed vitamin A (retinol, retinyl, and retinoyl acitate) found in liver and fortified foods (breakfast cereals and dietary supplements) to about 100% of the Daily Value (5,000 IU) (Recommendation, 1996).

VITAMIN D (CALCIFEROL)

Although vitamin D has been called a vitamin, in actuality, it is more appropriately classified as a **hormone.** Skin cells are able to make vitamin D when the precursor 7-dehydrocholesterol present in the skin is exposed to ultraviolet light or sunshine. Vitamin D from food, ergocalciferol (vitamin D_2) or cholecalciferol (vitamin D_3), is biologically inert. Further processing occurs in the liver with the conversion of vitamin D_2 or D_3 into 25-hydroxycholecalciferol (calcidiol) and a final change to the active form of 1,25 dihydroxycholecalciferol (calciferol) by the kidney (Fig. 7–3).

Physiologic Roles

Vitamin D is intricately related to calcium and phosphorus, each being required for optimal utilization of the other. The primary role of vitamin D is mineralization of bones and teeth and regulation of blood calcium and phosphorus levels. It functions with the parathyroid and thyroid (calcitonin) hormones to regulate intestinal absorption of calcium and phosphorus, enhance renal calcium and phosphorus reabsorption, and regulate skeletal calcium and phosphorus reserves.

Vitamin D may also be involved in the

Unchecked by an antioxidant, the free radicals can damage both the structure and function of cell membranes. Currently it is uncertain whether beta-carotene or some other factor in fruits and vegetables is anticarcinogenic. Supplementation is not advisable other than increasing consumption of fruits and vegetables as indicated in the Dietary Guidelines and Food Group Pyramid.

Requirements

The RDA for vitamin A is 1,000 mcg RE for men and 800 mcg RE for women. The need for vitamin A is increased during periods of rapid growth, when gastrointestinal problems affect its absorption or conversion, and in hepatic diseases that limit vitamin A storage or conversion of beta carotene to its active form.

Average intake in the United States meets the RDA. Inadequate intake occurs in lower socioeconomic groups as a consequence of less vegetable and fruit intake.

Sources

Vitamin A, as preformed retinol, is found in milk fat and butter (sometimes retinol is added to skim milk and margarine), eggs, meat, cod liver oil, and liver. Beta-carotene or provitamin A is also present in yellow, orange, and green leafy vegetables (spinach, turnip greens, broccoli) (Table 7–2). Beta-carotene is deep-red in pure form and derives its name from carrots, from which it was first isolated. Chlorophyll covers up the carotenoids in green vegetables. Most yellow, orange, and dark-green fruits and vegetables are high in carotene or vitamin A content. The deeper the color, the more vitamin A activity.

Absorption and Excretion

Absorption is optimal when body stores are depleted and when optimal amounts of other interrelated nutrients are present. The presence of vitamin E and the hormone thyroxine also enhance vitamin A utilization.

The liver stores approximately 90% of vitamin A. Adequate serum proteins are necessary to mobilize vitamin A from the liver.

Hyper- and Hypo- States

TOXICITY

When present in high concentrations, unbound vitamin A causes damage to cell membranes, especially in red blood cells and **lysosomes.** Large amounts of vitamin A supplements can exceed the storage capacity of the liver; free vitamin A enters the blood stream and exerts toxic effects on cell membranes.

Maternal consumption of vitamin A supplements both before conception and during the first trimester of pregnancy has been associated with fetal birth defects. Babies born to women taking vitamin A supplements at levels at or above 3,000 mg RE were more likely to have defects that originated in the cranial neural crest than babies whose mothers consumed 1,500 mg RE from supplements per day (Rothman et al., 1995). Toxicity is evident in infants by bulging of the fontanelle as a result of increased cerebrospinal fluid pressure. Other clinical symptoms include headache; vomiting; diplopia; **alopecia;** dryness of the mucous membranes; reddened gingiva; thinning of the epithelium; cracking and bleeding lips; and increased activity of osteoclasts, which will lead to decalcification, desquamation, bone growth retardation, softening of the skull, and liver damage. Toxicity symptoms usually appear only when excessive intakes, or more than 10 times the RDA, occur over a sustained period of time.

Toxicity from excessive intake of food sources is possible but does not occur too often. Beta-carotene is much less toxic than vitamin A. The body only converts the amount of carotenoids it needs into vitamin A. Even though they are not toxic, overconsumption may result in *hypercarotenemia,* yellow pigmentation of the skin occurring first on the palms of the hands and soles of the feet, caused by carotene storage in fatty tissue. This condition subsides when ingestion of beta-carotene is diminished.

TABLE 7–2   *Food Sources of Vitamin A*

Food	Portion	Vitamin A (RE)	Beta-Carotene (RE)	Calories (per serving)
Beef liver	3 oz	9,018	0	137
Baked sweet potato	1	2,487	14,920	117
Raw carrots, shredded	½ c	1,547	9,280	24
Mangos	1	806	805	135
Cooked spinach	½ c	798	4,788	29
Butternut squash, baked	½ c	718	4,305	41
Cooked dandelion greens	½ c	615	610	18
Cantaloupe	½ c	516	3,096	56
Cooked collard greens	½ c	509	3,051	31
Dried apricots	½ c	471	2,823	155
Cooked turnip greens	½ c	396	0	14
Raw spinach	1 c	376	2,256	12
Baked winter squash	½ c	365	357	40
Papaya	1 c	282	1,692	55
Cooked mustard greens	½ c	212	211	11
Cooked broccoli	½ c	175	1,050	26
Skim milk	1 c	150	0	86
Romaine lettuce	1 c	146	19	9
Butter	1 Tbsp	105	11	100
Raw apricot	1	92	553	17
Whole milk	1 c	92	NA	150
Whole egg	1	84	NA	77
Half and half cream	¼ c	79	NA	79
Canned oysters	3 oz	77	0	59
Tomato	1	76	139	26

NA, not available.

Nutrient data from Nutritionist IV software, FirstData Bank; San Bruno, CA. From Davis JR, Sherer K. *Applied Nutrition and Diet Therapy for Nurses,* 2nd ed. Philadelphia: W.B. Saunders, 1994.

DEFICIENCY

Inadequate dietary intake is the primary reason for vitamin A deficiency, found most commonly in children under 5 years of age. It may also result from chronic fat malabsorption. Vitamin A deficiency is rarely seen in the United States, but is a major nutritional problem in developing countries. Mild vitamin A deficiency, directly associated with at least 16% of all deaths in children 1 to 6 years of age in Asia, may be related to depressed immune response.

Inadequate vitamin A intake results in degen-eration of epithelial cells in the eye and cessation of tear secretion. Lids are swollen and sticky with pus, and eyes are sensitive to light in **xerophthalmia,** sometimes resulting in permanent blindness. The first symptom of xerophthalmia is night blindness, followed by the occurrence of xerotic spots on the conjunctiva, called Bitot's spots. These ulcers of the eye may spread and result in blindness if left untreated (Fig. 7–2).

Degeneration of epithelial cells results in dry, scaly skin caused by an inability to produce mucus. This occurs not only in epithelial cells, but also in the intestines and lungs. **Xeroderma** can progress until the whole body is covered with flaky, scaly skin similar to dandruff. It is followed by *follicular hyperkeratosis,* in which the skin is like goose flesh on the buttocks and arms.

Keratinization may also affect the respiratory and gastrointestinal tracts. In both areas, degen-eration of epithelial cells results in increased infections.

Severe vitamin A deficiency may result in *enamel hypoplasia* and defective dentin formation in developing teeth. Enamel hypoplasia involves defects in the enamel matrix and incomplete

calcification of the enamel and dent lose their ability to arrange the mal parallel linear formation, resu eration and atrophy of ameloblas deposition of dentine is thus altere tal animals, enamel hypoplasia ca tation of severe and prolonged vitan (Sweeney & Shaw, 1988). Som vitamin A-deficient infants have sh ties in the enamel consistent with experimental animals. Based on stu in developing countries with vitami and protein-energy malnutrition, it

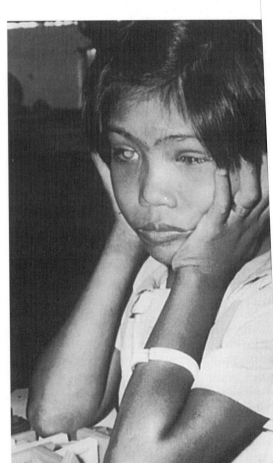

FIGURE 7–2 **Blindness from xerophthalmia. If this girl had been given food containing vitamin A, she need not have lost her sight. (Courtesy of WHO/Helen Keller International.)**

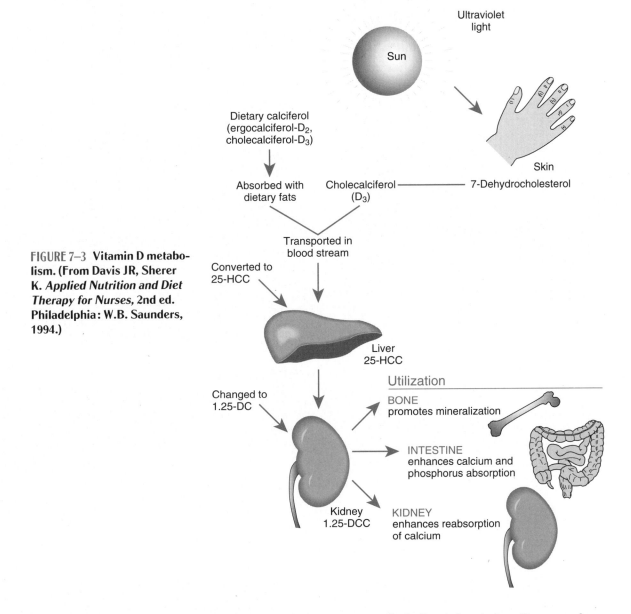

FIGURE 7–3 **Vitamin D metabolism. (From Davis JR, Sherer K. *Applied Nutrition and Diet Therapy for Nurses,* 2nd ed. Philadelphia: W.B. Saunders, 1994.)**

functioning of cells involved in **hematopoiesis,** the skin, cardiovascular function, and immune responses.

Requirements

The Food and Nutrition Board has determined that an adequate intake of vitamin D for all persons younger (including infants) than 51 years of age is 5 mcg (200 IU); an adequate amount for males and females between 51 and 70 years of age is 10 mcg (400 IU), with the amount increasing to 15 mcg for those over 70 years of age.

Vitamin D requirement is difficult to determine. When sufficient sunlight is available, people do not require an exogenous source of vitamin D. However, because many Americans have limited exposure to sunlight and many factors can interfere with ultraviolet light-dependent synthesis of vitamin D in the skin, vitamin D is considered an essential dietary nutrient.

Sources

SUNSHINE

The body's ability to produce enough vitamin D (sometimes called the sunshine vitamin) from sunlight is the reason the sun has been known as a source of health. Most people experience an increase in vitamin D during the summer months, with a lower amount during the winter because of less sun exposure. By age 70, the skin generally produces vitamin D at only half the level that it did at age 20.

In addition to geographic and seasonal factors, ultraviolet light from the sun may be blocked by air pollution, clothing, synthetic sunscreens, and indoor lifestyles. The use of sunscreens and moderation in sun exposure are important to protect against skin cancer.

FOOD

Even though adequate quantities of this vitamin may be derived from exposure to sunlight, additional food sources are necessary in most cases. Natural content of vitamin D in foods is limited and variable; food tables do not normally list vitamin D content. A diet composed of the best (unfortified) food sources of vitamin D would supply only slightly more than 2.5 mcg daily.

Foods are not legally required to be fortified, but about 98% of the milk in the United States is fortified to provide 10 mcg cholecalciferol (400 IU) per quart. Milk fortification is prevalent because of its popular consumption among children, and the calcium and phosphorus content of milk is beneficial for absorption and utilization of vitamin D. Because fortification is optional, it cannot be taken for granted.

Other foods, such as margarine, infant cereals, prepared breakfast cereals, chocolate beverage mixes, and cocoa, may also be fortified (Table 7–3). Nutrition labels can be used to assess daily intake of vitamin D; this information plus the amount of exposure to sunlight must be considered before considering vitamin D supplements.

Absorption

As with other nutrients, optimal absorption occurs when all closely interrelated nutrients (particularly calcium) are present in sufficient quantities. Conversely, diets high in fiber can result in less vitamin D absorption.

TABLE 7–3   *Food Sources of Vitamin D*

Food	Portion	Vitamin D (mcg)	Calories (per serving)
Broiled herring	3 oz	15	134
Broiled salmon	3 oz	11	155
Fortified milk	1 c	2.6	86–150
Margarine	1 T	1.5	50
Egg yolk	1	0.6	59

Nutrient data from Nutritionist IV software, FirstData Bank; San Bruno, CA. From Davis JR, Sherer K. *Applied Nutrition and Diet Therapy for Nurses,* 2nd ed. Philadelphia: W.B. Saunders, 1994.

Hyper- and Hypo- States

TOXICITY

Vitamin D toxicity is a disease of the twentieth century. When synthetic vitamin D supplements are taken by mouth in milligram amounts for weeks or months, toxicity signs occur. Calciferol poisoning can result in enhanced bone resorption, leading to deposition of calcium in soft tissues and irreversible kidney and cardiovascular damage. Without detection of symptoms and immediate reduction of the vitamin D source, permanent damage will result.

The most common reason for vitamin D toxicity is prolonged intake of pharmacologic doses. Toxicity from excessive vitamin D may arise when a concentrated calciferol preparation is mistakenly given. An infant given a commercial formula and a vitamin supplement can easily ingest two to four times the RDA of vitamin D.

DEFICIENCY

Signs of deficiency are commonly found in children because of increased requirements and decreased stores, and in elderly patients consuming inadequate diets with little exposure to sunshine. Plasma vitamin D is significantly lower in older patients than in a younger population; it is consistently higher for men than women among the elderly. In older patients, vitamin D and calcium supplements may be recommended by a physician to prevent osteoporosis. When supplementation is recommended, care must be used to prevent toxic overdoses.

Vitamin D deficiency affects skeletal structure in both children and adults. Laboratory values indicating serum calcium or phosphorus above or below normal values, the failure of bones to grow properly in length, and x-ray films showing abnormal **epiphyses** of the bones indicate deficiencies (Fig. 7–4). Because vitamin D is intricately related to calcium and phosphorus functions, a change in any of these three nutrients affects the others.

RICKETS The name *rickets* came from the word "wrikken," meaning to bend or twist. Rickets, caused by vitamin D deficiency, usually occurs in children between 1 to 3 years of age and is characterized by weak bones. Rachitic deformities such as bowlegs or knock-knees develop. The epiphyses of bones do not develop normally in children, so bones are twisted and warped. Other bone changes include a row of bead-like protuberances on each side of the narrow, distorted chest (pigeon breast) at the juncture of the ribs and costal cartilage (rachitic rosary) (Fig. 7–5). A narrow pelvis, making future childbearing difficult in women, is also observed.

Rickets develops during a time of extremely rapid growth when patients have had only a brief period to acquire vitamin D stores. Adequate intake of vitamin D during pregnancy and lactation is important because vitamin D can be passed from the mother to the infant before birth and in breast milk. Rickets is rare in the United States but occasionally occurs among African Americans, especially Muslims, because of dietary restrictions and traditional apparel that almost completely covers the body.

The alveolar bone is affected just like other bones in the body when rickets occurs. The trabeculae of the alveolar bone have wide osteoid borders and the number and size of the trabeculae are decreased (Sweeney & Shaw, 1988). Delayed dentition and small size molars are also seen in vitamin D deficiency.

OSTEOMALACIA Vitamin D deficiency in adults is called **osteomalacia;** it is also intricately related to calcium intake. Osteomalacia is characterized by decreased bone mineralization or softening of the bones, which may lead to deformities of the limbs, spine, thorax, and pelvis. The main symptoms are skeletal pain and muscle weakness, resulting in kyphosis or uneven gait. Oral manifestations include loss of the lamina dura around the roots of the teeth. The condition is more prevalent in women of childbearing age with calcium depletion due to multiple pregnancies or inadequate intake or in women who have little exposure to the sun.

ENAMEL HYPOPLASIA A small number of patients with evidence of rickets develop enamel hypoplasia as a result of vitamin D deficiency. Usually these changes are only visible with the aid of a microscope, or clinical assessment with careful exploration of the tooth surface using a sharp explorer. Whether these teeth are more susceptible to dental caries is uncertain. The enamel does not appear to be weakened, but the rougher surface may facilitate adherence of dental plaque and food residue. In severe cases of vitamin D deficiency, a **calciotraumatic line** may develop (Sweeney & Shaw, 1988).

Dental Hygiene Considerations

- Assess for vitamin D toxicity and deficit, especially in young children, pregnant and lactating women, and the elderly.
- Vitamin D supplements should be given only in prescribed dosage because patients vary widely in their susceptibility to vitamin D toxicity. Do not recommend that clients buy vitamin D supplements.
- If supplemental doses of vitamin D are used, cloudiness or a red color of the urine may indicate toxicity, and should be brought to the physician's attention.
- Conditions that may lead to vitamin D deficiency include any abnormalities that (1) interfere with intestinal absorption (e.g., diarrhea, steatorrhea, celiac disease, and biliary obstruction), and (2) abnormalities in calcium balance and bone metabolism caused by disease states such as renal failure. Evaluate the patient's health status for risk of vitamin D deficiency.
- Clients not exposed to sunlight should be monitored for adequate vitamin D intake

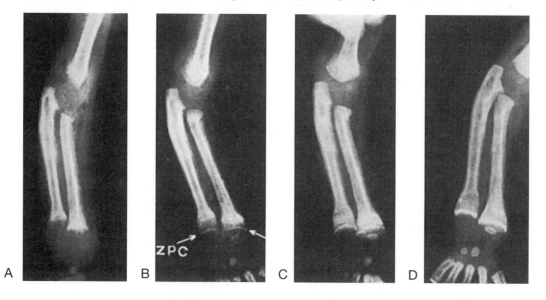

FIGURE 7–4 **(A) Active rickets; cupping and fraying of distal ends of radius and ulna; double contour along lateral outline of radius (periosteal osteoid). The two dense zones in the shaft of the ulna are calluses of greenstick fractures. (B) Healing rickets after 12 days of treatment with vitamin D. Zones of preparatory calcification; above them in the rachitic metaphyses, there is beginning calcification. (C) Healing rickets after 18 days of treatment. The zones of preparatory calcification are well defined, and the rachitic metaphyses appear well calcified. The epiphysis of the radius has become visible. (D) Healing rickets after 29 days of treatment. Zones of preparatory calcification, rachitic metaphyses, and shafts have become united. (From Behrman RE, Vaughan VC. *Nelson Textbook of Pediatrics.* 15th ed. Philadelphia: W.B. Saunders, 1996.)**

A   B   C   D

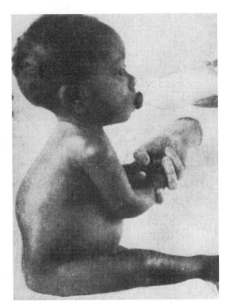

A

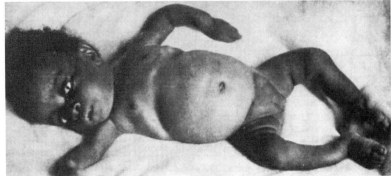

B

FIGURE 7-5 (A) Rachitic spinal curvature, well marked when the child is sitting. (From Behrman RE, Vaughan VC. *Nelson Textbook of Pediatrics.* 12th ed. Philadelphia: W.B. Saunders, 1983.) (B) Deformities in rickets, showing curvature of the limbs, potbelly, and Harrison groove. (From Behrman RE, Vaughan VC. *Nelson Textbook of Pediatrics,* 15th ed. Philadelphia: W.B. Saunders, 1996.)

and/or supplementation to maintain adequate vitamin D stores. Evaluate patient's living environment or hobbies to determine exposure to sunlight.

● Determine the use of sunscreens. Consistent use of sunscreens may contribute to vitamin D deficiency in some patients.

℞ Anticonvulsant drugs, such as phenytoin and phenobarbital, inactivate vitamin D, directly affecting skeletal and intestinal metabolism to cause osteomalacia. If a client is taking these drugs over a long period, vitamin D supplements may be beneficial, as well as some daily exposure to the sun.

Nutritional Directions

◆ The bright sunlight between 11 AM and 2 PM offers maximum conversion. As little as 10 to 15 minutes for exposure to the sun results in adequate conversion for light-skinned people.

◆ Vitamin D may be important for the maintenance of teeth in children (Sweeney & Shaw, 1988).

◆ Toxicity may result from excessive intakes of fortified foods or from not taking vitamin D supplements as prescribed.

VITAMIN E (TOCOPHEROL)

Four different tocopherols are collectively called vitamin E. Biologic activity of the tocopherols varies; alpha-tocopherol is the most potent.

Physiologic Roles

Vitamin E is the most important fat-soluble antioxidant. Vitamin E protects the integrity of normal cell membranes and effectively prevents hemolysis of red blood cells, and also protects vitamin A and unsaturated fatty acids from oxidation. Vitamin E supplementation has been shown to improve immune response in healthy elderly patients; this effect may be mediated by increases in **prostaglandins** that enhance growth of white blood cells. These functions will promote resistance of the periodontium to inflammation. Serum tocopherol (vitamin E) levels may be associated with cancer risk; this is further discussed in Health Application 7.

Requirements

The RDA for vitamin E is 10 mg alpha-tocopherol (α-TE) for men and 8 mg for women. High intakes of polyunsaturated fatty acids increase the vitamin E requirement. Most polyunsaturated oils also contain vitamin E, but if systemic stores are low or when chemical processes have destroyed vitamin E, the requirement is increased.

Sources

Vitamin E is available from vegetable oils and margarine made from them, whole-grain or fortified cereals, wheat germ, nuts, green leafy vegetables, and some fruits, such as apples, apricots, and peaches. Meats, fish, and animal fats contain very little vitamin E. Table 7–4 shows the amounts of vitamin E and linoleic acid in some foods. These nutrients are available in similar proportions.

Absorption and Excretion

Absorption of vitamin E is relatively inefficient, ranging from 20% to 80% in healthy individuals. Efficiency of absorption depends on the body's ability to absorb fat and appears to decline as the amount of dietary vitamin E increases.

Hyper- and Hypo- States

Lack of research on excessive amounts of vitamin E prevents prediction of toxic levels; however, vitamin E is relatively nontoxic. Oral vitamin E supplementation results in few side effects even at doses as high as 3,200 mg/day (Bendich & Machlin, 1988). As a result of numerous claims promoting the benefits of vitamin E in a variety of disorders, many patients take vitamin E supplements well in excess of the RDA. Individuals who benefit from vitamin E supplementation are prema-

ture infants, infants, children or adults who cannot absorb fats and oils because of diseases in the gastrointestinal tract, and individuals with conditions such as sickle cell anemia and benign but painful lumps in the breast.

Since vitamin E is widely distributed in foods, dietary deficiencies seldom occur if a well-balanced, varied diet is consumed.

Dental Hygiene Considerations

- Vitamin E may help the immune system function better so assess intake of vitamin E in immunocompromised clients.
- It is a misnomer to call vitamin E the "reproduction vitamin" because all vitamins are necessary for reproduction, and vitamin E is useless in the treatment of sterility, prevention of abortion, or treatment of toxemia during pregnancy.
- Vitamin E supplementation is not recommended for those with vitamin K deficiency or with known coagulation defects, or those receiving anticoagulation therapy, because it can interfere with vitamin K activity.
- ℞ Vitamin E supplementation depresses response to iron therapy, so if iron supplements are needed, discuss the interaction and advise the client to check with his or her physician or registered dietitian about possibly discontinuing vitamin E supplements until improvement is observed in iron status.

Nutritional Directions

- ◆ When oils are reused in frying, heavy losses of vitamin E occur.
- ◆ An increase in fruit and vegetable selections would provide more low-fat sources of vitamin E.
- ◆ High levels of vitamin E supplementation should be taken only with proper medical supervision. Advise clients to limit vitamin E supplements to less than 100 IU/day unless they are instructed otherwise by their physician (Stephens et al., 1996).

TABLE 7–4 *Food Sources of Vitamin E*

Food	Portion	Vitamin E (mg)	Alpha-Tocopherol (mg)	Linoleic Acid (gm)	Calories (per serving)
Sunflower seeds	¼ c	19	18	12	205
Corn oil	1 Tbsp	11	1.9	7.9	120
Mayonnaise, low-calorie	1 Tbsp	8.1	2.9	NA	40
Commercial mayonnaise	1 Tbsp	8.0	2.9	5.2	99
Almonds	¼ c	8.0	7.8	3.4	192
Salad dressings (vinegar/oil, French, Russian, blue cheese, thousand island, sesame seed, Italian)	1 Tbsp	7–8	0.6–0.9	2.6–4*	60–77*
Cooked sweet potato	½ c	7.6	7.5	0.2	172
Cooked lima beans	½ c	6.9	0	0.1	95
Margarine	1 Tbsp	6.5	1.6	4.7	100
Walnuts	1 Tbsp	6.1	0.3	10.5	190
Pecans	¼ c	5.4	0.8	4.3	180
Safflower oil	1 Tbsp	5.2	4.6	10.1	120
Peanuts	¼ c	4.2	2.5	5.6	209
Whipped margarine	1 Tbsp	4.2	1.1	2.1	70
Mixed nuts	¼ c	4.1	2.1	3.6	204
Bran cereal	½ c	3.9	0.6	NA	106
Cashews	¼ c	3.8	0.2	2.6	197
Peanut butter	1 Tbsp	3.2	1.1	2.3	94
Cooked spinach	½ c	3.1	1.9	0.01	29

NA, not available.

*Lower calories and linoleic acid if reduced- or low-calorie products are used.

Nutrient data from Nutritionist IV software, FirstData Bank; San Bruno, CA. From Davis JR, Sherer K. *Applied Nutrition and Diet Therapy for Nurses*, 2nd ed. Philadelphia: W.B. Saunders, 1994.

VITAMIN K

Three forms of vitamin K, a fat-soluble vitamin, have been identified, all belonging to a group of chemical compounds known as quinones. The naturally occurring vitamins are K1 (phylloquinone) which occurs in green plants, and K2 (menaquinone), which is formed by *Escherichia coli* bacteria in the large intestine and is found in animal tissues. The fat-soluble synthetic compound menadione (K3) is two to three times as potent as the natural vitamin.

Physiologic Roles

Vitamin K-dependent proteins have been identified in bone, kidney, and other tissues. These proteins bind calcium and may be involved in bone crystalline formation. Vitamin K functions principally as a catalyst for synthesis of blood-clotting factors primarily in maintaining prothrombin levels.

Requirements

The RDA for adult men is 80 mcg and for women is 65 mcg. With the exception of females between 25 and 30 years of age, Americans consume vitamin K within the RDA (Booth et al., 1996).

Sources

Even though limited amounts of vitamin K are stored in the body, a shortage of vitamin K is unlikely because it is derived from both food and microflora in the gut. Green leafy vegetables are high in vitamin K, but meats and dairy products provide significant amounts (Table 7-5).

Bacterial flora in the jejunum and ileum synthesize vitamin K and provide about half of the body's requirement. However, synthesis of vitamin K by intestinal bacteria does not provide adequate amounts of the vitamin; that is, a restriction of dietary vitamin K can alter clotting factors.

Absorption and Excretion

Vitamin K absorption decreases with high levels of vitamin E supplementation. Small amounts of vitamin K stores have a rapid turnover. Ordinarily 30% to 40% of the amount absorbed is excreted via bile into the feces as water-soluble metabolites, with approximately 15% excreted in the urine.

Hyper- and Hypo- States

No toxicity symptoms have been documented from oral intake of vitamin K. Synthetic menadione, however, may cause toxic effects.

Primary vitamin K deficiency is uncommon, but disease or drug therapy may cause deficiencies. Any condition of the biliary tract affecting the flow of bile prevents vitamin K absorption. Vitamin K deficiency is common in celiac disease and sprue (which affect absorption in the small intestine), and other diarrheal diseases (such as ulcerative colitis) as a result of malabsorption. In vitamin K deficiency or in those taking anticoagulants, blood

TABLE 7–5 *Food Sources of Vitamin K*

Food	Portion	Vitamin K (mcg)	Calories (per serving)
Cooked Brussels sprouts	½ c	287	33
Cooked spinach	½ c	142	29
Raw cabbage	½ c	52	8
Milk	1 c	10	86–150

Nutrient data from Nutritionist IV software, FirstData Bank; San Bruno, CA. From Davis JR, Sherer K. *Applied Nutrition and Diet Therapy for Nurses,* 2nd ed. Philadelphia: W.B. Saunders, 1994.

clotting time is delayed, increasing risk of bleeding problems.

Newborn infants may develop hemorrhagic disease secondary to vitamin K deficiency because the gut is sterile during the first few days after birth. Newborn infants are usually given a single dose of vitamin K intramuscularly immediately after birth to prevent hemorrhage.

Dental Hygiene Considerations

- Excessive amounts of vitamin A and/or vitamin E have a detrimental effect on vitamin K. Discourage the use of vitamins A and E if the client is prone to vitamin K deficiencies.
- Vitamin K should never be confused with the symbol "K" used to designate potassium or kosher foods. If information is confusing or unclear, double-check with physician or registered dietitian.
- ℞ Vitamin K may be used prophylactically prior to oral surgery to prevent prolonged bleeding in clients who have a condition that inhibits clotting.
- ℞ Frequently, blood thinning agents may be discontinued for several days prior to oral surgery to prevent excessive bleeding, or the client may be hospitalized for a few days.

- ℞ Cholestyramine prescribed for hyperlipidemia binds with bile salts. The presence of bile is required for vitamin K absorption. Therefore, clients being treated with this drug are at risk of vitamin K deficiency, so assess for any bleeding problems such as petechiae (pinpoint, flat red spots) or ecchymosis (bruising).
- ℞ Antibiotic therapy inhibits vitamin K-producing intestinal microflora and appears to be a factor in the origin of vitamin K deficiency, especially with impaired hepatic or renal function.
- ℞ Patients receiving warfarin (Coumadin) may develop serious hemorrhaging problems if high intakes of vitamin E are taken simultaneously.

Nutritional Directions

- A lack of vitamin K may lead to bleeding problems.
- Vitamin K is stable to heat, so cooking does not affect vitamin K content of foods.
- ℞ Large amounts of vitamin K-rich foods are contraindicated for clients on dicumarol or warfarin therapy.

VITAMIN C (ASCORBIC ACID)
Physiologic Roles

Vitamin C functions as an antioxidant in numerous reactions in the body. As a coenzyme, it has numerous metabolic roles. It is important in the production of **collagen,** which plays a vital role in wound healing. Vitamin C strengthens tissues and promotes capillary integrity. Vitamin C facilitates development of red blood cells by enhancing iron absorption and utilization. It also aids the body in utilization of folate and vitamin B_{12}. It has a coenzymatic function in the metabolism of amino acids and biosynthesis of thyroxine, epinephrine, bile acids, and steroid hormones. Vitamin C can also affect immune responses via functions of

leukocytes and macrophages. During the development of connective tissue, bones, and teeth, vitamin C is important in the formation of **fibroblasts,** osteoblasts, and odontoblasts.

Based on epidemiologic evidence, ascorbic acid intake may be associated with a lower risk of gastric and esophageal cancer. More details on the role of vitamin C as an antioxidant are found in Health Application 7.

Requirements

The RDA for adults is established at 60 mg daily. The requirement for vitamin C is increased under many situations in which it is directly involved (e.g., stress, healing, and infections). It is detrimentally affected by many drugs (e.g., tobacco, alcohol, oral conceptives, and aspirin) that increase requirements. Smokers may benefit from an intake of 200 mg vitamin C. Some experts believe that the daily RDA for vitamin C is too low, but amounts above 200 mg/day are excreted, indicating a saturation of vitamin C at that level (Levine et al., 1996).

Sources

The RDA can usually be met by choosing one serving of foods known as excellent sources (citrus fruits, cantaloupe, green pepper, broccoli, Brussels sprouts, strawberries, and mango). Good sources include peaches, cabbage, potatoes, sweet potatoes, and tomatoes; at least two servings of these sources may be required to meet the RDA (Table 7–6).

TABLE 7–6 *Food Sources of Vitamin C*

Food	Portion	Vitamin C (mcg)	Calories (per serving)
Hot chili peppers	½ c	182	30
Guava	1	165	46
Currants	½ c	102	36
Grapefruit	1	91	74
Kiwi	1	75	46
Raw sweet pepper	1	66	20
Fresh orange juice	½ c	62	56
Cooked broccoli	½ c	58	22
Mango	1	57	135
Tomato paste	½ c	56	110
Cooked brussels sprouts	½ c	48	30
Frozen orange juice	½ c	48	56
Navel orange	½ c	47	38
Canned hot chili peppers	½ c	46	17
Cranberry juice	½ c	45	72
Raw kohlrabi	½ c	43	19
Papaya	½ c	43	27
Strawberries, fresh	½ c	43	22
Raw cauliflower	½ c	36	12
Cantaloupe	1 c	34	28
Baked sweet potato	1	28	172
Collard greens	½ c	23	31
Tomato juice	½ c	22	21
Cooked asparagus	½ c	22	25
Raw cabbage	½ c	21	11
Baked potato	1	20	145

Nutrient data from Nutritionist IV software, FirstData Bank; San Bruno, CA. From Davis JR, Sherer K. *Applied Nutrition and Diet Therapy for Nurses,* 2nd ed. Philadelphia: W.B. Saunders, 1994.

Hyper- and Hypo- States

Scurvy, caused by vitamin C deficiency, is characterized by gingivitis, **petechiae,** follicular hyperkeratosis, fatigue, and depression, and cessation of bone growth (Fig. 7–6). Inadequate amounts of vitamin C during tooth development may result in **scorbutic** changes in the teeth because of changes in the ameloblasts and odontoblasts. Ameloblasts and odontoblasts atrophy, and there is a decrease in their orderly polar arrangement in a vitamin C-deficient environment. Any new dentin deposits forming at this time are similar to osteodentin; the pulp also atrophies and is hyperemetic. Dentin deposits completely cease in severe vitamin C deficiencies, with hypercalcification of predentin. Dentinal tubules also lack their normal parallel arrangement. In scorbutic adults, the dentin reabsorbs and is porotic.

Gingivitis caused by ascorbic acid deficiency

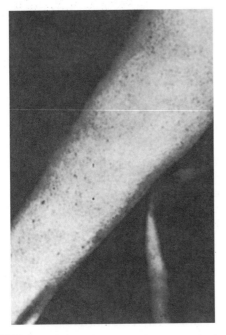

FIGURE 7–6 **Perifollicular hemorrhages on the leg of a 16-year-old boy with scurvy. (From Merck Report, May 1956, West Point, PA: Merck & Co., Inc.)**

also affects the periodontium, resulting in loosened teeth that may exfoliate. This effect is probably related to weakened collagen secondary to vitamin C deficiency.

Supplemental amounts of vitamin C can cause gastrointestinal distress and interfere with vitamin B_{12} absorption. Vitamin C intake above 1,000 mg daily results in urinary excretion of oxalate and urate and could increase risk of kidney stones (Levine, 1996).

Dental Hygiene Considerations

- Elderly clients, especially those who live alone or who avoid acidic foods to control esophageal reflux, those undergoing peritoneal dialysis or hemodialysis, smokers, and drug abusers are at greatest risk to become scorbutic. Therefore, assess for deficiency: periodontal disease, deep red to purple gingiva, bleeding upon probing, reported nose bleeds, melena (vomitus or stools containing blood), petechia (especially lower legs and back).

- In clients taking large doses of vitamin C, a sudden reduction in vitamin C may lead to scurvy. Intake should be gradually tapered.

- Evaluate the amount of vitamin C supplements taken. If vitamin C intake is high, vitamin B_{12} deficiency could occur.

- Chewable vitamin C tablets and vitamin C syrup are associated with enamel erosion and dentin hypersensitivity.

- ℞ Steroids, antibiotics, and salicylates can increase excretion of vitamin C.

Nutritional Directions

- Deficiency symptoms may develop within 60 to 90 days after total dietary elimination of vitamin C.

- Storage is important to prevent oxidation of vitamin C. Fruit juices kept in an airtight container that is appropriate for the amount stored retain more vitamin C. For example, two cups of juice in a pint container with an airtight lid protects the vitamin C content better than a pint of juice in a gallon container.

◆ Clients who smoke need 200 mg rather than 60 mg of vitamin C.

◆ Ascorbic acid is another name for vitamin C.

◆ Megadoses of vitamin C (500 mg or greater/day) can interfere with vitamin B$_{12}$ utilization.

◆ Sudden elimination of high intakes of vitamin C can result in deficiency symptoms known as *rebound scurvy.*

HEALTH APPLICATION 7

Update on Vitamin C and Other Antioxidants

Much has been learned about the function of vitamin C and E, beta-carotene, and the minerals selenium, zinc, copper, and manganese in their role as antioxidants. Antioxidants may be important in prevention of heart disease, cancer, age-related eye disease, and other chronic conditions associated with aging. Ascorbic acid is one of the strongest antioxidants and radical scavengers and acts as a primary defense against free radicals in the blood. However, the connections between vitamin C and these processes remains to be established. Research has shown that vitamin C and other antioxidants in amounts above the RDA are desirable, especially if this is achieved by improving food choices. Nutrients with antioxidant properties, such as vitamins C and E, beta-carotene, and monounsaturated fatty acids, are being studied for their ability to reduce susceptibility of low-density lipoproteins to oxidation, thereby increasing the risk of cholesterol deposits in the arteries.

For cancer prevention, retinoids and carotenoids may act at different stages of cancer development. Retinoids inhibit tumor formation. Functioning as antioxidants, carotenoids may prevent the induction of cancer. Vitamin E is also protective against cancer because of its antioxidant properties. Vitamin E can also prevent the toxic effects of ozone on the lung.

Only vitamin E reduces risk of oral cancer significantly. However, multivitamins usually contain 30 IU of vitamin E; this amount may not be adequate to reduce risk. At M.D. Anderson Cancer Center in Houston, oral precancers are treated with 400 IU vitamin E (Benner et al., 1993). Topical vitamin E has been effective in treating chemotherapy-induced mucosites in clients with cancer (Wadleigh et al., 1992).

Epidemiologic evidence of a protective effect of vitamin C for cancer is strong. Vitamin C, in its role as an antioxidant and free radical scavenger, acts to regenerate active vitamin E in cell membranes. Similar to vitamin E, vitamin C can act as a trap for nitrite, accounting for reduced risk of cancers of the oral cavity, esophagus, larynx, stomach, and pancreas in individuals who customarily eat fruits and vegetables containing vitamin C. Several studies have found that vitamin C-rich foods are more protective against lung cancer than foods containing beta carotene.

Vitamin C and E are both effective in preventing oxidation of lung lipids caused by pollutants and tobacco smoke, but vitamin C is more effective in preventing oxidation by nitrates, and vitamin E is more effective against ozone. Current RDAs are inadequate for maximum protection against air pollution levels.

Evidence is accumulating that high intakes of antioxidant vitamins by increasing fruit and vegetable intake may protect against age-related cataracts. Research also supports an association between antioxidant status and age-related macular degeneration, but this association may not be causal.

Indeed, antioxidants may counteract the effects of cell damage produced by metabolic reactions and environmental factors such as pollution, smoking, and toxic chemicals in the diet. Recommendations for supplemental amounts of these nutrients should be reserved for claims that have been well substantiated with clinical trials that prove cause and effect and explore related side effects. In fact, one study failed to prove that beta-carotene supplements reduced incidence of cancer in male smokers (Alpha-Tocopherol, 1994).

High levels of intake of most of the antioxidants are well tolerated by most individuals, but several known factors must be considered before recommending supplements. Toxic effects occur with less than 10 times the RDA for vitamin A; organ damage and deaths have been reported. Vitamin E supplements can antagonize vitamin K activity, especially in those undergoing treatment for blood clotting disorders. Adverse effects of vitamin C include diarrhea, hypoglycemia, increased risk of kidney stones, and dependency or rebound effect. Although vitamin C increases iron absorption, large amounts decrease availability of vitamin B_{12} and copper. Erosion and hypersensitivity of tooth enamel are unique adverse effects of chewable vitamin C tablets. Possibly further unexplored interactions may occur with other nutrients and drugs that would be affected by large amounts of antioxidants. If the consumer chooses to take vitamin C supplements, there is no benefit in taking more expensive ones, such as those containing bioflavonoids, over simple ascorbic acid.

In conclusion, the Dietary Guidelines for Americans to emphasize consumption of fruits and vegetables, and the goal of *Healthy People 2000* to increase the consumption of fruits and vegetables to five servings a day are simple keys to help prevent several chronic diseases. Advice to patients should be to eat a healthy diet that includes more fruits and vegetables, especially those that are high in vitamin C, E, and beta-carotene, and caution about taking megadoses of vitamins and minerals since side-effects can occur. Adequate intake ideally should be in the form of improving dietary selections rather than supplements because as-yet unidentified components present in food may be beneficial and protective.

CASE APPLICATION FOR THE DENTAL HYGIENIST

A healthy client asks your advice about taking vitamin C supplements to prevent periodontal disease. She is not sure what foods she should eat or what to look for if an excess or deficiency develops.

Nutritional Assessment

- Income.
- Living arrangements, cooking and storage facilities.
- Tobacco and other drug use.
- Knowledge level about vitamin C.
- Beliefs about water-soluble vitamins.
- Physical status, especially any bleeding problems.
- Use of any over-the-counter or physician-prescribed supplements/medications.
- Emotional state.

Nutritional Diagnosis

Health-seeking behavior related to inadequate/insufficient knowledge about vitamin C.

Nutritional Goals

Client will consume foods high in vitamin C and state beliefs/information about vitamin C.

Nutritional Implementation

Intervention: Teach the following about vitamin C: (1) functions, (2) requirements, (3) sources.
Rationale: This provides the client with a sound knowledge base about vitamin C.

Intervention: Explain hyper- and hypo- vitamin C states.
Rationale: Diarrhea, hypoglycemia, oxaluria, and rebound effect may occur with megadoses.

Large amounts of vitamin C decrease absorption of vitamin B_{12}. Because vitamin C helps maintain capillary integrity, a reduction of vitamin C will cause bleeding problems. Following large doses, scurvy may develop unless the amount is gradually decreased.

Evaluation

The client should consume citrus fruits, strawberries, cantaloupes, and mangos. Additionally, the client states that supplements are not necessary for vitamin C and large doses may interfere with absorption of other nutrients, or that if she does develop any bleeding problems, she will seek help. Lastly, the client should verbalize information concerning excesses and deficiencies of vitamin C.

Student Readiness

1. How do water-soluble vitamins differ from fat-soluble ones? What do these differences mean as you choose foods for your own menu? What do these differences mean as you teach clients about nutrition?

2. Which fat-soluble vitamins are the most toxic? What are the symptoms of toxicity? What treatment is recommended for each?

3. A client asks why food is fortified with vitamin D. How would you respond?

4. Plan a one-day menu that meets the RDA for vitamin E.

5. Keep a record of your food intake for one day. Use a table of nutrient values of foods to determine your vitamin A intake. Was your diet adequate? What are some food choices you could make for improvement?

6. Prepare a menu for one day that provides adequate amounts of vitamins A and D. Eliminate all sources of milk products and canned fish. What does this do to vitamin D intake? Now remove various types of egg products, green leafy vegetables, and dark-yellow vegetables and see the effect on the vitamin A content of the meal plan.

7. Most of the fat-soluble vitamins are found in fat sources; yet the current Dietary Guidelines for Americans restricts fat intake to inhibit cardiovascular disease. Discuss the impact of these guidelines on nutritional status if adequate precursor vitamin sources are not consumed.

8. Justify the rationale of vitamin D supplementation of milk products in the United States.

9. What is the role of vitamin A in cancer and what foods are advocated to prevent this condition?

10. Name the deficiency and toxicity conditions associated with vitamin A, D, K, and C.

11. What two types of cancer have been associated with vitamin C consumption? Name five foods other than oranges that are good sources of vitamin C.

12. As a group, discuss the pros and cons of the controversial issue of mandatory food labeling on nutrition supplements.

References

The Alpha-Tocopherol, Beta-Carotene Cancer Prevention Study Group. The effect of vitamin E and beta-carotene on the incidence of lung cancer and other cancers in male smokers. *N Engl J Med* 1994; 330(15):1029–1035.

Bendich A, Machlin JJ. Safety of oral intake of vitamin E. *Am J Clin Nutr* 1988; 48(3):612–619.

Benner SE et al. Regression of oral leukoplakia with alpha-tocopherol: A community clinical oncology program chemoprevention study. *J Natl Cancer Inst* 1993; 85(1):44–47.

Booth SL et al. Food sources and dietary intakes of vitamin K_1 (phylloquinone) in the American diet: Data from the FDA total diet study. *J Am Diet Assoc* 1996; 96(1):149–154.

Dawson-Hughes DB et al. Rates of bone loss in postmenopausal women randomly assigned to one of two dosages of vitamin D. *Am J Clin Nutr* 1995; 61(5):140–145.

Esterbauer H et al. Role of vitamin E in preventing the oxidation of low-density lipoprotein. *Am J Clin Nutr* 1991 Jan; 53(Suppl):314S-21S.

Hennekens CH et al. Lack of effect of long-term supplementation with beta carotene on the incidence of malignant neoplasms and cardiovascular disease. *N Engl J Med* 1996; 334:1145–1149.

Jacques PF, Chylack LT Jr. Epidemiologic evidence of a role for the antioxidant vitamins and carotenoids in cataract prevention. *Am J Clin Nutr* 1991; 53(Suppl): 352S-355S.

Kushi LH et al. Dietary antioxidant vitamins and death from coronary heart disease in post-menopausal women. *N Engl J Med* 1996; 334(18):1156–1162.

Levine M et al. Vitamin C pharmacokinetics in healthy volunteers: evidence for a recommended dietary allowance. *Proc Nat Acad Sci* 1996; 93(8):3704–3709.

Recommendations for vitamin A intake. *FDA Consumer* 1996; 30(1):4.

Robertson J et al. A possible role for vitamins C and E in cataract prevention. *Am J Clin Nutr* 1991; 53(Suppl): 346S-351S.

Rothman KJ et al. Teratogenicity of high vitamin A intake. *N Engl J Med* 1995; 333(21):1369–1373.

Smigel K. Vitamin E moves on stage in cancer prevention studies. *J Nat Cancer Institute* 1992; 84(13):996–997.

Stephens NG et al. Randomized controlled trial of vitamin E in patients with coronary disease: Cambridge Heart Antioxidant Study (CHAOS). *Lancet* 1996; 347(9004):781–786.

Sweeney EA, Shaw JH. Nutrition in relation to dental medicine. *In* Shils ME, Young VR (eds): *Modern Nutrition in Health and Disease,* 7th ed. Philadelphia: Lea & Febiger, 1988, 1069–1091.

Wadleigh RG et al. Vitamin E in treatment of chemotherapy-induced mucosites. *Am J Med* 1992; 92(5):481–484.

Chapter 8

Minerals Essential for Calcified Structures

OBJECTIVES

The Student Will Be Able To:

- List the minerals found in collagen, bones, and teeth and their main physiologic roles and sources.
- Describe causes and symptoms of mineral excess or deficits.
- Discuss the role of water fluoridation in the prevention of dental caries.
- Describe advantages and disadvantages of mineral supplementation.
- Discuss dental hygiene considerations for clients regarding calcium, phosphorus, magnesium, and fluoride.
- Describe nutritional directions for clients regarding calcium, phosphorus, magnesium, and fluoride.

GLOSSARY OF TERMS

Osteoblasts   cells associated with production of collagen and, ultimately, bone

Apatite   a calcium phosphate complex that forms crystalline salts within the matrix of bone and teeth

Osteoid   young bone that has not undergone calcification

Amorphous   having no definite form

Osteoclasts   resorbed bone in microscopic cavities

Compressional forces   actions in which the pressure attempts to diminish a structure's volume, which usually increases density

Tensional forces   actions in which the pressure stretches or stains the structure

Odontoblasts   connective tissue cells that deposit dentin and form the outer surface of the dental pulp

Bioavailability   the amount of nutrient available to the body based on its absorption

Tetany   a neuromuscular disorder of uncontrollable muscular cramps and tremors

Osteoporosis   an age-related disorder characterized by decreased bone mass, causing bones to be more susceptible to fracture

Equivocal evidence   results of studies in which an association between administration of a chemical and a particular tumor response is uncertain

Test Your NQ (True/False)

1. Meats are good sources of phosphorus. T/F
2. The only nutrients essential for strong healthy bones are calcium and phosphorus. T/F
3. Bone meal or dolomite is a good calcium supplement. T/F
4. Systemic fluoride causes changes in tooth morphology that increases caries resistance. T/F
5. To obtain adequate calcium, a teenager needs to drink 2 cups of milk a day. T/F
6. Water fluoridation is economically inefficient because very little of the water is actually consumed. T/F
7. All women should take calcium supplements to prevent osteoporosis. T/F
8. Calcium absorption is increased when a sugar is present. T/F
9. Caffeine intake may decrease calcium loss. T/F
10. All bottled waters contain fluoride. T/F

BONE MINERALIZATION AND GROWTH

Calcified structures in the body, the bones, and teeth, are composed of a matrix of both organic and inorganic substances. Tooth dentin and cementum, as well as bone, originate with a protein matrix, or collagen deposition. Collagen is present throughout the periodontium as the primary connective tissue fiber in the gingiva and the major organic constituent of alveolar bone. Collagen is continuously being remodeled throughout growth and development. Defective collagen synthesis will affect formation of bones and teeth.

The organic matrix of bone is 90% to 95% collagen fibers, which are secreted by **osteoblasts.** Formation of collagen requires the presence of a variety of substances, including protein, vitamin C, and the minerals iron, copper, and zinc. Once collagen is formed, **apatite,** a calcium phosphate complex, automatically crystallizes adjacent to the collagen fibers.

Osteoids are formed rapidly; most develop into the finished product, hydroxyapatite crystals.

Immediately following collagen formation, *mineralization* begins. Mineralization is the deposition of inorganic elements (minerals) on an organic matrix (mainly composed of protein in combination with some polysaccharides and lipids). In addition to calcium and phosphorous, numerous other minerals, especially magnesium, sodium, potassium, and carbonate ions, are incorporated into the mineral matrix.

Adequate nutritional components are necessary during both collagen formation and mineral deposition phases to prevent structural imperfections. The crystalline mineral matrix provides great compressional strength similar to marble. The combination of collagen and crystalline mineral matrix forms a material somewhat resembling reinforced concrete.

The skeleton is constantly growing, changing, and remodeling itself. About 0.4% to 10% of total bone calcium remains in an **amorphous** form. This calcium is a reserve source that can be rapidly utilized when serum calcium levels decrease. Osteoblasts deposit fresh calcium salts where new stresses have developed and where **osteoclasts** are removing calcium deposits. Bone absorption by osteoclasts is controlled by the parathyroid hormone. The rate of osteoblast and osteoclast activity is normally in equilibrium except during periods of growth. In senior citizens, bone resorption may exceed mineralization, thus causing osteoporosis.

This dynamic state accommodates the changing demands of the body. Bone strength is adjusted in proportion to the degree of stress on the bone. Continual physical stress stimulates calcification and osteoblastic deposition of bone.

FORMATION OF TEETH

Teeth are composed of three calcified tissues: enamel, dentin, and cementum. Enamel and dentin are principally composed of hydroxyapatite crystals similar to those in bone. Approximately 20% of dentin, cementum, and bone is organic material, principally collagen; only 1% of the enamel is organic material. Dentin lacks osteoblasts and osteoclasts found in bone; enamel and dentin do not contain blood vessels or nerves. As with bone, the mineral crystallization structure makes teeth extremely resistant to **compressional forces;** collagen fibers make them tough and resistant to **tensional forces.**

Once the tooth has erupted, no more enamel is formed, but mineral exchanges do occur slowly in response to the oral environment. Changes in mineral composition of enamel occur by exchange of minerals in the saliva rather than from the pulp cavity. Minerals such as fluoride, sodium, zinc, and strontium can replace calcium ions. Carbonate can be substituted for phosphate; carbonate and fluoride can be substituted for hydroxyl ions. These changes may change the solubility of apatite. Despite the fact that changes can occur in enamel composition, the enamel maintains most of its original mineral components throughout life.

The crystalline structure of enamel is one of the most insoluble and resistant proteins known. This special protein matrix in combination with a crystalline structure of inorganic salts makes enamel harder than dentin, comparable to the hardness of quartz. Enamel is more resistant to acids, enzymes, and other corrosive agents than dentin.

Dentin, the main tissue of the tooth, contains the same constituents as bone, but its structure is more dense. Its principal component is hydroxyapatite crystals embedded in a strong meshwork of collagen fibers. **Odontoblasts** line the inner surface of the dentin and provide nourishment for the dentin. The rate of deposition and absorption of minerals in the dentin is only one third that of bone (Guyton & Hall, 1996).

Cementum, which covers the dentin in the root area, is another bone-like substance, but because it contains less mineral, is softer than bone. It contains many collagen fibers that originate in the alveolar bone. Compressional forces cause the cementum to become thicker and stronger. Cementum exhibits characteristics more typical of bone than enamel and dentin. Minerals are absorbed and deposited at rates similar to that of alveolar bone.

Development of normal, healthy teeth is affected by metabolic factors, such as parathyroid hormone secretion, and availability of calcium, phosphate, vitamin D, protein, and many other nutrients. If these factors are deficient, calcification of teeth may be defective and abnormal throughout life.

INTRODUCTION TO MINERALS

Minerals are inorganic elements that have many physiologic functions. Numerous inorganic elements in the body account for only about 4% of total body weight, or 6 lbs for a 150-lb person. Minerals are subdivided into those required in larger amounts, i.e., major minerals, and those required in smaller amounts, i.e., micronutrients or trace elements (Table 8–1). Despite smaller amounts required, trace elements are just as important as major minerals.

Even in the United States, where food is abundant, many clients consume a diet inadequate in minerals. Intake of essential nutrients is assessed annually by the USDA. Reports have revealed low levels of calcium, magnesium, iron, zinc, copper, and manganese (i.e., less than 80% of the RDAs or below the ESADDI) for some of the RDA age-sex groups, but per capita availability of calcium, phosphorus, magnesium, iron, potassium, and zinc indicates adequate amounts are available (Putnam & Allshouse, 1993). Young children, teenage girls, and adult and elderly women are at risk of low intakes of calcium and iron. Copper intake is low for all groups (Putnam & Allshouse, 1993). Dietary inadequacies result in more harm to bone than tooth structure.

TABLE 8–1   *Mineral Elements in the Body*

Major Minerals (>100 mg/day)	Trace Elements (<100 mg/day)	Ultratrace Elements (No RDA)	Ultratrace Elements (Unknown Function or Contaminants)
Calcium (Ca)	Iron (Fe)	Boron (Bo)	Aluminum (Al)
Phosphorus (P)	Copper (Cu)	Arsenic (As)	Barium (Ba)
Sodium (Na)	Zinc (Zn)	Nickel (Ni)	Strontium (St)
Potassium (K)	Manganese (Mn)	Silicon (Si)	Mercury (Hg)
Magnesium (Mg)	Iodine (I)	Tin (Sn)	Silver (Ag)
Chlorine (Cl)	Molybdenum (Mo)	Vanadium (V)	Gold (Au)
Sulfur (S)	Fluorine (Fl)	Cadmium (Cd)	Antimony (Sb)
	Selenium (Se)	Lead (Pb)	Others
	Chromium (Cr)	Bromide	
	Cobalt (Co)	Lithium	

From Davis JR, Sherer K. *Applied Nutrition and Diet Therapy for Nurses,* 2nd ed. Philadelphia: W.B. Saunders, 1994.

CALCIUM
Physiologic Roles

At least 99% of the body's calcium is found in the skeleton and teeth. Calcium deposited in teeth remains permanently. However, calcium (as well as phosphorus) in the bone functions as a "savings account" for maintaining serum calcium levels. Only 1% of the calcium is found in blood, but as such, it controls body functions such as blood clotting, transmission of nerve impulses, muscle contraction and relaxation, membrane permeability, and activation of enzymes.

Saliva is supersaturated with calcium; thus saliva is a source of calcium to mineralize an immature or demineralized enamel surface and reduce susceptibility to caries. Both calcium and phosphate in saliva provide a buffering action to inhibit caries formation. This prevents dissolution of minerals in the enamel by plaque bacteria.

Requirements and Regulation

The DRI for calcium has been established at 1,000 mg/day for adults. During growth periods, from 9 to 18 years of age, the estimated requirement is higher (1,300 mg/day) because peak bone mass appears to be related to calcium intake during periods of bone mineralization. An intake of 1,400 mg calcium by 12-year-old girls resulted in 1.3% more bone deposition than in girls consuming about 960 mg/day (Lloyd et al., 1993). Women may continue to increase bone growth and density through their twenties but do not achieve the bone mass levels observed in most males. After age 35, and frequently during pregnancy and lactation, bone resorption exceeds formation, resulting in gradual loss of bone mass. This loss accelerates after menopause. The National Academy of Sciences has recommended that an adequate calcium intake for adults over 51 years of age is 1,200 mg/day. Osteoporosis, more prevalent in women than men, is a result of all these factors, combined with the longer lifespan of most females. In 1997, the Dietary Reference Intakes committee of the National Research Council reached a consensus regarding an adequate calcium intake to promote optimal skeletal health (National Research Council, 1997), as shown in Table 8–2.

CALCIUM BALANCE

Despite wide variations in calcium intake, serum calcium is relatively constant because each cell has a vital need for calcium. If the serum calcium level

TABLE 8–2   *Adequate Calcium Intake**

	mg/day
Infants (birth to 6 months)	210
Infants (6 to 12 months)	270
Children (1–3 years)	500
Children (4–8 years)	800
Adolescents (9–18 years)	1,300
Adults (19–50 years)	1,000
Adults over 51	1,200
Pregnancy and lactation	Same as for their age group.

*The observed average or experimentally set intake by a defined population or subgroup that appears to sustain a defined nutritional status, such as growth rate, normal circulating nutrient values, or other functional indicators of health. Adequate Intake (AI) is utilized if sufficient scientific evidence is not available to derive an estimated average requirement (EAR). For healthy breastfed infants, AI is the mean intake. All other life-stage groups should be covered at the AI value. The AI is not equivalent to an RDA.

From National Research Council Study Committee on the Scientific Evaluation of Dietary Reference Intakes, *Dietary Reference Intake for Calcium, Phosphorus, Magnesium, Vitamin D, and Fluoride.* Washington, DC: National Academy Press, 1997.

drops, bones are used as calcium reserves. When calcium withdrawal from bones exceeds deposits, calcium imbalance occurs. Decreased bone density caused by insufficient calcium is a slow process.

CALCIUM-TO-PHOSPHORUS RATIO

Serum levels of calcium and phosphorus are inversely related; this relationship is called the serum calcium-to-phosphorus ratio. If the calcium level goes up, the phosphorus goes down, and vice versa. This acts as a protective mechanism to prevent high combined concentrations with subsequent calcification of soft tissue and stone formation.

Sufficient phosphorus intake is necessary to decrease calcium loss with all intake levels. The ideal dietary calcium-to-phosphorus ratio for adults is 1 : 1; during periods of growth, a ratio of 1 : 1.5 is advisable. This ratio does not warrant as close attention under normal conditions as in disorders such as renal disease, when dangerously high levels of phosphorus and calcium may cause calcification in soft tissues.

Numerous studies have investigated the relationship of calcium to phosphorus ratios and alveolar bone resorption of edentulous clients. Additionally, calcium requirements are increased when dietary phosphate is high (as is typical of the American diet); therefore, a relationship may exist between calcium intake and edentulous ridge resorption.

Absorption and Excretion

Calcium balance, i.e., an intake that equals excretion, is not solely dependent on adequate calcium intake. Under normal conditions, less than one-third of the calcium consumed is absorbed.

Absorption occurs in the upper part of the intestine and is affected by many factors (Fig. 8–1). Calcium absorption from various dairy products is similar, whereas calcium present in dark green leafy vegetables is not readily absorbed. During periods of increased need, especially during growth and pregnancy and lactation, calcium absorption may increase to 50% of intake. Calcium absorption decreases with age, probably because of decreased gastric acidity. The rate of absorption is lowest in postmenopausal women because of diminished estrogen levels.

Although several plant foods contain large amounts of calcium, absorption is poor. Oxalates in vegetables and phytates from wheat bran bind calcium to reduce absorption, but they do not interfere with calcium absorption from other foods. Excessive dietary fiber (more than 35 gm/day) also interferes with calcium absorption.

Previously, many professionals in the scientific community believed that protein and phosphorus adversely affect calcium **bioavailability.** High-protein foods typically eaten in the United States have a high phosphorus content. The usual intake does not cause calcium loss, whereas a diet low in protein and phosphorus may have adverse effects on calcium balance in the elderly.

Sources

Milk and other dairy products supply most of the available calcium (Table 8–3). Not only are they the preferred source of calcium because of their high calcium content, but inherent lactose and other nutrient content enhances calcium absorption. In a study evaluating the effect of calcium supplementation compared to intake from dairy products, 11-year-old white girls consuming 1,200 mg calcium in the form of dairy products had an increased rate of bone mineralization (Chan et al., 1995). Table 8–4 lists portion sizes for various foods that provide approximately 300 mg of calcium. The amount of calcium available in the U.S. diet was 920 mg/day in 1994 (Zizza & Gerrior, 1995).

Consumers in the United States are spending millions of dollars annually on calcium supplements yearly. This strong trend toward the use of calcium supplements is especially evident in the older population. In addition to all the pharmaceutical products available, food manufacturers fortify products such as fruit juices, fruit-flavored drinks, and breakfast cereals and breads. Benefits may be less than expected, partly because of limited bioavailability of supplemental calcium. Of the supplements available, calcium citrate is best absorbed, but calcium carbonate, lactate, gluconate, phosphate, and citrate malate are all absorbed reasonably well. Calcium citrate malate (available in frozen orange juice and some fruit-flavored beverages) may be the most effective supplement available.

Hyper- and Hypo- States

Clinical conditions are associated with excesses and deficiencies of calcium. Hypercalcemia and hypocalcemic conditions (too much or too little

FIGURE 8–1 Calcium absorption and utilization. (From Davis JR, Sherer K. *Applied Nutrition and Diet Therapy for Nurses,* 2nd ed. Philadelphia: W.B. Saunders, 1994.)

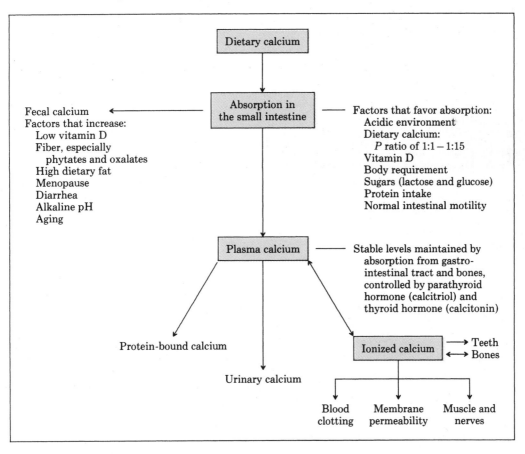

TABLE 8–3   *Calcium and Phosphorus Content of Selected Foods*

Food	Portion	Calcium (mg)	Phosphorus (mg)	Calories (per serving)
Romano cheese	3 oz	904	644	329
Swiss cheese	3 oz	815	512	320
Cheddar cheese	3 oz	611	434	341
American cheese	3 oz	521	632	317
Nonfat plain yogurt	1 c	452	355	127
Canned sardines	3 oz	325	417	177
Milk	1 c	300	232	86–150
Buttermilk	1 c	285	219	99
Canned salmon	3 oz	181	280	118
Low-fat cottage cheese	1 c	138	302	164
Turnip greens	½ c	125	28	25
Cooked spinach	½ c	123	51	21
Cooked oysters	3 oz	76	236	117
Cooked broccoli	½ c	36	46	22
Cooked shrimp	3 oz	33	116	84

Nutrient data from Nutritionist IV software, First Data Bank; San Bruno, CA. From Davis JR, Sherer K. *Applied Nutrition and Diet Therapy for Nurses,* 2nd ed. Philadelphia: W.B. Saunders, 1994.

calcium) are critical metabolic conditions and can lead to loss of consciousness, fatal respiratory failure, or cardiac arrest. These problems are seldom caused directly by calcium intake; how-

TABLE 8–4   *Calcium Equivalents*

The following foods contain approximately 300 mg calcium*:

  1 cup milk

  1½ oz cheddar cheese

  2 cups cottage cheese

  1 cup yogurt

  1½ slices processed cheese

  1½ cups ice cream

  1½ cups dark green leafy vegetables†

  4 oz salmon

  2½ oz sardines

*The RDA for calcium is 800 mg for persons 24 years and older.

†Calcium from vegetable sources is not as easily absorbed by the intestine and is not as effective in fulfilling calcium requirements.

From Davis JR, Sherer K. *Applied Nutrition and Diet Therapy for Nurses,* 2nd ed. Philadelphia: W.B. Saunders, 1994.

ever, bone density can be adversely related to intake.

HYPERCALCEMIA

Hypercalcemia is observed most frequently in infants between 5 and 8 months of age. It is caused by overdoses of cholecalciferol or excessive amounts of vitamin D preparations. Treatment involves providing a low-calcium diet with no vitamin D. Hyperparathyroidism, certain types of bone disease, vitamin D poisoning, sarcoidosis, cancer, and prolonged excessive intake of milk may cause adult hypercalcemia.

HYPOCALCEMIA

Hypocalcemia results in **tetany,** involving the muscles of the face, hands, feet, and eventually the heart. Depressed serum calcium levels may be caused by hypoparathyroidism, some bone diseases, certain kidney diseases, and low serum protein levels.

EXCESSIVE CALCIUM INTAKE

Excessively high calcium intake may cause constipation and inhibit iron and zinc absorption.

INADEQUATE CALCIUM INTAKE

Dietary deficiency of calcium is frequently observed. This can be attributed to (1) uninformed choices or not selecting adequate amounts, (2) the mistaken belief that adults do not need milk or that milk contributes too many calories, (3) economic hardships plus a lack of knowledge regarding inexpensive sources of calcium-rich foods, or (4) lactose intolerance in many people. In general, inadequate calcium intake affects bone mass more than tooth structure. Reduced calcium intake may result in increased dental caries during tooth formation and maturation. After tooth formation, calcium from diet does not affect caries rate.

Rickets, discussed in chapter 7 in connection with vitamin D deficiency, results in porous, soft bones. Rickets is the result of inadequate amounts of calcium deposits in the bone during childhood. Calcium intake may be adequate, but absorption is poor because of inadequate vitamin D.

Osteoporosis is caused by numerous factors, including decreased estrogen, inadequate calcium intake, and lack of weight-bearing activity. The relationship of calcium intake to bone density indicates a protective effect solely in women reporting high "lifetime" calcium intake, and not in women who increased intake only following menopause. Building bone during the formative years is the best insurance against osteoporosis. Oral signs of osteoporosis may be loss of calcium in the alveolar bone contributing to tooth exfoliation (Fig. 8–2). However, the condition usually goes undetected until pain or spontaneous fracture occurs. Osteoporosis is discussed further in Health Application 8.

Numerous scientists have investigated the role of dietary calcium in blood pressure regulation. Despite the fact that high blood pressure is more prevalent in clients with a low calcium intake, not all clients have the same response to calcium supplementation. Although some are responsive to calcium supplementation, others experience a rise in blood pressure. Because there is no way to predict blood pressure response, recommendation of calcium supplements to treat hypertension is inappropriate at this time.

Dental Hygiene Considerations

- Low serum calcium may be a result of a low serum protein or inadequate parathyroid hormone secretion. Correction of the primary problem is necessary rather than calcium supplementation.
- Lack of physical activity starts bone depletion immediately. In young people, recovery of calcium deposits is usually rapid, but elderly people may never regain bone density.
- No benefits have been observed for fracture healing when increased calcium or hormones are taken. Consumption of calcium in the amounts recommended in the RDA is appropriate.
- Hyperparathyroidism induces bone disease. Alveolar bone is especially at risk, exhibiting extensive bone resorption.
- Interventions for osteoporosis include encouraging calcium-rich foods and exercise.
- People who do not smoke use calcium more efficiently. If a client smokes, recognize that more calcium may be needed.
- Suggest alternatives for increasing calcium intake for clients with lactose intolerance.
- ℞ For older clients with decreased gastric acid, encourage calcium supplements with meals or a snack to enhance calcium absorption.

Nutritional Directions

- Adequate calcium and phosphorus intake daily is important to support bone formation and maintenance.
- Calcium supplement absorption can be enhanced if taken with some form of sugar; lactose, dextrose, or sucrose enhances its absorption.

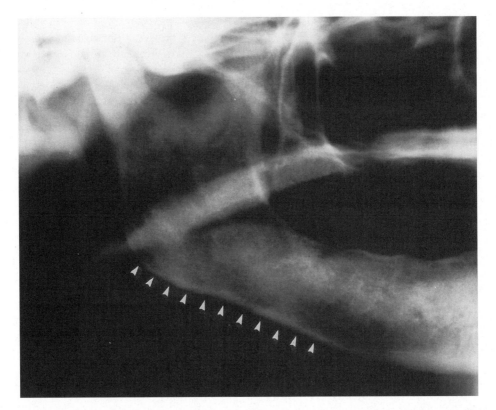

FIGURE 8–2   Radiographic appearance of osteoporosis affecting bone of the maxillofacial complex. This portion of a panoramic radiograph depicts thinning of the gonial and interior cortices of an edentulous mandible *(arrows)*. A slight increase in the general size of marrow spaces is also apparent. (Courtesy of BW Benson. DDS, MS; Associate Professor, Department of Diagnostic Sciences, The Texas A&M University System, Baylor College of Dentistry, Dallas, TX.)

◆ Evaluate calcium supplements for their solubility, which will affect absorption. For calcium to be absorbed from a supplement, the tablet must first dissolve. To measure how well a calcium tablet will dissolve in the body, drop a tablet in a solution of 4½ oz water and 1½ oz vinegar to produce an environment similar to that of the stomach. Stir occasionally. At least two-thirds of a high-quality tablet will dissolve within 30 minutes.

◆ Various supplements need to be evaluated for the amount of elemental calcium provided (actual amount of calcium in the supplement) and cost per tablet. Poor client compliance may be expected if several tablets are necessary, the supplement is too expensive, or it causes gastrointestinal problems. More than 500 mg per tablet may cause constipation. Refer clients who are appropriate candidates for calcium supplementation to a physician or registered dietitian.

◆ Weight-bearing exercise has a positive effect on normal calcium deposits in bone.

◆ If a client's usual calcium intake is low, encourage increased consumption of dairy products first if tolerated. If the client has an aversion to milk, powdered milk can be added to many items, or other high-calcium foods can be used.

◆ The use of dolomite as a calcium supplement is questionable. Dolomite is produced from the animal bones that have accumulated lead during their lifetime. Thus, prolonged use of bone meal can result in lead poisoning. A client must always question whether such supplements have appropriate sanitation and quality control.

℞ After menopause, calcium supplements have been shown to diminish bone loss when coupled with estrogen replacement therapy.

℞ Absorption of both calcium and tetracycline are decreased if taken concurrently.

℞ Antacids and corticosteroids increase urinary excretion of calcium.

PHOSPHORUS

Physiologic Roles

Phosphorus is the second most abundant mineral in the body, with about 85% in the skeleton and teeth. Its presence in all body cells is necessary for almost every aspect of metabolism, including (1) the transfer and release of energy stored as ATP; (2) the composition of phospholipids, DNA, and RNA; and (3) the metabolism of fats, carbohydrates, and proteins.

In the 1950s, animal studies indicated phosphates might be linked to dental caries; however, human studies have been inconclusive. No mechanism has been elucidated by which phosphates inhibit dental caries.

Requirements

The RDA of phosphorus for adults over 25 years of age is 700 mg. The ideal calcium to phosphorus ratio is 1:1. Because phosphorus is more readily available, intake is generally 1.5 times higher than calcium.

Absorption and Excretion

Approximately 60% to 70% of dietary phosphorus is absorbed in the jejunum. Its absorption can be inhibited by the same dietary factors that affect calcium absorption: phytate, excessive amounts of fats, iron, aluminum, and calcium. The kidneys excrete excessive amounts of phosphorus to maintain optimum body levels.

Sources

Phosphorus is so abundant in foods that deficiencies have not been observed. A diet adequate in calcium and protein will contain enough phosphorus because all three minerals are present in the same foods (see Table 8–2). In addition to milk products, meats are also a good source of phosphorus. Dietary restriction of phosphorus is extremely difficult because of its wide use as a food additive in baked goods, cheese, processed meats, and soft drinks.

Hyper- and Hypo- States

Hyperphosphatemia (serum level above 2.6 mg/dL) may occur in cases of hypoparathyroidism or renal insufficiency. Excessive amounts of phosphorus bind with calcium, resulting in tetany and convulsions.

Hypophosphatemia may occur with long-term ingestion of aluminum hydroxide antacids, which interfere with phosphorus absorption, or in certain stress conditions in which the calcium-to-phosphorus balance is disturbed. The principal clinical symptom of hypophosphatemia is muscle weakness. Even relatively small phosphorus depletions may cause increased calcium excretion, resulting in a negative calcium balance and bone loss. This may lead to failure of reparative dentin formation. The resultant wide dentinal tubules allow bacteria to enter the damaged enamel. Intestinal conditions, such as sprue and celiac disease, can result in phosphorus malabsorption deficiencies.

Dental Hygiene Considerations

- Low phosphate levels may occur in individuals with eating disorders (anorexia nervosa or bulimia) or those taking diuretics, or as a result of alcohol withdrawal. Monitor these clients for symptoms of deficiency.
- Any inhibitory effect of phosphorus in the dental caries process appears to be due to its topical availability on immature enamel rather than its systemic effect. Further research is needed in this area.
- Calcium, phosphate, and fluoride ions are lost during the demineralization or acid dissolution of the caries process; they can be redeposited in the enamel to remineralize

the tooth when no bacterial fermentation is occurring (DePaola et al., 1994).

- Low phosphate intake may lead to an increased rate of caries formation, but additional or supplemental phosphate may not be helpful in preventing dental caries.

Nutritional Directions

- Phosphorus is widespread in foods, and a deficiency is unlikely. Educate clients that the goal is to maintain an equal calcium-to-phosphorus ratio. For example, an excessive consumption of soft drinks (greater than two to three cans a day) in place of milk can interrupt the calcium-to-phosphorus balance.

MAGNESIUM

Physiological Roles

Bones contain almost two-thirds of the body's magnesium. It is the third most prevalent mineral in teeth, with dentin containing about two times the amount present in enamel. Magnesium has an important function in maintaining calcium homeostasis and preventing skeletal abnormalities.

Magnesium is vitally important to the structural integrity of heart muscle as well as other muscles and nerves. Its role in enzymes is fundamental to energy (ATP) production.

Requirements

The RDA for magnesium is 320 mg/day for women and 420 mg/day for men. Magnesium intake in the United States has been approximately 350 mg per day since 1986 (Putman & Allshouse, 1993). Magnesium deficiency has not been observed in healthy Americans (NRC, 1989).

Sources

Whole-grain products, nuts, beans, and green leafy vegetables are some of the best sources of magne-

sium (Table 8–5). Magnesium is part of the chlorophyll molecule (Fig. 8–3); therefore, green leafy vegetables are good sources. Bananas are a good source of magnesium. Enrichment does not replace the magnesium removed from refined grains.

Hyper- and Hypo- States

Because kidneys regulate plasma magnesium levels, toxicity has been associated with kidney failure. Magnesium supplementation in rats appears to increase the development of dental caries.

In certain diseases or under stressful conditions, deficiencies may occur. Magnesium in bone is not available to replace serum magnesium deficits. A deficiency may result from numerous disease states, including gastrointestinal abnormalities with diarrhea, renal disease, general malnutrition, and alcoholism or medications that interfere with magnesium conservation. Symptoms of a magnesium deficiency are neuromuscular dysfunction, personality changes, muscle spasms, convulsions (especially in infants), tremors, hyperexcitability, anorexia, nausea, apathy, and cardiac arrhythmias.

Dietary deficiencies may affect the teeth and

TABLE 8-5 *Magnesium Content of Selected Foods*

Food	Portion	Magnesium (mg)	Calories (per serving)
Sunflower seeds	¼ c	127	205
Sesame seeds	¼ c	126	206
Cashews	¼ c	89	197
Cooked spinach	½ c	79	21
Wheat germ	¼ c	69	104
Navy beans	½ c	54	130
Beet greens	½ c	49	20
Blackeyed/cowpeas	½ c	43	112
Baked potato	1	39	145
Sliced beets	½ c	32	26
Lima beans	½ c	29	85
Cooked shrimp	3 oz	29	84
Cooked broccoli	½ c	19	22

Nutrient data from Nutritionist IV software, First Data Bank; San Bruno, CA. From Davis JR, Sherer K. *Applied Nutrition and Diet Therapy for Nurses,* 2nd ed. Philadelphia: W.B. Saunders, 1994.

supporting structures. Changes in ameloblasts and odontoblasts result in hypoplasia of the enamel and dentin. Alveolar bone formation may be reduced, along with a widening of the periodontal ligament space and gingival hyperplasia.

Dental Hygiene Considerations

- Hypomagnesemia in about one-third of the infants born to diabetic mothers appears to be related to the severity of maternal diabetes and premature birth (Shils, 1988).

- ℞ Decreased food intake and/or impaired absorption and use of certain diuretics may be contributing factors to hypomagnesemia. Encourage a well-balanced diet with liberal intake of foods high in magnesium.

Nutritional Directions

- Diets high in unrefined grains and vegetables provide more magnesium than diets including a lot of refined foods, meats, and milk products.

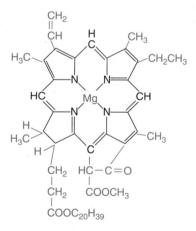

FIGURE 8-3 **Structure of chlorophyll. All chlorophyll molecules are essentially alike; they differ only in details of the side chains. Magnesium is basic to all chlorophyll molecules.**

FLUORIDE
Physiologic Roles

In a strict nutritional connotation, fluoride is not a nutrient essential for health. Even though fluoride is present in low concentrations in soft tissues, it does not have any known metabolic function. However, because of its notoriety as being beneficial to dental health, fluoride is considered a desirable element for humans. Saliva contains relatively low amounts of fluoride; the amount of fluoride ingested has little effect on salivary levels.

Fluoride is advantageous to dental health because of its systemic effects prior to tooth eruption and topical effects after tooth eruption (Fig. 8–4). The caries preventive properties of systemic and topical fluoride are cumulative.

Fluoride ions can replace hydroxyl ions in the hydroxyapatite crystal lattice. This fluoridated hydroxyapatite, or fluorapatite, is less soluble and makes the tooth more resistant to acid demineralization. Additionally, it enhances remineralization

FIGURE 8–4   Concentration gradient of fluoride in outer enamel from permanent and deciduous teeth, from area with 1 and 0.1 ppm of fluoride in the drinking water. (From Gron P. Inorganic chemical and structural aspects of oral mineralized tissues. In Shaw JH et al. (eds): *Textbook of Oral Biology*. Philadelphia: W.B. Saunders, 1978, 484–507.)

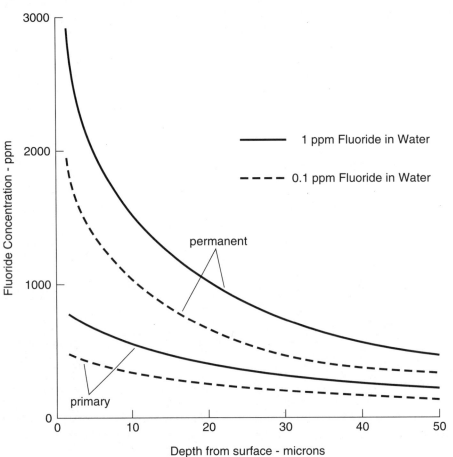

when the tooth is subject to the caries process (DePaola, 1991). Calcium and phosphate are present in saliva and plaque fluid at higher concentrations than fluoride. When small pits develop in the enamel, fluoride is believed to promote deposition of calcium phosphate to remineralize the enamel surface.

Another less well recognized effect of systemic fluoride is changes in tooth morphology which increases resistance of the tooth to adherence of dental plaque (DePaola, 1991). Numerous investigators have observed that in fluoridated areas, posterior teeth have a distinct gross morphology: surfaces are whiter and more reflective, cusps are rounder, and fissures more shallow and less penetrable (DePaola, 1991). Fluoride is more effective in the prevention of smooth surface than occlusal caries.

Fluoride may be passed from the mother and incorporated into developing fetal tooth buds. Fluoride during this stage is probably incorporated in the apatite crystals during formation. The Council on Dental Therapeutics of the American Dental Association and the Academy of Pediatrics believe additional research is needed in this area before recommending the use of a prenatal fluoride supplement.

Primary teeth benefit from the presence of fluoride during tooth development. Fluoride is present in the inner part of the enamel and dentin at lower concentrations; this occurs mainly during the amelogenesis/dentogenesis stage. Enhanced concentration in the surface enamel occurs during the maturation stage of tooth development. Fluoride can be readily incorporated into the apatite crystal from topically available fluoride during the maturation stage, but this reversible process is superficial rather than distributed throughout the enamel thickness, as shown in Figure 8–5.

The presence of fluoride in oral fluids also interferes with the demineralization process. In general, the presence of fluoride results in a less cariogenic environment. Topically available fluoride reduces dental caries by inhibiting demineralization, promoting remineralization, and interfering with the formation and function of acidogenic dental plaque bacteria. Higher concentrations of fluoride inhibit *Streptococcus mutans* in dental plaque and accelerate remineralization during early stages of enamel caries development (ten Cate & Featherstone, 1991). Lower levels of fluoride inhibit bacterial enzymes, reducing demineralization of enamel as a result of less acid production by bacteria (DePaola et al., 1994).

The protective effect of fluoride against caries is greatest during the first 8 years of life, but adults as well as children continue to benefit from consumption of fluoridated water. Systemic fluoride uptake by calcified tissues is high in infancy through age 16 when mineralization of unerupted permanent teeth occurs (ADA Council on Dental Therapeutics, 1994). When compared with healthy enamel, more fluoride is retained in demineralized enamel.

Fluoride is also incorporated into the matrix of bone mass, improving the strength of bone and decreasing bone resorption and bone solubility.

Requirements

Due to its toxicity, adequate intake of fluorine has been established at 3.1 mg/day for women and 3.8 for men. Average intake in the United States is between 0.9 mg/day in areas with nonfluoridated water and 1.7 mg/day in areas with fluoridation (0.7 to 1.2 ppm). A total daily intake of 0.05 to 0.07 mg/kg body weight is generally regarded as optimal (Stannard et al., 1990).

Absorption and Excretion

Most of the fluoride is absorbed in the stomach, with small amounts absorbed in the intestine. The rate and degree of absorption depends upon the solubility of the source and the amount ingested at a particular time. Absorption of fluoride from sodium fluoride in water is estimated to be 100%. Only 65% to 72% of the fluoride is absorbed when sodium fluoride is added to formula or milk (Spak et al., 1982). Protein-bound fluorine in foods is not as well absorbed.

Approximately 60% to 70% of fluoride intake is excreted by the kidneys; about 5% is excreted in the feces. Aluminum, as in aluminum-containing

Fluoride in: Cariostatic Mechanism

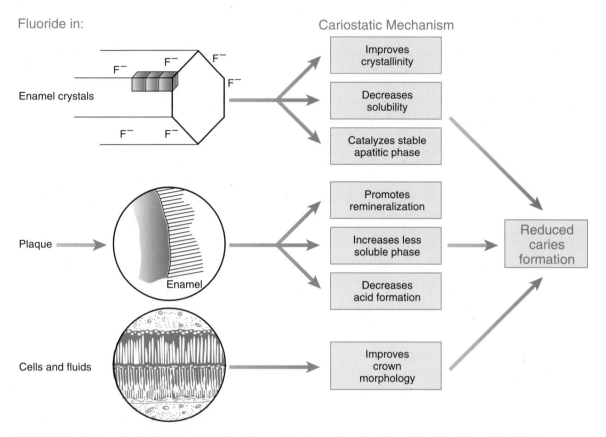

FIGURE 8–5   **Schematic illustration depicting the mechanisms of cariostatic action fluoride and their inter-relationship. (From Nikiforuk G. Mechanism of cariostatic action of fluorides. In Nikiforuk G (ed):** *Understanding Dental Caries Prevention: II.* **Basel, S. Karger.)**

antacids, can bind with fluoride and increase fluoride excretion in the feces.

Sources

WATER

Fluoride is available through community water supplies, food, beverages, dentifrices, and other dental products. Fluoridation of community water contributes to fluoride intake and is a practical, cost-effective means of achieving significant decreases in the prevalence of dental caries. More than 50% of daily fluoride intake is from water consumption (Stannard et al., 1990). To ensure that everyone receives adequate amounts of fluoride, the

National Research Council recommends that drinking water contain approximately 1 ppm fluoride (equivalent to 1 mg/L). In warmer climates where water consumption is higher, the optimal level of fluoride may need to be reduced to 0.6 to 0.7 ppm (Sweeney & Shaw, 1988).

In 1990, 42 of the largest cities in the United States added fluoride to municipal water supplies. Approximately 62% of the U.S. population now has access to floridated drinking water (CDC Fluoridation Census 1992, 1993); the revised goal, as stated by *Healthy People 2000* guidelines, targets 75% of the population. A 40% to 60% reduction in prevalence of caries has been observed in children with life-long exposure to optimally fluoridated water (0.7 to 1.2 ppm fluoride) and no other fluoride therapy. Longitudinal studies indicate a 40% to 70% reduction in decayed, missing, and filled teeth as a result of fluoridated water (ADA, 1989).

In contrast, many households and businesses are using bottled water because of concerns about contamination and poor quality control of public water supplies, and as a healthy alternative to soft drinks and alcoholic beverages. The U.S. FDA Safe Drinking Water Act stipulates bottled water can contain no more than 4.0 ppm of fluoride, but no minimal

TABLE 8–6   *Fluoride Content of Bottled Waters*

Water	Fluoride Content (ppm)
Aqua Cool	0.32
Artic Polar	0.70
Balsam Spring	0.16
Belmont Springs	0.12
Crystal Geyser	0.75
Evian	0.15
Heart of Tuscany	Less than 0.10
Hennizz	0.17
Ice Mountain	0.78
Naya	0.22
Neumasket	0.13
Perrier	0.31
Poland Springs	Less than 0.10
Ramlosa	1.25
Saratoga	0.20
Shaw's	0.20
Simpson Spring	0.14
Sparcal	0.33
Spring Hill Farm	0.14
Star	0.21
Stop & Shop	0.55
Tipperary	0.55
Triton Spring Water	0.14
Volvic	0.34

From Stannard J et al. Fluoride content of some bottled waters and recommendations for fluoride supplementation. *J Pedodontics* 1990; 14(2):103–107.

level is mandated. Bottled waters vary widely in fluoride content (from a low 0.10 ppm to a high of 1.25 ppm), as shown in Table 8–6. Fluoride concentrations are not indicated on the bottle. Fluoride binds to glass; therefore bottled water sold in glass bottles will have a slightly lower fluoride content than the original water (Stannard et al., 1990).

FOOD

Food is not a major source of fluoride for adults. All foods contain some fluoride, but the amounts provided in vegetables, meats, cereals, and fruits are insignificant, containing between 0.2 to 1.5 ppm of fluoride (Table 8–7). Seafood may contain 5 to 15 ppm fluoride. Tea provides approximately 0.1 mg fluoride per cup (even when fluoride-free water is used), but herbal tea has negligible fluoride. The process of mechanically deboning poultry results in the poultry containing a high concentration of fluoride.

Some infant foods are fortified with fluoride. Because of varied levels of fluoride in the water supply, in 1979 the amount of fluoride in infant formulas was reduced. Components in soy bind fluoride; therefore, soy-based formulas usually have higher fluoride levels than milk-based formulas.

Fluoride is added to 90% of all toothpastes in the United States; this is provided in a readily absorbable form (DePaola et al., 1994).

Hyper- and Hypo- States
FLUOROSIS AND BONE HEALTH

Mottling of tooth enamel results from overexposure (approximately three to four times the amount necessary to prevent caries) during tooth formation. Ameloblasts are extremely sensitive to excessive fluoride ingestion. Dental fluorosis is directly related to fluoride exposure during tooth development and cannot occur after tooth development has been completed. Fluorosed enamel contains a total protein content similar to that of normal enamel, but it contains a relatively high proportion of immature matrix proteins.

TABLE 8–7 *Fluoride Content of Selected Foods*

Food	Portion	Fluoride (mcg)	Calories (per serving)
Tea, brewed	8 oz	7600	2
Fish, smelt	3 oz	2041	170
Fish, mackerel	3 oz	1128	133
Fish, cod	3 oz	314	89
Potato	½ c	294	112
Cottage cheese	1 c	199	164
Fish, crab	3 oz	170	82
Spinach, cooked	½ c	95	27
Cheese—blue, cheddar, ricotta	3 oz	75	120–345
Pork and beans, canned	½ c	67	183
Onions, cooked	½ c	63	46
Split peas	½ c	60	115
Carrots, canned	½ c	49	28
Corn, canned	½ c	49	92
Almonds	¼ c	29	192

Nutrient data from Nutritionist IV software, First Data Bank; San Bruno, CA.

Mild to moderate enamel fluorosis on early-forming enamel surfaces was strongly associated with use of infant formula prior to 1979, before manufacturers began reducing and controlling the fluoride content of formula, frequent brushing, and appropriate use of fluoride supplements. Dental fluorosis varies from very mild cases characterized by whitish opaque flecks, to white or brown staining, to severe dental fluorosis with secondary, extrinsic, brownish discoloration and varying degrees of enamel pitting (Color Plates 2, 3, and 4). When drinking water contains 2 ppm or more of fluoride, teeth appear extremely white; brown stains appear when the fluoride level is greater than 4 ppm. Mild to moderate fluorosis is primarily cosmetic; severe dental fluorosis can result in increased caries rate.

The ingestion of large amounts of fluoride in adults can result in adverse effects on skeletal tissue and kidney function. At levels of more than 10 ppm, crippling skeletal fluorosis is common (CDC, 1991). These changes may gradually increase in severity, eventually resulting in a general increase in bone density and considerable calcification of ligaments in the neck and vertebral column. Eventually bones become brittle and break easily.

DENTAL CARIES

A lack of fluoride results in increased dental caries. The protective effect against caries is greatest during tooth formation. The American Dental Association and the American Academy of Pediatrics recommend exposure of the teeth to fluoride until calcification of all teeth is completed (about age 16). Dosages for fluoride supplements for children are presented in Table 12–4. Various conditions warrant fluoride treatment in adults.

Continued use of fluoridated water into adulthood may be beneficial in maintaining the integrity of teeth (Jong, 1991). The prevalence of coronal and root caries has consistently declined more (20% to 35%) in adults living in communities with optimally fluoridated water than in adults residing in cities with lower levels of fluoride in the water (Public Health Focus, 1992).

Safety

The addition of fluoride in the water supply continues to be opposed by a small vocal and aggressive minority of people in the United States. "Antifluoridation" groups have attempted to link water fluoridation to cancer, AIDS, Alzheimer's disease, and Down's syndrome, but scientific evidence to support their allegations has not been provided.

Fluoridation is one of the most thoroughly researched health issues in recent history. In 1990, the U.S. Public Health Service released findings of the National Toxicology Program in which **equivocal evidence** was found linking fluoride and cancer (CDC, 1991). No trends could be identified that were attributed to the introduction or duration of fluoride into drinking water. The report concluded that evidence of associations between fluoridated water and birth defects or problems of the gastrointestinal and genitourinary tracts, and respiratory system is lacking. Fluoridation does not increase the incidence or mortality rate of any chronic condition, including cancer, heart disease, intracranial lesions, nephritis, cirrhosis, or Down's syndrome.

In contrast, the committee, as well as most all professional health organizations, have concluded that results of numerous long-term community trials of adding fluoride to public water supplies at optimal levels verify the effectiveness, safety, and economy of this public health measure in reducing the prevalence of dental caries. Fluoridation of water is the most cost-effective method of preventing dental caries and provides the greatest benefit to those who can least afford preventive and restorative dentistry.

Dental Hygiene Considerations

- Educate clients about the purpose and value of fluoridation on oral health. Approximately one-third of American adults do not know why fluoridation of water is important.
- Contact the state or local water company to determine the fluoride content of the water

system. They can also analyze well water to determine fluoride content and may provide some general information about the fluoride content of well water in that area.

- Reliably estimate the total amount of fluoride the client consumes daily in foods and water. Since fluoride is available from multiple sources, the possibility of toxic levels should be considered when recommending fluoride supplements or providing treatment, especially for children.
- In many cases, total fluoride exposure appears to be higher than necessary to prevent tooth decay (CDC, 1991). No more than the amount of fluoride necessary to provide the desired effect should be used.
- Recommend fluoride supplements only when the fluoride level of the home water supply is known to be deficient.
- An increase in fluoride intake is beneficial during development of skeletal tissue and teeth. Encourage fluoride-fortified foods, water, or supplements for breast-fed infants, and fluoridated water for children and adolescents.
- Growth of cariogenic bacteria is reduced by the presence of fluoride. Suggest use of dentifrices or mouthwashes with fluoride for oral self-care.
- Educate young children to use only small (pea size) amounts of fluoridated dentifrices and to minimize swallowing toothpaste.
- ℞ If fluoride and calcium supplements are given concurrently, absorption of both is decreased.

Nutritional Directions

- Fluoridation of community water supplies is the most effective method of preventing dental caries, including coronal and root caries.
- To provide maximum benefits, systemic fluoride is important before tooth eruption,

possibly in utero, and until the last molar erupts, when development of unerupted permanent teeth is occurring.

♦ Fluoride supplementation is not recommended for infants under 6 months unless they are exclusively receiving ready-to-feed formula or are being breast-fed.

♦ If a child receives suboptimal levels of fluoride, an increase in dental caries may occur. Exposure to multiple sources of fluoride increases a child's risk of receiving too much fluoride and developing fluorosis.

♦ Fluoride supplements are not appropriate for those living in areas where the fluoride content of drinking water is 60% of the optimal for water fluoridation (Stannard et al., 1990).

♦ Topical availability of fluoride at low concentrations on a daily basis after tooth eruption is important to deter the development of dental caries.

♦ If caries susceptibility is high, professionally applied and self-applied home fluoride applications may be a component of the dental hygiene care provided.

♦ When bottled water is being used, obtain the fluoride content from the distributor.

♦ Studies have found no association between fluoride supplementation and cancer in humans.

℞ Aluminum antacids decrease fluoride absorption.

HEALTH APPLICATION 8

Osteoporosis

Osteoporosis is a common and costly disease. As many as 25 million Americans are affected by osteoporosis, which causes 1.5 million fractures annually and incurs a financial burden of between 10 and 18 billion dollars in medical charges (McBean et al., 1994). Fractures resulting from osteoporosis are a significant source of bone pain, disability, and disfigurement.

Genetic factors contribute significantly to attainment of peak bone mass. Fair-skinned underweight white women are at greatest risk for osteoporosis. Peak bone mass is achieved at approximately 35 years of age. After puberty, males have approximately 10% to 15% more bone mass than females, and blacks have approximately 10% more bone mass than do whites. Early menopause is a very strong predictor for the development of osteoporosis.

Other risk factors include calcium and vitamin D deficiency, immobilization, physical inactivity, alcoholism, cigarette smoking, and excessive exercise that produces amenorrhea. A physical environment that increases risk of slipping, and neuromuscular and visual problems may contribute to a fall, and consequently, a fracture. Excessive protein or caffeine intake may increase calcium loss in urine and enhance osteoporotic changes (McBean et al., 1994). Two commonly used medications have a documented effect on bone mineralization. Thiazide diuretics, principally used for blood pressure control, positively affect bone mineralization; glucocorticoids, used to reduce inflammation, adversely affect bone mineralization. A calcium and vitamin D deficiency early in life appears to negatively affect bone mineralization more than intake after age 35.

For individuals at risk for osteoporosis, an objective of treatment is to slow or stop the disease progression before irreversible structural changes have occurred. Classically, the regimen has included estrogen for postmenopausal females, calcium, vitamin D, exercise, and nutritional adjustments. Numerous theories proposing mechanisms for the effect of estrogen in reducing rate of bone loss have been inconclusive (Lindsay, 1991). Estrogen, if initiated, should be taken for at least 10 to 15 years. Stopping earlier seems to accelerate bone loss. A regimen of estrogen-progesterone-calcium retards bone loss and improves calcium balance better than calcium supplements alone.

Calcitonin, another drug approved for treatment of osteoporosis, inhibits osteoclast bone resorption. Salmon calcitonin serves as an alternative therapy when estrogen is contraindicated. Sodium fluoride and parathyroid hormone appear to increase bone mass.

Walking, weight-bearing exercise, or an active lifestyle is beneficial in prevention and treatment of osteoporosis. Physical exercise may increase bone mass to different extents in various parts of the skeleton. Adequate exposure to sunlight and vitamin D intake are also important.

The relationship between diet and bone maintenance or enhanced mineral content is not clear cut. A diet high in protein may increase urinary calcium, but the impact of this increased loss is unknown. Recent studies have not demonstrated a negative effect on calcium balance by increased protein or phosphorus intake. Also, fecal calcium excretion may increase if a high-fiber diet is followed. Higher amounts of calcium (above 1,000 mg calcium daily) provide a bone-protective effect, which is partly due to greater peak bone mass and partly due to protection against age-related bone loss.

On the other hand, adequate calcium intake at all stages of life, with a daily intake of a minimum of 1,000 mg for all healthy adults, continues to be emphasized. Calcium is not related to bone health but is necessary for healthy bones.

Despite extensive media coverage, about one-half of adult Americans consume less than 500 mg/day. Calcium intakes of 1,000 mg for adults and 1,200 mg for adults over 51 was recently endorsed by the National Academy of Sciences. Postmenopausal women not on estrogen replacement therapy should have 1,500 mg/day based on the Consensus Conference on optimal calcium intake (NIH Consensus Development Panel, 1994).

Dietary modifications for clients at risk include at least two servings of dairy products daily (to provide 75% of RDAs). For clients who have inadequate intake of milk or milk products (including those who are lactose intolerant), inclusion of calcium supplements may be indicated. Caffeine is used in moderation since caffeine increases calcium excretion. Herbal teas or decaffeinated drinks can be substituted. If the client consumes a high-fiber diet, calcium intake should be increased.

Clients who are trying to lower their cholesterol intake may inadvertently decrease calcium intake. Cholesterol can be reduced without adversely affecting calcium intake by following these guidelines: (1) substitute skim milk products and low-fat yogurts and cheeses for whole milk and cheeses, (2) increase daily intake of fruits, vegetables, and whole-grain products, (3) use unsaturated oils, such as safflower, sunflower, canola, corn, or olive, and (4) reduce (don't eliminate) red-meat intake.

CASE APPLICATION FOR THE DENTAL HYGIENIST

During Annie's routine dental exam, her mother asked whether she should start Annie (age 5) on a fluoride supplement. Annie's examination revealed a caries-free mouth. She brushes her teeth twice a day.

Nutritional Assessment

- Food consumption pattern
- Frequency of carbohydrate intake
- Fluoride content of water consumed; average amount of water/water-based beverages consumed
- Type and amount of toothpaste used

Nutritional Diagnosis

Health-seeking behaviors related to inadequate knowledge about fluoride supplementation.

Nutritional Goals

Client will practice good oral self-care and receive adequate fluoride to prevent dental caries.

Nutritional Implementation

Intervention: Explain the benefits of fluoride.
Rationale: Fluoride is advantageous to dental health because of its systemic effect prior to tooth eruption and topical effects after tooth eruption. The caries preventive properties of systemic and topical fluoride are additive.

Intervention: Discuss the toxic effects of fluoride.
Rationale: Dental fluorosis is directly related to the level of fluoride exposure during tooth development. It can also have adverse effects on bone structure.

Intervention: Assess current fluoride consumption from (1) food, (2) water supply, and (3) dentifrices.
Rationale: (1) All foods contain some fluoride, but the amounts provided in vegetables, meats, cereals, and fruits are insignificant unless large amounts of seafood, tea, or mechanically deboned poultry is consumed. (2) Water is usually the main source of fluoride, but some municipal water supplies and bottled water may contain negligible amounts of fluoride. (3) Fluoride is added to 90% of all dentifrices in the United States; many children swallow most of the toothpaste used.

Intervention: Show Annie and her mother how much toothpaste to use and discuss the importance of not swallowing the toothpaste.
Rationale: Because fluoride in toothpaste can be readily absorbed, toothpaste should not be swallowed to prevent harmful effects of systemically available fluoride.

Intervention: Encourage the client and her mother to consume a well-balanced diet and to limit snacking to two times a day.
Rationale: Not only is fluoride important, but other nutrients are also essential for dental health. Snacks, especially carbohydrate-containing foods, increase risk for dental caries.

Intervention: Suggest fluoride supplements only if fluoride intake appears to be low.
Rationale: In many cases, total fluoride exposure appears to be higher than necessary to prevent tooth decay. No more than the amount of fluoride necessary to provide the desired effect should be used.

Intervention: Recommend parental supervision and assistance of Annie's toothbrushing and flossing at least once daily.
Rationale: Monitoring the child's brushing technique and assisting with floss will ensure that effective plaque removal occurs once a day.

Evaluation

If the client and her mother can demonstrate the toothbrushing procedure, says she will brush her teeth after every meal, and will try to eat the foods her mother provides, and dental caries continue to be minimal, dental hygiene care was effective.

Student Readiness

1. A client claims that she dislikes milk. How would you advise her to obtain the needed calcium?
2. What are the main physiologic roles of calcium, phosphorus, magnesium, and fluoride?
3. How do minerals differ from vitamins?
4. How would you respond to a remark that milk is only for babies?
5. Discuss three dietary factors that affect calcium absorption.

6. Determine the level of fluoride in your community's drinking water. If an adult client (weight about 75 kg) is drinking only bottled water that does not contain fluoride and dislikes fish and tea, how much topical fluoride would be necessary to furnish the ESADDI for fluoride?

7. List five types of over-the-counter calcium supplements available. Evaluate these items for primary sources of calcium, elemental calcium per unit consumed, and how many tablets or units would have to be consumed daily to receive 1,000 mg of elemental calcium.

8. Discuss how to deal with a client who is opposed to fluoridation.

9. Why would you advise a client to obtain his/her mineral requirement from food sources rather than mineral supplements (unless ordered by the physician)?

Case Study

Mrs. J.M., a 69-year-old female, fell and fractured her hip 6 months ago. She admits she is taking calcium supplements occasionally when she can afford them. She does not like milk and has been unable to walk much since her fall.

1. What nutritional advice could you give her about her osteoporosis?

2. What is the RDA for calcium?

3. What foods could you suggest she consume to increase her calcium intake?

4. When should she take her calcium supplement to maximize its absorption?

5. What oral changes might you expect to find in your assessment?

6. What effect would increased vitamin D have on her condition?

References

American Dietetic Association (ADA). Position paper: The impact of fluoride on dental health. *J Am Diet Assoc* 1989; 89(7):971–974.

American Dental Association (ADA). Council on Dental Therapeutics. New fluoride schedule adopted. *ADA News* 1994:12–14.

Centers for Disease Control (CDC). Public Health Service report on fluoride benefits and risks. *JAMA* 1991; 266(8):1061–1062, 1066–7.

CDC Fluoridation Census 1992. Atlanta, Ga: US Dept of Health & Human Services 1993;iv–xiii.

Chan GM et al. Effects of dairy products on bone and bone composition in pubbertal girls. *J Pediatr,* 1995 Apr 126(4):551–6.

DePaola DP et al. Nutrition in relation to dental medicine. *In* Shils ME, Young VR (eds): *Modern Nutrition in Health and Disease,* 8th ed. Philadelphia: Lea & Febiger, 1994, 1007–1028.

DePaola PF. Reaction paper: The use of topical and systemic fluorides in the present era. *J Public Health Dent* 1991; 51(1):48–52.

National Research Council Study Committee on the Scientific Evaluation of Dietary Reference Intakes.

Dietary Reference Intakes for Calcium, Phosphorus, Magnesium, Vitamin D, and Fluoride, Washington, DC: National Academy Press, 1997.

Guyton AC, Hall JE. *Textbook of Medical Physiology,* 9th ed. Philadelphia: W.B. Saunders, 1996.

Jong AW. Duration of fluoride supplementation (questions and answers). *JAMA* 1991; 266(6):850.

Lindsay R. Estrogens, bone mass, and osteoporotic fractures. *Am J Med* 1991; 91(Suppl 5B):5B-10S-13S.

Lloyd T et al. Calcium supplementation and bone mineral density in adolescent girls. *JAMA* 1993; 270(7):841–844.

McBean LD, et al. Osteoporosis: Visions for care and prevention—a conference report. *J Am Diet Assoc* 1994; 94(6):668–671.

Public Health Focus: Fluoridation of community water systems. *MMWR Morb Mortal Wkly Rep* 1992; 41(21):372–375, 381.

Putnam JJ, Allshouse JE. Food consumption, prices, and expenditures, 1970–92. USDA, ERS, Statistical Bull No. 867. Washington, DC, 1993.

Spak CJ et al. Bioavailability of fluoride added to baby formula and milk. *Caries Res* 1982; 16(3):249–256.

Stannard J et al. Fluoride content of some bottled waters

and recommendations for fluoride supplementation. *J Pedodontics* 1990; 14(2):103–107.

Sweeney EA, Shaw HJ. Nutrition in relation to dental medicine. *In* Shils ME, Young VR (eds): *Modern Nutrition in Health and Disease.* Philadelphia: Lea & Febiger, 1988, 1069–1091.

Ten Cate JM, Featherstone JDB. Mechanistic aspects of the interaction between fluoride and dental enamel. *Crit Rev Oral Biol Med* 1991; 2(2):283–296.

Wardlaw, G. The effects of diet and life-style on bone mass in women. *J Am Diet Assoc* 1988; 88(1): 17–22, 25.

Zizza C, Gerrior S. The US food supply provides more of most nutrients. *Food Rev,* 1995; 18(1):40–45.

Chapter 9

Nutrients Present in Calcified Structures

OBJECTIVES

The Student Will Be Able To:

- List physiologic roles and sources of copper, selenium, chromium, and manganese.
- List ultratrace elements present in the body.
- List reasons why large amounts of one mineral may cause nutritional deficiencies of another.
- Apply dental hygiene considerations for trace elements present in calcified structures.
- Discuss nutritional directions for clients regarding the role of trace elements present in calcified structures.

GLOSSARY OF TERMS

Manganese madness   severe psychotic symptoms and neuromuscular symptoms that resemble those of parkinsonism

Stannous   containing tin

Osteodystrophy   abnormal bone development, similar to osteomalacia

ppb   parts per billion

Test Your NQ (True/False)

1. The National Research Council has established ESADDIs for copper, manganese, chromium, and molybdenum. T/F
2. Lead in dental enamel can be used to determine exposure to lead. T/F
3. Copper is important in the formation of collagen. T/F
4. Aluminum toxicity is a cause for Alzheimer's disease. T/F
5. Selenium functions as an antioxidant. T/F
6. Refined foods are a good source of trace minerals. T/F
7. Aluminum is cariogenic. T/F
8. The function of many trace elements present in enamel and dentin is unknown. T/F
9. Sugar is a good source of chromium. T/F
10. Selenium supplements are a good way to increase longevity. T/F

Very small amounts of several minerals are essential for optimal growth and development. Many of these ultratrace elements, listed in Table 9–1, are found in enamel and dentin. Despite the amount of a mineral the body needs, its presence determines whether or not the body can function normally. Their role may not be obvious as you clinically assess clients; nevertheless, clients with inadequate amounts may exhibit deficiency symptoms.

Estimated Safe and Adequate Daily Dietary Intakes (ESADDIs) have been established for several of these nutrients because data are so limited about human requirements and the amounts needed. Many may be toxic in larger amounts; hence safe ranges have been set.

Evidence has been presented suggesting that ultratrace minerals, especially arsenic, boron, nickel, and silicon, may be essential physiologically. Since no human deficiencies have been determined, their importance in humans can only be inferred from results of animal studies. Therefore, human requirements have not been quantified. If they are required, the amounts needed are easily met by naturally occurring sources in foods, water, and air. Other elements present in calcified structures, such as cadmium, lead, and tin, have no known function and may be contaminants.

TABLE 9–1   *Trace Element Concentrations in Human Enamel and Dentin*

	Enamel* (ppm)	Dentin* (ppm)
Aluminum	1.5–700	10–100
Boron	0.5–39	1–10
Cadmium	0.3–10	
Chromium	<0.1–100	1–100
Copper	0.1–130	0.2–100
Iron	0.8–200	90–1,000
Lead	1.3–100	10–100
Lithium	0.23–3.40	
Manganese	0.8–20	0.6–1,000
Molybdenum	0.7–39	1–10
Nickel	10–100	10–100
Selenium	0.1–10	10–100
Strontium	26–1,000	90–1,000
Sulfur	130–530	
Tin	0.03–0.9	
Vanadium	0.01–0.03	1–10
Zinc	60–1,800	

*mcg/gm dry wt.

Adapted from Gron P. Inorganic chemical and structural aspects of oral mineralized tissues. *In* Shaw JH et al. (eds): *Textbook of Oral Biology.* Philadelphia: W.B. Saunders, 1978, 484–507.

COPPER
Physiologic Roles

Copper is essential for formation of red blood cells and connective tissue. Its function as a catalyst is important in the formation of collagen from a precollagenous stage. Copper is a cofactor of many enzymes that function in oxidative reactions and production of *neurotransmitters* (including norepinephrine and dopamine), which transmit messages through the central nervous system.

Copper is readily incorporated into tooth enamel. Epidemiologic data suggest copper is cariogenic, but in bacteriologic studies, copper is cariostatic by reducing acidogenicity of plaque.

Requirements

The National Research Council has established the ESADDI of copper to be 1.5 to 3 mg/day for adults. The American food supply provides about 1.7 mg/day/person (Gerrior & Zizza, 1994).

Absorption and Excretion

Approximately one-third of dietary copper is absorbed, with absorption occurring in the stomach and duodenum. Absorption is enhanced by a low pH and decreased with large amounts of calcium and zinc. Copper is principally excreted through bile in feces.

Sources

Copper is widely distributed in foods. The richest sources include shellfish, oysters, crabs, liver, nuts, sesame and sunflower seeds, legumes, and cocoa.

Hyper- and Hypo- States

Copper toxicosis is seldom encountered. Copper taken orally is an emetic, and as little as 10 mg of oral copper can produce nausea. Serum copper levels are elevated in clients with rheumatoid arthritis, myocardial infarction, conditions requiring administration of estrogen, and pregnancy.

Wilson's disease represents a special metabolic disorder in which large amounts of copper accumulate in the liver, kidney, brain, and cornea. Copper concentration in the cornea leads to a characteristic brown or green ring called the Kayser-Fleischer ring.

Most copper deficiencies have been detected under unusual conditions, such as total parenteral nutrition or with zinc supplementation. Copper deprivation results in profound effects on the bones, brain, arteries, and other connective tissues, decreases hair and skin pigmentation and causes hematologic abnormalities such as a low white blood cell count. It is reasonable to assume that all the effects are ultimately due to an inadequate supply of copper needed for copper enzyme synthesis and activity.

Copper deficiency causes a variety of lesions within connective tissues and bone, such as failure to grow (in children), spontaneous fractures, osteoporosis, arthritis, arterial disease, and ultimately marked bone deformities with severe deficiency. These lesions have been attributed to abnormal formation of cross-linkages in collagen and elastin. Changes resemble those seen in vitamin C deficiency.

Dental Hygiene Considerations

- Anemia not corrected with iron supplements may be due to copper deficiency.
- ℞ Zinc supplements exceeding 1,500 mg/day decrease copper absorption, possibly leading to anemia-related fatigue.

Nutritional Directions

- High dietary fiber intakes increase the dietary requirement for copper.
- Large amounts of vitamin C supplements (1,000 mg) decrease serum bioavailability of copper.

SELENIUM

Physiologic Roles

Selenium functions mainly as a cofactor for an antioxidant enzyme that protects membrane lipids, proteins, and nucleic acids from oxidative damage. Selenium works hand in hand with vitamin E; a deficiency of either nutrient increases the requirement for the other. Although selenium has been suspected as a carcinogen, it may actually be an anticarcinogen.

Selenium is present in tooth enamel and dentin. It is probably incorporated into the enamel during amelogenesis; large amounts during tooth formation may be detrimental to the mineralization process.

Requirements

The RDA establishes the adult requirement at 70 mcg for men and 55 mcg for women. Selenium intake in the United States is believed to be adequate (Pennington & Young, 1991).

Sources

Animal products, especially seafood, kidney, liver, and other meats are rich in selenium. Selenium intake correlates closely with caloric and protein intake. Selenium in dairy products and eggs is more readily absorbed than from other foods.

Hyper- and Hypo- States

Both toxicity and deficiency have been seen in animals from irregular distribution of selenium in soil, but these are rarely seen in humans. Routine ingestion of 2 to 3 mg of selenium can cause toxic symptoms of nausea and vomiting, weakness, dermatitis, hair loss, and garlicky breath odor. Cirrhosis of the liver may also develop.

Animal studies indicate that excessive selenium may promote dental caries when given preruptively, whereas moderately high levels appear to have some cariostatic effects. Increased dental caries rates have been observed in areas where the food and water contain higher levels of selenium. Whether this is caused by a topical effect on dental plaque or the structural composition of the tooth is unknown.

In the People's Republic of China, an endemic cardiomyopathy is associated with severe selenium deficiency called Keshan disease. Fatality rate is as high as 80% in infants and children and in women of child-bearing age. Oral selenium prophylaxis is extremely effective in reducing, but not completely eliminating, Keshan disease.

Dental Hygiene Considerations

- Decreased selenium levels may cause heart damage, resulting in a heart attack.
- Selenium is essential for health, but it can also be toxic for humans.

Nutritional Directions

- Selenium supplements should not be taken by those with cancer unless specified by a physician because of possible toxicity.

CHROMIUM

Physiologic Roles

Chromium is involved in carbohydrate and lipid metabolism, especially in the utilization of glucose. Chromium is a cofactor for insulin, so a deficiency causes insulin resistance.

Requirements

The ESADDI of a healthy adult has been estimated to be between 50 and 200 mcg/day. Chromium is poorly absorbed; whether or not intestinal absorption compensates for increased demand is unclear.

Sources

Chromium is found in meats, whole-grain cereals, brewer's yeast, and meats. Refined cereals are depleted of chromium.

Hyper- and Hypo- States

Deficiency states are rare and slow to develop. Chromium toxicity has been caused by indus-

trial exposure, resulting in liver damage and lung cancer.

Dental Hygiene Considerations

- Assess clients employed in industry for chromium toxicity.
- Adequate amounts of chromium may improve glucose tolerance in some people with elevated blood glucose levels if their body still secretes insulin. However, it does not replace the need for insulin in most clients with diabetes mellitus.
- Serum chromium levels decline with age, possibly contributing to glucose problems seen in non-insulin-dependent diabetes mellitus.

Nutritional Directions

- Because sucrose consumption results in increased insulin levels, body chromium can be conserved by using table sugar in moderation.

♦ Do not take chromium supplements unless instructed by a physician. Currently, there is no evidence that any type of supplemental chromium can help with fat loss or muscle development, or will lower serum cholesterol or increase longevity (Mertz, 1994).

MANGANESE

Physiologic Roles

Manganese is essential in several enzyme systems, and is important for optimal bone matrix development, prevention of osteoporosis, insulin production, and other metabolic functions.

Requirements

The ESADDI is 2 to 5 mg/day. Average intake for adults is 2 to 3 mg/day (Pennington & Young, 1991). The absorption of iron and manganese is inversely proportional, so a large amount of one causes a reduction in the other.

Sources

Foods high in manganese are whole-grain cereals, legumes, and leafy vegetables. The bioavailability of manganese from meats, milk, and eggs makes these important sources despite their smaller quantities.

Hyper- and Hypo- States

Manganese dust can be an environmental hazard. Miners have developed a syndrome similar to Parkinsonism called **"manganese madness."**

Manganese deficiencies have never been reported in those consuming a normal diet. Signs of deficiency include abnormal formation of bone and cartilage, growth retardation, congenital malformations, impaired glucose tolerance, and poor reproductive performance.

An increased concentration of manganese in saliva plaque and enamel are associated with increased caries. Studies have not clarified whether this association is due to incorporation of manganese in enamel or its effects on oral bacteria.

Dental Hygiene Considerations

● Inhaling manganese dust can be toxic. Clients whose occupation increases inhalation of manganese (i.e., factory workers or coal miners) may exhibit psychotic symptoms or symptoms similar to Parkinson's disease.

Nutritional Directions

♦ Phytate and fiber in bran, tannins in tea, and oxalic acid in spinach inhibit absorption of manganese.
♦ Manganese should not be confused with magnesium.

MOLYBDENUM

Molybdenum functions as an enzyme cofactor. Molybdenum, a trace element present in teeth, may inhibit caries formation. However, studies with people and animals have been inconsistent and molybdenum is not recommended clinically for prevention of dental caries. No mechanism has been proposed for how molybdenum could inhibit caries formation, but rodent studies suggest that molybdenum affects crown morphology.

Legumes, whole-grain cereals, and many vegetables are good sources. The ESADDI for molybdenum is 75 to 250 mcg.

Except for deficiency reported during administration of total parenteral nutrition, molybdenum deficiency has not been documented in the United States.

Dental Hygiene Considerations	*Nutritional Directions*
• Consumption of large quantities of molybdenum may result in copper deficiency, making the client prone to anemia.	◆ Milk and whole grains are good sources of molybdenum.

ULTRATRACE ELEMENTS

Many ultratrace elements have been studied for their potential influence on dental caries. Results of research investigations are complicated by many factors. Nevertheless, some studies suggest relationships between some of these trace elements and the development of caries in humans or animals; further research is warranted to determine the mechanism of their effects.

More attention has been given to ultratrace elements as contaminants in the environment and foods. Some are considered to have no harmful effects and are used therapeutically, such as aluminum in antacids.

Boron

Boron has a direct effect on metabolism of calcium, phosphorus, or magnesium and may be needed to maintain membrane structure. Inadequate amounts of vitamin D increases boron requirement. Boron is necessary for the development and maintenance of strong healthy bones.

Boron is principally present in foods of plant origin, especially fruits, vegetables, nuts, and legumes.

Boron deficiency affects mineral metabolism. Clients with disturbed mineral metabolic disorders of unknown etiology, such as osteoporosis, may be deficient in boron.

Nickel

The physiologic role of nickel is still unclear. Nickel deficiency results in suboptimal growth in animals. Inadequate nickel alters trace-element composition of bone and impairs iron utilization.

Good sources of nickel include dried beans and peas, grains, nuts, and chocolate.

Silicon

Silicon contributes to the structure and resilience of collagen, elastin, and polysaccharides. Silicon is present in tooth enamel in larger amounts than most other trace elements, but its function, if any, is unknown. Deficiencies in animal studies result in depressed collagen in bone and long-bone abnormalities, resulting in malformed joints and defective bone growth.

Tin

Tin has no known function in development or maintenance of bone, but it may affect bone metabolism because tin accumulates in bone. The absorption of tin can alter utilization of calcium and zinc, affecting bone growth and maintenance. Animal studies have shown that a high level of tin in the diet results in decreased collagen synthesis and decreased compressive strength of bones. Although results of studies have not been consistent, several investigators believe that **stannous** fluoride exhibits more cariostatic activity than other fluoride compounds by reducing plaque accumulation and gingivitis.

Most Americans consume only small amounts of tin daily as most foods contain trace amounts of tin. Foods packed in tin cans that are totally coated with lacquer contain very little tin, but acidic foods, such as pineapple and orange juice and tomato sauce, not packed in cans coated with lacquer contain significant amounts of tin. Stannous chloride is approved for use as a food additive, and stannous fluoride is the active ingredient in some self-applied dentifrices and mouth rinses.

Aluminum

Aluminum probably is not an essential nutrient; in fact, its presence in the body appears to be harmful. Under normal conditions, very little aluminum is absorbed; the kidneys excrete about the same amount as is absorbed.

Aluminum accumulates in bone and has been observed to cause **osteodystrophy** in clients who have received aluminum from routes other than through the gastrointestinal tract. Water used in intravenous solutions and dialysis fluid is contaminated with aluminum. The kidneys are frequently unable to remove the daily load of aluminum presented in individuals receiving these fluids, causing undesirable effects. Efforts are being made to lower aluminum content of these fluids. However, aluminum accumulation can still occur through oral ingestion of aluminum hydroxide antacids and from the diet.

Aluminum is also present in all dental tissues. Dental caries may be reduced because aluminum enhances the uptake and retention of fluoride and enhances the cariostatic activity of fluoride. Solubility of enamel is decreased, and dental plaque formation and acidogenicity is inhibited by aluminum.

Lead

Much information is available about the harmful effects of lead in the body but little is known about its beneficial role or its essentiality. Lead is more readily absorbed from the gastrointestinal tract during infancy and early childhood than in adulthood; thus children are more susceptible to lead exposure. Nutritional status can influence susceptibility to lead toxicity.

A large proportion of absorbed lead is incorporated into the skeleton and teeth. Lead deposited in the enamel matrix has been associated with pitting hypoplasia. The amount of lead in shedded deciduous teeth can be used as an index of lead exposure. The effect of lead stored in the bones and teeth is unknown.

The federal government has enacted legislative measures to decrease lead exposure. Currently most domestic food processors do not use lead-soldered cans, but canned goods imported into the United States may still be made with lead solder. The Environmental Protection Agency (EPA) has reduced the allowable lead in drinking water from 50 parts per billion (**ppb**) to 5 ppb. As a result of these regulatory measures, National Health and Nutrition Examination Surveys show average blood levels dropped 78% between 1976 and 1991. Lead is ingested from toddlers' normal hand-to-mouth activities; in older children, playing with dirt or lead-contaminated objects may result in lead ingestion.

Inorganic lead can have detrimental effects on the body. Even low levels of lead exposure may impair intellectual performance. As serum lead levels rise, general cognitive, verbal, and perceptual abilities are increasingly affected by slower learning aptitudes, which appear to be irreversible. Lead toxicity is most pronounced in children and fetuses because it can damage the central nervous system and kidneys. Lead also decreases normal production of red blood cells.

Lithium

Lithium is another ultratrace element found in calcified structures. As lithium accumulates in animal bones, the calcium content of bone decreases. When this substitution is made in apatite of bone and teeth, the structure and solubility properties are changed. A decreased calcium-to-phosphorus ratio of apatite caused by lithium substitution is accompanied by an increase in acid solubility.

Vanadium

Studies on the essentiality of vanadium have been inconsistent in their findings. Most research has not found that vanadium deficiency consistently impairs any biologic function in animals. Vanadium is readily incorporated into areas of rapid mineralization of bones and tooth dentin, but its role in bones and teeth is unknown.

The cariostatic effect of vanadium has been studied. Although an inverse correlation between vanadium content in drinking water and caries incidence was observed in one study, animal experiments are inconclusive in their results. It has been hypothesized that vanadium may exchange for phosphorus in the apatite tooth substance.

Dental Hygiene Considerations

- Boron deficiency signs may be related to abnormalities in vitamin D, calcium, phosphorus, or magnesium levels.
- Aluminum is a cariostatic agent, especially in combination with fluoride.

Nutritional Directions

- A diet low in boron increases calcium excretion, so clients with osteoporosis should be encouraged to consume more fresh fruits and vegetables.
- Acidic foods and foods with high nitrate content can accumulate very high levels of tin if stored in opened cans in the refrigerator for more than 3 days.
- Consumption of a variety of foods and fluids helps obtain these trace minerals.
- Unrefined foods generally provide more trace minerals than do highly refined foods.
- Supplements of these trace elements are not encouraged until further research is performed.
- Some bone meal sold in health food stores for calcium supplementation contains dangerous amounts of lead.
- Dental amalgam, a mixture of several metals (mercury, silver, tin, and copper), does not compromise the health of most people. The small amounts of mercury vapor released from amalgams could cause allergic reactions in a very small minority. Despite anecdotal reports of improvement upon amalgam removal, there is no evidence that removing amalgam has a beneficial effect on health. The removal process itself may possibly expose the client to additional mercury (Subcommittee on Risk Management, 1993).

HEALTH APPLICATION 9

Alzheimer's Disease

Alzheimer's disease is the major cause of dementia in the elderly. It is a slowly progressive disease, characterized by deterioration of judgment, orientation, memory, personality, and intellectual capability, with a usual duration of 6 to 10 years between onset and death.

Although much has been learned about the disease, a specific cause has not been determined. Similarities observed between aluminum toxicity and Alzheimer's disease led to the hypothesis that dietary or environmental aluminum might be involved. As a result, the public was advised, especially by lay people, that aluminum cookware could be toxic. Chelation therapy was advocated to remove aluminum from the body as an unorthodox treatment for Alzheimer's. However, brain lesions and neurotransmitter changes seen in aluminum toxicity and Alzheimer's are different. In contrast to subtle cognitive changes associated with Alzheimer's disease, aluminum toxicity presents with motor dysfunction.

It is currently believed that aluminum accumulates secondary to a neurochemical defect. Nutritional deficiencies have been shown to cause changes in the brain similar to those found in Alzheimer's. But those with Alzheimer's disease are typically well-nourished initially, and eating patterns appear better than in those without the disease (Root & Longenecker, 1988).

Numerous nutritional therapies have been studied without effective results. Trials of lecithin and choline have not shown any improvement in cognitive function or slowing the rate of progression of the disease. However, lecithin or choline along with medications that activate the parasympathetic fibers system have caused some improvement in those with Alzheimer's disease.

Alzheimer's disease has significant effects on nutritional status. Initially, individuals with Alzheimer's may have problems with food purchasing and preparation. Appetite and food intake fluctuate with mood swings and increasing confusion. They may forget when they last ate, skipping some meals and sometimes eating meals twice. Changes in food preferences may be tied into decreases in olfactory function. Sweet and salty foods are preferred.

During the middle phase of the illness, Alzheimer's sufferers become agitated and may pace all night, increasing caloric expenditure. Weight loss is common. Energy requirements may increase by as much as 1,600 Cal/day, and frequent snacking is necessary to maintain body weight. Due to abnormal sleep patterns, caffeine may need to be withheld since caffeine is a central nervous system stimulant.

Appetite is usually good, but caloric intake is usually inadequate to maintain body weight unless snacks and/or liquid nutritional supplements are provided. Food hoarding or failure to chew food sufficiently increases the risk of choking. Ability to use utensils deteriorates. Finger foods may be more appropriate as they allow self-feeding to continue. Foods requiring cutting up should be presented already cut. Serving foods one at a time will help decrease confusion. A larger midday meal is recommended when cognitive abilities are at their peak.

During the final stage, which is characterized by severe intellectual impairment, food may not be recognized and may be refused. Enteral feedings are usually indicated to maintain nutritional status as a result of this impaired cognition.

CASE APPLICATION FOR THE DENTAL HYGIENIST

A young female executive confides in you that she always feels tired and sometimes finds it difficult to get through the day. When you bring up the subject of nutrition, she tells you that she read a book about the importance of minerals and began taking supplements approximately 1 year ago. These self-prescribed supplements include selenium and zinc. She also takes a daily supplement of vitamin C. She is concerned about a lack of energy, which she relates to her poor eating habits. Meals are frequently missed or eaten at her desk.

Nutritional Assessment

○ Willingness to learn.
○ Knowledge level regarding food consumption guidelines such as the Food Guide Pyramid and Dietary Guidelines for Americans.
○ Desire for improving nutritional and general health.
○ Cultural or religious influences.

○ Knowledge of the physiologic roles of vitamins and minerals.
○ Recognition of the interactive effects of vitamins and minerals, especially when taken in excess of the RDA.

Nutritional Diagnosis

Health-seeking behaviors related to inadequate knowledge of optimal nutrition, healthy eating habits, and the deleterious effects associated with consumption of excess vitamins and minerals.

Nutritional Goals

Client will use the dietary guidelines and food pyramid to improve her eating pattern and dietary intake of nutrient-dense foods. Client will recognize the health risks associated with improper supplementation and will decrease reliance on nutritional supplements.

Nutritional Implementation

Intervention: Review the Dietary Guidelines for Americans and discuss how these guidelines support healthy eating habits and disease prevention.

Rationale: Healthy dietary practices can improve energy reserves and overall nutritional status.

Intervention: Encourage consumption of a variety of foods from each of the five main food groups.

Rationale: A nutritious diet is composed of a variety of foods which together supply all the essential nutrients needed for good health.

Intervention: Review serving sizes and emphasize more servings of foods that are nutrient dense and low in calories. Encourage a meal timetable that is planned according to each day's schedule.

Rationale: Eating an inadequate number of calories from foods that are limited in nutrients can contribute to fatigue and poor nutrition. Scheduled mealtimes throughout the day will help to supply an adequate number of calories when appropriate serving sizes of nutritious food are selected.

Intervention: Describe the body's metabolic need for vitamins and minerals. Advise the client that a well-balanced diet can supply all the nutrients needed without supplementation.

Rationale: Vitamins and minerals are required for normal metabolic and physiologic functions. When taken in excess of the RDA, in the form of supplements, some nutrients can be harmful.

Intervention: Describe the interaction of zinc supplementation with copper absorption and relate to the symptom of fatigue. Inform the client that large amounts of vitamin C in excess of the RDA may decrease the availability of copper in the blood. List the toxic effects of selenium.

Rationale: Since most minerals are supplied by a varied diet, supplementation can result in toxic levels and harmful nutrient interactions.

Intervention: Advise the client to see her physician if fatigue persists or worsens.

Rationale: Poor dietary intake may act as a contributing factor to fatigue when the actual cause may be related to a systemic disease or condition.

Evaluation

The client will improve dietary habits by planning meals and snacks each day. Meal planning will accommodate the client's work schedule. The client will use the Food Guide Pyramid and the Dietary Guidelines to improve the nutritional quality and quantity of her diet. Client can state the symptoms associated with large quantities of zinc, selenium, and vitamin C and will stop taking supplements. Persistent or worsening symptoms of fatigue will prompt the client to seek the advise of a physician.

Student Readiness

1. Why has the National Research Council established ESADDIs rather than RDAs for most of the trace elements?

2. List all the nutrient interactions indicated in this chapter that decrease absorption or altered metabolism of another. Why would a dental hygienist advise a client to obtain mineral requirements from food sources rather than mineral supplements (unless ordered by a physician)?

3. Which trace minerals incorporated into enamel are beneficial? Which weaken the tooth or make it more susceptible to tooth decay?

4. Which element is involved in insulin metabolism? Why would you discourage the use of sugar and refined cereals for diabetic clients?

5. If a client is concerned about obtaining adequate amounts of trace elements, what are some suggestions that a dental hygienist can make?

6. Name some minerals that may be useful as well as toxic to clients.

References

Gerrior SA, Zizza C. Nutrient content of the U.S. food supply 1909–90. USDA, Home Economics Research Report #52, 1994.

Mertz W. Chromium in human nutrition: A review. *J Nutr* 1993; 123(4):626–633.

Pennington JAT, Young BE. Total diet study nutritional elements, 1982–1989. *J Am Diet Assoc* 1991; 91(2): 179–183.

Root EJ, Longenecker JB. Nutrition, the brain and Alzheimer's disease. *Nutr Today* 1988; 23(4):11–18.

Subcommittee on Risk Management. Dental amalgam: A public health service strategy for research, education, and regulation. US Public Health Service, 1993.

Chapter 10

Vitamins Required for Oral Soft Tissues and Salivary Glands

OBJECTIVES

The Student Will Be Able To:

- Describe oral soft tissue changes that occur in a B-complex deficiency.
- Differentiate between scientific facts versus food fads concerning vitamins.
- Discuss the role and sources of vitamin B_{12} for vegetarians.
- Compare and contrast the function, sources, surpluses or toxicities, and associated symptoms of vitamins and minerals important for healthy oral soft tissues.
- Identify dental hygiene considerations for vitamins closely involved in maintaining healthy oral soft tissues.
- Discuss nutritional directions for vitamins closely involved in maintaining healthy oral soft tissues.
- Describe the association between beriberi and alcoholism.
- Identify the most prominent oral signs of iron-deficiency anemia.

GLOSSARY OF TERMS

Signs   objective evidence of disease that is perceptible to the clinician

Symptoms   subjective evidence of abnormality as perceived by the client

Pyogenic   producing pus

Fungating   producing fungus-like growth

Filiform papillae   smooth thread-like structures on the dorsum of the tongue that are covered by a nonkeratinized epithelium

Fungiform papillae   knob-like structures on the tongue scattered throughout the filiform papillae

Thiaminase   an active enzyme that inactivates thiamin

Nystagmus   involuntary rapid movement of the eyeball

Ataxia   a gait disorder characterized by uncoordinated muscle movements

Cheilosis   cracks and sores around the corners of the mouth; the skin is scaly with red lesions

Glossitis   inflammation of the tongue

Stomatitis   inflammation of the oral mucosa

Severe sensory neuropathy   impairment of the ability to sense touch, vibration, temperature, and pinprick

Myelin   lipid substance that insulates nerve fibers and affects transmission of nerve impulses

R-binder   protein produced by the salivary glands necessary for absorption of vitamin B_{12}

Achlorhydria   decreased production of hydrochloric acid in the stomach

Glossopyrosis   pain, burning, itching, and stinging of the tongue with no apparent lesions

Avidin   a biotin-binding glycoprotein substance present in raw egg white

Test Your NQ (True/False)

1. Milk is a good source of riboflavin. T/F
2. Vitamin B_6 is the sunshine vitamin. T/F
3. Beriberi is caused by niacin deficiency. T/F
4. Strict vegetarians may be prone to vitamin B_{12} deficiency. T/F
5. Complaints of flushing and intestinal disturbances are symptoms of thiamin toxicity. T/F
6. A smooth purplish red or magenta tongue may be observed in clients with vitamin B_6 deficiency. T/F
7. Whole grains are rich in thiamin. T/F
8. Carrots are a good source of folate. T/F
9. Thiamin requirement is determined by one's caloric requirement. T/F
10. The first signs of a nutritional deficiency often occur in the oral cavity. T/F

PHYSIOLOGY OF SOFT TISSUES

The oral cavity can reflect systemic disease before other **signs** and **symptoms** become evident; it may also cause systemic problems by affecting one's nutrient intake. The oral cavity is the site of a wide variety of systemic disease manifestations for several reasons: (1) it has a rapid cellular turnover rate, (2) it is under constant assault by microorganisms, and (3) it is a trauma-intense environment.

The systemic circulation provides nutrients and removes metabolic waste products from underlying structures and the salivary glands via the blood supply.

Changes in color, size, shape, texture, and functional integrity of the oral tissues often reflect systemic nutritional disorders. Signs and symptoms in soft oral tissues can be caused by deficiencies of many of the B-complex vitamins, iron, vitamins C and K, iron, and protein (Table 10–1). Nutritional deficiencies result in similar oral signs and symptoms such as pain, erythema, atrophy of tissues, and infection. **Pyogenic** and **fungating** microorganisms cause local infections in cracked epithelial surfaces.

Approximately 90% of the saliva is produced and secreted by three paired sets of major salivary glands: the parotid, submandibular, and sublingual glands. Additionally, the lips and inner lining of the

TABLE 10–1   *Vitamins and Minerals Required for Healthy Oral Soft Tissues*

Water-Soluble Vitamins	Fat-Soluble Vitamins	Minerals
B Vitamins	Vitamin A	Iron
Thiamin		Zinc
Riboflavin		Iodine
Niacin		
Vitamin B_6		
Folate		
Vitamin B_{12}		
Pantothenic acid		
Biotin		
Vitamin C		

cheeks are equipped with hundreds of minor salivary glands.

Saliva keeps surfaces of the oral cavity healthy and lubricated, and is necessary to maintain functional integrity of taste buds. Solid substances must first be dissolved in saliva to be tasted. Healthy adults produce approximately 1.0 to 1.5 L of saliva per day. *Sympathetic* impulses influence salivary composition; *parasympathetic* stimulation increases the amount of saliva secreted. Sympathetic autonomic nerves stimulate the body in times of stress and crisis. Parasympathetic autonomic nerves balance or slow down impulses from sympathetic nerves.

Compared to plasma, saliva is *hypotonic,* with its main constituent being water. Hypotonic solutions have a lesser solute concentration than plasma. It contains more than 20 proteins and glycoproteins, and many electrolytes, including sodium, potassium, calcium, chloride, bicarbonate, inorganic phosphate, magnesium, sulfate, iodide, and fluoride. Saliva functions as a *buffer* to maintain pH in the mouth. Buffering substances increase their acid or alkali content to change the pH of the solution. The pH of unstimulated saliva is approximately 6.1, but this can increase to 7.8 at high flow rates. Antimicrobial properties of saliva provide protection as well as remove toxins such as tobacco smoke.

The entire oral cavity is lined with a nonkeratinizing mucosa, except for the hard palate, the dorsum of the tongue, and the gingivae that surround the teeth, which are covered with a keratinizing epithelium. The oral cavity may contain antigenic substances; the oral mucosa separates a potentially adverse environment from underlying connective tissue.

Mucosal cells have a very rapid turnover rate, resulting in a complete turnover in 3 to 5 days. Rapid generation of new cells in the oral epithelia provides replacement tissue for trauma resulting from friction of the teeth and mastication. Additionally, the hundreds of cells in the **filiform papillae** and **fungiform papillae** are in constant transition, from their anabolism until their catabolism.

Most of the taste buds are located on the lateral walls of the foliate and circumvallate papillae and on dorsal surfaces of the fungiform papillae of the tongue. A loss of fungiform and foliate papillae leads to loss of taste buds and changes in taste acuity.

Many filiform papillae cover the anterior two-thirds of the tongue. If the filiform papillae become denuded or atrophied, the tongue appears red and pebbled, or has a strawberry appearance. Fungiform papillae are bright red because of a rich vascular supply. Keratinized cells normally cover the fungiform papillae on the tongue surface. Chronic severe nutrient deficiencies will result in loss of fungiform papillae and a smooth red tongue.

Dental Hygiene Considerations

- Because of the rapid turnover rate of oral tissues, the first signs of nutritional deficiency are frequently evident in the oral cavity. The glossal epithelium is usually the first to be affected, followed by areas around the lips. Assess clients for oral signs of nutritional deficiencies.

- The tongue may become edematous as a result of disease or nutritional deficiency.

- Angular cheilitis (also called *cheilosis*) and glossitis are commonly associated with deficiencies of several B-complex vitamins.

- Saliva aids in the ability to speak properly, swallow, and taste foods.

- The composition of saliva influences systemic nutrition by affecting taste and determining what foods will be consumed.

- Nutrient intake does not appear to have significant effects on salivary composition except with severe malnutrition. On the other hand, saliva secretion can be affected by the types of food consumed, i.e., salivary flow is decreased when only liquids are consumed.

- Xerostomia (dry mouth) may result in increased incidence of caries, stomatitis, and gingival inflammation, and greater susceptibility to oral infections (see chapter 18).

- Saliva may be used to diagnose some local and systemic diseases and heavy-metal toxicity, such as mercury toxicity.
- ℞ Salivary secretion is controlled primarily by cholinergic parasympathetic nerves; therefore clients taking anticholinergic medications (which usually contain atropine) will exhibit decreased salivary flow. These medications may be prescribed for bradycardia (low heart rate), diarrhea, peptic ulcers, and occasionally asthma.

Nutritional Directions

- ◆ Saliva helps maintain the integrity of the teeth, tongue, and mucous membranes of the oral and oropharyngeal areas.
- ◆ Nutritional abnormalities affect oral soft tissues in a variety of ways.

THIAMIN (VITAMIN B₁)
Physiologic Roles

Thiamin functions as a coenzyme in metabolism of energy nutrients via the Krebs cycle to produce energy. This role makes it crucial for normal functioning of the brain, nerves, muscles, and heart. However, the main effects of thiamin deficiency are disturbances of carbohydrate metabolism, which is impossible without thiamin. Thiamin is also a necessary component in the synthesis of niacin and helps regulate appetite. It is a constituent of enzymes that degrade sucrose to organic acids that can ultimately dissolve tooth enamel.

Requirements

Because thiamin is involved in utilizing carbohydrates as calories, the requirement is based on total caloric need. The RDA for adults is 0.5 mg/1,000 Cal, or a minimum intake of 1 mg/day for clients consuming less than 2,000 Cal/day. Participation in rigorous physical activity utilizes more energy, so more thiamin is required. Also, requirements are increased by pregnancy, fever, hyperthyroidism, cardiac conditions, and alcoholism.

Sources

Thiamin is widely distributed in foods, and intake of a variety of foods, including whole grains or enriched grains, can ensure adequate amounts (Table 10–2). Approximately 40% of thiamin intake is provided by grain products or unrefined and enriched cereals and grains. In the meat group, pork is an exceptionally good source. Other good sources include nuts and legumes.

Hypo- States

Thiamin is required for metabolism of carbohydrates, proteins, and fats; therefore, a wide range of symptoms develops with insufficient intake. Primary dietary deficiency usually occurs in developing countries, where polished rice is the staple diet. In developed countries, thiamin deficiency is secondary to alcoholism, ingestion of raw fish containing microbial **thiaminases,** chronic febrile states, and total parenteral nutrition. Cooking deactivates thiaminases. Thiamin deficiency may also occur in malnourished homeless people and Southeast Asian immigrants to the United States.

Thiamin is called the "morale vitamin" because short-term deficiency causes clients to become depressed, irritable, anorexic, fatigued, and unable to concentrate. The brain and central nervous system (CNS), almost entirely dependent upon glucose for energy, are seriously impaired when thiamin is not available.

Severe thiamin deficiency results in beriberi, which causes extensive damage to the nervous and cardiovascular systems. *Beriberi* means "I cannot"; clients with this severe thiamin deficiency cannot move easily. The classic chronic form of beriberi presents with impairment of both sensory and motor function without involvement of the CNS. Other symptoms include muscular wasting (dry beriberi), edema (wet beriberi), deep muscle

TABLE 10–2   *Thiamin Content of Selected Foods*

Food	Portion	Thiamin (mg)	Calories (per serving)
Brewer's yeast	1 Tbsp	1.3	25
Lean broiled pork chop	3 oz	0.83	218
Sunflower seeds	¼ c	0.82	205
Baked ham	3 oz	0.62	151
Wheat germ	¼ c	0.54	103
Cooked oatmeal	1 c	0.26	145
Cooked Eastern oysters	3 oz	0.25	117
Green peas, frozen	½ c	0.23	63
Black beans	½ c	0.21	114
Baked acorn squash	½ c	0.17	58
Baked potato	1	0.16	145
Cooked split peas	½ c	0.15	115
Kidney beans	½ c	0.14	113
Watermelon	1 c	0.13	51
White bread	1	0.12	67
Orange	1	0.11	62
Lean broiled sirloin steak	3 oz	0.11	176
Whole-wheat bread	1	0.10	69
Peanuts	¼ c	0.09	209
Baked winter squash	½ c	0.09	40
Blackeyed/cowpeas	½ c	0.08	80

Nutrient data from Nutritionist IV software, First Data Bank; San Bruno, CA. From Davis JR, Sherer K. *Applied Nutrition and Diet Therapy for Nurses,* 2nd ed. Philadelphia: W.B. Saunders, 1994.

pain in the calf, peripheral paralysis, tachycardia, and an enlarged heart.

Whether or not a thiamin deficiency is evident in oral tissues is controversial. Some clinicians have associated a flabby, red, and edematous tongue with thiamin deficiency (see Color Plate 5). The fungiform papillae enlarge and become hyperemic and gingival. Tissues sometimes present an "old rose" color.

Beriberi associated with alcoholism is characterized by mental confusion, **nystagmus,** and **ataxia.** These symptoms occur most frequently in malnourished alcoholics. Alcohol intake increases thiamin requirement; also, total nutrient intake is usually poor in alcoholics. Early diagnosis is essential to initiate thiamin therapy early in the

course of the disease and to prevent permanent damage and death.

Dental Hygiene Considerations

- A careful dietary history, including a clinical assessment of the oral cavity, alcohol consumption, and activity level, helps identify early stages of thiamin deficiency.

- Vitamin deficiencies seldom occur in isolation. If a deficiency is suspected, symptoms of other vitamin B deficiencies may also be present.

- Because thiamin is essential for carbohydrate metabolism, a thiamin deficiency is closely linked to aberrations of brain function. For clients who are confused or have altered thought processes, assess nutrient intake.

- Carbohydrate loading or a very high-carbohydrate diet and high physical activity slightly increase the thiamin requirement. (Generally increased intake results in increased thiamin consumption.)
- Although immediate clinical response to thiamin therapy is often dramatic, ultimate recovery may be incomplete, and relapses may occur, especially if precipitating factors persist.

Nutritional Directions

- Raw fish contains an active enzyme, thiaminase, which destroys thiamin.
- Baking soda added to cooking water to enhance the color of vegetables destroys thiamin.
- Overcooking and high temperatures destroy thiamin.
- ℞ Antacids reduce utilization of thiamin.
- ℞ Some diuretics can increase thiamin excretion.

RIBOFLAVIN (VITAMIN B₂)

Physiologic Roles

Riboflavin functions as a coenzyme in the metabolism of carbohydrate, protein, and fat to release cellular energy. Closely related to the metabolism of protein, all conditions requiring increases in protein (e.g., burns or growth spurts) lead to additional riboflavin requirements. Riboflavin is also essential for healthy eyes and maintenance of mucous membranes. Along with thiamin, riboflavin is necessary for synthesis of niacin.

Requirements

The National Research Council has recommended a minimum intake of 1.2 mg/day for all adults (0.6 mg/1,000 Cal), with an allowance of 1.7 mg for men and 1.3 mg for women. This level is influenced by individual caloric requirements. Additionally, when nitrogen balance is positive, more riboflavin is retained.

Sources

Although milk and milk products are excellent sources of riboflavin, approximately 30% of the dietary intake is furnished by foods in the grain group (Table 10–3). Meat, poultry, and fish also provide about one-fourth of the dietary requirement.

Hypo- States

The body carefully guards its limited riboflavin stores. Even in severe deficiency as much as one-third of the normal amount is present in the liver, kidney, and heart. Primary riboflavin deficiency is uncommon but is encountered in those with multiple nutrient deficiencies as a result of poor nutrient absorption or utilization. Since riboflavin is essential to the functioning of vitamin B₆ and niacin, riboflavin deficiency will lead to symptoms related to secondary deficiency of these nutrients.

Symptoms associated with riboflavin deficiency include angular **cheilosis, glossitis,** dermatitis, and anemia (see Color Plate 6). These symptoms may be observed within 8 weeks when intake has been inadequate. Along with angular cheilosis, the lips may become extremely red and smooth. Fungiform papillae become swollen and slightly flattened and mushroom shaped during early stages of riboflavin deficiency; the tongue has a pebbly or granular appearance. Severe chronic deficiencies lead to progressive papillary atrophy and patchy, irregular denudation of the tongue. The tongue may become purplish red or magenta colored because of vascular proliferation and decreased circulation. In more advanced cases, the entire tongue may become atrophic and smooth

TABLE 10–3   *Riboflavin Content of Selected Foods*

Food	Portion	Riboflavin (mg)	Calories (per serving)
Beef liver	3 oz	3.48	137
Braunschweiger sausage	3 oz	1.30	305
Ricotta cheese	1 c	0.46	340
Cheddar cheese	1 c	0.42	455
Milk	1 c	0.41	86–150
Buttermilk	1 c	0.38	99
Low-fat cottage cheese	1 c	0.37	164
Brewer's yeast	1 Tbsp	0.34	25
Cooked Eastern oysters	3 oz	0.28	117
Almonds	¼ c	0.25	192
Baked lean pork loin	3 oz	0.22	204
Cooked spinach	½ c	0.21	21
Cooked beet greens	½ c	0.21	20
Canned salmon	3 oz	0.16	118
Raw mushrooms	½ c	0.16	9
Beef, lean	3 oz	0.15	151
Turkey breast	3 oz	0.11	115
Cooked asparagus	½ c	0.09	25
Cooked broccoli	½ c	0.08	26

Nutrient data from Nutritionist IV software, First Data Bank; San Bruno, CA. From Davis JR, Sherer K. *Applied Nutrition and Diet Therapy for Nurses,* 2nd ed. Philadelphia: W.B. Saunders, 1994.

(see Color Plate 7). These symptoms, especially glossitis and dermatitis, may actually be secondary to vitamin B_6 deficiency.

Dental Hygiene Considerations

- Hyperthyroidism, fevers, the added stress of injuries or surgery, and malabsorption syndromes increase riboflavin requirements. Assess clients with these conditions for signs of deficiency: cheilitis, papillary atrophy, glossitis, and dermatitis.
- Congenital facial abnormalities may occur if the mother is deficient in riboflavin at the time of conception.
- Bilateral cheilosis may not be riboflavin deficiency; improperly constructed dentures and aging also may contribute to cheilosis.
- ℞ Phenothiazines and antibiotics increase

excretion of riboflavin, so monitor for a deficiency in those clients on long-term therapy.

Nutritional Directions

- Enriched products provide more riboflavin than their whole-grain counterparts.
- Lighted display cases have the potential to cause decomposition of riboflavin when milk is marketed in translucent plastic containers.
- A mixed diet that contains a pint of milk and 4 to 6 oz of meat daily ensures an adequate riboflavin supply.
- Vegans are at risk of developing riboflavin deficiency.
- Toxicity symptoms are not observed with oral consumption of riboflavin.

NIACIN

Physiologic Roles

The term *niacin* is loosely used to refer to two compounds, nicotinic acid and nicotinamide. Both compounds are utilized by the body. Niacin is crucial as a coenzyme in energy (ATP) production. It functions with riboflavin in glucose production and metabolism and is also involved in lipid and protein metabolism.

Niacin is essential for growth of cariogenic oral microorganisms. It also functions in enzymes involved in the microbial degradation of sucrose to produce organic acids.

Requirements

The body obtains niacin not only directly from the diet, but also indirectly from conversion of an amino acid, tryptophan, and possibly also from synthesis by intestinal microorganisms. RDAs are given in terms of niacin equivalents (NE) that include dietary sources of niacin plus its precursor, tryptophan. Approximately 1 mg of niacin may be formed from 60 mg of dietary tryptophan. Niacin requirements are related to caloric intake. The RDA niacin equivalent for adults is between 13 and 19 mg (6.6 mg/1,000 Cal) daily.

Sources

Tryptophan is found mainly in milk, eggs, and meats. Niacin is widely distributed in plant and animal foods. Good sources include meats, cereals, legumes, seeds, and nuts (Table 10–4). The RDA for niacin equivalents is easily met with foods high in niacin plus those having tryptophan. Approximately 65% of the niacin in the U.S. diet is provided from meat, milk, and eggs.

TABLE 10–4 *Niacin Content of Selected Foods*

Food	Portion	Niacin (mg)	Calories (per serving)
Beef liver	3 oz	9.12	137
Baked chicken breast	3 oz	6.65	156
Broiled halibut	3 oz	6.06	119
Broiled lean lamb chop	3 oz	5.57	200
Canned salmon	3 oz	5.56	118
Turkey, white meat	3 oz	5.35	168
Peanuts	¼ c	5.15	212
Canned tuna	3 oz	4.93	116
Sardines	3 oz	4.47	177
Broiled lean sirloin	3 oz	3.65	176
Brewer's yeast	1 Tbsp	3.00	25
Turkey, dark meat	3 oz	3.00	188
Cooked shrimp	3 oz	2.20	84
Baked potato	1	2.18	145
Peanut butter	1 Tbsp	2.09	94
Wheat germ	¼ c	2.00	104

Nutrient data from Nutritionist IV software, First Data Bank; San Bruno, CA. From Davis JR, Sherer K. *Applied Nutrition and Diet Therapy for Nurses,* 2nd ed. Philadelphia: W.B. Saunders, 1994.

Hyper- and Hypo- States

Supplemental doses of nicotinic acid (3 to 6 gm/day) have been recommended to lower serum cholesterol and triglyceride levels. (Nicotinamide will not function in this role.) The use of 250 mg of nicotinic acid daily results in the vitamin functioning as a vasodilator, producing flushing of the skin, nausea, itching, tachycardia, fainting, and blurred vision. Because the body is able to store some niacin, larger doses may lead to serious problems, including abnormal liver function and gout (see Nutrition Update 10).

Niacin deficiency is usually associated with a maize (corn) diet, since corn products contain all the essential amino acids except tryptophan. This increases the body's requirements for tryptophan and niacin. The deficiency is also seen in alcoholics, but is unlikely in individuals who consume adequate protein levels. Niacin deficiency results in degeneration of the skin, gastrointestinal tract, and nervous system, a condition known as *pellagra.* Symptoms of pellagra have been referred to as "the 3 D's—dermatitis, diarrhea, and depression or dementia." The term *pellagra* is derived from the Latin word for animal hide; the skin may be rough and look like goose flesh. The most striking and characteristic sign of pellagra is a reddish skin rash, especially on the face, hands, or feet, that is always bilaterally symmetrical (i.e., it appears on both sides of the body at the same time) (Fig. 10–1). It flares up when the skin is exposed to strong sunlight. Neurologic symptoms include depression, apathy, headache, fatigue, and loss of memory. If untreated, death may occur.

Deficiency also affects mucous membranes: (1) painful **stomatitis** causes diminished food intake; (2) lesions in the gastrointestinal tract result in diarrhea and less vitamin absorption. Pellagrous glossitis begins with swelling of the papillae at the tip and lateral borders of the tongue. The tongue becomes painful, scarlet, and edematous. Atrophic changes involve loss of the filiform and fungiform papillae, and the tongue becomes smooth and shiny. The mucosa is also reddened. Fissures occur in the epithelium and along the sides of the tongue; these become infected rapidly. The gingivae may become inflamed, resembling that found in acute necrotizing ulcerative gingivitis (see Color Plate 8). (Dreizen, 1971). The corners of the lips are initially pale; fanlike fissuring occurs that radiates into the perioral epithelium and may leave permanent scars.

Dental Hygiene Considerations

- Assess clients, especially alcoholics and immigrants, for oral signs of niacin deficiency: complaints of a nonspecific burn-

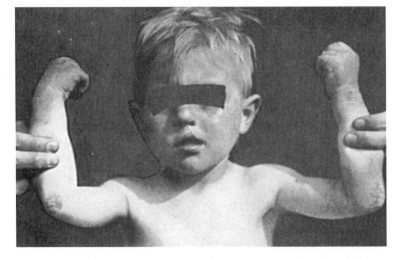

FIGURE 10–1 **Pellagra in a 3-year-old boy: lesions on the hands and elbows and an early lesion over the nose and malar eminences. (From Behrman RE, Vaughan VC.** *Nelson Textbook of Pediatrics.* **14th ed. Philadelphia: W.B. Saunders, 1992.)**

ing sensation through the oral cavity; smooth, shiny, bright red tongue swollen at the tip and lateral margins; stomatitis and red and inflamed marginal and attached gingiva.

- Niacin and thiamin may affect the appetite; however, weight-conscious clients should not avoid these vitamins. Evaluate beliefs concerning these two vitamins.
- The presence of niacin may stimulate cariogenic oral flora, thus playing a role in the dental caries process when it is available.

R Prolonged treatment with isoniazid for tuberculosis may lead to niacin deficiency. Therefore, niacin supplements may be prescribed by the physician to prevent deficiency.

Nutritional Directions

- Clients should understand that a frequent side effect of a therapeutic dose of nicotinic acid is flushing. This should be discussed with the physician.
- *Nicotinic acid* and *niacinamide* are correct terms for niacin and should not be confused with nicotine.

VITAMIN B$_6$ (PYRIDOXINE)

Vitamin B$_6$ is the term commonly used for this group of three compounds, pyridoxine, pyridoxal, and pyridoxamine. All three forms can be utilized by the body in their roles as coenzymes.

Physiologic Roles

Several essential roles for vitamin B$_6$ have been identified. In addition to (1) its role as a coenzyme in protein metabolism, vitamin B$_6$ plays a part in (2) conversion of tryptophan to niacin, (3) hemoglobin synthesis, (4) synthesis of unsaturated fatty acids from essential fatty acids, (5) energy production from glycogen, and (6) proper functioning of the nervous system including brain cells.

Requirements

The current RDA for vitamin B$_6$ is 2.0 mg/day for men and 1.6 mg/day for women. The requirement for vitamin B$_6$ increases with protein intake because of its major role in amino acid metabolism. Limited amounts of vitamin B$_6$ are produced by microorganisms in the digestive tract.

Sources

Beef, poultry, fish, and pork are good sources of vitamin B$_6$. Other good sources include some fruits, nuts, whole-grain products, and vegetables (Table 10–5). Foods from animal and plant sources provide 48% and 52% of the total vitamin B$_6$ intake, respectively.

Absorption and Excretion

Absorption of vitamin B$_6$ differs from other B-complex vitamins. All three forms of the vitamin are converted to an absorbable form by an intestinal enzyme. Body stores are small, and repletion is gradual.

Hyper- and Hypo- States

Numerous studies have been presented regarding the benefits of providing supplemental amounts of vitamin B$_6$ in coronary heart disease, cancer, and premenstrual syndrome. Because of inconsistent findings, supplemental amounts are not currently recommended. Acute pyridoxine toxicity is uncommon; however, routine consumption of megadoses (more than 2 gm for 2 months or more) has documented side effects such as ataxia and **severe sensory neuropathy,** and, in some instances, bone pain and muscle weakness. In most cases, complete recovery occurs with discontinuation of megadose supplementation.

Deficiency rarely occurs alone; vitamin B$_6$

TABLE 10–5   *Pyridoxine (Vitamin B₆) Content of Selected Foods*

Food	Portion	Pyridoxine (mg)	Calories (per serving)
Beef liver	3 oz	0.77	137
Banana	1	0.66	105
Navy peas	½ c	0.53	113
Baked potato	1	0.47	145
Baked chicken breast	3 oz	0.47	168
Sunflower seeds	¼ c	0.45	205
Salmon	3 oz	0.39	157
Turkey	3 oz	0.39	145
Tuna fish	3 oz	0.37	116
Wheat germ	¼ c	0.37	103
Watermelon	1 c	0.23	51
Cooked spinach	½ c	0.22	21
Baked flounder	3 oz	0.20	99
Brewer's yeast	1 Tbsp	0.20	25
Cantaloupe	1 c	0.18	56
Pinto beans	½ c	0.13	118
Cauliflower	½ c	0.13	15
Cooked asparagus	½ c	0.13	23

Nutrient data from Nutritionist IV software, First Data Bank; San Bruno, CA. From Davis JR, Sherer K. *Applied Nutrition and Diet Therapy for Nurses,* 2nd ed. Philadelphia: W.B. Saunders, 1994.

deficiency is most commonly observed along with several other B vitamins. Clinical signs include CNS abnormalities or epileptiform convulsions, dermatitis with cheilosis and glossitis, impaired immune responses, and anemia. Pyridoxine deficiency-induced glossitis is denoted by pain, edema, and papillary changes. Initially, the tongue has a scalded sensation, followed by reddening and hypertrophy of the filiform papillae at the tip, margins, and dorsum. The filiform papillae remain as red dots but may not be visible because of swelling of the tongue; the fungiform papillae are obvious as hypertrophied red knobs (Dreizen, 1984).

A mother's body stores of vitamin B₆ are critical to the well-being of her newborn infant. Oral contraceptive agents (OCAs) taken before conception may lower maternal vitamin B₆ levels during pregnancy and in breast milk. A daily intake of 2 mg of vitamin B₆ may be recommended for women taking OCAs, especially if a pregnancy is planned in the near future.

Dental Hygiene Considerations

- Clients may present with pain of the tongue which precedes redness and swelling of the tip of the tongue. Eventually atrophy of papillae results in a smooth, purplish tongue. Angular cheilitis, oral ulcers, and stomatitis may also be noted.

- Intake of this vitamin may decrease with increasing age, poor education, and lower income status. Therefore, encourage foods high in vitamin B₆ and monitor for deficiency signs and symptoms.

- In animal studies, the presence of pyridoxine alters oral flora and reduces dental caries incidence.

℞ Use of drugs that affect the metabolism of vitamin B_6 warrants vitamin B_6 supplementation to avoid secondary vitamin B_6 deficiency. These drugs include isoniazid and cycloserine (for tuberculosis), penicillamine (for Wilson's disease, lead poisoning, kidney stones, arthritis), and oral contraceptive agents.

℞ Excessive pyridoxine can reduce clinical benefits of levodopa therapy in Parkinson's disease. Encourage client to limit intake of foods fortified with vitamin B_6 and avoid vitamin B_6 supplements. If the desired effects of the drug are not seen or if over-the-counter supplements are being taken, refer the client to the physician.

Nutritional Directions

- Vitamin B_6 supplements should not be taken unless ordered by a physician.
- If supplements are needed, signs and symptoms will improve within 1 week.
- Adequate daily intake of vitamin B_6 is important.
- Vitamin B_6 is removed during grain processing and not replaced during enrichment; therefore, whole-grain breads and cereals are better sources.

FOLATE/FOLIC ACID

The generic term *folate* encompasses several compounds that have nutritional properties similar to those of folic acid. Several different metabolically active forms have been identified.

Physiologic Roles

Folate functions as a coenzyme for approximately 20 enzymes. As such, it has an important role in synthesis of RNA and DNA. It functions in conjunction with vitamins B_{12} and C in maintaining normal levels of mature red blood cells. Purine, pyrimidine, methionine, and choline synthesis are interrelated with vitamin B_{12}.

Requirements

The RDA is 200 mcg for adult males and 180 mcg for females. Folate requirements are increased during periods of growth and development, such as adolescence, pregnancy, and lactation, because of its role in DNA formulation.

Sources

Rich sources of folate include liver, green leafy vegetables, legumes, and some fruits (grapefruit and oranges), as shown in Table 10–6. The FDA has mandated that by 1998, manufacturers must fortify enriched bread, pasta, and cereal products with specific amounts of folic acid.

Absorption and Excretion

Dietary folates must undergo some changes for their absorption. The intestinal enzyme that accomplishes this requires a slightly acidic pH and is activated by the presence of zinc. Naturally occurring folate is not always as well absorbed as supplements, and persons needing larger amounts may need a supplement in addition to fortified folate-rich foods (Cuskelly, 1996).

Hyper- and Hypo- States

In large doses, folate may cause kidney damage and mask symptoms of vitamin B_{12} deficiency. The FDA recommends less than 1 mg (or 1,000 mcg) of folate daily to avoid toxicity.

Folate deficiency, the most common vitamin deficiency among the B-complex vitamins, may occur secondary to excessive alcohol consumption, gastrointestinal disease, or medications that interfere with folate absorption and/or metabolism (Table 10–7).

TABLE 10–6 *Folate Content of Selected Foods*

Food	Portion	Folate (mcg)	Calories (per serving)
Brewer's yeast	1 Tbsp	313	25
Beef liver	3 oz	184	137
Pinto beans	½ c	147	118
Cooked spinach	½ c	131	21
Cooked asparagus	½ c	89	22
Sunflower seeds	¼ c	82	205
Romaine lettuce	1 c	76	9
Orange juice	½ c	55	56
Dry roasted peanuts	¼ c	53	214
Sliced beets	½ c	45	26
Cooked broccoli	½ c	39	22
Navy beans	½ c	33	113
Cooked turnip greens	½ c	33	25
Cooked cauliflower	½ c	32	15
Cantaloupe	1 c	27	56
Egg, poached	1	18	74
Banana	1	22	105
Wheat germ	1 Tbsp	20	26
Baked potato	1	14	145
Peanut butter	1 Tbsp	13	94

Nutrient data from Nutritionist IV software, First Data Bank; San Bruno, CA. From Davis JR, Sherer K. *Applied Nutrition and Diet Therapy for Nurses,* 2nd ed. Philadelphia: W.B. Saunders, 1994.

Deficiency symptoms first appear in rapidly dividing cells, such as in the gastrointestinal tract, red blood cells (RBCs), and white blood cells. RBCs do not develop normally; they become pale and extremely large (megaloblastic) yet cannot transport oxygen to cells, a condition known as *megaloblastic anemia.* Folic acid deficiency during pregnancy is associated with an increased risk of spina bifida and other neural tube defects and may reduce heart disease risk (Boushey et al., 1995). Approximately 1 million persons in the United States, mostly elderly, suffer from a form of megaloblastic anemia known as *pernicious anemia* (Anonymous, 1993).

Glossitis is usually present in persons with folic acid deficiency. The tongue becomes fiery red and papillae are absent (see Color Plate 9). Marked chronic periodontitis with loosening of the teeth may occur (see Color Plate 10). Folic acid deficiency impairs immune responses and resistance of the oral mucosa to penetration by pathogenic organisms such as *Candida.*

TABLE 10–7 *Drugs That May Negatively Affect Folate Status**

Anticonvulsants

Oral contraceptives

Analgesics

Cancer chemotherapeutic agents

Anti-inflammatory agents

H$_2$-receptor blockers

Antacids

*Nutritional status may be negatively affected because of interference with folate absorption and/or metabolism.

From Davis JR, Sherer K. *Applied Nutrition and Diet Therapy for Nurses,* 2nd ed. Philadelphia: W.B. Saunders, 1994.

Dental Hygiene Considerations

- Evaluate oral status for folate deficiency. Observe for swelling and pallor or reddening of the tip of the tongue (depending on the degree of anemia) with atrophy of filiform papillae, reddening of the fungiform papillae at the tip and laterally, and formation of small ulcers. Posterior progression eventually leads to complete atrophy of the filiform papillae and the formation of bright red spots (fungiform papillae). Cheilitis and painful ulcerations of the buccal mucosa and palatal and gingival epithelia may also occur.

- Factors that increase the metabolic rate, such as infection and hyperthyroidism, or that increase the cellular turnover rate, such as a malignancy, increase folate requirement. Assess for folate intake by questioning about dietary intake.

- Folic acid supplementation may improve resistance to the development of periodontal inflammation.

- ℞ Folate absorption decreases when folate is given with anticonvulsants and OCAs.

Increased gingival inflammation has been associated with OCAs. Encourage women taking birth control pills to increase their consumption of folate-rich foods.

℞ Phenytoin (Dilantin) is associated with gingival overgrowth. Folate supplementation reduces the severity and incidence of this overgrowth. However, clients taking anticonvulsants should be carefully monitored if folate supplements are prescribed because high intakes can decrease effectiveness of the medication.

Nutritional Directions

- ◆ Folate may be called *folic acid* or *folacin*.
- ◆ Prolonged cooking destroys folate.
- ◆ Folate is easily destroyed by food processing; raw vegetables provide more folate than cooked ones.
- ◆ Daily intake of 0.4 mg folic acid before and during early pregnancy reduces the risk of neural tube defects by approximately 60% (Werler et al., 1993).
- ◆ Orange juice is a good source of folate since vitamin C protects it from deterioration.

VITAMIN B$_{12}$

Vitamin B$_{12}$, or *cobalamin,* represents a complex group of compounds that contain cobalt. (The only known function of cobalt is as an integral component of vitamin B$_{12}$.) It is the only vitamin that contains a mineral.

Physiologic Roles

Vitamin B$_{12}$ functions as a coenzyme in conjunction with folate metabolism in nucleic acid synthesis. It also functions in the catabolism of certain amino acids and fatty acids. Vitamin B$_{12}$ is essential for making red blood cells and for myelin synthesis.

Requirements

The RDA for adults is small, 2 mcg daily. A high vitamin B$_{12}$ intake results in accumulation in the

liver with increasing age, but this may be desirable because serum vitamin B$_{12}$ levels decline in the elderly because of lower absorption rates.

Sources

Microorganisms (bacteria, fungi, and algae) can synthesize vitamin B$_{12}$. Vitamin B$_{12}$ is not found in plants unless they are contaminated by microorganisms (legumes and root vegetables). More than 80% of dietary vitamin B$_{12}$ is provided by meat and animal products (Table 10–8). Gastrointestinal flora produce small amounts of absorbable vitamin B$_{12}$.

Absorption and Excretion

Vitamin B$_{12}$ from food is released from its polypeptide linkages by gastric acid and enzymes in

TABLE 10–8   *Vitamin B$_{12}$ Content of Selected Foods*

Food	Portion	Vitamin B$_{12}$ (mcg)	Calories (per serving)
Beef liver	3 oz	60.5	137
Cooked Eastern oysters	3 oz	32.5	117
Fortified oak flakes	1 c	2.5	177
Cooked lean beef	3 oz	2.2	175
Cooked shrimp	3 oz	1.3	84
Protein fortified low-fat milk	1 c	1.1	137
Broiled lean pork chop	3 oz	0.8	295
Whole egg	1	0.4	74
Baked chicken breast	3 oz	0.3	168
Cheddar cheese	1 oz	0.2	114

Nutrient data from Nutritionist IV software, First Data Bank; San Bruno, CA. From Davis JR, Sherer K. *Applied Nutrition and Diet Therapy for Nurses,* 2nd ed. Philadelphia: W.B. Saunders, 1994.

the stomach and intestine. Free vitamin B$_{12}$ combines with salivary **R-binder** in the stomach. In the small intestine, trypsin (pancreatic enzyme) removes the R-binder, and vitamin B$_{12}$ combines with *intrinsic factor,* secreted by the parietal cells in the stomach. Absorption of vitamin B$_{12}$ occurs at specific receptor sites in the ileum and is possible only if it is bound to intrinsic factor. The vitamin is recycled from bile and other intestinal secretions. Excessive amounts are bound to a protein and stored for up to 3 to 4 years in the liver, or they are excreted.

Hyper- and Hypo- States

No benefits are seen from large quantities of vitamin B$_{12}$, but no harmful effects have been observed either. Injections of vitamin B$_{12}$ are popular treatments for fatigue and weakness, but few individuals meet accepted medical criteria for its use.

A deficiency of vitamin B$_{12}$ is rarely caused by insufficient dietary sources unless strict vegan diets are followed. Lack of intrinsic factor is the primary cause of deficiency. Pernicious anemia (a megaloblastic anemia) occurs frequently in the elderly relative to **achlorhydria** and decreased synthesis of

intrinsic factor by the parietal cells. Deficiency symptoms develop very slowly.

Initial oral symptoms of vitamin B$_{12}$ present with **glossopyrosis,** followed by swelling and pallor with eventual disappearance of the filiform and fungiform papillae. The tongue may be completely smooth, shiny, and deeply reddened (see Color Plate 11). Bright-red, diffuse, excruciating painful lesions may occur in the buccal and pharyngeal mucosa and undersurface of the tongue (Dreizen, 1971). An oral examination may reveal stomatitis or a pale or yellowish mucosa.

Neurologic symptoms occur as a consequence of demyelination of the nerves. Deficiency symptoms are rapidly corrected with vitamin B$_{12}$ injections.

In a totally vegan community, children with vitamin B$_{12}$ deficiency may have stunted growth. Other symptoms include *anorexia,* altered taste sensation, abdominal pain, and general weakness.

Dental Hygiene Considerations

● Assess for oral signs of deficiency: signs and symptoms of vitamin B$_{12}$ deficiency are similar to those of folic acid deficiency, except that burning tongue pain precedes physical signs of vitamin B$_{12}$ deficiency.

- Without R-binder and/or intrinsic factor, absorption of vitamin B_{12} is drastically reduced. Thus, clients with xerostomia may have poor absorption of vitamin B_{12}.
- Concomitant ingestion of megadoses of ascorbic acid via foods or tablets can destroy substantial amounts of vitamin B_{12} and produce vitamin B_{12} deficiency. If the client is prone to or has vitamin B_{12} deficiency and takes large amounts of vitamin C supplements, advise him or her to decrease vitamin C intake to approximate RDA levels.

- Clients who have had permanent gastric surgery or ileal damage require monthly injections of vitamin B_{12} for life.

Nutritional Directions

- Because vitamin B_{12} is found only in meat products, vegans (i.e., strict vegetarians) require vitamin B_{12}-fortified foods or a daily supplement.
- Vitamin B_{12} shots are not a panacea for "tired blood."

PANTOTHENIC ACID
Physiologic Roles

Pantothenic acid is similar to the other B vitamins in its metabolic roles. Pantothenic acid plays a key role in carbohydrate, fat, and protein metabolism. Additionally, it is important in synthesis and degradation of triglycerides, phospholipids, and sterols, and in formation of certain hormones and nerve-regulating substances.

Requirement

In 1989, the National Research Council subcommittee concluded that there is insufficient evidence to establish a RDA for pantothenic acid. Thus, an ESADDI of 4 to 7 mg/day was established for adults.

Sources

Pantothenic acid is synthesized by most microorganisms and plants. It is particularly abundant in animal foods, legumes, and whole-grain cereals. Bacteria in the digestive tract also produce

pantothenic acid. The usual intake of pantothenic acid in the United States is reported to be 5 to 10 mg/day.

Hypo- States

Naturally occurring dietary deficiency of pantothenic acid has not been documented.

Dental Hygiene Considerations

- Pantothenic deficiency rarely occurs alone but may occur along with other B-vitamin deficiencies.
- Pantothenic acid may help in wound healing, so ensure that clients facing oral or periodontal surgery are eating a well-balanced diet.

Nutritional Directions

- Distribution of this vitamin is widespread.
- Diets including whole-grain unprocessed foods contain more pantothenic acid.

BIOTIN
Physiologic Roles

Biotin functions as a coenzyme in metabolism of carbohydrate, protein, and fat.

Requirements

The dietary requirement of biotin is uncertain because intestinal microflora synthesize it. The

TABLE 10–9   *Biotin Content of Selected Foods*

Food	Portion	Biotin (mcg)	Calories (per serving)
Cooked cauliflower	½ c	10.7	15
Egg, poached	1	10.0	74
Brewer's yeast	1 Tbsp	6.4	25
Watermelon	1 c	6.4	51
Peanut butter	1 Tbsp	6.4	94
Cooked spinach	½ c	5.7	21
Cantaloupe	1 c	4.8	56
Banana	1	4.6	105

Nutrient data from Nutritionist IV software, First Data Bank; San Bruno, CA. From Davis JR, Sherer K. *Applied Nutrition and Diet Therapy for Nurses,* 2nd ed. Philadelphia: W.B. Saunders, 1994.

ESADDI for biotin has been established at 30 to 100 mcg for adults.

Sources

While biotin is widely distributed in foods, its availability is low compared to that of other water-soluble vitamins (Table 10–9). Rich sources of biotin include egg yolk, liver, and cereals. Microflora in the gastrointestinal tract probably provide part of the body's needs.

Hypo- States

Biotin deficiency can be produced by the ingestion of **avidin.** Avidin is denatured by heat; therefore, cooked egg white does not present a problem. Twenty-five to 30 egg whites per day can produce anorexia, nausea, vomiting, glossitis, pallor, depression, and a dry scaly dermatitis.

Oral signs of biotin deficiency are pallor of the tongue and patchy atrophy of the lingual papillae.

While the pattern resembles geographic tongue, it is confined to the lateral margins or is generalized to the entire dorsum.

Dental Hygiene Considerations

- Assess clients for signs of deficiency: glossitis, lingual and mucous pallor, papillae atrophy.
- ℞ Antibiotics reduce the production of biotin by intestinal bacteria.

Nutritional Directions

- Drinking or eating large amounts of raw egg whites over a long period of time may lead to biotin deficiency.
- Eggs should be cooked to decrease avidin's binding capacity and to minimize the danger of salmonella poisoning.
- A balanced diet that includes a variety of foods will contain adequate amounts of biotin.

OTHER VITAMINS

As you have already learned, most nutrients perform more than one physiologic function. Although one nutrient may appear to be more important in calcified structures, and of lesser importance in oral soft structures, its roles actually are equally important. The following nutrients have been discussed in previous chapters, but they have important functions in soft oral tissues that the dental hygienist should not overlook.

Vitamin C

Vitamin C is involved in improving the host defense mechanism by ensuring optimal activity of white blood cells. Thus, it has an important role in protecting soft oral tissues from infections caused by bacterial toxins and antigens as well as protecting tooth enamel from plaque microorganisms.

Vitamin C's role in collagen formation is well known. Vitamin C deficiency causes weakened collagen, leading to gingivitis and poor wound healing (see Color Plate 12).

Vitamin A

Vitamin A, necessary for maintaining the integrity of epithelial tissues, is a significant factor in the development and maintenance of salivary glands. Large amounts of vitamin A have an antikeratinizing effect on epithelial cells. Vitamin A increases synthesis of cellular proteins that stimulate growth and influence metabolism.

Vitamin A deficiency produces squamous metaplasia with keratin production in the duct cells of salivary glands. This results in decreased salivary secretion and xerostomia. Oral and oropharyngeal cancers have been associated with vitamin A deficiency in humans.

Vitamin E

As discussed in Chapter 7, cell membranes contain polyunsaturated fatty acids that are susceptible to peroxidation. Vitamin E plays a major role as an antioxidant to neutralize free radicals, especially in membranes that contain a large proportion of unsaturated fatty acids. Not only does it prevent inflammation of the periodontium, but it promotes the integrity of cell membranes of the mucosa. Low plasma vitamin E levels are highly correlated with atrophy of filiform papillae of the tongue (Drinka et al., 1993).

Dental Hygiene Considerations

- One of the first signs of vitamin C deficiency is increased susceptibility to infections. During later stages, the gingivae become reddened and swollen, and bleed easily; also collagenous structure is weakened and wound healing is slow.
- Vitamin C supplementation has been shown to decrease permeability of the sulcular epithelium and to increase collagen synthesis.
- Parotid gland enlargement has been associated with deficiencies of vitamins A and C and protein malnutrition.
- Vitamin A has been used to treat oral mucosal conditions characterized by hyperkeratosis, but its efficacy in this problem is controversial.
- Vitamin A deficiency may result in retarded epithelialization and slow wound healing.

Nutritional Directions

- Foods rich in antioxidants (vitamins A and E, and carotene) may suppress chemically induced neoplasias in the mouth, esophagus, and stomach.
- Vitamin C functions in maintaining the health of the gingivae, thereby maintaining periodontal health. A varied and adequate diet including at least one food high in vitamin C each day will provide adequate amounts.

HEALTH APPLICATION 10

Supplements

Approximately 38% of all Americans consume dietary supplements, with an expenditure of $2.92 billion in 1990 (Federal Register, 1993). Dietary supplements include 3,400 different products, such as vitamins, minerals, protein, amino acids, herbs, lipid supplements, dietary fiber, and other chemical compounds that have biologic activity. These supplements are subject to misrepresentation and misuse because they are so misunderstood by most consumers. Supplements have been marketed as enhancing sexual potency, controlling premenstrual syndrome, and more recently, boosting the immune system. About 20% of vitamins and dietary supplements make unsubstantiated claims or are not proven as safe (Federal Register, 1993).

Clients become their own diagnosticians by self-prescribing vitamin supplements. They usually do not consult a physician and thus may delay seeking medical attention for various health problems. Many clients consider vitamins safe to take in any amount, but each year, thousands of vitamin-poisoning cases occur, especially in children. The potencies of these self-prescribed supplements vary widely, containing insignificant amounts to more than 5,000% of the RDI per tablet. Vitamins A, B_6, C, D, and several minerals (zinc and selenium) have the highest potential for toxicity. A dietary or medical history should include queries about any dietary supplements. Clients may also be taking amino acid and folic acid supplements and/or unconventional items or herbal products described as "natural."

The American Medical Association (AMA, 1987) recommends that doses of supplemental vitamins should range from 50% to no more than 150% of the RDI. Use of vitamin preparations containing more than two times the RDI for any vitamin should be limited to the treatment of specific circumstances under medical supervision.

According to the American Medical Association (1987) and the American Dietetic Association (Position of the ADA, 1996), nutrient supplementation can be helpful in meeting the RDA in specific conditions:
1. Vitamin D, for those with limited milk intake and sunlight exposure.
2. Calcium, with lactose intolerance or allergies to dairy products.
3. Folic acid, for women of child-bearing age who consume limited amounts of fruits, leafy vegetables, and legumes.
4. Multivitamin and mineral supplements, for those following severely restricted weight loss diets.
5. Supplemental vitamin B_{12}, for strict vegans who eliminate all animal products.

Iron supplementation during pregnancy is routinely used. For clients who choose to self-prescribe supplements, low levels of nutrients that do not exceed the RDA are recommended (Position of the ADA, 1996).

Public-health nutrition will be served best by the insistence on a scientifically sound basis for vitamin supplementation and therapy. Despite the consensus of popular opinion, healthy clients do not need vitamin supplements if they eat a well-balanced diet using a variety of foods. Obtaining nutrients from dietary sources rather than by supplementation reduces the potential for both nutrient deficiencies and excesses. Numerous components in foods that may reduce disease risk have not been completely identified; this emphasizes the fact that nutrition may not be benefitted by manipulating the food supply or by supplementation at this time (Position of the ADA, 1996).

If a client insists on supplements, a single supplement providing both vitamins and minerals in quantities that do not exceed the RDIs may be allowed. Store brands of vitamins are often identical to name brands; expensive supplements are no better than less costly supplements. Except for vitamin E, "natural" vitamins are no more beneficial than synthetic vitamins. (An all-natural vitamin E should only contain d-alpha-tocopherol). Dietary supplements should be suggested by physicians or registered dietitians who are aware of current scientific knowledge and have assessed the client's dietary and nutritional status (Position of the ADA, 1996).

Megadoses of vitamins with intakes of 20 to 600 times the RDAs are sometimes advocated. Vitamin *megadosage* is defined as a dosage more than 10 times greater than the RDA. A megadose of a vitamin is actually a misnomer because the amounts at megadose levels are so high that a vitamin is functioning as a drug rather than as a nutrient. A well-established principle of pharmacologic therapy is that all substances are potentially toxic at large enough doses.

The AMA Council on Scientific Affairs (AMA, 1987) states megadose vitamin therapy is based only on anecdotal or nonscientific evidence. This can contribute to false hopes and needless financial expenditure, and may invoke direct toxic effects or hinder the metabolic interactions among vital nutrients.

CASE APPLICATION FOR THE DENTAL HYGIENIST

A young mother of a 3-year-old says she has heard that she should be taking folic acid supplements because she is considering discontinuing her birth control pills. She is concerned about the effects of the birth control pills on her nutritional status and their effect on a fetus should she become pregnant.

Nutritional Assessment

○ Types of foods consumed
○ Knowledge base of foods rich in folic acid
○ Current use of any dietary supplements
○ Motivation to change eating habits
○ Knowledge of physiologic values and absorption of folic acid

Nutritional Diagnosis

Health-seeking behavior related to nutritional status and effects on fetus.

Nutritional Goals

Client will consume foods rich in folic acid and ask her gynecologist about the need for taking a multivitamin supplement or a folic acid supplement.

Nutritional Implementation

Intervention: Evaluate the oral area for symptoms of folate deficiency.
Rationale: This will help determine whether or not she is currently deficient and help determine whether or not she should consult her physician immediately.

Intervention: Teach the following about folate: (1) different names used, (2) functions, (3) requirements, and (4) sources.
Rationale: This provides the client with a sound base of knowledge about folic acid.

Intervention: Discuss symptoms of folic acid deficiency and harmful effects of too much folic acid.
Rationale: While it is important that the client obtain adequate amounts of folic acid to prevent neural tube defects, too much can also be harmful.

Intervention: Discuss the stability of folate during cooking and processing.
Rationale: Knowing that folate can easily be destroyed during food preparation allows the client to make decisions based on her eating habits that would determine whether or not her diet would provide adequate amounts of folate.

Intervention: Explain that her requirement for folic acid is increased because of the birth control pills and because of the needs of the fetus and other physiologic changes that occur early during the pregnancy.
Rationale: This knowledge will help her realize the importance of changing dietary patterns consistently.

Evaluation

The client should increase her intake of folate-rich foods (cereal products that are fortified with folate; oranges; liver; raw, green, leafy vegetables). Additionally, she consults her gynecologist before discontinuing the OCA and begins taking a multivitamin as instructed by the physician. She can state why she has an increased requirement for folic acid and why it is important not to take excessive amounts.

Student Readiness

1. Name the two water-soluble vitamins most involved in the metabolism of fats, proteins, and carbohydrates to form energy (ATP) through the Krebs cycle.
2. Match the conditions associated with the appropriate vitamin deficiency:

Thiamin	Cheilosis
Riboflavin	Scurvy
Iodine	Pellagra
Niacin	Megaloblastic anemia
Vitamin B_{12}	Beriberi
Ascorbic acid	Graves' disease

3. Why is it important that water-soluble vitamins be consumed daily?
4. Define "vitamin megadose." What are the disadvantages of taking vitamin megadoses?
5. Name three foods that are good sources of each of these nutrients: thiamin, riboflavin, vitamin B_{12}, and folate.
6. What would you teach a vegetarian about vitamin B_{12}?
7. Discuss why signs and symptoms of deficiencies of water-soluble vitamins appear periorally. List signs and symptoms of deficiencies you should be alert for and list vitamins that might be implicated.
8. What recommendations could you offer to a client to ensure the availability of folate? Why is folate so important during pregnancy?
9. Evaluate five of the stress or megavitamin supplement preparations in a drugstore or health food store. List the amounts of vitamin C, niacin, and vitamin B_6 (pyridoxine) in them, and compare those amounts to the RDAs for children under 10 years of age, males 19 to 24, and females 25 to 50 years of age.

CASE STUDY

A 32-year-old male presents with the following symptoms: swollen tongue with reddening at the tip, small oral ulcerations, and gingival hyperplasia. The client is being treated with long-term anticonvulsant medication.

1. Is a dietary assessment indicated? Explain your answer.
2. What are the possible effects of the client's medication on his nutritional and oral status?
3. If a deficiency exists, which vitamins/minerals are most likely deficient? Why?
4. Which types of foods and food preparation methods should be suggested? Why?
5. What advice should you give regarding oral care?

References

American Medical Association (AMA) Council on Scientific Affairs. Vitamin preparations as dietary supplements and as therapeutic agents. *JAMA* 1987; 257(14):1929–1936.

Anonymous. FDA to make hard decision on folic acid. *Science* 1993 Aug 27; 261:118.

Boushey CJ et al. A quantitative assessment of plasma homocysteine as a risk factor for vascular disease. Probable benefits of increasing folic acid intakes. *JAMA* 1995; 274(13):1049–1057.

Cuskelly GJ. Effect of increasing dietary folate on red-cell folate: implications for prevention of neural tube defects. *Lancet* 1996; 347(9002): 657–659.

Dreizen S. Oral indications of the deficiency states. *Postgrad Med* 1971, 49(1):97–102.

Dreizen S. Systemic signs—significance of glossitis. *Postgrad Med* 1984; 75(4):207–214.

Drinka PJ et al. Nutritional correlates of atrophic glossitis: Possible role of vitamin E in papillary atrophy. *Am J Coll Nutr* 1993; 12(1):14–20.

Federal Register. DHHS, FDA, 1993 June 18.

McKenney JM et al. A comparison of the efficacy and toxic effects of sustained versus immediate release niacin in hypercholesterolemia patients. *JAMA* 1994; 271(9):672–677.

Position of the American Dietetic Association: Vitamin and mineral supplementation. *J Am Diet Assoc* 1996; 96(1):73–77.

Werler MM et al. Periconceptional folic acid exposure and risk of accurrent neural tube defects. *JAMA* 1993; 269(10):1257–1261.

Chapter 11

Water and Minerals Required for Oral Soft Tissues and Salivary Glands

Test Your NQ (True/False)

1. Thirst is the primary regulator of fluid intake. T/F
2. Meats are more than half water. T/F
3. Water is the most abundant component in the body. T/F
4. Heme iron is provided by meat sources and is more readily absorbed than iron from vegetable or grain products. T/F
5. Normal fluid requirements include 10 to 12 cups of fluid daily. T/F
6. The RDA for sodium is 5,000 mg/day. T/F
7. Taste alteration is a symptom of zinc deficiency. T/F
8. Potassium is principally found in extracellular fluid. T/F
9. Broccoli is a good source of potassium. T/F
10. Oral pallor is associated with iodine deficiency. T/F

Water and several mineral elements are essential for maintenance of healthy oral tissues and even tooth enamel. Visual signs on gums, mucous membranes, and salivary glands are less obvious than those observed with the B-vitamin complex and vitamin C deficiencies previously discussed. Nevertheless, water and several minerals have a significant effect on the integrity of the oral cavity, and ultimately, nutritional status. Oral problems associated with hyper- or hypo- states may not be critical immediately, being slower to develop. For instance, chronically decreased salivary flow attributable to inadequate body fluids may lead to rampant tooth decay and eventually loss of teeth.

WATER

Water is the most abundant component in the body. At birth, water constitutes approximately 75% to 80% of body weight. Because such a large percentage of the infant body is water, fluid loss is more significant in infants than in adults. Total body water decreases with age, representing just 50% to 60% of the total body weight of an adult. Adipose tissue contains less water than does muscle; thus, a person with a large amount of fat has a lower percentage of total body water. Women's bodies, with inherently larger fat stores, contain less water as compared to men, who have a higher percentage of lean muscle tissue.

Body fluids are distributed intracellularly and extracellularly. *Intracellular fluid* (ICF), which constitutes 60% of the body's fluid weight, includes all the fluid within cells, chiefly the cells of muscle tissue. *Extracellular fluid* (ECF) consists of fluid outside the cells. Fluid compartments are separated from one another by the presence of semipermeable membranes. These membranes serve as barriers by preventing movement of certain substances; however, they do not completely isolate the compartments. Water is essentially unrestricted in its movement from compartment to compartment. Certain **solutes,** such as glucose, amino acids, and oxygen, also cross membranes freely. The cellular membranes thus allow the maintenance of solute concentration by their selectivity.

When two compartments are separated by semipermeable membranes and the movement of some solutes is restricted, **osmosis** will occur. Osmotic pressure within the body serves to equalize the solute concentration of intracellular and extracellular fluids by shifting small amounts of water in the direction of the higher concentration of solute, as shown in Figure 11–1.

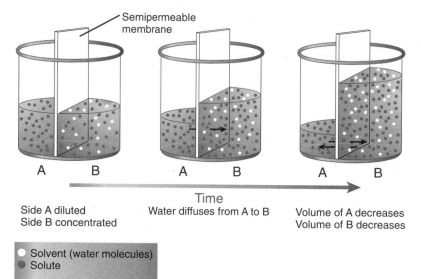

Semipermeable membrane

FIGURE 11–1 **Osmotic pressure.**

Time

Side A diluted
Side B concentrated

Water diffuses from A to B

Volume of A decreases
Volume of B decreases

○ Solvent (water molecules)
● Solute

Physiologic Roles

Water has several important physiologic roles: (1) it acts as a solvent, enabling chemical reactions to occur by actually entering into some reactions, such as hydrolysis; (2) it maintains the stability of all body fluids, as the principal component and medium for fluids (blood and lymph), secretions (saliva and gastrointestinal fluids), and excretions (urine and perspiration); (3) it enables nutrients to be transported to the cells and provides a medium for excretion of waste products; (4) it acts as a lubricant between cells to permit movement without friction; and (5) it regulates body temperature by evaporating as perspiration from the skin. Negative fluid balance has serious detrimental effects on many physiologic functions. A few days without water can be fatal.

Requirements and Regulation

An intake of approximately 2,500 to 3,000 ml (approximately 10 to 12 cups) of fluid is required daily for metabolic needs and to compensate for daily losses. Water is lost through a variety of routes: (1) urination, (2) perspiration, (3) expiration, and (4) defecation. Urine production depends on the amount of fluid intake and the type of diet

eaten; however, waste products must be kept in solution; minimum urine output to eliminate waste products is 400 to 600 ml/day.

Water losses in the form of sweat can vary greatly. A rise in body temperature is accompanied by increased sweating and respiration. Strenuous exercise can greatly affect the amount of water lost through the skin. Vapor in expired air varies with the rate of respiration. The presence of respiratory inflammation also elevates the respiration rate. Approximately 100 to 200 ml of water are lost each day in feces; this is dramatically increased in persons with diarrhea.

Water losses result in stimulation of water intake via thirst and decreased kidney output to maintain fluid balance. Saliva may also help maintain water balance because saliva flow is reduced in dehydration, leading to drying of the mucosa and the sensation of thirst.

Normal fluid requirements, shown in Figure 11–2, can be drastically changed in different climatic environments, with various exercise levels, and with illnesses that result in or are accompanied by diarrhea or vomiting. The body cannot store water, so the amount lost must be replaced.

Thirst is the primary regulator of water intake. When as little as 2% of body water is lost, *osmoreceptors* are stimulated, creating a physiologic desire to ingest liquids. Osmoreceptors in the hypothalamus are sensitive to changes in serum osmolality levels. Stimulation of osmoreceptors not only causes thirst, but also increases the release of *antidiuretic hormone* (ADH) from the pituitary gland (Fig. 11–3). ADH causes the body to retain fluid by decreasing urinary output.

Conversely, if there is too much water in the body, ADH secretion is inhibited, and excess water is eliminated.

Decreased blood volume also stimulates the release of renin, which leads ultimately to increased release of aldosterone by the adrenal cortex. This results in retention of sodium and water by the kidneys.

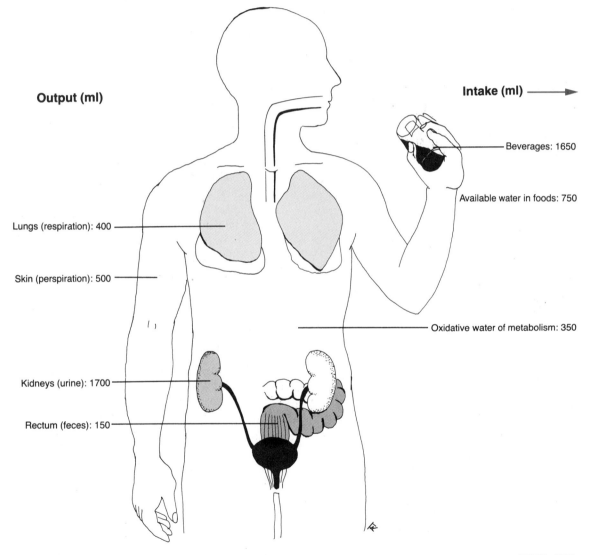

Output (ml)

Lungs (respiration): 400

Skin (perspiration): 500

Kidneys (urine): 1700

Rectum (feces): 150

Intake (ml) ⟶

Beverages: 1650

Available water in foods: 750

Oxidative water of metabolism: 350

TOTAL: 2750

TOTAL: 2750

FIGURE 11–2 **Fluid intake and output. (From Davis JR, Sherer K. *Applied Nutrition and Diet Therapy for Nurses,* 2nd ed. Philadelphia: W.B. Saunders, 1994.)**

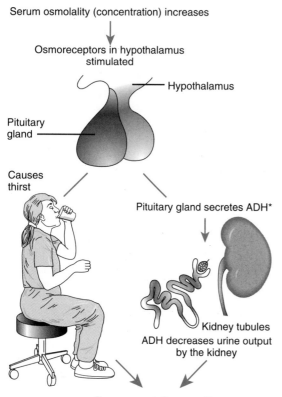

Serum osmolality (concentration) increases

Osmoreceptors in hypothalamus stimulated

Hypothalamus

Pituitary gland

Causes thirst

Pituitary gland secretes ADH*

Kidney tubules
ADH decreases urine output by the kidney

Serum osmolality normalizes

*ADH—antidiuretic hormone

FIGURE 11–3 **The role of osmoreceptors and antidiuretic hormone in fluid balance.**

Absorption

No digestion is necessary for water absorption; it is transported fully in both directions across the intestinal mucosa by osmosis. As much as 1 L can be absorbed from the small intestine in 1 hour. Normally almost all the fluid is reabsorbed, with only about 100 to 200 ml excreted in the feces daily.

Sources

During the process of metabolism, both liquids and solid foods provide water. Surprisingly, some fruits and vegetables have a higher percentage of water than milk, and meats are more than half water (Table 11–1). Water that is liberated in the

process of metabolism is also available to the body. Metabolism of fat produces approximately twice as much water as the metabolism of protein and carbohydrate; about 300 to 350 ml/day are supplied from this process.

Hyper- and Hypo- States

Regulation of fluid intake and fluid excretion by the kidneys usually maintains fluid balance in the body. However, imbalances may occur. *Fluid volume excess* (FVE) is the relatively equal gain of water and sodium in relation to their losses; *fluid volume deficit* (FVD) results from relatively equal losses of sodium and water.

FLUID VOLUME EXCESS

Fluid volume excess mainly occurs in ECF compartments secondary to an increase in total body sodium content (Fig. 11–4). Because water follows sodium, an excess of sodium leads to an increase in total body water. Excess fluid moves into the *interstitial* compartments, located between cells and in body cavities such as the joints, pleura, and gastrointestinal tract, causing edema.

Congestive heart failure, chronic renal failure, chronic liver disease, and high levels of steroids

TABLE 11–1   *Percentage of Water in Foods*

Food	Percent Water
Fruits and vegetables	70–99
Milk	88
Eggs	75
Cooked meats	50–70
Hard cheese	37–40
Bread	35
Margarine and butter	16
Nuts	5
Dry cereals and crackers	4
Shortening, oils, and sugar	0

Data from *Nutritive Value of Foods,* U.S. Department of Agriculture, Home Garden Bull. No. 72, Washington, DC, 1964.

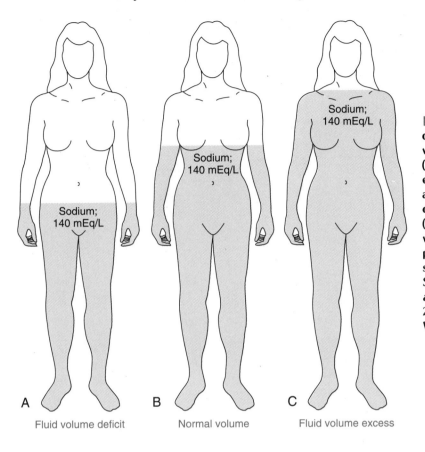

A Fluid volume deficit

B Normal volume

C Fluid volume excess

FIGURE 11–4 **Fluid-volume disturbances. As compared with (B) normal body fluids, in (A) fluid volume deficit (FVD), equal percentage of water and sodium losses occur, producing an isotonic depletion. In (C), fluid volume excess, both water and sodium are retained, producing an isotonic expansion. (Redrawn from Davis JR, Sherer K. *Applied Nutrition and Diet Therapy for Nurses,* 2nd ed. Philadelphia: W.B. Saunders, 1994.)**

may predispose to FVE because of sodium retention. Diseases that cause a loss of protein and lower serum albumin levels (malnutrition and renal diseases) may contribute to FVE because the osmotic forces ordinarily exhibited by proteins and albumin are lacking.

Common manifestations of FVE include rapid weight gain, puffy eyelids, distended neck veins, and elevated blood pressure. **Peripheral** edema is observed.

Treatment involves correction of the underlying problems, or therapy for the specific disease. Treatment may involve fluid and/or sodium restriction, or use of diuretics.

FLUID VOLUME DEFICIT

In FVD, the sodium-to-water ratio remains relatively equal; thus, ADH and aldosterone secretions are not activated. Prolonged inadequate fluid intake can result in FVD. However, FVD is usually associated with excessive loss of fluids from the gastrointestinal tract (vomiting, diarrhea, drainage tubes), urinary tract (diuretics, **polyuria**), or skin (sweating). Fever increases utilization of electrolytes, increases fluid losses in expired air, and causes **diaphoresis.**

Decreased food and fluid intake can result from anorexia, nausea, and fatigue. Other less obvious reasons are an inability to (1) obtain water, such as with impaired movement; (2) activate the thirst mechanism, as in **hypodipsia;** or (3) swallow, as in neuromuscular problems or unconsciousness. Occasionally excessive fluid losses occur with prolonged exercise.

Common characteristics of FVD include weight loss, hypotension, and orthostatic hypotension. Classic signs are dry tongue with **longitudinal**

fissures, xerostomia, shrinkage of oral mucous membranes, decreased skin turgor, dry skin, and decreased urinary output. A diminished salivary flow is associated with inadequate fluid intake. Treatment involves replacing lost fluid. If FVD is mild, oral fluids are likely to be sufficient, but intravenous solutions are needed with significant FVD.

Dental Hygiene Considerations

- Direct measurement of the total amount of body water is not possible. Evaluation of physical signs of fluid deficit or excess is vital to diagnosis and treatment.

- Assess clients for puffy eyelids or distended neck veins; question if they have observed recent weight changes, and if they have had their blood pressure checked by a physician recently.

- Observe for dry tongue with longitudinal fissures, xerostomia or shrinkage of oral mucous membranes, adequacy of salivary flow, decreased skin turgor, and dry skin. Inquire about frequency and amount of urine output and fluid intake.

- Salivary flow measurements may be indicated for clients who present with FVD.

- Decreased fluid reserves in geriatric clients and the greater surface area to body mass in infants place these groups at greater risk for FVD.

- Rapid weight changes generally indicate loss/gain of water rather than fatty tissue; a loss/gain of 480 ml (2 cups) of fluid is equivalent to a loss/gain of 1 lb.

- Because of the oral mucosa's sensitivity to the body's fluid volume, increases and decreases in body fluid will affect the fit of a denture.

Nutritional Directions

- Encourage clients experiencing a "dry mouth" to increase fluid intake and salivary production by chewing sugarless gum.

- Beverages containing caffeine increase urine production.

- The water supply and use of water softeners are "hidden" sources of sodium that may make edema worse.

- High-protein diets, as when principally protein foods are eaten and fruit and vegetable intake is deficient, require larger amounts of water to eliminate the higher levels of urinary waste products.

- Because of fluid loss through perspiration, clients need to drink fluid during exercise. (Loss of 1 lb of body weight during exercise means 2 cups of water have been lost.) Plain cool water is recommended.

ELECTROLYTES

Electrolytes are compounds or ions that dissociate in solution; they are also known as *cations* if they have a positive charge, and *anions* if negatively charged. Cations include sodium, potassium, calcium, and magnesium; anions include chloride, bicarbonate, and phosphate. Because the electrolyte concentration in plasma is so low, it is expressed as milliequivalents per liter (mEq/L). Electrolytes are important in both water balance and acid-base balance.

Electrolyte distribution is different in ICF and ECF compartments. The principal cation in plasma and interstitial fluid is sodium; the principal anion is chloride. The principal cation in ICF is potassium; the principal anion is phosphate. The major difference between intravascular and interstitial fluid is the large amount of protein in the former. Because sodium and potassium are the major cations, these will be discussed in greatest detail.

SODIUM

Physiologic Roles

Important physiologic roles of sodium include (1) maintaining normal ECF concentration by affecting the concentration, excretion, and absorption of potassium and chloride, and water distribution; (2) regulating acid-base balance; and (3) facilitating impulse transmission in nerve and muscle fibers. Sodium is present in calcified structures in the body; its function in bones and teeth is unclear. It is also present in saliva. Sodium concentration in saliva determines one's recognition of salt in food.

Requirements and Regulation

Because sodium is so readily available in foods, no RDA has been established. The National Research Council estimates a safe minimum intake might be set at 500 mg/day. This amount is increased in the face of abnormal losses. Sodium regulation involves several mechanisms. To keep the ECF concentration normal, the sodium-potassium pump is constantly moving sodium from the cell to the ECF. Aldosterone released by the adrenal cortex results in sodium reabsorption or excretion by the kidneys depending on the body's need (Fig. 11–5). The kidneys can adjust sodium excretion to match sodium intake despite great variations in intake. Thus, if serum sodium is high, aldosterone is inhibited and sodium is excreted; the opposite is true for depressed serum sodium levels.

The most recent Dietary Guidelines for Americans recommends limiting sodium intake to less than 3,000 mg/day. Daily Values on food labels are based on a recommended intake of no more than 2,400 mg daily. Currently, the average daily sodium intake for adults is 3,400 mg from food consumption; discretionary sodium (added in cooking or at the table) increases intake about 15%, with the resulting total nearly 4,000 mg daily (Statement, 1995). The FDA and the National High Blood Pressure Education Program Coordinating Committee (Statement, 1995) believe that lowering dietary sodium intake to the recommended amounts will reduce the population's mean blood pressure; doing so is safe and not associated with adverse effects.

Sources

About 10% of the sodium consumed comes from the natural content of foods and fluids regularly ingested (Statement, 1995). Sodium is a natural constituent of most foods (Table 11–2); animal foods such as meat, saltwater fish, eggs and dairy products, and some vegetables (beets, carrots, celery, spinach, and other dark-green leafy vegetables) contain appreciable amounts of sodium. Processed foods provide approximately 75% of sodium intake (Statement, 1995). "Hidden" sources include drinking water; baking powder; baking soda; dentifrices, including tooth pastes containing baking soda or sodium fluoride; antibiotics; chewing tobacco; and over-the-counter medications (antacids, cough medicines, laxatives).

Hyper- and Hypo- States

Serum sodium concentration is an index of water deficit or excess, not an index of sodium levels of the body. Sodium levels in the blood are significantly higher than potassium because sodium is the major cation in intravascular fluid. **Hypernatremia** and **hyponatremia** are usually a result of hormonal imbalances or increased fluid losses or retention. "True" hypernatremia or hyponatremia, or imbalances caused by too much or too little sodium intake, rarely occurs in adults. If renal and hormonal mechanisms for sodium retention and excretion function efficiently and water intake is adequate, the amount of dietary sodium causes little change in total body sodium; sodium fluctuations do affect plasma volume.

HYPERNATREMIA

A gain of sodium in excess of water, or loss of water in excess of sodium, can predispose to hypernatremia. Because water and sodium are closely related,

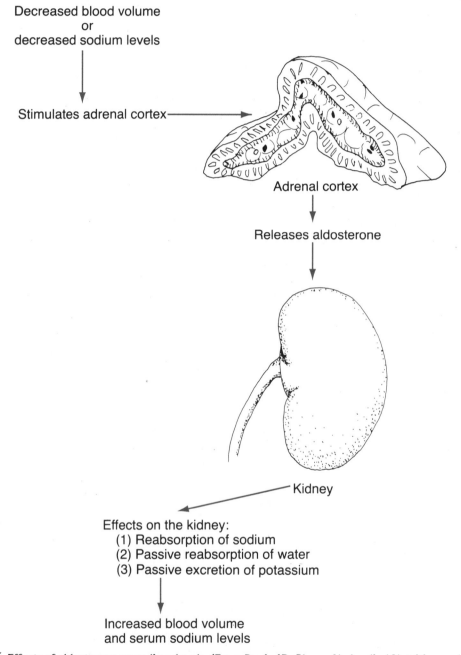

Decreased blood volume
or
decreased sodium levels

Stimulates adrenal cortex

Adrenal cortex

Releases aldosterone

Kidney

Effects on the kidney:
  (1) Reabsorption of sodium
  (2) Passive reabsorption of water
  (3) Passive excretion of potassium

Increased blood volume
and serum sodium levels

FIGURE 11–5 Effects of aldosterone on sodium levels. (From Davis JR, Sherer K. *Applied Nutrition and Diet Therapy for Nurses,* 2nd ed. Philadelphia: W.B. Saunders, 1994.)

TABLE 11–2   *Sodium Content of Food**

Foods	Approximate Sodium Content (mg)	Comments
Breads, Cereals, and Grain Products		
Cooked cereal, pasta, rice (unsalted)	Less than 5 per ½ cup	Unprocessed grains are naturally low in sodium.
Ready-to-eat cereal	100–360 per oz	Ready-to-eat cereals vary widely in sodium content: some have no salt added at all; others are higher in sodium than most breads.
Bread, whole-grain or enriched	110–175 per slice	
Biscuits and muffins	170–390 each	
Vegetables		
Fresh or frozen vegetables (cooked without added salt)	Less than 70 per ½ cup	Most canned vegetables, vegetable juices, and frozen vegetables with sauce are higher in sodium than fresh or frozen ones cooked without added salt.
Vegetables, canned or frozen with sauce	140–460 per ½ cup	
Fruit		
Fruits (fresh, frozen, or canned)	Less than 10 per ½ cup	Fresh, frozen, and canned fruits and fruit juices are low in sodium.
Milk, Cheese, and Yogurt		
Milk and yogurt	120–160 per cup	A serving of milk or yogurt is lower in sodium than most natural cheeses, which vary widely in their sodium content. Processed cheeses, cheese foods, and cheese spreads contain more sodium than natural cheeses. Cottage cheese falls somewhere between natural and processed cheeses.
Buttermilk (salt added)	260 per cup	
Natural cheeses	110–450 per 1½-oz serving	
Cottage cheese (regular and low-fat)	450 per ½ cup	
Process cheese and cheese spreads	700–900 per 2-oz serving	
Meat, Poultry, and Fish		
Fresh meat, poultry, finfish	Less than 90 per 3-oz serving	Most fresh meats, poultry, and fish are low in sodium; canned poultry and fish are higher. Most cured and processed meats, such as hot dogs, sausage, and luncheon meats, are even higher in sodium because sodium is used during processing to preserve them.
Cured ham, sausages, luncheon meat, frankfurters, canned meats	750–1350 per 3-oz serving	
Fats and Dressings		
Oil	None	
Vinegar	Less than 6 per Tbsp	
Prepared salad dressings	80–250 per Tbsp	
Unsalted butter or margarine	1 per tsp	
Salt pork, cooked	360 per oz	

Table continued on following page

TABLE 11–2 *Sodium Content of Food* * *(Continued)*

Foods	Approximate Sodium Content (mg)	Comments
Condiments		
Catsup, mustard, chili sauce, tartar sauce, steak sauce	125–275 per Tbsp	
Soy sauce	1,000 per Tbsp	
Salt	2,000 per tsp	
Snack and Convenience Foods		
Canned and dehydrated soups	630–1300 per cup	Most "convenience" foods are quite high in sodium. Frozen dinners and combination dishes, canned soups, and dehydrated mixes for soups, sauces, and salad dressings, contain a lot of sodium. Condiments such as soy sauce, catsup, mustard, tartar sauce, chili sauce, and pickles and olives are also high in sodium.
Canned and frozen main dishes	800–1400 per 8-oz serving	
Unsalted nuts and popcorn	Less than 5 per oz	
Salted nuts, potato chips, corn chips	150–300 per oz	
Deep-fried pork rind	750 per oz	Many low-sodium or reduced-sodium foods are available as alternatives to those processed with salt and other sodium-containing ingredients. Check the label for the sodium content of these foods.

*The ranges are rough guides: individual food items may be higher or lower in sodium.

From U.S. Department of Agriculture, Human Nutrition Information Service. *Nutrition and Your Health, Dietary Guidelines for Americans: Avoid Too Much Sodium.* Home and Garden Bull No. 232-6 Washington DC. 1986.

From Davis JR, Sherer K. *Applied Nutrition and Diet Therapy for Nurses,* 2nd ed. Philadelphia: W.B. Saunders, 1994.

a change in one causes a change in the other. Thus, hypernatremia can be associated with FVD or FVE.

Water deprivation (unconscious, debilitated individuals or infants), insensible water loss (exposure to dry heat, sweating, hyperventilation), and watery diarrhea lead to loss of water in excess of sodium. Infants are more prone to watery diarrhea, whereas elderly clients are susceptible to water deprivation. If **polyuria** is not balanced with increased water intake, hypernatremia may occur.

Symptoms of hypernatremia are a result of fluid moving from the ICF to the ECF in an attempt to equalize sodium and water balance. This movement of fluid causes atrophy of tissue cells. Cells in the central nervous system shrink, producing hallucinations, disorientation, lethargy, and possibly coma. Other signs are extreme thirst; dry, "sticky"

tongue and oral mucous membranes; fever; and convulsions. A sticky tongue can be identified by slowly rolling a tongue depressor over the lateral side of the tongue; tacky filiform stick to the tongue depressor, and then will rise up. The standard treatment is to gradually lower the sodium concentration using intravenous solutions.

HYPONATREMIA

Hyponatremia may develop when sodium losses exceed water losses or when fluids are retained, leading to a greater concentration of water than sodium. Because of the decrease in ECF concentration, sodium moves from the ECF to the ICF and water enters the ICF, causing cellular edema. This can cause problems especially in the cranium where there is no room for expansion. Sodium deficiency may lead to a decrease in salivary flow or a decrease in sodium concentration of saliva.

Heat exhaustion in unacclimatized individuals may result from sodium deficit. Hyponatremia may also occur in those who drink excessive quantities of water as part of a psychiatric disorder or when excessive amounts of diuretics are given. Hyperglycemia may precipitate hyponatremia because the elevated blood glucose level draws water into the vascular space (edema), causing a dilutional effect.

Early symptoms of hyponatremia are nausea and abdominal cramps. Other symptoms—headache, confusion, lethargy, and coma—are the result of cellular edema. Even though there is cellular edema, peripheral edema is not present. This is because the water is primarily retained within cells rather than in the interstitial compartment.

Chronic hyponatremia is usually well tolerated; thus, it may or may not be treated, depending on the precipitating cause and severity.

Dental Hygiene Considerations

- The normal sodium requirement for healthy adults is 200 to 250 mg/day. With heavy perspiration and during lactation, requirements are increased. Even in these conditions, 2,000 mg/day is sufficient to prevent hyponatremia.
- Assess clients for signs and symptoms of hypernatremia (thirst; dry, sticky tongue; dry mouth) and hyponatremia.
- The salt recognition threshold is determined by sodium concentration of saliva, i.e., the lower the level of sodium in the saliva, the easier it will be for one to detect a small amount of salt in food.
- A low salt recognition threshold is desirable for clients who need to curtail salt intake for health reasons; but in the hyponatremic, diminished salt consumption could further contribute to sodium depletion.
- Sodium deficiency may lead to a decreased salivary flow rate.

Nutritional Directions

- Stress the importance of appropriate sodium intake, as recommended by the physician.
- Dietary sodium restriction is rarely the cause of hyponatremia. Sodium depletion may occur in combination with excessive losses due to vomiting, diarrhea, surgery, or profuse perspiration from exercise or fever.
- To convert milligrams of sodium to milliequivalents, divide the number by 23 (the atomic weight of sodium). For example, 1,000 mg of sodium ÷ 23 = 43 mEq of sodium.
- Table salt is not the same thing as sodium. Table salt is 40% sodium and 60% chloride. 1 tsp salt is equivalent to 2,000 mg of sodium.
- Explain the "hidden" sources of sodium when indicated.
- A high-sodium food is considered as one containing 500 to 700 mg of sodium per serving. Consumption of one high-sodium food daily is within moderation.

POTASSIUM

Physiologic Roles

Potassium has the following important physiologic roles: (1) maintains cell (ICF) concentration; (2) directly affects muscle contraction (especially cardiac) and electrical conductivity of the heart; (3) facilitates transmission of nerve impulses; and (4) regulates acid-base balance.

Requirements and Regulation

Similar to sodium, there is no RDA for potassium. The minimum requirement to maintain normal body stores and normal plasma concentration is 1,600 to 2,000 mg/day. Potassium deficiency rarely occurs from a normal American diet because potassium is present in practically all foods.

The sodium-potassium pump regulates potassium levels. Depending on cellular needs, potassium is constantly moving either into or out of cells.

Aldosterone indirectly affects potassium serum levels. If aldosterone is released, sodium is reabsorbed but potassium is excreted. Subsequently, if aldosterone is inhibited, potassium is retained in the body (see Fig. 11–5). Approximately 80% of ingested potassium is excreted in the urine. The rest is lost through feces or sweat.

Sources

Sources of potassium are naturally available from foods and fluids regularly ingested (Table 11–3). Processed foods usually contain lower levels of potassium than fresh products. Potassium supplements (oral and intravenous) are another source.

Hyper- and Hypo- States

Minor deviations in serum potassium levels can be life-threatening. Abnormal levels are referred to as *hyperkalemia* or *hypokalemia.*

TABLE 11–3   *Potassium Content of Selected Foods*

Food	Portion	Potassium (mg)	Calories (per serving)
Dried apricots	½ c	896	155
Baked potato	1	844	220
Dried prunes	½ c	600	193
Cantaloupe	1 c	494	56
Dried pears	½ c	480	236
Banana	1	451	105
Baked winter squash	½ c	448	40
Cooked fresh spinach	½ c	420	21
Dried peaches	½ c	413	100
Pinto beans	½ c	400	118
Milk	1 c	377	86–150
Kidney beans	½ c	357	113
Lima beans	½ c	347	85
Broiled sirloin steak	3 oz	343	176
Blackeyed/cowpeas	½ c	319	112
Stewed tomatoes	½ c	305	33
Split peas	½ c	296	115
Baked butternut squash	½ c	291	41
Cooked beets	½ c	265	26
Orange juice	½ c	237	56
Cooked fresh broccoli	½ c	227	22
Cooked frozen zucchini	½ c	217	19
Cooked cauliflower	½ c	200	15
Cooked asparagus	½ c	196	25
Watermelon	1 c	186	51

Data from Nutritionist IV software, First Data Bank; San Bruno, CA. From Davis JR, Sherer K. *Applied Nutrition and Diet Therapy for Nurses,* 2nd ed. Philadelphia: W.B. Saunders, 1994.

HYPERKALEMIA

Hyperkalemia has three causes: (1) impaired renal excretion, (2) increased shift of potassium out of cells, and (3) increased potassium intake. Acute or chronic renal failure impairs potassium excretion, resulting in potassium being retained in the body. This is logical because 80% is excreted through the kidneys. Increased serum potassium levels can result from an increased dietary intake, excessive administration of potassium supplements orally or intravenously, or excessive use of potassium-containing salt substitutes. Burns, trauma, crushing injuries, increased catabolism, and acidosis cause potassium to leave the cell and enter the blood stream.

Hyperkalemia is life-threatening because cardiac arrest can occur. Elevated potassium levels are irritating to the body; symptoms include muscle weakness (the first sign), tingling and numbness in extremities, diarrhea, bradycardia, abdominal cramps, confusion, and electrocardiographic changes. Treatment for hyperkalemia involves potassium restriction or using medications to remove potassium.

HYPOKALEMIA

Excessive loss or inadequate intake of potassium can result in hypokalemia. Potassium loss occurs through the gastrointestinal and renal tracts, and by excessive sweating. Because potassium is contained in gastric and intestinal secretions, vomiting and diarrhea may cause hypokalemia. Some potassium is lost through sweat; excessive perspiration can lead to hypokalemia. Drugs, such as the diuretics, furosemide and hydrochlorothiazide, and the antibiotics, carbenicillin and Amphotericin B are the major offenders.

Potassium is the major ICF cation; deficits can affect every body system. Death from cardiac or respiratory arrest can occur. Clinical manifestations are anorexia, absence of bowel sounds, muscle weakness in the legs, leg cramps, and electrocardiographic changes. Information concerning dietary measures to increase potassium intake should be provided to those at risk of hypokalemia, as shown in the Guidelines for Increasing Potassium Intake.

Guidelines for Increasing Potassium Intake

- Increase intake of high-potassium fruits and vegetables (apricots, raisins, citrus fruits, bananas, tomatoes and tomato products, green leafy vegetables (broccoli, Brussels sprouts, parsley, spinach), carrots, potatoes (white and sweet), and corn.
- Use whole-grain products.
- Include adequate amounts of high-protein foods (2 to 3 cups of milk/milk products; 4 to 6 oz meat).
- Use minimal amounts of water in cooking foods.
- Utilize all liquids from cooked fruits, vegetables, and meats in soups, gravies, or sauces.
- Use a potassium-containing salt substitute.
- Make an economical high-potassium, low-calorie food supplement by combining vegetable scraps that are ordinarily discarded (e.g., carrot or potato peelings, celery stalks, outside pieces of lettuce, cabbage, and snipped ends from green beans; the addition of parsley will make it especially high in potassium), covering them with water and simmering them for about 1 hour; strain and season to taste. This broth can be served hot or cold or substituted for water in many recipes.

From Davis JR, Sherer K. *Applied Nutrition and Diet Therapy for Nurses,* 2nd ed. Philadelphia: W.B. Saunders, 1994.

Dental Hygiene Considerations

- Be aware of factors that can cause potassium to elevate or decrease.

Nutritional Directions

- Stress the importance of appropriate potassium intake.
- Read labels; salt substitutes may be high in potassium. Consult a physician or dieti-

tian before using potassium-containing salt substitutes.

℞ Encourage clients taking potassium-wasting diuretics to consume high-potassium foods if they are not taking a potassium supplement.

CHLORIDE

Physiologic Roles

Chlorine is the primary anion connected with sodium in extracellular fluid to help maintain extracellular fluid balance, osmotic equilibrium, and electrolyte balance. Large concentrations of chloride are present in gastric secretions, which are important for protein digestion and creating an acidic environment to inhibit bacterial growth and enhance iron and calcium absorption.

Requirements and Regulation

The National Research Council has determined that estimated minimal chloride intake should be 750 mg for adults. Chloride intake and losses closely parallel those of sodium.

Sources

Most chloride intake is from salt or sodium chloride. Therefore sources of chloride are the same as those for sodium, including processed foods. Water is an additional source of chloride.

Hyper- and Hypo- States

Toxicity from chloride is virtually nonexistent.

Conditions associated with sodium depletion, such as heavy persistent sweating, chronic diarrhea, or vomiting, may precipitate hypochloremia and an acid-base imbalance.

IRON

Physiologic Roles

Every cell contains iron; approximately 4 gm (less than 1 tsp) are present in the entire body. Iron is a major component of hemoglobin, which transports oxygen from the lungs to the tissues, including the oral soft and hard tissues. It also catalyzes many oxidative reactions within cells and participates in the final steps of energy metabolism. Other roles include (1) conversion of beta-carotene to vitamin A, (2) synthesis of collagen, (3) formation of purines as part of nucleic acid, (4) removal of lipids from the blood, (5) detoxification of drugs in the liver, and (6) production of antibodies.

Lactoferrin, a salivary glycoprotein, is capable of binding iron. It has an antibacterial action by competing with iron-requiring organisms in the mouth for limited amounts of available iron.

Requirements

The recommendations are 15 mg/day for women and 10 mg/day for men. The RDA is higher for women than for men because women lose blood during menstruation. During the reproductive phase of a woman's life, iron loss is at least double that of a man or of a postmenopausal woman. Iron requirements also increase during times of impaired absorption (diarrhea), the increased need for oxygen transport and energy production prompted by physical activity, and other periods of rapid growth. The RDA is based on the approximation that 10% of dietary iron is absorbed. The demand for iron replenishment is constant because cells are continually being replaced; the life of a red blood cell is 120 days. When a cell dies, iron is released and transported to various storage sites for iron.

Absorption and Excretion

Similar to calcium, iron is poorly absorbed. Most of the iron in food is in the oxidized form of ferric iron (Fe^{+++}). Gastric acid in the stomach helps promote iron absorption. By binding to **transferrin,** a continuous supply of iron may be transported through the body since transferrin functions to recycle the iron that is present.

Absorption of *heme iron* parallels the body's need; absorption of *nonheme iron* is dependent on intraluminal and meal composition as well as physiologic need. Heme iron is provided by meat sources that contain hemoglobin from red blood cells and myoglobin from muscle molecules. Non-heme iron is present in eggs, milk, and plants. Acidic conditions enhance iron absorption, but calcium and manganese interfere with its absorption. Factors affecting iron absorption are listed in Figure 11–6.

Combinations of food can enhance iron absorp-

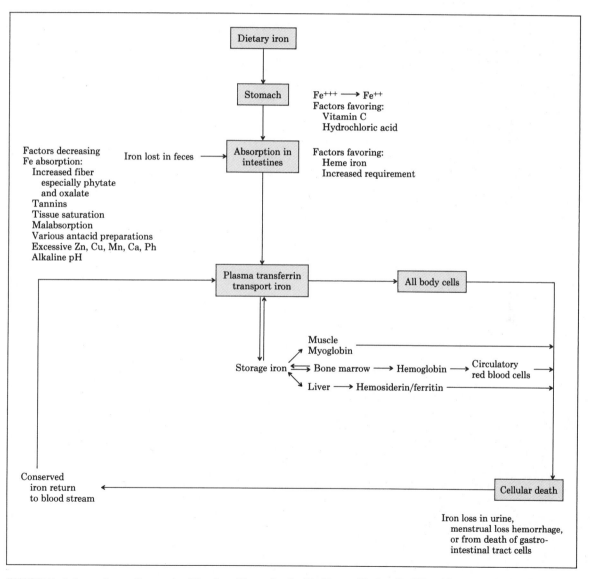

FIGURE 11–6 Iron absorption and utilization. (From Davis JR, Sherer K. *Applied Nutrition and Diet Therapy for Nurses,* 2nd ed. Philadelphia: W.B. Saunders, 1994.)

tion. A meal of roast beef (rich in iron) with potatoes (rich in vitamin C) and a tossed green salad (rich in folate) will increase iron absorption.

Sources

Iron is probably the most difficult mineral to obtain in adequate amounts in the American diet. Although liver is often considered the best source of iron,

meats (especially beef), egg yolk, dark-green vegetables, and enriched breads and cereals all contribute significant amounts (Table 11–4).

Hyper- and Hypo- States

The body cannot easily eliminate excess iron; this may explain why iron absorption rates are poor. It is unusual for the body to overcome its regulation

TABLE 11–4   *Iron Content of Selected Foods*

Food	Portion	Iron (mg)	Calories (per serving)
Cooked oysters	3 oz	11.4	117
Beef liver	3 oz	5.8	137
Spinach, cooked	½ c	3.2	21
Blackstrap molasses	1 Tbsp	3.2	45
Dried apricots	½ c	3.1	155
Lean beef sirloin	3 oz	2.9	176
Cooked shrimp	3 oz	2.6	84
Navy beans	½ c	2.6	113
Lean round steak	3 oz	2.5	163
Kidney beans	½ c	2.3	115
Lean rib lamb chop	3 oz	1.9	200
Ground hamburger	3 oz	1.8	231
Sauerkraut	½ c	1.7	22
Cooked oatmeal	½ c	1.6	145
Seedless raisins	½ c	1.5	218
Prune juice	½ c	1.5	91
Veal-rib cut	3 oz	1.2	185
Chicken leg	3 oz	1.2	157
Green peas	½ c	1.3	63
Whole-wheat bread	1 slice	0.9	67
Lean ham	3 oz	0.8	134
Lean pork loin chop	3 oz	0.8	218
Bologna, pork	3 oz	0.7	210
Broccoli	½ c	0.6	26
White tuna	3 oz	0.5	116
Chicken breast	3 oz	0.4	67
Cod fish	3 oz	0.4	89
Peanut butter	1 Tbsp	0.3	94

Data from Nutritionist III software, First Data Bank; San Bruno, CA. From Davis JR, Sherer K. *Applied Nutrition and Diet Therapy for Nurses,* 2nd ed. Philadelphia: W.B. Saunders, 1994.

of intestinal absorption. Iron overload can occur, however, if ingestion of iron is extremely elevated. *Hemosiderosis,* a hereditary disorder, occurs when excessive iron in the storage form, known as **hemosiderin,** accumulates in the body. This may occur with (1) excessive iron intake, (2) multiple blood transfusions, and (3) a failure to regulate absorption. Inexpensive red wines contain wide variations in iron content (10 to 350 mg/L) and have been associated with hemosiderosis. In its initial stage it is difficult to diagnose because of its resemblance to other conditions that have fatigue and general weakness as symptoms.

Elevated iron stores have been associated with increased risk of coronary heart disease and cancer. More studies are needed to confirm these findings. Iron supplements should not be taken indiscriminately without a comprehensive laboratory workup.

Iron-deficiency anemia continues to be a worldwide problem. A deficiency can lead to various symptoms, such as microcytic anemia, fatigue, faulty digestion, blue sclerae, pale conjunctivae, and tachycardia. Iron-deficiency anemia may be caused by inadequate dietary intake of iron; accelerated iron demand; increased iron losses; and inadequate absorption secondary to diarrhea, decreased acid secretions, or antacid therapy. Iron deficiency is frequently the result of postnatal feeding practices and has a serious impact on growth and on mental and psychomotor development in infants and children.

The most prominent oral signs of iron deficiency include pallor, angular cheilitis, and glossitis (see Color Plate 13). Oral candidiasis is frequently associated with iron deficiency.

Dental Hygiene Considerations

- Despite the prevalence of iron-deficiency anemia, supplements are not recommended without laboratory testing to indicate a deficiency.
- The most prominent sign of iron deficiency in the oral cavity is pallor and swelling of the tongue. The client may also complain of soreness and burning of the tongue. Atrophic changes progress from a patchy denudation of papillae to a smooth, reddened tongue.
- Hemosiderosis is common among chronic alcoholics, usually men, who may drink more than 1 L of inexpensive wine daily. Do not recommend iron-rich and iron-fortified foods to clients with hemosiderosis.
- Few clients realize the potential danger from ferrous sulfate supplements. Iron-containing supplements are the leading cause of poisoning deaths in children under 6 in the United States. The American Association of Poison Control Centers reports that between 1986 and 1994, 38 children between the ages of 9 months and 3 years died as a result of accidentally swallowing iron-containing products (Hingley, 1996). Encourage storage of iron supplements in a place inaccessible to children.

Nutritional Directions

- A vitamin C-rich food with supplements or with meals will increase absorption of iron, especially nonheme iron. Take iron with orange juice or tomato juice or vitamin C-enriched juices such as apple juice.
- If nonheme-containing grains or vegetables are consumed with small amounts of heme iron, absorption of the nonheme iron doubles.
- Coffee and tea decrease iron absorption. No decrease in iron absorption occurs when coffee is drunk 1 hour before a meal.
- Keep iron supplements out of reach of children.
- Maintain good oral hygiene practices when iron supplements are taken to prevent extrinsic staining of teeth. The abrasive effect of baking soda can help reduce staining. Liquid forms for iron can be taken through a straw.

℞ Avoid taking iron supplements with milk and calcium supplements because calcium interferes with iron absorption. (Only calcium carbonate does not affect absorption of iron.)

ZINC

Physiologic Roles

Zinc is a cofactor in over 120 enzymes that perform a variety of functions affecting cell growth and replication; sexual maturation, fertility, and reproduction; night vision; immune defenses; and taste and appetite. Zinc is required for DNA, RNA, and protein synthesis. It is in this role that zinc is essential for bone growth and mineral metabolism. Zinc-containing enzymes are important in collagen synthesis and bone resorption and remodeling.

Requirements

The National Research Council has recommended a daily intake of 15 mg for men and 12 mg for women. Although some concerns have been expressed about marginal intakes, zinc deficiencies

TABLE 11–5   *Zinc Content of Selected Foods*

Food	Portion	Zinc (mg)	Calories (per serving)
Eastern oysters	3 oz	155	117
Pacific oysters	3 oz	14.1	69
All bran cereal	1 c	11.2	212
Broiled lean sirloin	3 oz	5.5	176
Beef liver	3 oz	5.2	137
Lean veal chop	3 oz	5.1	185
Lean hamburger patty	3 oz	4.6	231
Lean lamb chop	3 oz	4.5	200
Wheat germ	¼ c	3.5	101
Cheddar cheese	1 oz	2.6	341
Lean pork chop	3 oz	2.5	218
Chicken leg	3 oz	2.4	158
Lean ham	3 oz	2.2	134
Pork bologna	3 oz	1.7	210
Canned clams	3 oz	1.0	38
Milk	1 c	1.0	121
Whole egg	1	0.6	74
Cod fish	3 oz	0.5	89
Whole-wheat bread	1 slice	0.5	67
Baked potato	1	0.5	145
Chicken breast	3 oz	0.4	67

Data from Nutritionist IV software, First Data Bank; San Bruno, CA. From Davis JR, Sherer K. *Applied Nutrition and Diet Therapy for Nurses,* 2nd ed. Philadelphia: W.B. Saunders, 1994.

have not been reported in Americans consuming a variety of foods.

Absorption and Excretion

Bioavailability of zinc varies widely; approximately 25% to 40% of dietary zinc is absorbed. Absorption is highly dependent upon several factors, including body size; total dietary zinc; and the presence of other potentially interfering substances, such as calcium, fiber, and phosphate salts. Higher-quality protein improves zinc absorption. Many substances in plant products (fiber, phytate) interfere with zinc absorption.

Zinc is lost in the feces. Abnormal losses from diarrhea or ileostomies increase zinc requirements.

Sources

Protein-rich foods are good sources of zinc. Lamb, beef, crustaceans (especially oysters), eggs, and peanuts contain significant amounts of zinc (Table 11–5).

Hyper- and Hypo- States

Consumption of high levels of zinc normally causes vomiting and diarrhea, epigastric pain, lethargy, and fatigue, but can result in renal damage, pancreatitis, and even death. Supplementation is recommended only under medical supervision.

In developing countries, severe zinc deprivation has been related to excessive consumption of inhibitors, which adversely affect zinc absorption, rather than inadequate zinc intake. Individuals at particular risk of zinc deficiency include those whose zinc requirements are relatively high (such as during periods of rapid growth), the elderly, total vegetarians whose diet consists primarily of cereal protein and/or is generally nutrient deficient, and those with severe malabsorption (diarrhea) or other chronic health problems (Table 11–6).

Oral manifestations of zinc deficiency include changes in the epithelium of the tongue, such as

TABLE 11–6   *Causes of Zinc Deficiency*

Dietary Deficiency
Poor food selection (especially typical of edentulous patients)
Poor appetite
Total parenteral nutrition
Decreased Absorption
High fiber
High phytate
High dietary iron/zinc ratio
Pica or geophagia
Malabsorption syndromes
Alcoholic cirrhosis
Pancreatic insufficiency
Chronic renal disease
Increased Loss
Thiazide diuretics
Alcoholism
Oral penicillamine therapy
Genetic Disorders
Acrodermatitis enteropathica
Sickle-cell disease
Thalassemia

From Davis JR, Sherer K. *Applied Nutrition and Diet Therapy for Nurses,* 2nd ed. Philadelphia: W.B. Saunders, 1994.

thickening of epithelium, and increase of cell numbers, and flattened filiform papillae.

Zinc deficiency in humans is associated with loss of taste acuity, poor appetite, and impaired wound healing. Decreased linear growth and hypogonadism in adolescent boys are principal manifestations of zinc deficiency. Zinc deficiency also results in congenital defects such as skeletal abnormalities, especially cleft palate and lips. Collagen synthesis defects are seen in zinc-deficient animals. Even when adequate amounts of zinc are provided for an extended time, abnormalities in mineral metabolism are not completely reversed. When zinc deficiency is diagnosed, zinc supplementation is vital.

Dental Hygiene Considerations

- Adverse effects have been reported with chronic consumption of 15-mg zinc supplements; these doses are approximately 100% of the RDA.
- Clients with abnormalities of taste due to zinc deficiency may respond to supplementation, but additional zinc is not effective in reversing abnormal taste acuity associated with other conditions.
- Supplementation in zinc-depleted clients is beneficial for wound healing but unnecessary for healthy individuals.
- Zinc supplementation interferes with utilization of iron and copper and adversely affects high-density lipoprotein levels. Do not advocate use of zinc indiscriminately.

- Reduced food intake associated with zinc deficiency may impair growth of the parotid gland.

Nutritional Directions

- Relatively small amounts of animal protein can significantly improve bioavailability of zinc from a legume-based meal.
- Fruits and vegetables are low in zinc, whereas peanuts and peanut butter are high.
- Meats are the preferred source of zinc because of its bioavailability.
- No evidence exists that zinc supplementation increases virility and improves sex drive.
- If a well-balanced diet is consumed, zinc supplements are rarely needed and may be harmful.

IODINE

Physiologic Role

Iodine is a part of thyroxine, the hormone secreted by the thyroid gland. Thyroxine regulates the basal metabolic rate; an altered metabolic rate will affect other nutrient requirements.

Requirements

The adult RDA for iodine is 150 mcg daily. Because iodine is related to the metabolic rate, needs are increased during periods of accelerated growth, especially during pregnancy and lactation.

Sources

The only natural source of iodine is seafood and plants grown near the ocean. The best safeguard for an adequate intake is the use of iodized salt.

Hyper- and Hypo- States

Very high levels of iodine may cause adverse effects in some individuals. Excessive amounts of iodine can result in enlargement of the thyroid gland similar to the condition produced by deficiency. Thyroiditis, hypothyroidism, hyperthyroidism, **goiter,** and sensitivity reactions have occurred in relation to excessive iodine intake through foods, dietary supplements, topical medications, and iodinated contrast media.

Iodine deficiency has virtually been eliminated in the United States because of iodine fortification of salt. A deficiency may cause profound metabolic and emotional influences ranging from a mild deceleration of catabolic functions, with sensitivity to cold, dry skin, mildly elevated blood lipids, to mild depression of mental functions. Endemic goiter occurs where the soil and/or water is low in iodine content (Fig. 11–7).

With insufficient iodine intake, the thyroid cannot produce adequate amounts of thyroxine. The pituitary gland continues to secrete thyroid-stimulating hormone, resulting in further hypertrophy and engorgement of the thyroid gland. Goiter is usually associated with iodine deficiency but may be caused by excessively large intake of **goitrogens.** Cabbage, cauliflower, Brussels sprouts, broccoli, kale, raw turnips, and rutabagas contain goitrogens.

Goiter is the main disorder resulting from

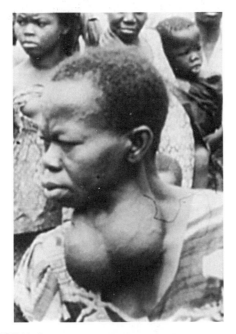

FIGURE 11-7 **Goiter resulting from iodine deficiency. (Courtesy of Food and Agricultural Organization Liaison Office with the United Nations. UN Headquarters Room DC-1125, New York, NY. Photo by Marcel Ganzin.)**

low-iodine intake. Other iodine-deficiency disorders include stillbirths, abortions, and congenital anomalies; endemic *cretinism,* usually characterized by mental retardation and deaf mutism related to fetal iodine deficiency; and impaired mental function. Children born to mothers with severe iodine deficiency have delayed eruption of primary and secondary teeth. Craniofacial growth and development are altered; malocclusion is common (Dreizen, 1989).

Dental Hygiene Considerations

- Assess clients for possible thyroid problems. Enlargement of the thyroid gland can indicate hyperthyroidism or hypothyroidism. Refer these clients to a physician.
- Severe hypothyroidism is termed *myxedema,* and hyperthyroidism is also called *Graves' disease.*

Nutritional Directions

- Sea salt has been advocated by health-food promoters, but much of the iodine is lost in processing.
- Prior to purchase, confirm from package labeling that the salt selected is iodized.

HEALTH APPLICATION 11

Hypertension

Hypertension is a condition defined as a persistent elevation of systolic blood pressure above 140 mmHg in clients less than 45 years of age (greater than 150 mmHg in those over 45), and diastolic pressure above 90 mmHg. For every increment of blood pressure above normal levels, there is a commensurate increase in risk of cardiovascular complications (Joint National Committee, 1988). Hypertension may result in myocardial infarction, cerebrovascular accident, and congestive heart failure. Uncontrolled hypertension can affect blood vessels of the eyes, kidneys, and nervous system. Hypertension cannot be cured, but it can be controlled. Weight loss of over 10 lbs is as effective at lowering blood pressure as pharmacologic treatment and potentiates drug effects (Trials, 1992).

Hypertension has been called mankind's most common disease. Approximately one in five adult Americans has hypertension. Hypertension is about twice as common among blacks as whites; chances of developing the disease increase with age.

Causes

Elevation of blood pressure is related to the degree of obesity. Body fat deposited in the trunk increases risk for developing essential hypertension independent of the overall level of obesity, whereas peripherally deposited fat does not. *Essential hypertension* is elevated blood pressure of unknown cause.

The beneficial effect of caloric restriction on blood pressure is seen before weight loss is significant. Greatest reductions in blood pressure occur during the first half of weight loss (Schotte & Stunkard, 1990). Approximately 50% of all hypertensive cases could be prevented entirely with weight control.

Hypertension is virtually unheard of in societies where sodium intake is low. Unlike cultures with low salt usage, all populations that use salt see blood pressure rise with age. Likewise, individuals originally from populations with low blood pressure who have become acculturated to Western civilization often develop higher blood pressure as they age. On the other hand, those who consume comparable amounts of salt do not have the same probability of developing hypertension. Genetic factors may make some more sensitive to salt intake, but there is no clear-cut method of identifying salt sensitivity. Even an individual with normal blood pressure can be salt sensitive.

Despite the fact that sodium restriction does not always result in lower blood pressure, the consensus from a survey of studies is that sodium reduction lowers mean blood pressure (Cutler et al., 1991). Sodium restriction (less than 2 gm/day) enhances effectiveness of diuretics and other pharmacologic treatments.

High potassium intake has a protective effect against hypertension. Potassium increases urinary sodium excretion. Customary high-sodium, low-potassium diets consumed when most foods are highly processed may be detrimental to normal blood pressure regulation. Potassium supplementation does not alleviate the need for pharmacologic therapy even with a sodium-restricted diet, but increasing dietary potassium intake from natural foods may decrease the amount of medication needed (Siani et al., 1991).

Dietary modifications will lower blood pressure for many with mild-to-moderate hypertension. Weight control and reduced sodium intake are not only useful initial therapies, but they also enhance antihypertensive effect of drugs (Treatment, 1991). Other dietary considerations include adequacy of potassium, magnesium, and calcium intake, dietary fat intake, and limited use of alcohol (see the Guidelines for Nonpharmacologic Management of Hypertension).

Guidelines for Nonpharmacologic Management of Hypertension

◆ Control weight.
  1. Weight loss to within 15% of desirable weight for obese persons.
  2. Weight loss to ideal body weight (IBW) for overweight persons.
  3. Maintenance of IBW for persons with normal weight.
     ◆ Limit sodium intake to 2 to 3 gm daily.
     ◆ Maintain recommended calcium intake.
     ◆ Increase intake of fresh fruits and vegetables to increase dietary fiber and potassium.
     ◆ Lower total fat intake to 30% of total calories, with 10% from saturated fats.
     ◆ Consume fatty fish (mackerel, herring, salmon, etc.) several times a week to provide omega-3 fatty acids and to help lower saturated fat intake.
     ◆ Consume a well-balanced diet utilizing a variety of foods to ensure adequate intake of magnesium.
     ◆ Restrict alcohol intake to one to two drinks daily or less.
     ◆ Do not use potassium, calcium, or magnesium supplements unless recommended by the physician/dietitian.
     ◆ Avoid tobacco.
     ◆ Participate in some type of relaxation therapy.
     ◆ Participate in a regular aerobic exercise program. Initiate an exercise program gradually.

From Davis JR, Sherer K. *Applied Nutrition and Diet Therapy for Nurses*, 2nd ed. Philadelphia: W.B. Saunders, 1994.

The American Heart Association recommends less than 3,000 mg sodium daily. Salt is not added at the table, but foods can be lightly salted in cooking. Foods high in salt—pickles, olives, bacon, ham, chips, canned soups, salted nuts, and crackers—are omitted. Some prepared foods and fast foods are limited or omitted (see Table 11–7 and the Guidelines for No-Extra-Salt Diets).

Guidelines for No-Extra-Salt Diets

The object of this restriction is to limit the amount of sodium intake to between 4 and 5 gm (170 to 220 mEq) daily by (1) avoiding foods that are concentrated sources of sodium and (2) not adding salt to foods.

1. Avoid adding salt to food at the table.
2. Use small amounts of salt in food preparation: 1/4 tsp of salt/lb of meat; 1/8 tsp salt/serving of cooked cereal and vegetables.
3. Avoid the following high-sodium processed foods:
   - ◆ *Meats:* Smoked, cured, salted or canned meats, fish, or poultry, including bacon, chipped beef, corned beef, cold cuts, ham, frankfurters, and sausages; sardines, anchovies, and marinated herring; pickled meats or eggs.
   - ◆ *Dairy products:* Processed cheese, blue cheese, buttermilk.
   - ◆ *Vegetables:* Sauerkraut, pickled vegetables prepared in brine, commercially frozen vegetable mixes with sauces.
   - ◆ *Breads and cereals:* Breads, rolls, and crackers with salted tops.
   - ◆ *Soups:* Canned soups, dried soup mixes, broth, bouillon (except salt-free).
   - ◆ *Fats:* Salad dressings containing bacon bits, salt pork, dips made with instant soup mixes and processed cheese.
   - ◆ *Beverages:* Commercially softened water, cocoa mixes, club soda, sports drinks, tomato or vegetable juice.
   - ◆ *Miscellaneous:* Casserole and pasta mixes; salted chips, popcorn, and nuts; olives; commercial stuffing; gravy mixes; seasoning salts (garlic, celery, onion), lite salt, monosodium glutamate; meat tenderizer; catsup, prepared mustard, prepared horseradish, soy sauce.

From Davis JR, Sherer K. *Applied Nutrition and Diet Therapy for Nurses,* 2nd ed. Philadelphia: W.B. Saunders, 1994.

In general, when sodium must be restricted, hidden sources of sodium should be considered: (1) sodium bicarbonate and other sodium products used as leavening agents; (2) sodium benzoate as a preservative in margarine and relishes; (3) sodium citrate and monosodium glutamate enhance flavors in gelatin desserts, beverages, and meats; and (4) sodium bicarbonate or sodium fluoride added to dentifrices or used in place of commercial dentifrices and mouth rinses. Some medications add significant amounts of sodium, particularly when taken regularly and frequently, such as antacids, laxatives, and cough medicines. Thus, teaching clients to read labels is important

TABLE 11–7   *Levels of Dietary Sodium Restriction*

		Sodium Content	
	Condition	mEq/day	mg/day
No added salt	Mild hypertension; mild fluid retention	174	4,000
Mild restriction	Hypertension; cirrhosis with ascites	87	2,000
Moderate restriction	Congestive heart failure	43	1,000
Severe restriction	Congestive heart failure: cirrhosis with massive ascites	22	500

From Davis JR, Sherer K. *Applied Nutrition and Diet Therapy for Nurses,* 2nd ed. Philadelphia: W.B. Saunders, 1994.

TABLE 11-8   *Herbs and Spices to Complement Foods*

Food	Herbs/Spices
Soups	Bay, tarragon, marjoram, parsley, rosemary
Poultry	Garlic, oregano, rosemary, sage
Beef	Bay, chives, cloves, cumin, garlic, hot pepper, marjoram, rosemary
Lamb	Garlic, marjoram, oregano, rosemary, thyme (make little slits in lamb to be roasted and insert herbs)
Pork	Coriander, cumin, garlic, ginger, hot pepper, pepper, sage, thyme
Cheese	Basil, chives, curry, dill, fennel, garlic, marjoram, oregano, parsley, sage, thyme
Fish	Dill, fennel, tarragon, garlic, parsley, thyme
Fruit	Cinnamon, coriander, cloves, ginger, mint
Bread	Caraway, marjoram, oregano, poppy seed, rosemary, thyme
Vegetables	Basil, chives, dill, French tarragon, marjoram, mint, parsley, pepper, thyme
Salads	Basil, chives, French tarragon, garlic, parsley, rocket-salad, sorrel (these are best used fresh or added to salad dressing, otherwise, use herb vinegars for extra flavor)

Adapted from Shimizu HH. Do yourself a flavor. *FDA Consumer.* U.S. Department of Health and Human Services. Pub. No. 84-2192, 1984.

From Davis JR, Sherer K. *Applied Nutrition and Diet Therapy for Nurses,* 2nd ed. Philadelphia: W.B. Saunders, 1994.

when intake is curtailed. A product can be labeled low sodium if it contains less than 140 mg per serving.

In spite of reduced-sodium diets being used so frequently, they are difficult to follow, partly because they are bland and tasteless. Americans are accustomed to higher amounts of salt on foods and may be unaware of the myriad spices other than salt that can be used as flavor enhancers (Table 11–8). If a high salt intake has been established, sodium intake can gradually be decreased. The preferred salt level will decrease after about 3 months of moderately lowered intake. This can possibly be explained by there being lower concentrations of sodium in saliva, which diminishes one's desire for salt.

Increasing intake of fresh fruits and vegetables is usually beneficial. These items are not only low in calories and sodium, but also high in potassium and fiber.

Adequate amounts of calcium should be included in the diet. Even if cholesterol intake is restricted, avoidance of dairy products and possible dietary deficiency of calcium is undesirable.

CASE APPLICATION FOR THE DENTAL HYGIENIST

An elderly client presents with complaints of a dry mouth and sore tongue. He states he has not been thirsty, and intake has been poor for 4 days. His physician recently prescribed a diuretic for hypertension and told him to eliminate salt. He complains "nothing tastes good."

Nutritional Assessment

- Oral mucous membranes, tongue characteristics
- Fluid likes and dislikes
- Mental changes

Nutritional Diagnosis

Fluid volume deficit related to diuretic and poor fluid/food intake.

Nutritional Goals

Client will have good skin turgor and moist oral mucous membranes, and will increase his intake of liquids and food.

Nutritional Implementation

Intervention: Explain the need for fluid intake.
Rationale: Knowledge and involvement in care will increase compliance.

Intervention: Encourage the client to drink his favorite fluids, preferably water, on a regular schedule.
Rationale: The client is more apt to drink his favorite fluid and in doing so will replace fluids lost as a result of the diuretic.

Intervention: Identify methods to increase salivary flow and oral lubrication.
Rationale: The client can increase his degree of oral comfort and promote healing of soft tissue.

Intervention: Explain the importance of oral hygiene and how to perform oral self care thoroughly and safely.
Rationale: Less saliva allows more food debris to remain on the teeth, which would increase risk of dental caries. Because the oral mucosa and gingival tissues are more susceptible to trauma, an extra-soft bristle brush may be appropriate for plaque removal, and the client should be cautioned against aggressive oral hygiene, such as flossing.

Intervention: Explain why foods without salt do not taste good and how his tastes will gradually improve.
Rationale: Most Americans consume about three times the amount of sodium needed. The sodium concentration in saliva determines a client's recognition of salt in food; higher levels of sodium in saliva means higher levels of sodium are needed for the sodium to be detected. The preferred salt level will decrease after about 3 months of moderately lowered intake.

Intervention: Discuss types of dentifrices consistent with the physician's order to eliminate salt.
Rationale: Sodium bicarbonate or sodium fluoride are added to some dentifrices and mouth rinses; these would increase his sodium intake, especially if oral hygiene is practiced several times a day and the client ingests the dentifrice or mouth rinse.

Evaluation

Desired outcomes include the client's consumption of 8 to 10 cups of preferred beverage a day, moist oral mucous membranes, and no dental caries.

Student Readiness

1. Define intracellular and extracellular fluid. What are the principal electrolytes found in each?

2. Write down your daily intake of fluid. How does this compare with the required intake?

3. Fluid is essential for survival. Discuss the advantages and disadvantages of intake of water versus other fluids such as milk, carbonated beverages, tea, and coffee.

4. List five clinical observations that are indicative of fluid volume deficit. What type of medication is frequently prescribed that affects hydration status?

5. What can cause hypernatremia and hyponatre-

mia? Why is altering the salt intake of these clients not usually the mode of treatment?

6. What can cause FVD or FVE?

7. What is the general effect of food processing on the sodium and potassium content of foods?

8. Explain the physiologic change that occurs when salt intake is decreased and why adding large amounts of salt to foods is unwise. Would you consider salt addictive?

9. Discuss dental hygiene interventions for iron-deficiency anemia. Discuss factors affecting iron absorption.

10. A client asks you why he has to take zinc when his iron stores are depressed. How would you respond?

11. Which two nutrients discussed are important for collagen formation?

12. Name the electrolyte(s) or mineral(s) discussed in this chapter associated with the following symptoms:

Shrinkage of mucus   Enlargement of
    membranes   thyroid
Thirst   Poor wound healing
Oral pallor   Swollen tongue
Taste abnormalities   Appetite
Lethargy

13. The Dietary Guidelines for Americans and the American Heart Association recommend restricting red meat in the diet. Their recommendations also include increasing fiber from cereal and vegetable sources to help reduce blood lipid levels. Discuss how these two recommendations affect the known deficiency of iron stores in the U.S. population in general. Would you anticipate that long periods of compliance with cholesterol-reducing protocols might necessitate iron supplements in affected individuals?

CASE STUDY

A 17-year-old boy presents with complaints of dry mouth, difficulty in swallowing food, dry sticky tongue, and dry skin. The client reports that he has just recovered from the flu that was accompanied by diarrhea and vomiting. In addition, he informs you that he is currently in training for an athletic competition and exercises 3 to 4 hours a day. A 24-hour diet recall reveals that the client's fluid intake includes 24 to 32 ounces of caffeinated soft drinks without ice, no other beverages, and a high protein intake.

1. What other information should you obtain from the client's dietary intake?

2. Could the client's oral symptoms be attributed to his current fluid intake?

3. Is salivary analysis indicated for this client?

4. What suggestions could you make that would improve/increase his fluid intake?

5. What oral self-care practices would you recommend to relieve his oral discomfort and facilitate swallowing?

CASE STUDY

A 15-year old girl comes into the dental office reporting a history of iron-deficiency anemia. She has clinical symptoms typical of this anemia: glossitis, smooth shiny red tongue, and painful cracks at the corners of her mouth. Her physician has prescribed ferrous sulfate and zinc to correct this deficiency.

1. When evaluating dietary intake, what are some foods you would need to watch for to assess iron intake?

2. If the client is having problems with ferrous sulfate (constipation, nausea), would it be advisable to resolve the anemia by just increasing iron intake? Why or why not?

3. Why has the physician ordered zinc supplements?

4. What should you tell her about iron from plant or animal foods?

5. What can she do to help increase absorption of iron?

References

Cutler JA et al. An overview of randomized trials of sodium reduction and blood pressure. *Hypertension* 1991; 17(1 Suppl):I27–I33.

Dreizen S. The mouth as an indicator of internal nutritional problems. *Pediatrician* 1989; 16(3-4): 139–146.

Hingley AT. Preventing childhood poisoning. *FDA Consumer* 1996; 30(2):7–11.

Joint National Committee. The 1988 Report of the Joint National Committee on detection, evaluation, and treatment of high blood pressure. *Arch Intern Med* 1988; 148(5):1023–1038.

Schotte DE, Stunkard AJ. The effects of weight reduction on blood pressure in 301 obese patients. *Arch Intern Med* 1990; 150(8):1701–1704.

Siani A et al. Increasing the dietary potassium intake reduces the need for antihypertensive medication. *Ann Intern Med* 1991; 115(10):753–759.

Statement from the National High Blood Pressure Education Program Coordinating Committee. Coordinated by the National Heart, Lung and Blood Institute, National Institutes of Health. Approved March 30, 1995.

Treatment of Mild Hypertension Research Group. The treatment of mild hypertension study: A randomized, placebo-controlled trial of a nutritional hygienic regimen along with various drug monotherapies. *Arch Intern Med* 1991 Jul; 151(7):1413–1423.

Trials of Hypertension Prevention Collaborative Research Group. The effects of nonpharmacologic interventions on blood pressure of persons with high normal levels. *JAMA* 1992; 267(9):1213–1220.

Section II

CONSIDERATIONS OF CLINICAL NUTRITION

Chapter 12

Nutritional Requirements Through the Life Cycle and Eating Habits Affecting Oral Health

The Student Will Be Able To:

- Describe the procedure for introducing solid foods after the initial stage of feeding by bottle or breast.
- Discuss ways to handle typical nutritional problems that occur during different stages of the life cycle.
- Know dental hygiene considerations of nutritional needs during different stages of the life cycle.
- Identify nutrition education needs for clients in different stages of the life cycle.
- Discuss physiologic changes that alter the infant, adolescent, and elderly client's nutritional status.
- Discuss differences in amounts of nutrients needed by elderly clients as compared with younger adults.
- Describe factors that influence the food intake of older clients.
- Discuss dietary changes that could be made to provide optimum nutrient intake for elderly clients.

GLOSSARY OF TERMS

Recumbent lying down

Streptococcus mutans cariogenic bacterium

Cleft lip/palate split where parts of the upper lip or palate fail to grow together

Food jags refusing to eat anything except one food for several days

Bruxism clenching and grinding of teeth that erodes and diminishes the height of dental crowns

Sealants a clear or shaded plastic material that is applied to the occlusal surfaces of permanent teeth

Homeostatic mechanisms   the body's ability to correct nutritional imbalances, for instance, decreased nutrient intake accompanied by an increase in absorption or efficiency or use

Renal failure   an inability of the kidneys to maintain normal function of excreting toxic waste materials

Taste threshold   the lowest concentration at which taste can be detected

Anosmia   loss of smell

Hypogeusia   loss of taste

Xerostomia   dry mouth or lack of salivation

Dysphagia   difficulty with swallowing

Atrophic gastritis   chronic stomach inflammation with atrophy of the mucous membrane and glands and diminished hydrochloric production

Nocturia   excessive urination at night

Incontinence   inability to control urinary excretion

Test Your NQ (True/False)

1. Commercial infant formulas are fairly standardized in their nutrient content. T/F
2. Nutritional needs for a client aged 51 are different from those for an 81-year-old. T/F
3. Solid foods should be introduced at 6 weeks of age. T/F
4. Orange juice is the first fruit juice to offer an infant. T/F
5. New denture wearers should introduce meats first, followed by beverages or liquid intake. T/F
6. Toddlers may refuse to eat anything except one food for several days. T/F
7. Healthy elderly women require increased amounts of iron. T/F
8. Energy requirements decrease with age. T/F
9. Self-medication with vitamins is a healthy practice for the elderly. T/F
10. During adolescence, more nutrients are required than during any other stage of life. T/F

Many of the nutritional objectives established by the federal government for a healthier America by the year 2000 (discussed in chapter 1) are specifically targeted to managing problems encountered by various age groups and stages throughout the lifespan. Achievement of these goals will be a major milestone for the optimal health of infants and children and thereby affect the health and life span of older Americans.

GROWTH

Growth is the definitive test of health and is used as the single most sensitive and specific indicator of nutritional status. Increasing size results in greater nutritional requirements, but the need for calories per kilogram decreases as one grows. It is important that dental hygienists who work with infants and children be familiar with normal growth and developmental patterns that reflect adequacy of nutritional intake. The birth weight of an infant doubles in 4 months (from 7½ to 14 lbs), and by 1 year, it has usually tripled. The growth spurt then slows down, and the infant gains only another 4 to 6 lbs until 2 years old.

Length or height is increased by 50% by 1 year

of age and doubles by age 4. (Since the infant is unable to stand, **recumbent** length is measured.) One half of adult height is achieved by age 2½ to 3 years of age. In the normally growing child, height increases parallel that of weight, with rapid increases during adolescence. The end of this adolescent growth spurt is signaled by slowing of growth, completion of sexual maturation, and closure of the epiphyses of long bones.

NEWBORNS

Not only health at birth, but also future life-long health depends on loving care and feeding of the newborn by the mother or caretaker. The infant is normally able to thrive on human milk or commercially available formulas, but many of the physiologic systems are immature at birth. Because of the small stomach capacity, frequent feedings are needed.

Infant Nutritional Requirements

Adequate nutrition is more important during infancy and childhood than any other stage of the life cycle. As might be expected from the rapid growth rate, energy requirements are much higher than for an adult: 90 to 120 Cal/kg/day versus 30 to 40 Cal/kg/day. Additionally, infants have a higher resting metabolic rate, and intestinal absorption is relatively inefficient.

The RDA for protein is 13 gm daily. This translates to about 1.6 to 2.2 gm/kg body weight. As a result of immature renal function, total protein should not exceed 20% of the calories. Both breast milk and commercial formulas provide about 50% of the calories from fat to supply the high caloric needs.

Breast Milk

Human milk is unique in nutrients and contains other substances such as enzymes, hormones, and growth factors. Breast milk is normally thin with a slightly bluish color.

The overall composition of breast milk is relatively constant, regardless of the nutritional status of the mother. Compared with cow milk, human milk is high in lactose and relatively low in protein. Specific protein fractions synthesized in the breast tissue help protect against gastrointestinal infections.

Breast milk contains principally unsaturated fatty acids; saturated fatty acids are lower than in cow milk. Lipase enzyme inherent in breast milk improves fat digestion. Human milk is relatively high in cholesterol and more than half the calories in breast milk come from fat. Despite numerous studies, it is uncertain whether human milk has a beneficial or adverse effect on the development of heart disease.

The relatively low mineral content of human milk is ideal for the infant's immature kidneys. Although the iron content is low, approximately 50% to 75% is absorbed. Because of the high bioavailability of iron, additional sources of iron are unnecessary during the infant's first 4 to 6 months.

Breast milk is adequate to meet the infant's needs for at least 4 months. Supplemental foods during that time may reduce iron absorption. Between 4 to 6 months, iron-rich foods or a daily low-dose oral iron supplement should be initiated.

Commercial Formulas

Although nutrients differ slightly for various brands, all commercial formulas comply with standards set by the Infant Formula Act established in 1980 (Table 12–1). Infant formulas are similar to breast milk. Human milk is very complex, and its exact chemical makeup is unknown. Adequate nutrients are provided in an appropriate caloric concentration (about 20 Cal/oz). Nonfat cow's milk is the basis for most infant formulas, modified to ensure that the performance of formula-fed infants (growth, absorption of nutrients, gastrointestinal tolerance, and reactions in blood) will match that of breast-fed infants.

TABLE 12–1 *Recommended Dietary Allowances for Infants Compared with Nutrient Content of Human Milk, Cow Milk, and Infant Formula*

Nutrient	Recommended Dietary Allowances*		Human Milk† (per liter)	Cow Milk‡ (per liter)	Average Commercial Formula
	0 to 6 Months	6 to 12 Months			
Calories	108/kg	98/kg	750	670	680
Protein (gm)	2.2/kg	1.6/kg	11	20	15
Fat (gm)			45	36	36
Cholesterol (mg)			238	119	160
Calcium (mg)**‖	210	270	295	1220	500
Phosphorus (mg)**‖	100	275	143	935	300
Iron (mg)	6	10	0.2	0.5	12/1.4§
Sodium (mEq)	5	8.7	6.6	21	10
Potassium (mEq)	12.8	17.9	13	11	20
Renal solute load (mOsm/L)			79	221	150

*Data from National Research Council, *Recommended Dietary Allowances,* Washington, DC: National Academy Press, 1989.

†Data from Souci SW, et al. *Food Composition and Nutrition Tables 1986/87,* 3rd ed. Stuttgart: Wissenschaftliche Verlagsgesellschaft, 1986.

‡Whole milk (3.5% fat content).

§Level depends on whether iron fortified or not.

**From Food and Nutrition Board, National Academy of Science. Dietary Reference Intakes for Calcium, Phosphorus, Magnesium, Vitamin D, and Fluoride. Washington, DC: National Academy Press, 1997.

‖Adequate intake.

From Davis JR, Sherer K. *Applied Nutrition and Diet Therapy for Nurses,* 2nd ed. Philadelphia: W.B. Saunders, 1994.

As established by the guidelines of the American Academy of Pediatrics, the electrolyte, mineral, and vitamin contents are similar. Adequate amounts of these nutrients (except for fluoride and iron) are furnished if the infant receives 150 to 180 mL/kg/day. Fluoride is not added to formulas because of high variability of fluoride in the water supply. Because of the incident of municipal water contamination with the parasite *Cryptosporidium* in Milwaukee in 1993, the American Academy of Pediatrics Committee on Nutrition recommends boiling all water given to the infant for 1 to 2 minutes even if it is to be added to formula (Stehlin, 1996).

Infant formulas are so well balanced that the only supplement of real concern is iron. Iron-fortified formulas are recommended after 2 to 3 months of age.

Commercial formulas are more appropriate for infants than cow or goat milk. Malnutrition has been reported in infants fed home-recipe formulas. This may be related to variations in nutrient composition or unsanitary handling practices that may result in frequent infections or gastrointestinal disorders. Numerous specialized formulas are available for infants with special metabolic problems or intolerance problems, such as Lofenalac (Mead Johnson) for phenylketonuria or Meat Base Formula (Gerber) for cow milk intolerance. Soy-based formulas are probably the more frequently used specialized formula for infants unable to tolerate normal formulas. Infant formulas can be discontinued at about 1 year of age, but the milk provided thereafter should be whole milk. Special toddler formulas are available. While they are nutritionally good and do not need refrigeration, they are not necessary.

Infant Feeding Practices

Contrary to rigid feeding schedules enforced in the past, infants today are generally fed on demand, when they are hungry. A pattern usually develops within about 2 weeks, with the infant eating six times daily at 4-hour intervals. Gradually a pattern of feeding will evolve, allowing both infant and parents to sleep through the night. The position for bottle-feeding is as much like that of breast-feeding as possible (Fig. 12–1). Touching helps to strengthen feelings of love, security, and trust, and is as important as the nutrients in the formula. The infant should never be left alone with the bottle propped during feedings.

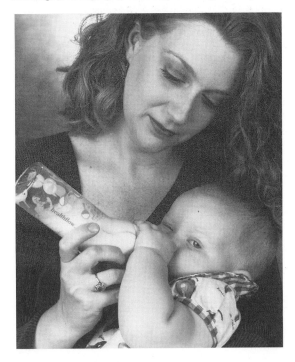

FIGURE 12–1 Mother feeding her infant with a bottle. New bottles allow feeding the baby in a more natural position, similar to the positioning for breast feeding. (Photography courtesy of Doug Davis.)

NEUROMUSCULAR MATURATION

Consideration of the developmental stage of the infant is necessary for a successful feeding regimen. Nutrition is related to neuromuscular maturation, especially for infants (Table 12–2).

Suckling is replaced with sucking by 4 months of age, when the orofacial muscles are used with the mouth more pursed, and the tongue moving back and forth. This backward movement of the tongue makes the smacking noises that occur.

A forward motion of the tongue and dropping the mandible is typical during the first 3 months. If semisolid foods are offered at this time, the tongue will force the food out. No discriminating taste is occurring, just reflex action.

The sucking motion becomes developed enough for the infant to eat and handle semisolid foods from a spoon around 4 to 6 months of age. This correlates with development of fine, gross, and oral motor skills to consume foods added to provide caloric and nutrient intake (see Table 12–2). If foods are not added by 6 months of age, growth may drop below the growth curves.

About 6 to 8 months of age, infants develop the ability to receive food and pass it between the gums in a chewing motion. By 7 months, infants can chew, so pureed foods are not required; some variety of texture is mandatory if infants are going to accept unfamiliar foods later in life. Unless textured foods are offered, the development of oral musculature may be slow or delayed, affecting the child's speech.

INTRODUCTION OF FOODS

Numerous false assumptions are associated with the introduction of solid foods. Despite the fact that many parents introduce solid foods during the first month, no nutritional advantage is associated with this practice. The most common reason for early feeding is to help the infant sleep through the night. This will naturally occur between 1 to 3 months of age, with girls sleeping through the night earlier than boys. This is a developmental milestone not related to what is fed.

Disadvantages in starting semisolid foods too early are (1) unnecessary costs, (2) high probability

TABLE 12–2   *Developmental Milestones in Feeding*

Stage/Age	Reflexes and Developmental Landmarks	Appropriate Nourishment
Newborn (Birth to 10 days)	Rooting reflex Sucking Puts hand or thumb in mouth	Colostrum or infant formula
Infant		
2 weeks to 3 months	Tonic neck reflex present Head control poor Bite reflex (stimulation to gums elicits a bite and release pattern) Recognizes feeding position and begins sucking and mouthing when placed in position	Breast milk or formula Begin fluoride supplement unless water contains fluoride
3 to 4 months	Development of mature suck and head control Rooting and bite reflex fade Suckle-swallow interferes with taking solid food	Breast milk or formula
4 to 6 months	Helps hold bottle Munching pattern begins Development of palmar grasp Able to bring objects to mouth and bite them Drooling (due to teething)	Semisolid or pureed foods; add 1 food at a time, beginning with rice cereal, strained vegetables, thin strained meats and fruits Provide at least 32 oz formula Begin iron supplement or fortified formula
6 to 9 months	Strong sucking pattern (less jaw movement) Gag reflex fades Holds bottle alone Develops inferior pincer grasp Able to self-feed by securing large pieces with a palmar grasp Lateral jaw movements Rotary chewing begins Can voluntarily release and resecure objects	Finger foods such as arrowroot biscuits, oven-dried toast, zwieback (foods should be soluble) Increase variety of textures (junior type or diced foods) Breast milk or fortified infant formula Fluoride supplement
9 to 12 months	Bites foods Grasps bottle and foods and brings them to the mouth Able to drink from a cup that is held Finger feeds with pincer grip Rotary chewing pattern Reaches for spoon	Same as above Fluoride supplement Breast milk or fortified infant formula (if homogenized milk is used, not >65% of total kilocalorie intake)

TABLE 12–2   *Developmental Milestones in Feeding* (Continued)

Stage/Age	Reflexes and Developmental Landmarks	Appropriate Nourishment
Infant *Continued*		
12 to 15 months	Messily attempts to use cup and spoon	Provide foods that adhere to spoon when scooped (mashed potatoes, applesauce, cooked cereal and cottage cheese)
		Homogenized milk
15 to 24 months	Walks alone	Chopped fibrous meats, e.g., a roast or steak
	May seek and get food independently	Solid foods
	Uses spoon to self-feed	
	Holds glass with both hands	Introduce raw vegetables and fruits gradually
	More skilled at cup and spoon feeding	
	Names food, expresses preferences; prefers unmixed foods	Foods of high nutrient value should be available
	Experiences food jags	Balanced food intake should be offered, but the child should be allowed to develop transitory food preferences
	Appetite appears to decrease	
		Homogenized milk

From Davis JR, Sherer K. *Applied Nutrition and Diet Therapy for Nurses,* 2nd ed. Philadelphia: W.B. Saunders, 1994.

of overfeeding, (3) effects on the immature digestive system, (4) increased risk of development of food allergies, (5) reduction of milk intake in lieu of a less nutritionally complete, adequate food, (6) decreased iron absorption, and (7) decreased absorption of energy and nitrogen.

Following the introduction of foods between 4 and 6 months, formula intake should remain around 32 oz daily. Foods should be presented to the infant with a spoon, never in a bottle.

Because of the possibility of a food allergy, only one new food should be introduced at a time. A waiting period of at least 7 days is recommended to observe for allergic reactions following the introduction of a new food. Early exposure to *allergens,* foreign substances or antigens that induce immunoglobulin E antibody production and stimulate an allergic reaction, in foods and in breast milk may increase the risk of allergic disorders in infants. Foods most commonly causing allergies include milk, soy, peanuts, egg whites (including ice cream), wheat, and chocolate. Therefore, it is advisable to not introduce these foods until after 9 to 12 months of age.

The recommended order of introduction for vegetables, meats, and fruits varies among pediatricians. Some advise the introduction of vegetables after cereals, then meats followed by fruits. Because sweet flavors are well accepted, the other foods are offered first. Preference for sweet foods is an innate desire.

Gradually, junior-type foods with a few lumps are introduced to initiate some chewing. The presence of a few teeth does not mean the infant is ready to actually masticate foods. Certain vegetables are more difficult to digest and are introduced after 1 year of age: cucumbers, onions, cabbage, and broccoli. Commercial baby food may be used, but foods from the family menu can be pureed for use. Avoid adding sugar to foods or products that contain large amounts of sugar.

When semisolid foods are introduced, the goal should be to include all food groups as soon as possible to assure a well-balanced diet

(Table 12–3). Guidelines for feeding infants to provide a balance of nutrients are similar to the Dietary Guidelines for Americans, except for limiting fat and cholesterol content.

SUPPLEMENTS

If iron-fortified formula is not used, iron supplementation is recommended for formula-fed infants after 4 months of age, breast-fed infants at 4 to 6 months of age, and preterm infants after 2 months of age. Iron supplementation (usually ferrous sulfate or ferric ammonium citrate) is ordinarily given as liquid drops or fortified cereals.

Systemically, fluoride supplementation is recommended for infants and children to increase the strength and acid resistance of developing tooth enamel. Thus, fluoride supplements are encouraged with ready-to-feed formulas. Infants receiving formulas reconstituted from a powder should be given fluoride supplements if the water supply is not fluoridated. As shown in Table 12–4, vitamin supplements containing fluoride may be prescribed by a physician or dentist.

Dental Hygienist Considerations

ASSESSMENT

- *Physical*—infant's developmental stage, neuromuscular development, age.

- *Dietary*—parent's knowledge of bottle feeding and feeding solid foods, source of iron, fluoride, and use of other supplements.

INTERVENTIONS

- Avoid recommending sugar-free foods, especially those containing sorbitol. This sugar substitute is a known cause of diarrhea in infants and children.

Nutritional Directions

- For the first months of life, 32 oz/day of formula will satisfy full-term infants.
- The practice of bottle propping should be avoided.
- The rate of growth is faster during infancy than at any other stage of life. Fats, a concentrated source of energy, are needed to support this rapid growth (40% to 50% of the total calories is recommended).
- Despite growing concerns over heart disease, cholesterol intake is important during the early developmental stages of infancy. There is little basis for recommending changes in fat intake before age 2.
- Store all vitamin/mineral supplements in a safe place from children; between 1986 and 1994, 38 children between 9 months and

TABLE 12–3   *Recommended Food Intake for Good Nutrition According to Food Groups*

Food Group	Serving Size	Servings/day	1 yr	2–3 yr	4+ yr
Bread, cereal, rice, pasta	1 slice 1 oz (cereal)	6–11	1–2	2–4	3–11
Vegetables	½ cup	3–5	½	1	3–5
Fruit	1 apple, banana	2–4	½	1	2–4
Milk, cheese	1 cup 1½ oz cheese	2–3	½	1	1–3
Meat, poultry, etc	2–3 oz	2–3	½–1	½–1	1–3

After age 2 yr, fats, oils, and sweets should be consumed sparingly.

C = 1 cup or 8 oz or 240 mL

Tbsp = tablespoon (1 Tbsp = 15 ml = ½ oz).

Nelson WE ed: *Nelson Textbook of Pediatrics.* 15th ed. Philadelphia: W.B. Saunders, 1996.

TABLE 12–4   *Dietary Fluoride Supplement Dosage Recommendations**

	Parts Per Million (ppm) of Fluoride in Water Supply		
Age of Child	Less than 0.3	0.3 to 0.7	Greater than 0.7
Birth to 2 years	0.25 mg/day	0	0
2 to 3 years	0.50 mg/day	0.25 mg/day	0
3 to 14 years†	1.00 mg/day	0.50 mg/day	0

The recommended dosage of a fluoride supplement varies with the fluoride content of the water and the age of the child. Contact your local water company or health department to determine the level of fluoride in the water.

*Recommended by the Council of Dental Therapeutics of the American Dental Association and by the Committee on Nutrition of the American Academy of Pediatrics.

†The American Academy of Pediatrics recommends providing tablets through at least age 16.

Reproduced by Permission of *Pediatrics* V 95, pg 777 Copyright 1995.

3 years of age died from iron overdose (Hingley, 1996).

◆ Reduced-fat milk is inappropriate for children under age 2.

◆ Honey is not appropriate for children under 1 year of age because botulism may occur.

◆ Advise parents to try not to show any dislike for a new food being served.

◆ Warn parents that supplements containing fluoride should never be added to milk; fluoride binds with milk and soy proteins, decreasing availability of fluoride significantly.

◆ Toddlers learn about food by touching/playing with it. Allow this to occur by offering finger foods.

Oral Problems in Infants

BABY BOTTLE TOOTH DECAY

A leading oral health problem among children under the age of 3 is baby bottle tooth decay (BBTD), also known as nursing bottle caries. This nutritional disease, associated with inappropriate feeding practices, is characterized by early rampant decay (Fig. 12–2). Treatment of BBTD is costly, requiring extensive extractions and/or restorations and causing serious future oral health problems and unnecessary suffering. Severe cases are treated under general anesthesia in a hospital. Since it is preventable and easily diagnosed in later stages, health care professionals and caregivers need to watch for early warning signs and detect the disease.

CONTRIBUTING FACTORS. The decay is created when a sweetened liquid (fruit juice, milk, sweetened water) pools around the teeth for extended periods of time while a child is sleeping. This will lead to demineralization of the enamel. Night-, nap- and frequent daytime bottle feedings are all factors related to BBTD. Excessive breast feeding, particularly when the infant sleeps with the mother and nurses as desired throughout the night, can also result in BBTD.

As the child sleeps, the cleansing action of saliva is diminished because of reduced salivary flow. The ultimate effect is poor clearance of the liquid. Also, the natural or artificial nipple rests on the palate during sucking, allowing the liquid to pool around the maxillary incisors. The position of the tongue covers and protects the mandibular incisors from the sweetened liquid (Table 12–5). Since the disease state follows the eruption pattern, the first molars will be affected next, then the canines. Children with BBTD are also at higher risk of interproximal decay as they grow older.

A second contributing factor to BBTD is infection with ***Streptococcus mutans.*** Colonization of *S. mutans* occurs after the infant's teeth erupt. Therefore, the teeth provide a surface for colonization of the pathogen, not the oral mucosa.

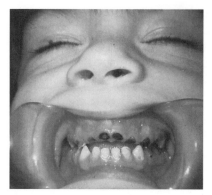

FIGURE 12–2 **Baby bottle tooth decay. (Courtesy of Alton McWhorter, DDS, MS, Associate Professor Pediatric Dentistry; The Texas A&M University System, Baylor College of Dentistry, Dallas, TX.)**

Infection with *S. mutans* occurs through transmission of the pathogen from the caregiver to the infant. This occurs when sharing utensils or other objects contaminated with saliva. The infant is

TABLE 12–5 *Sources of Fermentable Carbohydrates for Infants*

Liquids
Milk, cow, flavored, breast
Commercial infant formulas
Unsweetened fruit juice
Sweetened fruit juice and fruit drinks
Sweetened soft drinks
Sodas
Any sugar-sweetened beverages, such as sugar or corn syrup added to water
Other Sources
Some infant foods
Medication
Use of sweets to comfort or reward infant, such as pacifier dipped in honey
Infant cereals, teething biscuits, crackers
Dry cereals
Arrowroot biscuits and other cookies, pretzels
Fruits

more likely to be infected if the caregiver has a high level of *S. mutans*. The addition of frequent or prolonged exposure to a fermentable carbohydrate will inoculate *S. mutans*. Destruction of the tooth surface begins and can ultimately progress to rampant caries and abscesses.

COUNSELING. Begin dietary counseling as soon as the dental team is apprised of the pregnancy. Obtain diet histories of both parents to reveal cariogenic eating patterns that can be transferred to the newborn infant. An analysis of the frequency of fermentable carbohydrate intake and oral hygiene habits can be instrumental to creating an awareness of a potential problem for the parent (see chapter 16). Intercepting and modifying damaging health practices prior to birth can prevent BBTD and possibly the development of caries later.

Dental Hygienist Considerations

ASSESSMENT

- *Physical*—cursory exam to detect decalcification or carious lesions in the teeth.
- *Dietary*—parental knowledge of BBTD and what causes it; parental preferences for sweets; sharing of utensils contaminated with saliva; use of bottle propping, especially at night; use of corn syrup in the water bottle; dipping the bottle nipple or pacifier in honey or molasses.

INTERVENTIONS

- Educate all expectant parents and parents of infants about techniques for avoiding BBTD: when feeding an infant, hold the child and bottle; avoid bottle propping or using the bottle as a pacifier at bedtime.
- Wean the child from the bottle at about 12 months of age.
- Educate the parents about BBTD when (a) carious lesions are initially noted in a young child, (b) a child over 1 year of age is given a nighttime bottle, (c) either parent has active caries or dentures, and/or (d) sweets are used to comfort or reward the infant.

Nutritional Directions

- Terminate nighttime bottles or fill with water, or use a pacifier.
- Do not let infant suck the bottle unattended.
- Explain the importance of deciduous teeth (appearance, speech, ability to eat).
- Discuss the role of sugars, including sugar in milk, in the decay process.
- Explain methods of oral hygiene care for infants.
- Describe disadvantages of rampant decay in an infant (discomfort, future dental phobia, infection, cost, tongue-thrust habit).

CLEFT PALATE/LIP

In the United States, 1 infant out of every 700 (approximately 5,000 children) is born with a **cleft lip/palate** each year. Scientists believe that any number of factors, such as malnutrition, drugs, disease, or heredity, may cause this condition.

Feeding the infant with a cleft palate, with or without a cleft lip, presents unique problems. The length of time needed for feedings to provide adequate nutrients can be exhaustive for both mother and infant. Because of the opening between the roof of the mouth and the floor of the nasal cavity, the negative pressure needed for sucking cannot be created (Fig. 12–3). However, breast feeding can usually be successful; the infant adapts by squeezing or chewing the nipple.

Special devices are available if necessary. These are recommended when more than 1 to 1½ hours are required per feeding. The infant is held in a sitting position to prevent the formula from entering the nose. As soon as possible, spoon feeding is introduced. In severe cases, a prosthesis is made when the child is older (Fig. 12–4).

Patience is required, and extra time for feeding must be allowed to provide needed nutrients. The Suggestions for Feeding an Infant with Cleft Palate offers some tips for feeding techniques to provide nutrients while minimizing risks.

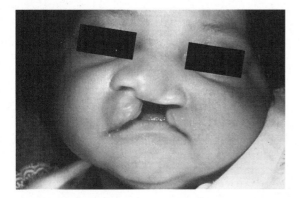

FIGURE 12–3 **Cleft lip/palate. (Courtesy of Nancy Sue Seale, DDS, MSD, Professor and Chairman, Department of Pediatric Dentistry, The Texas A&M University System, Baylor College of Dentistry, Dallas, TX.)**

Suggestions for Feeding an Infant with Cleft Palate

- Enlarging the hole in the nipple of the infant's bottle enables him or her to get milk more easily
- Boiling new nipples before use softens them
- Mixing pureed foods (fruits, vegetables, meats) with milk or broth makes a thinner consistency so they may be fed from a bottle with an enlarged hole in the nipple
- Frequent burping aids in releasing excessive air intake
- To pervent regurgitation, the older child should be taught to eat slowly and to take small bites
- Using a straw helps some children take liquids more easily
- Feeding the child with a cleft palate takes longer than feeding a normal child; the mother needs to allow the necessary time. Fatigue on the part of the parent may interfere with the child's receiving adequate nourishment

Adapted from Nizel AE. *Nutrition in Preventive Dentistry Science and Practice,* 2nd ed. Philadelphia: W.B. Saunders, 1981.

From Davis JR, Sherer K. *Applied Nutrition and Diet Therapy for Nurses,* 2nd ed. Philadelphia: W.B. Saunders, 1994.

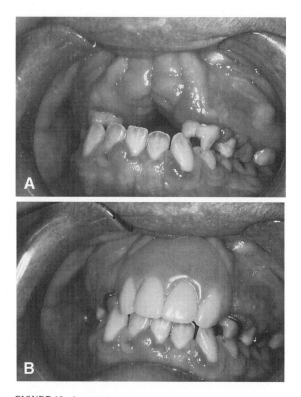

FIGURE 12–4   **(A) Cleft palate (B) Cleft palate with removable prosthesis. (Courtesy of Kathleen B. Muzzin, RDH, MS, Clinical Associate Professor, Caruth School of Dental Hygiene, The Texas A&M University System, Baylor College of Dentistry, Dallas, TX.)**

Dental Hygienist Considerations

ASSESSMENT
- *Physical*—cleft palate/lip aspiration.
- *Dietary*—feeding technique and past experiences in feeding infants.

INTERVENTIONS
- Explain that the principal problem is a lack of normal suction, but that by using some different feeding techniques, the infant can obtain adequate nutrients.
- These infants should be fed slowly at a 60° to 80° angle following guidelines in Suggestions for Feeding an Infant with Cleft Palate.

Nutritional Directions

- Introduce spoon feeding as soon as possible.
- Oral skills will develop after surgery to correct the problem.
- Acidic and spicy foods may irritate the delicate tissue in the cleft area.
- Young children with cleft palate are at increased risk for choking on foods that may slip into the trachea.
- Because of the increased incidence of enamel hypoplasia, encourage meticulous oral hygiene practices and limited cariogenic food or liquids to avoid carious lesions at these sites.
- Refer parents to the American Cleft Palate Association for literature and to local support groups.

TODDLER AND PRESCHOOL CHILDREN

Poor nutritional status (as measured by growth rate and biochemical indices) is generally more prevalent in lower socioeconomic groups, in which the amounts and variety of foods may be limited. Approximately 10% of all children, regardless of socioeconomic background, may be iron deficient. Zinc and calcium are also frequently deficient in the diet.

Because of high activity level, basal metabolic rate, and growth, the caloric requirement is relatively high, roughly 1,000 calories plus 100 calories per year of life. The high calcium requirements are generally met with formula through age 1, and with whole milk from age 1 to 2. Skim milk may be introduced after the second birthday. The RDAs for major nutrients are listed in Table 12–6.

During preschool years, life-long habits and food attitudes are formed that will to some extent affect health throughout life. A variety of foods should be available that provide the needed nutrients (see Table 12–6). A basic understanding of the nutrient content of foods, the role of foods in health, and food-related behaviors for these age groups is important for parents to promote food habits that are conducive to adequate nutrient intake. Foods are not only important for their relationships to health, but also contribute to social and personal pleasures.

Parental attitudes, eating habits, and food choices are the most influential factors in the child's food preferences. Foods that are disliked by one or both parents are not served often or may not be served at all. Additionally, children model themselves after their parents and tend to enjoy foods their parents like. When planning menus, the child's food preferences must be considered; but parents can control the options. Without appropriate guidance, young children will not independently make healthy food choices; therefore, the parents' role is to offer nutritious foods. Children can choose how much or even whether they will eat the food that has been provided. Feeding problems can result when either the parent or the child crosses this line of responsibility. The best predictor of a child's ability to regulate energy intake is parental control

of feeding. Children who had less ability to self-control energy intake had mothers who were more controlling of the child's food intake (Johnson & Birch, 1994). More food is eaten by the child when the family eats together, rather than just offering food for the child to eat alone.

Food jags are common and are a way to assert independence. This typical developmental stage is temporary. The food obsession may cause parental concern, but overreaction may prolong rather than correct such behaviors.

Toddlers (1 to 3 Years Old)

During the second year of life, development of fine motor skills results in toddlers learning to feed themselves. Although this is a messy learning process, it is a transitional period that will stabilize by age 2. Finger feeding may be preferred to spoon feeding; some finger foods should be provided at every meal. A cup can be manipulated by the toddler by about 18 months of age. Rotary chewing skills will develop in the second year. Until then, finely chopped meats are more popular.

Toddlers prefer regularity, so eating at the same time is desirable and helps control appetite. Regular meals also help to avoid fatigue, which can interfere with emotions as well as appetite. Tired children eat poorly. If the child has been very active, a short rest

TABLE 12–6   *Recommended Dietary Allowances for Selected Nutrients for Children Through Adolescence*

Nutrient	Children 1–3	Children 4–6	Children 7–10	Boys 11–14	Girls 11–14	Boys 15–18	Girls 15–18
Calories	1,300	1,800	2,000	2,500	2,200	3,000	2,200
Protein (gm)	16	24	28	45	46	59	44
Vitamin C (mg)	40	45	45	50	50	60	60
Calcium (mg)*†	500	800	1,300	1,300	1,300	1,300	1,300
Iron (mg)	10	10	10	12	15	12	15

*From Food and Nutrition Board, National Academy of Science. Dietary Reference Intakes for Calcium, Phosphorus, Magnesium, Vitamin D, and Fluoride. Washington, DC: National Academy Press, 1997.

†Adequate intake.

Data from National Research Council Subcommittee on the 10th edition of the RDAs. *Recommended Dietary Allowances.* 10th ed. Washington, DC: National Academy Press, 1989.

period before the meal will improve the child's intake.

Refusing to eat is a way to attract attention. Appetites are erratic and unpredictable. Parents should not force children to eat when they are not hungry. When well-balanced meals are provided, caloric intake at any given meal varies greatly, but compensation at subsequent meals results in little variability in total energy intake. If sufficient amounts are not eaten at the meal, parents may limit snacking or provide nutrient-dense snacks. Snacks can contribute significantly to adequate nutrient intake.

Small amounts of food should be offered several times a day. Serving sizes should be based on appetite, but initially about 1 Tbsp can be offered for each year of age. A good rule to follow in menu planning for children is one tart, one mild, and one crispy food. Brightly colored foods are especially appealing to children.

Preschool Children (4 to 6 Years Old)

Preschoolers are relatively independent at the table and can feed themselves. Certain factors need to be considered to make the mealtime pleasant rather than an ordeal. By allowing children to eat with adults, they will imitate others in both manners and food habits. Parental insistence on proper utensil usage, manners, and other demands that are inappropriate for this age group may result in less food intake. Parents need to ignore some inappropriate mealtime behaviors and focus on positive nonmealtime activities. Conversation and role modeling can reinforce appropriate eating behavior and promote food intake.

Snacks are still important for adequate nutrient intake. Some wholesome snacks enjoyed by this age group include cheese cubes, fresh fruit, raw vegetable sticks, milk or yogurt, and fruit juices.

Few children eat the recommended five servings of fruits and vegetables daily. Strong-flavored vegetables (overcooked cabbage and onions) are generally disliked but are more popular if served raw. Crisp, raw vegetables are well accepted. Tough stringy fibers, such as those in celery or string beans, should be removed. Since these children still enjoy eating with their fingers, cutting fruits and vegetables into small pieces increases their acceptance. Preschoolers generally prefer their foods separate; casseroles and stews may not be well accepted. Foods that can be easily chewed are more readily accepted.

Dental Hygienist Considerations

ASSESSMENT
- *Physical*—socioeconomic level, child's age, developmental level.
- *Dietary*—eating environment, frequency of meals and snacks, quantity of foods consumed, adequacy of intake, parental beliefs/preferences about food.

INTERVENTIONS
- Encourage eating meals at regular times. Serve food shortly after being seated to avoid restless behavior.
- If sufficient amounts are not eaten, limit snacking or provide nutrient-dense snacks; offer cheese cubes, fresh fruit, raw vegetable sticks, milk or yogurt, fruit juices; whole grain cereals and bread.
- Clarify any misconceptions that may interfere with a child's ability to consume foods that meet their nutrient needs for growth and development, such as "healthy foods do not taste good" or "healthful eating means eliminating all high-fat foods."

Nutritional Directions

- Offer new foods frequently; introduce one new food at a time with a familiar food to get more acceptance. The child is expected to taste each food that is prepared and served; but the taste may be very small.
- It is believed that atherosclerosis begins in childhood and that a reduction of dietary fats (especially saturated) and cholesterol after the second birthday decreases the risk of this disease. However, undue restriction

of fat intake could possibly compromise a child's growth and development and potentially lead to eating disorders or unhealthy attitudes about food.

♦ If the child is allowed to snack too frequently, he or she may not ever become hungry.

♦ Food, especially sweet foods, should not be used as a bribe or reward.

♦ Children should not be made to clean their plates.

♦ Present disliked foods in a matter-of-fact manner, serving small portions (1 to 2 tsp); discard without comment if the child does not eat them.

♦ Successful feeding of children may be best accomplished by providing a variety of healthful foods and allowing them to eat without coercion. Without some guidance, however, children may fill up on calorie-dense foods that do not provide adequate amounts of other nutrients.

Oral Problems of Toddlers and Preschool Children

DENTAL CARIES

Most children experience dental disease, and a few experience high rates of caries. Since tooth formation begins before birth and is not completed until about 12 years of age, the actual structure of the tooth is affected by food intake during this time. Poorly developed teeth are more susceptible to decay later in life.

A clear relationship has been shown between nutritional deficiency during tooth development and tooth size, tooth formation, time of tooth eruption, and susceptibility to caries. One occurrence of mild to moderate malnutrition during the first year of life is associated with increased caries in both the deciduous and permanent teeth later in life (Alvarez, 1995). Calcium, along with vitamin D, must be present for proper calcification of the dentin and normal enamel. Vitamin D is critical to tooth development; later deficiency can promote tooth decay.

A reduction in the prevalence of dental caries and remineralization of teeth are observed when 1 ppm of fluoride in drinking water is present during tooth formation. Excessive fluoride in water can cause permanent mottling of teeth. A 60% reduction of caries is gained by using fluoridated water during earlier growth periods. Topical administration of fluoride to teeth can also result in reduction of tooth decay.

Food selection and patterns of consumption influence oral health. Use of a toothbrush with dental floss, fluoride toothpaste, and sealants cannot completely control caries formation. Cariogenicity of food is influenced by the presence of fermentable carbohydrates, physical properties, and the frequency of consumption (see chapter 16).

Dental Hygienist Considerations

ASSESSMENT

● *Physical*—condition of oral cavity, presence of dental caries.

● *Dietary*—intake of fermentable carbohydrates, frequency of snacking, calcium and vitamin D intake, source of fluoride.

INTERVENTIONS

● Stress the importance of providing adequate amounts of protein, vitamins C, A, and C, calcium, phosphorus, and fluoride during the formation and calcification of teeth.

● Provide nutritious snacks such as cheese cubes or raw vegetables. Fibrous foods promote salivary flow and buffering capacity of saliva.

● Provide an opportunity to brush the teeth after eating; if not possible, rinse mouth with water.

Nutritional Directions

♦ Vitamin D-fortified milk and cheeses not only provide nutrients needed for healthy teeth, but also are noncariogenic.

♦ If the water supply is not fluoridated, a fluoride supplement should be provided as described earlier in the chapter. Also, encourage the use of fluoridated toothpastes.

♦ An examination and topical fluoride in the dental office are recommended every 6 to 12 months.

♦ Limit sticky carbohydrate foods such as candies, cookies, crackers, pastries, and raisins between meals. These contribute to dental caries by their carbohydrate content, physical properties, and frequency of consumption.

SPECIAL-NEEDS CHILDREN

Health conditions, such as mental retardation of unknown origin, cerebral palsy, Down syndrome, infantile autism, and muscular dystrophy have significant oral health and oral hygiene implications. Mastication and swallowing problems occur in all these conditions except Down syndrome. Some children with oral-motor problems can improve; others cannot.

Children with cerebral palsy and Down syndrome may practice **bruxism.** Loosened teeth interfere with the child eating chewy foods such as meats. Children with cerebral palsy, Down syndrome, and mental retardation are likely to have abnormal sensory input and muscle tone. Difficulties with sucking, swallowing, spoon-feeding skills with semisolid or solid foods, chewing development, and independent feeding are common. Tongue thrust associated with many of these conditions results in significant food waste and may jeopardize nutritional status.

Dental problems may become exaggerated in these children as a result of difficulty in maintaining good oral hygiene, the child's unique dietary habits and patterns, and the influences of their prescribed medications. Such problems include oral infections, dental caries, and periodontal disease.

The dental hygienist may become involved in team treatment of these children. Treatment is individualized, depending on the potential capabilities and skills of the child. Nutrition intervention for feeding skill difficulties is to assist in planning diets that are easiest for the client to eat and still meet their nutritional needs.

SCHOOL-AGE CHILDREN (7 TO 12 YEARS OLD)

These middle childhood years are the result of early growth and development; reserves are laid down for upcoming rapid adolescent growth. New activities and new friends begin to influence choices and broaden one's horizons. The child will be exposed to different foods and food patterns and begin to accept more foods. These new ideas may affect food choices at home.

Almost all foods are liked; vegetables are the least favorite. Planning menus around food groups is important to include all the necessary nutrients. Foods containing mostly sugars or fats need not be eliminated, but they should not replace recommended amounts from the food groups. The appetite is usually good; but food habits and intake may suffer because children do not take time for meals (15 to 20 minutes). Enforcement of a specific amount of time at the table may prevent the child from forming the habit of eating too fast. Poor appetite may be caused by stresses, such as schoolwork and emotional difficulties.

Students are ravenous after school. Although bakery products, soft drinks, candy, and chips are favorites, nutritious snacks are preferable. More access to money and influence of peers and mass media may result in expenditures at fast-food restaurants and from vending machines. These foods are usually high in fat, salt, and sugar.

The number of children who are overweight has almost doubled in the last 25 years. Weight loss or gain reflects inadequate or excessive intake, which should be balanced with an appropriate amount of exercise. In addition to children watching television, they are now spending more hours in front of a computer screen. The goal for obese children is weight maintenance or reduction in the rate of weight gain while height increases. By "growing into their weight," body fat decreases without compromising lean body mass and growth.

This age range also generally marks the exfoliation of all or most of the primary teeth and the eruption of most of the permanent teeth. This is significant since the application of topical fluoride now becomes as effective as systemic fluoride administration. To provide maximum protection, systemic fluoride is recommended through age 14 for those in nonfluoridated or inadequately fluoridated areas. Systemic fluoride is effective during the mineralization phase of erupting teeth and prior to eruption. Application of **sealants** act as a barrier protecting the decay-prone areas of the teeth from plaque and acid.

Dental Hygienist Considerations

ASSESSMENT
- *Physical*—schoolwork or emotional difficulties, activity level, sports interests.

- *Dietary*—nutrient/fluid intake, appetite, food preferences and eating patterns, child's/parent's beliefs about nutrition.

INTERVENTIONS
- Have nutritious snacks readily available.
- Do not recommend weight-reduction diets for overweight children.
- Evaluate for maximum fluoride protection, particularly for erupting and newly erupted teeth.

Nutritional Directions

- Children involved in meal preparation are more likely to eat the food they prepare and to be aware of what is in the food.
- Have nutritious foods available for snacks, such as dried fruits, yogurt, popcorn, low-fat cheese, or dry roasted seeds or nuts.
- Encourage appropriate oral hygiene techniques.

ADOLESCENTS

Major biologic, social, psychological, and cognitive changes occur during adolescence. Because of these changes, 17% of U.S. teenagers are considered to be at nutritional risk. It is not surprising that many adolescents consume less than adequate amounts of nutrients, and fitness levels are declining. Rapid growth rates cause them to be particularly susceptible to nutrient deficiencies. Many of their eating practices place them at risk for developing chronic diseases later in life.

Growth and Nutrient Requirements

Growth of long bones, secondary sexual maturation, and fat and muscle deposition create an increased nutrient requirement. Although the RDAs provide recommended nutrient intakes by chronologic age, nutrient needs closely parallel physical development. For instance, adolescent girls need to increase their energy intake sooner and decrease it more quickly than boys because of earlier onset of

puberty and lower total body weight once adulthood is reached. Adolescent boys have greater nutritional needs than adolescent girls because of growth rates and body composition changes (see Table 12–6). A 15-year-old boy requires 3,000 calories as compared with 2,200 calories for a 15-year-old girl.

The need for calcium and iron is of particular importance. Forty-five percent of adult skeletal mass is formed during adolescence (National Dairy Council, 1996); calcium needs are greater than at any other time of life. Calcium intake during adolescence promotes calcium retention and bone mineral density. Adequate calcium intake is important for achievement of peak bone mass. An increase in calcium intake by adolescent females from 800 to 1,300 mg/day may increase hip bone density 6%.

The expansion of blood volume, and increase in red cell mass and muscle mass especially in boys, and the need to replace iron losses associated with menstruation in girls require increased iron. Participation in sports activities leads to red blood cell destruction. Poor dietary habits result in inadequate folate, riboflavin; vitamins B_6, A, and C, iron; and calcium intake.

Influential Factors on Eating Habits

Complex external factors, such as family, peers, mass media, and economic and sociocultural factors, and internal factors, such as physiologic needs, body image, self-concept, food preferences, and personal values/beliefs toward health and nutrition all influence food choices. Probably the strongest influential factor among teenagers is peer pressure. Not only are food choices affected, but also the times available to eat may be determined by group activities. Eating is an important part of socialization and exerting one's independence.

Most adolescents are stressed because of continual changes. Sexuality, body image, scholastic and athletic pressures, relationships with friends and relatives, finances, career plans, and ideologic beliefs may cause conflicts as adolescents try to understand their identity. The presence of stress can decrease the utilization of several nutrients, particularly vitamin C and calcium.

Increasing numbers of children and adolescents are overweight. Adolescents, especially girls, are often obsessed about their body image and a desire to be thin. They are eager to try fad diets and other unsafe weight-loss methods which may be inadequate in nutrients. This is unfortunate because nutrients during this period are necessary to build and strengthen their bodies to last a lifetime. Obesity, anorexia nervosa, and bulimia are serious health concerns amenable to early treatment. Oral problems associated with eating disorders are discussed in chapter 15. Prevention may be the only successful treatment in some cases.

Favorite food choices are carbonated beverages, milk, steak, hamburgers, pizza, spaghetti, chicken, french fries, ice cream, oranges, orange juice, apples, and bread. Vegetables are not popular. Milk consumption is being replaced by carbonated beverages, especially in adolescent girls.

About 25% of an adolescent's calories come from high-calorie, low-nutrient dense foods, making overeating easy. Such problems as excessive intake of sodium, sugar, and fat; inadequate fiber; frequent snacking and skipping meals; eating on the run; and reliance on convenience and fast foods are accentuated during this time.

Fast-food restaurants, vending machines, and convenience stores fit adolescents' busy, active lifestyles. Fast foods are acceptable nutritionally when consumed in moderation as a part of a well-balanced diet. Lower-calorie items and a wider variety of selections now on the menu, such as salad and low-fat milkshakes, can contribute to nutrient requirements without providing excessive calories.

Snacking is often essential for meeting daily energy and nutrient needs, especially when the adolescent is physically active or in a growth period. These snacks can offer significant nutrients and can be improved with the substitution of a milkshake for a cola, or by adding orange juice.

Nutrition Counseling

The best tactic for nutrition counseling among adolescents is to appeal to their physical image or their muscular development for sports. The earlier information is presented, the more likely it is to be accepted and used later in life. In helping adolescents improve their eating patterns, the best approach is to praise good food choices, ignore those that are neutral, and discourage harmful practices. By presenting nutrition and health information in terms relevant to adolescent lifestyles and personal interests, health professionals can help teenagers understand how current eating and exercise habits affect their current and future health.

Dental Hygienist Considerations

ASSESSMENT
- *Physical*—activity level, growth spurt, use of illicit drugs, body image, self concept, influence of peer pressure, stress level.
- *Dietary*—adequacy of nutrient intake based on the Food Guide Pyramid; use of fast foods, convenience foods or vending ma-

chines; food preferences and personal values/beliefs toward health and nutrition; alcohol intake.

INTERVENTIONS

- Encourage use of calcium-containing foods.
- Praise good eating patterns; help modify foods and suggest substitutions.
- Determine the frequency, quantity, and form of cariogenic foods.

Nutritional Directions

- Teenagers should be aware of long-term risks and benefits of good nutrition, but the best approach is to focus on the short-term benefits of eating well.
- Restriction of calorie intake during the rapid growth period will compromise lean body mass accumulation despite a seemingly adequate protein intake (which is used for energy instead of growth).
- Intense physical activity can cause increased urinary loss of calcium and red blood cell destruction.
- Snacking can have a positive influence on the overall nutritional status of the teenager. Parents can stock the kitchen with nutritious snack foods, such as cooked meats, raw vegetables, milk, cheese, fruit, nuts, peanut butter, raisins, and popcorn to encourage good eating habits.
- Use of dietary supplements by most adolescents is not needed.

MATURITY IN THE LIFE SPAN

Major shifts in the age of the population are affecting American health care needs. Compared with 1988, when there were 30 million people aged 65 years and older (10% of the population), this population is expected to increase to approximately 39 million people (16%) by 2010 (U.S. Bureau of the Census, 1989; 1990). Improved medical care and good nutrition since infancy have helped us increase our life span; it is now important to increase the quality of that life.

Nutrition Screening Initiative

Malnutrition in the elderly usually occurs gradually. By the time it is recognized, full-blown medical problems are present that could have been avoided by correcting a lifestyle issue with simple measures. Up to 65% of clients admitted to acute-care hospitals and 50% of nursing home clients are at risk of malnutrition (Silver, 1991). Approximately 85% of our geriatric population have chronic diseases and conditions that increase their risk of poor nutritional status (Committee, 1986).

A multidisciplinary project of the American Dietetic Association, the American Academy of Family Physicians, and the National Council on Aging has launched a Nutrition Screening Initiative (NSI) to identify people at nutritional risk before significant deterioration of health. A checklist of key *risk factors* (major identifiable biologic or environmental circumstances or events that increase risk and suggest special care and attention) of poor nutritional status in persons over age 65 is given in Figure 12–5. This simple checklist, requiring only a few minutes to complete, is accompanied by a discussion of warning signs. Since food intake is directly related to oral problems, one of the questions in the initial screening inquires about oral problems affecting intake. These risk factors are used by clients to help determine whether a professional should be consulted. If so, the professional can further assess whether and to what extent nutritional well-being is impaired and what measures should be implemented before the situation becomes severe (Fig. 12–6).

Level 1 screening is designed to be administered in community settings by trained health workers. If indicated, these clients are referred to a physician or dietitian, or to other preventive interventions (economic assistance, shopping, transportation assistance, and so forth). Level 2 screening is the most comprehensive NSI tool and is designed for health

Determine Your Nutritional Health

The warning signs of poor nutritional health are often overlooked. Use this checklist to find out if you or someone you know is at nutritional risk.

Read the statements below. Circle the number in the yes column for those that apply to you or someone you know. For each yes answer, score the number in the box. Total your nutritional score.

	YES
I have an illness or condition that made me change the kind and/or amount of food I eat.	2
I eat fewer than 2 meals per day.	3
I eat few fruits or vegetables, or milk products.	2
I have 3 or more drinks of beer, liquor or wine almost every day.	2
I have tooth or mouth problems that make it hard for me to eat.	2
I don't always have enough money to buy the food I need.	4
I eat alone most of the time.	1
I take 3 or more different prescribed or over-the-counter drugs a day.	1
Without wanting to, I have lost or gained 10 pounds in the last 6 months.	2
I am not always physically able to shop, cook and/ or feed myself.	2
	TOTAL

Total Your Nutritional Score. If it's—

0-2	*Good!* Recheck your nutritional score in 6 months.
3-5	You are at moderate nutritional risk. See what can be done to improve your eating habits and lifestyle. Your office on aging, senior nutrition program, senior citizens center on health department can help. Recheck your nutritional score in 3 months.
6 or more	You are at high nutritional risk. Bring this checklist the next time you see your doctor, dietitian, or other qualified health or social service professional. Talk with them about any problems you may have. Ask for help to improve your nutritional health.

FIGURE 12–5 Determining nutritional health: Checklist for the "warning signs" of poor nutritional health. (Reprinted with permission by the Nutrition Screening Initiative, a project of American Academy of Family Physicians, American Dietetic Association, and National Council on the Aging, Inc., and funded in part by a grant from Ross Products Division, Abbott Laboratories.)

professional use generally requiring physician and dietetic or health care team involvement.

The general consensus is that "prevention of malnutrition is better than treatment during a crisis" (Davies, 1988). Most elderly clients can be motivated to make changes that will affect their health if the information is presented with an understandable rationale.

Physiologic Factors Influencing Nutritional Needs and Status

Many organ functions begin to decline with age, some as early as age 30; these physiologic changes may significantly influence nutritional require-ments of elderly people. **Homeostatic mechanisms** decline with age, and the precarious physiologic balance may be upset by disease; physical and/or mental disabilities; and environmental, economic, and social disabilities. Yet chronologic age and functional capacity do not always correlate.

In addition to the functional decline of many body organs, which may affect absorption, transportation, metabolism, and excretion of nutrients, food intake may be affected by age-related physiologic changes as well. Impairment of visual, auditory and olfactory sensory organs is common. Poor vision makes food preparation difficult and even hazardous in some cases, and may be responsible for senior citizens not identifying contaminated foods, which could lead to food-borne illnesses. Poor hearing increases isolation and decreases socialization.

ORAL CAVITY

Several physiologic changes in the oral cavity are significant factors in nutritional status. A progressive decline in gustatory and olfactory sensitivity, one's perception, or even the sensations in one's mouth affects food choices and quantity since "nothing tastes good." **Renal failure** and certain medications also lead to deterioration of taste sensitivity or perception. The **taste threshold** is high for the basic sensations as sweet, salty, sour, and bitter. Elderly persons may confuse taste

sensations, describing sour foods as metallic and salty foods as tasteless. Foods may be overly seasoned with salt or sugar as a consequence of **anosmia** and **hypogeusia.** Losses in salt or sugar perception make it difficult for some to comply with a low-sodium or diabetic diet. Other seasonings can be used to help replace the taste of salt or sugar.

Many commonly used medications, especially diuretics, antidepressants, and hypnotics, cause **xerostomia,** which compromises oral processing of foods and utilization of nutrients. Xerostomia affects about 72% of the elderly and has significant detrimental effects on nutrient intake (Loesche et al., 1995). Xerostomia causes difficulties with chewing and starting a swallow. Geriatric clients

FIGURE 12–6 **Schematicim: a practical approach to nutritional screening. (Reprinted with permission by the Nutrition Screening Initiative, a project of American Academy of Family Physicians, American Dietetic Association, and National Council on the Aging, Inc., and funded in part by a grant from Ross Products Division, Abbott Laboratories.)**

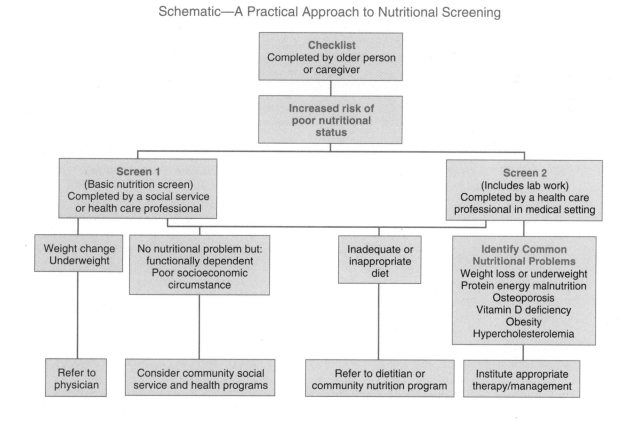

Schematic—A Practical Approach to Nutritional Screening

with xerostomia are more likely to omit crunchy foods such as vegetables, dry foods such as bread, and sticky foods such as peanut butter (Loesche et al., 1995). In conjunction with poor fluid intake, the elderly may become more susceptible to caries associated with the aging process.

Food selection is highly correlated with dentition. By age 65, an estimated 41% of Americans are completely edentulous (Carlos & Wolfe, 1989), and dental caries, including root surface caries, and destructive periodontal disease are widespread.

Periodontal disease, occurring in more than 90% of elderly people, is partially responsible for loss of teeth. A 1986 survey by the National Institutes of Dental Research representing more than 4 million retired individuals revealed an average loss of 11 teeth (NIDR, 1987). Calcium is readily mobilized from trabecular bone. A negative calcium balance results in loss of calcium from the maxilla and mandible, which are primarily trabecular bone. Normally alveolar bone is maintained in response to occlusal forces associated with chewing. Bone resorption accelerates and bone height rapidly diminishes in edentulous clients. If severe mandibular resorption occurs, it is very difficult to construct a well-fitting dental prosthesis.

Generally, clients who wear dentures have reduced masticatory efficiency—75% to 85% less than with natural teeth (Martin, 1991). Clients with seriously compromised natural dentition, periodontal health conditions, edentulous areas, or ill-fitting appliances tend to alter their food choices to reduce chewing or fear of choking. Consumption of some meats and fresh fruits and vegetables may decrease for choices that are softer. In comparison with younger individuals with no dental problems, magnesium, fluoride, and folic acid intake is significantly below the RDA. After edentulous persons fully adjust to new dentures, caloric intake increases, but magnesium, folic acid, fluoride, zinc, and calcium levels in their diet continue to be low. Weight changes, often occurring in the elderly, can be a reason for an ill-fitting dental appliance.

Unfortunately, many elderly individuals or their families do not believe that the cost of a new or replaced appliance is warranted because of their perceived life expectancy. Figure 12–7 compares improperly fitted dentures with correctly fitting ones in the same person. Even though they have dentures, some may not wear them, or they may not be able to chew because of a periodontal condition.

The prevalence of root caries is much higher in elderly adults than among younger adults: a 1985 survey by the National Institutes of Dental Research in 1985 revealed that over 60% of elderly adults have root caries. Recession of gingival tissues exposes root surfaces of teeth to the oral environment. The lack of a protective enamel layer on the root of the tooth makes it highly susceptible to dental caries.

GASTROINTESTINAL TRACT

Changes in esophageal motility and deterioration of nerve function may cause **dysphagia.** This frequently observed disorder increases risk of aspiration pneumonia and morbidity from inadequate nutrition. Persons with swallowing problems eat slowly and may not be able to consume adequate amounts.

Diminished hydrochloric acid secretion may affect absorption of calcium, iron, and vitamin B_{12}. **Atrophic gastritis** and **achlorhydria** (frequently observed in elderly persons) result in pernicious anemia because vitamin B_{12} cannot be separated from the food protein as a result of decreased gastric acid. Additionally, the lack of acid permits overgrowth of bacteria that utilize much of the available vitamin B_{12}.

Constipation may be a consequence of altered gastrointestinal motility, along with loss of bowel muscle tone, inadequate food and fluid intake, low-fiber diets, and inactivity. Additional causes include chronic laxative use and some medications, especially analgesics, antihypertensives, and narcotics. Constipation can be corrected by increasing fiber-containing foods, fluid intake, and activity level. Irritant laxatives should be avoided. A serious consequence of constipation is fecal impaction, which may result from impairment of rectal sensation and abnormalities of motor function related to medications or disease.

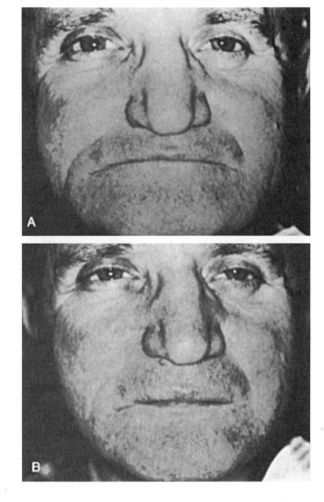

FIGURE 12–7 **A: Geriatric client wearing dentures with incorrect occlusal vertical dimensions; note overclosure. B: Same client with correct occlusal vertical dimension; note improvement in facial appearance. (From Nizel AE.** *Nutrition in Preventive Dentistry: Science and Practice.* **2nd ed. Philadelphia: WB Saunders, 1980.)**

RENAL SYSTEM

As a consequence of aging and certain chronic conditions (diabetes, hypertension, and atherosclerosis), renal function progressively declines. Drug and metabolic waste excretion and urine concentration are decreased.

THIRST MECHANISMS

Decreased thirst sensations are associated with aging. Fluid intake may not increase automatically to offset increased water losses from the compromised kidney; therefore, elderly persons are prone to dehydration.

Fever, which can lead to mild dehydration in healthy individuals, may result in severe dehydration in the elderly. Increased water intake should be encouraged.

MUSCULOSKELETAL SYSTEM

Bone **resorption** progresses rapidly in the elderly. Trabecular bone loss may be associated with physical inactivity, unavailability of calcium (inadequate dietary intake, imbalance in calcium to phosphorus ratio, and decreased calcium absorption), changes in hormones affecting calcium metabolism, and altered vitamin D metabolism associated with impaired renal function. Bone loss increases susceptibility to fractures and possible disability. Osteoporosis or shortening and outward bowing of the spine may develop.

Lean body mass declines, whereas adipose tissue increases. Persons with decreased lean body mass may have fragile esophageal tissues. Decreases in vital proteins result in an inability to respond to a physiologic injury or insult and declining function of many organ systems. Muscle mass can be preserved by increasing physical activity.

Basal metabolic rate decreases with less muscle mass (see Figs. 6–2 and 12–8). In older individuals, the basal metabolic rate may be as much as 10% to 12% below the level of 20-year-olds (see chapter 6).

Socioecoonmic and Psychological Factors

ECONOMIC FACTORS

Most retired people live on fixed incomes significantly lower than when they were employed. Poverty is estimated to be double the rate observed in younger adults; 25% of those living independently have an annual income under $10,000 (Nutrition Screening, 1990). Inflation, failing health, and medical bills can have a devastating effect on fixed incomes. The food budget frequently suffers and is a risk factor for inadequate nutrition. For example, fresh fruit and vegetable choices may be curtailed because of their high cost. Title III Nutri-

tion Programs for the Elderly (congregate dining and Meals on Wheels) are available to improve the nutrition and health status of the elderly and possibly prevent or postpone more expensive services of long-term care institutions. High-quality, nutritious meals are furnished free to the elderly who qualify or at a minimal charge for all senior citizens.

SOCIAL FACTORS

An inability to drive or access to transportation affects utilization of health services and availability of food. Approximately one-third of non-institutionalized persons over 65 live alone (Nutrition Screening Initiative, 1990). Those who live with another person and are socially active tend to consume a larger variety of foods. An inactive person who lives alone may lack motivation to prepare well-balanced meals, especially if appetite is poor.

PSYCHOLOGICAL FACTORS

Apathy and depression can predispose elderly persons to decreased appetite and interest in food. Depression is difficult to distinguish from symptoms related to the stresses of later life—illness and changes in lifestyle. Depression may be considered by some as a natural and inevitable component of aging; therefore treatment may not be obtained. Loneliness is related to dietary inadequacies.

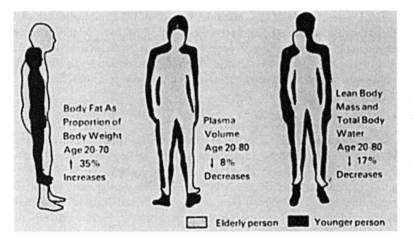

FIGURE 12–8 **Changes in the body with aging. (From Vestal RE. Drugs and the Elderly. NIH Publication No. 79-1449. Washington, DC: U.S. Department of Health, Education and Welfare, 1979.)**

TABLE 12-7   *Reasons for Drug Abuse*

Client Factors
Giving incomplete drug history to all the physicians consulted
Altering dosages—larger amounts taken to relieve symptoms
Being overly concerned about health (conviction that he or she is suffering from a serious ailment or preoccupied with daily bowel movements)
Mismanaging drugs—not taken as scheduled, leading to increased or decreased frequency (increases with number of drugs taken concurrently)
Sharing drugs with others
Being influenced by advertisements

Health Care Provider Factors
Prescribing medicines by several physicians
Improperly prescribing dosage in relation to client's current weight and renal function
Failing to correlate current drug usage to symptoms
Inappropriately using drugs to control client behaviors (sedatives and tranquilizers)
Inadequately reviewing care plans by nurses

Adapted from Roe DA. *Geriatric Nutrition.* 2nd ed. Englewood Cliffs, NJ: Prentice-Hall, 1987.

Other Factors Influencing Nutritional Status

Often, the existence of two or more chronic diseases, such as diabetes, renal disease, or heart disease, occurs in the elderly. Dietary restrictions associated with management of these diseases can be confusing; improper food selection or fear of choosing the wrong foods may be a factor for inadequate nutrition. The result of certain treatments, such as with cancer, can affect eating by creating loss of appetite, nausea and vomiting, diarrhea or constipation, xerostomia, or changes in the taste of food.

Approximately 45% of elderly clients living independently take multiple prescription drugs that can interfere with appetite and nutrient absorption (Nutrition Screening Initiative, 1990). Medications are likely to be used excessively or misused (Table 12–7).

Although drug-nutrient interactions can compromise anyone's nutritional status, these problems are accentuated in the elderly. Physiological and pathophysiologic changes, such as decreased hepatic and renal clearance, result in greater variability and less predictability of the drug's effects.

Nutrient Requirements

RDAs

Metabolism to maintain body functions requires all the same nutrients, but nutrient amounts may need to be adjusted in the elderly because of stress and diseases of aging. Current RDAs provide guidelines for nutrient requirements of adults over 51. Elderly individuals differ from one another more than any other group. The general consensus is that dietary needs of persons between 50 and 60 years of age are different from those over 70, but inadequate information was available in 1989 for the National Research Council to establish a different RDA. Per the RDA, nutrient allowances are the same as for adults 23 to 50 years of age except for caloric requirements, the B vitamins closely associated

TABLE 12–8   *National Academy of Sciences—National Research Council Recommended Dietary Allowances, Revised 1989*

	Men	Women
Age (yr)	51+	51+
Weight (kg)	77 (170 lb)	65 (143 lb)
Height (cm)	173 (68 in.)	160 (63 in.)
Protein (gm)	63	50
Fat-Soluble Vitamins		
Vitamin A (mcg retinol equivalents)	1,000	800
Vitamin E (mg α-tocopherol equivalents)	10	8
Vitamin D (mcg cholecalciferol)	5	5
Water-Soluble Vitamins		
Ascorbic acid (mg)	60	60
Folacin (mcg)	200	180
Niacin (mg)	15	13
Riboflavin (mg)	1.4	1.2
Thiamin (mg)	1.2	1
Vitamin B_6 (mg)	2	1.6
Vitamin B_{12} (mcg)	2	2
Vitamin K (mcg)	80	65
Minerals		
Calcium (mg)*†	1,200	1,200
Phosphorus (mg)*†	700	700
Iodine (mcg)	150	150
Iron (mg)	10	10
Magnesium (mg)	350	280
Zinc (mg)	15	12
Selenium (mcg)	70	55

*From Food and Nutrition Board, National Academy of Science. Dietary Reference Intakes for Calcium, Phosphorus, Magnesium, Vitamin D, and Fluoride. Washington, DC: National Academy Press, 1997.

†Adequate intake.

Adapted from National Research Council Subcommittee on the Tenth Ediction of the RDAs: *Recommended Dietary Allowances.* 10th ed. Washington, DC: National Academy Press, 1989.

with energy intake (thiamin, riboflavin, and niacin), and a lower iron allowance for women because of menopause (Table 12–8). Current data suggests that the RDAs established in 1989 underestimated adequate intakes for riboflavin, vitamin B_6, folic acid, vitamin B_{12}, vitamin D, and calcium (Russell, 1997).

FLUIDS

Fluid intake is of particular concern because elderly persons are susceptible to fluid imbalances secondary to the physiologic changes previously discussed. Certain chronic illnesses (heart and kidney disease) lead to impairment of various homeostatic mechanisms controlling water balance. Seemingly mild stresses—such as the presence of fever, infection, or diarrhea, or the use of diuretics—can upset the normal homeostasis. Dehydration is probably the primary cause of confusion in the hospitalized elderly. In normal situations, six to eight glasses of fluids per day are recommended.

Adequate fluids must be provided for both normal and abnormal fluid losses. An elderly client may intentionally restrict fluids because of nocturia, incontinence, or having to request assistance to be toileted. Soups, juices, milk products, decaffeinated soft drinks, tea, and coffee can enhance fluid intake since plain water is not highly favored by elderly clients.

ENERGY

Recommended energy intake reflects average requirements of groups of people and actually varies significantly with clients, depending on the amount of lean body mass and activity level. The RDA for clients over 51 has been lowered to 2,300 for men and 1,900 for women (or 30 Cal/kg). This decrease of calories from the younger age group is related to a lower basal metabolic rate and physical activity.

PROTEIN

An intake of 12% to 14% or more of the energy needs should come from protein foods, or a minimum of 50 gm in a 1,900-calorie diet. An allowance of 0.8 to 1 gm/kg appears to be adequate. Added stress from surgery, infection, injury, gastrointestinal disease, or routine drug usage increases catabolism, thereby increasing dietary protein requirements. Inadequate monetary resources to purchase meat products is a principal reason elderly persons consume less protein.

CARBOHYDRATE

Because carbohydrates have not been identified as essential nutrients, there is no RDA for simple or complex carbohydrates. Currently, approximately 45% of the calories are from carbohydrate. A larger amount of complex carbohydrates is advisable since tolerance of simple sugars diminishes with aging. This also increases vitamin and mineral intake as well as dietary fiber, which contributes to enhanced bowel motility.

FAT

The upward adjustment of carbohydrate is balanced with the need for less dietary fat. According to Dietary Guidelines for Americans, less than 30% of the energy requirement should come from fat (USDA, USDHHS, 1990). However, the benefit of decreasing cholesterol and fat intake to lower serum cholesterol levels in clients over 70 is not established.

MINERALS

Dietary mineral intake may need to be adjusted, based on assessment of the client's nutritional status. Excess or even normal dietary levels can have deleterious consequences in certain diseases, particularly chronic illness such as hypertension or congestive heart failure. On the other hand, rigid and severe restrictions may seriously affect food acceptance. Thus, individualization is crucial.

Elderly clients (especially women) usually have a negative calcium balance and lose bone mass, leading to spontaneous fractures. Inadequate calcium intake is possibly one reason for this, but genetic, hormonal, and environmental factors are also important. Decreased physical activity contributes to calcium loss over the years. The combined use of alcohol, antacids, and drugs also disturbs calcium reserves (see chapter 8).

Milk provides needed calcium. However, regular consumption of milk is difficult to accomplish because of its expense and the frequent trips needed to purchase it. Dry milk, while less palatable than regular milk, can be incorporated into many foods without deleterious effects on taste. Additionally, some persons have difficulty obtaining adequate calcium because of lactose intolerance.

Age-related diseases (osteoporosis, arthritis) are major contributors to iron deficiency. Many gastrointestinal diseases can significantly reduce dietary iron absorption, and gastrointestinal bleeding increases iron losses. Therapeutic drug use can markedly alter dietary iron utilization.

Dietary zinc appears to be closely related to energy intake and can be adequate with careful food selection on a modest calorie intake. Older adults seem to consume only marginal amounts of zinc (less than 45% of the RDA) because of lower protein consumption. In addition, intestinal absorption is decreased in those over 65 years of age. Numerous health problems are associated with zinc deficiency, including hypogeusia, poor appetite, delayed wound healing, and depressed immune function. Even though zinc supplementation is popular, self-medication with amounts above the RDA (15 mg) may be harmful, as discussed in chapter 11. A physician's diagnosis and recommendation should be obtained.

FAT-SOLUBLE VITAMINS

Absorption of vitamin A is increased with age, but intake is usually below the RDAs. Vitamin A stores may become depleted in elderly persons stressed by disease and malnutrition and with cirrhosis, alcoholism, and chronic gastrointestinal disorders.

Vitamin D status may be compromised in the elderly, especially if chronically ill and/or institutionalized. A deficiency may be the result of several causes: dietary insufficiency, malabsorption, kidney disease, and inadequate exposure to sunlight. Vitamin D stores decline with age, particularly in those unable to go outdoors. Additionally, aging appears to reduce conversion of vitamin D precursors to the active form both in the skin and by the kidneys. Since adequate vitamin D nutriture is required for optimal absorption of calcium, inadequate intake affects bone mineralization. For this reason, the Food and Nutrition Board recommends increasing vitamin D intake to 10 mcg daily for 51 to 70 year olds and 15 mcg for those over 70.

WATER-SOLUBLE VITAMINS

Many elderly persons have low plasma and tissue levels of ascorbic acid. This is generally considered to be a consequence of inadequate intake or increased requirement related to routine medications. Several epidemiologic studies have shown

that cataract formation is delayed in those with higher intakes of vitamin C.

Neurologic symptoms similar to dementia may result from deficiencies of vitamins B_6, B_{12}, and folate. Diets are reported to be marginal. Normal folate nutriture can be maintained despite low folate intake and malabsorption (secondary to atrophic gastritis), possibly as a result of increased bacterial folate synthesis in the upper gastrointestinal tract. With increasing age, serum levels of pyridoxal (vitamin B_6) phosphate decrease. Altered vitamin B_6 metabolism could necessitate a higher requirement. Economic factors and chewing problems may negatively affect meat consumption, thus negatively affecting vitamin B_6 and B_{12} intake. Cobalamin (vitamin B_{12}) may be less available in the elderly because of atrophic gastritis and bacterial overgrowth. Studies have reported decreased symptoms (confusion, disorientation, and neurologic problems) in those treated with vitamin B_{12}. In addition to these neurologic symptoms, metabolic abnormalities also occur before serum B_{12} concentrations are low; anemia occurs only in severely B_{12} depleted individuals (Allen & Casterline, 1994).

Eating Patterns

DEFICIENCIES

Numerous surveys, including the 10-State Nutrition Survey, the Health and Nutrition Examination Survey (HANES), and USDA food consumption studies have clearly shown that persons 50 years of age and older consume less food than younger adults. Inadequate amounts of water and nutrients are consumed both in the community and in institutions.

Dairy products, fruits, and vegetables are frequently lacking in the diet, especially for those living alone. The choice of softer food usually results in a decrease in protein and intake of more fat and simple carbohydrates. Snacks are popular, averaging two per day (afternoon and evening). These may provide important additional energy, but they are often high only in carbohydrate, particularly sucrose. In general, those with less education and income; the housebound, especially those living alone; those with physical disabilities, depression, and other mental disorders; those with recent drastic lifestyle changes; and those who do not have regularly cooked meals are considered to be at risk of developing malnutrition.

SUPPLEMENTS

Milk-based food supplements, such as an instant breakfast mix, are economical and can help prevent nutrient deficiencies. A tasty supplement can augment overall nutrient intake to maintain nutritional status. On the other hand, commercial liquid nutrition supplements, such as Ensure (Ross) and Sustacal (Mead Johnson), are more convenient and may be preferred.

Dental Hygienist Considerations

ASSESSMENT

- *Physical*—visual appraisal of weight status, chronic disease, dentures, swallowing process, xerostomia, condition of oral cavity and gingiva; dry mucous membranes; financial status, socioeconomic status, mental status, educational level, psychological status; types of drugs taken, including over-the-counter drugs and aspirin use.
- *Dietary*—adequacy of nutrients and fluid intake based on the Food Guide Pyramid; motivation to eat and drink; beliefs and attitudes about foods or products to delay the aging process; multivitamin/mineral use.

INTERVENTIONS

- Encourage new denture wearers to swallow liquids with the dentures first, then to chew soft foods, and, last, to bite and masticate regular foods. It is easier to master the complex masticatory movements in this order and protects the mouth from becoming sore.
- Wearing new dentures, especially by edentulous postmenopausal women, may promote positive calcium balance and decrease alveolar resorption with calcium supplements.

- For edentulous clients, inquire about the preferred texture of food. Do not assume edentulous clients require pureed foods; because of lack of visual appeal and flavor, appetite may become depressed if only these foods are offered.
- Encourage clients to eat slowly and to chew the food well.
- Encourage nutrient-dense foods, especially for clients who have a low-calorie intake.
- Suggest enriched or fortified cereals or to increase intake of iron and other nutrients.
- Encourage milk and milk-product consumption or discuss adding dry milk into foods.
- Often health care providers recommend lemon glycerin swabs to moisten oral tissues in clients with xerostomia. Because lemon is an acid that may cause decalcification of the teeth, and glycerin is a form of alcohol that can create a dryer mouth, a better alternative would be to moisten a swab with water and apply it to the dry mucosa.
- Avoidance of certain food categories (such as fresh fruit and vegetables and meats) because of masticatory difficulties may aggravate other nutrition-related problems if these foods are major sources of vitamins and minerals.

Nutritional Directions

- A well-balanced diet following the Dietary Guidelines for Americans may delay the symptomatic aging process.
- Factors that slow the aging process include regular exercise, abstinence from smoking, and reducing stress.
- Less muscle tissue and a lower activity level result in a reduced caloric requirement.
- Physical training enhances muscle strength and preserves muscle mass.
- If xerostomia is present, use artificial salivas, gum, or hard, sugarless candies; practice

frequent oral hygiene care; and drink adequate fluids.

♦ For clients with compromised natural dentition or xerostomia, suggest including fluids, sauces, or gravies with each meal to make chewing easier. However, do not let beverages interfere with food intake.

♦ Nutrition counseling by a Registered Dietitian can provide information on consuming adequate amounts of high-quality protein to help clients living on a limited budget and offer alternatives to eating problems.

♦ Discuss economical fruit, vegetable, and meat selections (see chapter 14).

♦ Encourage wise selections of convenience foods. Explain how to read food labels to make selections that are appropriate for restricted diets or to provide a well-balanced diet.

♦ Adequate fluid intake is beneficial in preventing and treating constipation.

♦ Vitamin supplements over 100% of the RDIs should be taken only if there is a specific need or if recommended by a physician.

♦ Use of vitamin and mineral supplements does not eliminate the need to consume a nutritionally balanced diet, nor do they protect against the development of chronic diseases associated with inappropriate food intake.

♦ Encourage consumption of a vitamin C-rich food daily.

♦ Review economical sources of folate and cooking practices to retain folate.

℞ Excess supplementation of vitamins and minerals may cause more problems with hypervitaminosis and detrimental effects on other nutrients. For instance, zinc supplements can result in copper imbalance and reduce high-density lipoprotein cholesterol levels.

HEALTH APPLICATION 12

Considerations Regarding Nutrient Requirements for Growth, Development, and Future Health

The Food Guide Pyramid, discussed in chapter 1 (Fig. 1–4), is the basis for meeting nutritional requirements of growing children. Portion sizes are adjusted based on children's smaller size and physiologic needs, and in some instances the number of servings from a particular food group varies from an adult's needs. The key message of the Food Guide Pyramid, variety, moderation, and balance in food choices, applies to childhood nutrition.

Dietary Guidelines for Children

Pediatricians and nutrition experts have not reached a consensus on the issue of appropriate dietary guidelines for children. They are concerned with two goals: (1) providing adequate calories and nutrients to support growth and development, and (2) reducing the risk of diet-related chronic diseases later in life. While most are basically in agreement on the goals, making the necessary dietary changes would not guarantee the positive outcomes desired and could potentially have some negative effects.

The energy needs of children and adolescents are high to support growth and development (Fig. 12–9). Many children consume less calories per day than the RDAs. At the same time, childhood obesity in the United States is increasing. Whether the RDAs for energy requirements of children are too high or whether other factors, such as genetic and environmental or decreased physical activity, are the cause has not been determined.

Younger children need to eat foods with high nutrient and energy density because they are unable to eat large quantities of food at any particular time. Because of their extra nutrient needs for growth and development, dietary deficiencies develop more quickly and have more severe consequences than adults.

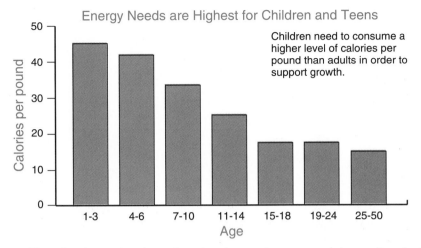

Energy Needs are Highest for Children and Teens

Children need to consume a higher level of calories per pound than adults in order to support growth.

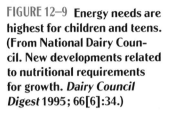

FIGURE 12–9 **Energy needs are highest for children and teens. (From National Dairy Council. New developments related to nutritional requirements for growth.** *Dairy Council Digest* **1995; 66[6]:34.)**

The basic reasoning for implementing the Dietary Guidelines for fat and cholesterol is based on the assumption that childhood obesity and/or cholesterol levels will continue into adulthood. Based on current knowledge, it is uncertain whether a modification of food choices during childhood will prevent future chronic disease or whether most children will be able to meet energy and nutrient requirements on a reduced-fat diet. Additionally, the effect of implementing a reduced-fat diet during childhood on the incidence of eating disorders is unknown.

In the Bogalusa Heart Study, a greater percentage of the children consuming less than 30% of their calories from fat did not meet the RDAs for numerous vitamins and minerals compared to children whose intakes were not modified (i.e., intake of more than 40% of calories from fat) (Nicklas et al., 1992). Even without making any changes in eating habits, many children's nutrient intake fails to meet the RDAs, especially for calcium, vitamin B_6 and zinc. Intake of these and other nutrients is frequently affected when fats are reduced because of a reduction in intake of milk and meat products. A severe reduction in fat has resulted in delayed growth and puberty.

The American Health Foundation (AHF) recently recommended that a reasonable goal for dietary fiber intake during childhood and adolescence may be approximately equivalent to the age of the child plus 5 gm/day. This formula (age + 5) represents a level that would provide health benefits, such as normal laxation, without compromising mineral balance or caloric intake in children over 2 years of age. Based on this formula, minimal dietary fiber intake would be 8 gm/day for a 3-year-old and would gradually increase to 20 gm/day for a 20-year-old. The gradual increases are consistent with current guidelines for adult dietary fiber intake (25 to 35 gm/day). The amount of dietary fiber recommended for children under 2 years of age is still being debated.

CASE APPLICATION FOR THE DENTAL HYGIENIST

A 75-year-old edentulous client is not eating because he states he has difficulty chewing and food does not taste good. He has lost 14 lbs (usual weight, 170 lbs) and dislikes a lot of red meat and milk.

Nutritional Assessment

○ Height, weight, ideal body weight, % weight loss
○ Nutrient/fluid intake in relation to RDAs
○ Medications
○ Alterations in taste or smell
○ Support group, significant others, living arrangements, social support
○ Psychological status

Nutritional Diagnosis

Altered nutrition: less than body requirements related to taste changes and chewing difficulty.

Nutritional Goals

Client will consume a well-balanced diet (based on the Food Guide Pyramid) and verbalize ways to increase protein and calcium intake.

Nutritional Implementation

Intervention: Encourage small, frequent meals.
Rationale: This helps the elderly client consume adequate amounts of nutrients by decreasing fatigue and feelings of fullness that may occur with larger meals.

Intervention: Suggest use of spices such as pepper, thyme, and basil.
Rationale: These spices may improve the taste of foods since an elderly client's taste thresholds are altered.

Intervention: Encourage fluids with meals.
Rationale: This will make chewing easier.

Intervention: Examine and question about the fit of the prosthesis. Clinically, conduct an intraoral and extraoral examination, especially noting any deviations from normal of the underlying tissue.
Rationale: The weight change may have created a loose-fitting denture and ultimately difficulty in chewing. An ill-fitting denture may also result in weight loss.

Intervention: Emphasize use of eggs, turkey, chicken, fish, meats marinated in wine or vinegar, and soy products such as tofu and bacon bits.
Rationale: Since he does not like red meats, the client may obtain needed protein in a more acceptable manner.

Intervention: Emphasize the use of low-fat or nonfat dairy products, such as yogurt, cream cheese, cheese, or frozen yogurt.
Rationale: Since he does not like milk, these foods are alternatives to supply the needed calcium.

Intervention: Encourage adding powdered milk to soups, sauces, cereals, and casseroles.
Rationale: These are methods to increase both protein and calcium consumption.

Intervention: Encourage the client to walk outdoors for 10 to 20 minutes daily and to eat foods that require more chewing, such as lettuce salads, raw carrots, and cabbage.
Rationale: Exercise is important to maintain bone density in the mandible and throughout the body. Calcium absorption, dependent on vitamin D, can be obtained through sunshine.

Intervention: Suggest mixing meat with vegetables.
Rationale: Since he enjoys vegetables, this form may be more palatable for him and will thus enhance protein intake.

Intervention: Refer the client to Meals on Wheels or another federally funded program (food stamps), community meals centers, or church-sponsored centers.
Rationale: Anorexia may be due to a lack of socialization during mealtimes.

Evaluation

The client should be eating at least 75% of the number of food servings from the Food Guide Pyramid and steadily gain weight until desired body weight is achieved. Other behaviors, such as consuming yogurt, eggs, fish, and dry milk in foods, will increase calcium and protein intake.

Student Readiness

1. Plan meals for 1 day for a family with a 2-year-old toddler, a 10-year-old boy, and a 15-year-old girl.
2. Discuss feeding a newborn infant from birth to age 1.
3. What is considered normal weight for a newborn infant?
4. Describe your approach to counseling an expectant parent about BBTD.
5. A mother wants to know why snacks are needed and which ones to give her preschooler to lessen the risk of developing dental cavities. What would you tell her?
6. A mother tells you that since her child is hyperkinetic she is going to stop all sugar. How would you respond?
7. Plan a day's menus for an elderly edentulous client.
8. What are some vitamin and mineral deficiencies that might influence mental attitudes of elderly clients?
9. Discuss reasons elderly clients might not eat adequately.
10. Visit a group meal program. Review the menu and discuss beneficial effects of the program's various activities.
11. List nutritional interventions to help a healthy elderly client with full dentures to eat.
12. Observe the staff at an extended-care facility and note positive activities related to maintaining good oral health and those that can be improved.

CASE STUDY

Mrs. C. is at her 6-month recall and brags about her 6-month old daughter, Jennifer. Jennifer weighed 7 lbs at birth and now weighs 15 lbs. She was bottle-fed from birth. At 3 months, Mrs. C. introduced cereals, but Jennifer has resisted all attempts to increase her solid food intake. She is allowed to go to sleep with a bottle and is often propped up in her crib with a bottle at the day care center.

1. What additional assessment data would you need?
2. Is Jennifer's weight gain within the expected range?
3. How much should she gain in the next 6 months?
4. What tentative dental hygiene diagnosis could you derive?
5. The dental hygienist encourages Jennifer's mother to discontinue the habit of allowing her to go to sleep with a bottle and to request that the day care center do the same. Why?
6. The physician recommends that solid foods be introduced gradually to Jennifer. What foods should be introduced first?
7. When will Jennifer be old enough for finger foods?
8. Why should honey be withheld until 1 year of age?

CASE STUDY

A 75-year-old man widowed for 2 years is seen in the health-care clinic for decreased intake. He states that nothing tastes good. He is on a limited, fixed income from Social Security. He has lost 6 lbs within the last year. His current weight is 130 lbs, height is 5'7". He is edentulous and refuses to get dentures because he feels he is "too old."

He fixes a bologna sandwich occasionally, but mostly eats frozen food dinners. He thinks meats and fruits are too expensive to buy and states that "they spoil before I can eat them." He will eat overcooked vegetables in the summer because a neighbor shares products from his garden. He does not want to use any community resources because he does not "want a handout."

1. Explain why "food does not taste good."
2. What psychological and social factors may influence his dietary patterns?
3. What are some practical ways to increase protein and calcium in his diet?
4. How could you address his attitude of not wanting to accept "a handout"?

5. What medical and dental information should you assess on this man to determine nutritional status?

6. What are the strengths and weaknesses of his diet?

7. What behaviors would indicate this client is meeting his nutritional needs?

Case Study

R.J. is a large 16-year-old male (6'4", 190 lbs) who has complained to you about pain from dental caries. He is active in athletics in school and has a part-time job. You determine from his dietary history that his appetite is very good and that his nutrient intake is adequate, except for vegetables. Snacking, principally soft drinks, candy, and cookies, constitutes almost 50% of his total caloric intake.

1. How would you counsel R.J.? What motivational factors would you consider for him?

2. What are some dental hygiene nutritional diagnoses/goals and interventions for Raymond?

3. What further data are needed for a complete assessment?

4. When having R.J. choose better snack options, what are some that you would recommend?

Case Study

Norma returns for a 6-month recall. Since her last check up, this 17-year-old female has developed 12 new dental caries in the lower anterior teeth. Norma's parents are in their 50's. Her father has lost numerous teeth as a result of periodontal disease and her mother is completely edentulous. Norma has no medical problems other than rhinitis (inflammation of the nasal mucous membranes secondary to allergies), which causes her to breath through her mouth much of the time. The oral examination showed normal color and tone of the oral mucosa, tongue, and gingivae. Her decayed, missing, filled rate was 17. She reports eating a varied well-balanced diet except for fruit and vegetable intake. Because of the dryness in her mouth, she relies heavily on cough drops and chewing gum.

1. What is a possible cause of these new dental caries?

2. What suggestions would you give her to relieve mouth dryness?

3. Based on her dietary habits, what nutrient appears to be inadequate?

References

Allen LH, Casterline J. Vitamin B_{12} deficiency in elderly individuals: Diagnosis and requirements. *Am J Clin Nutr* 1994; 60(1):12–14.

Alvarez JO. Nutrition, tooth development, and dental caries. *Am J Clin Nutr* 1995; 61(2):4105–4165.

Carlos JP, Wolfe MD. Methological and nutritional issues in assessing the oral health of aged subjects. *Am J Clin Nutr* 1989; 50 (5 Suppl):1210–1218.

Committee on Education and Labor. Compilation of the Older Americans Act of 1965 and related provisions as amended through December 29, 1981. Washington, D.C., 97th Congress, 1986.

Davies L. Practical nutrition for the elderly. *Nutr Rev* 1988; 46(2):83–108.

Department of Health and Human Services (DHHS), Public Health Service, National Institutes of Health,

National Heart, Lung, and Blood Institute, National Cholesterol Education Program. Report of the expert panel on blood cholesterol levels in children and adolescents. NIH Publication No. 91-2732, 1991.

Hingley AT. Preventing childhood poisoning. *FDA Consumer* 1996; 30(2):7–11.

Johnson SL, Birch LL. Parents' & childrens' adiposity and eating style. *Pediatrics* 1994; 94(11):653–661.

Loesche WJ et al. Xerostomia, xerogenic medications, and food avoidances in selected geriatric groups. *J Am Geriatrics Soc* 1995 Apr; 43(4):401–407.

Martin W. Oral health in the elderly. *In* Chernoff R, ed. *Geriatric Nutrition: The Health Professional's Handbook.* Gaithersburg, MD: Aspen, 1991: 107–182.

National Dairy Council. Teens at risk: Nutrition issues for the 90's. *Dairy Council Digest* 1996; 67(3): 13–18.

National Institute of Dental Research (NIDR). Oral Health of U.S. Adults: The National Survey of Oral Health in U.S. Employed Adults and Seniors: 1985–86. Washington, D.C. GPO, USDHHS 1987. NIH Publication No. PHS 87–2868.

Nicklas TA et al. Dietary fiber intake of children and young adults: The Bogalusa Heart study. *J Am Diet Assoc* 1995; 95(2):209–214.

Nicklas TA et al. Nutrient adequacy of low fat intakes for children. The Bogalusa Heart study. *Pediatrics* 1992; 89(2):221–228.

Nieves JW et al. Teenage and current calcium intake are related to bone mineral density of the hip and forearm of women aged 30–39 years. *Am J Epidemiol* 1995; 141(4):342–351.

Nutrition Screening Initiative Survey. Washington, D.C.: Peter D Hart Research Associates; February 1990.

Russell R. New views on the RDAs for older adults. *J Am Diet Assoc* 1997; 97:515–518.

Saldanha LG et al. Fiber in the diet of US children: Results of national surveys. *Pediatrics* 1995; 98(2): 994–1001.

Silver AJ. Assessing the nutritional status of the elderly. *J Am Diet Assoc* 1991; 91 (Suppl 9):A156.

Stehlin IB. Infant formula: Second best but good enough. *FDA Consumer* 1996 June; 30(5):17–20.

US Bureau of the Census. *Statistical Abstract of the United States: 1990.* 110th ed. Washington, D.C.: US Government Printing Office, 1990.

US Bureau of the Census. Projections for the Population of the United States by Age, Sex and Race, 1989 to 2080. Current Population Report Series. P–25, No. 1018, Washington, D.C., 1989.

US Department of Agriculture (USDA), US Department of Health and Human Services (USDHHS). *Dietary Guidelines for Americans.* 3rd ed. Home and Garden Bulletin No. 232. Washington D.C.: US Government Printing Office, 1990.

Chapter 13

Nutritional Requirements Affecting Oral Health in Females

OBJECTIVES

The Student Will Be Able To:

- List nutrients that are usually supplemented during pregnancy and lactation.
- Recommend some changes in food intake during pregnancy and lactation to provide adequate nutrients.
- List high-risk factors for pregnancy.
- Recognize dental hygiene considerations for clients who are pregnant or breastfeeding.
- Identify nutritional directions for the above clients.

GLOSSARY OF TERMS

Low birth weight   weighing less than 5½ lbs (2,500 gm)

Premature   born before the state of maturity, occurring with a gestational age (length of pregnancy) of less than 37 weeks

Gravida   pregnant woman; 3 would reflect that a woman has been pregnant three times regardless of the outcome of the birth

Primigravida   woman in her first pregnancy

Phenylketonuria   an inborn error of metabolism

Nutritional insult   deficiency or excessive amounts of specific nutrients

Nutrient-dense   containing a high percentage of nutrients in relation to the number of calories it provides

Anencephaly   absence of a major portion of the brain and skull

Erythropoiesis   the formation of red blood cells

Pica   abnormal consumption of specific food and nonfood substances, such as dirt, clay, starch, or ice

Test Your NQ (True/False)

1. All efforts should be made to satisfy a pregnant woman's food cravings because cravings reflect an innate need for certain nutrients. T/F
2. The fetus is nourished from the mother's nutrient stores. T/F

3. Following a pregnancy, most mothers have at least one cavity because calcium was pulled from teeth for use by the developing fetus. T/F

4. A woman should eat twice as much food when she is pregnant because she is eating for two. T/F

5. Women should gain 22 to 27 lbs during a pregnancy. T/F

6. Vitamin A is the only nutrient that warrants global supplementation during pregnancy. T/F

7. Virtually all women can produce enough milk. T/F

8. Breast milk that is too thin must be nutritionally inadequate. T/F

9. If the breast milk supply is inadequate, a feeding should be omitted to have more milk available later. T/F

10. WIC is a governmental program that provides supplemental foods for women, infants, and children. T/F

HEALTHY PREGNANCY

Although there is no specific definition of a healthy pregnancy, the health of both mother and infant is important. In addition to continued preservation of the mother's physical health, emotional and psychological welfare is also important. The goals for an infant are that he or she be full-term (born between the 39th week and 41st week of gestation) and mature (weighing more than 6 lbs) (IM, 1990). **Low-birth-weight** (LBW) and **premature** infants have more abnormalities as well as increased morbidity (infections and illnesses) and mortality and decreased mental performance. Primary factors for success are preconceptional nutritional status, appropriate weight gain, and adequate intake of essential nutrients during pregnancy. Apparently if the mother's nutritional status is poor, the placenta does not perform its function well.

A classic report published in 1970 by the National Academy of Sciences established a basis for increased nutritional requirements during pregnancy. This was followed with further recommendations regarding weight gain and nutrient supplements published in *Nutrition During Pregnancy* (IM, 1990). This information was compiled by separate subcommittees that evaluated available scientific information to establish guidelines for optimal outcomes.

Factors Affecting Fetal Development

PRECONCEPTIONAL NUTRITIONAL STATUS

Maternal health and fetal growth and development are affected by nutrient intake not only during the pregnancy, but prior to conception as well. Numerous pregnancies with less than a year between pregnancies deplete nutritional reserves. A recent history of oral contraceptive use indicates an increased need for vitamins C, B_6, and B_{12}, and folate. Because of the rapid development of body parts and organs during the first trimester, birth defects are likely to occur if usual dietary habits are poor or if drugs are used during this critical period. However, infant birth weights are affected more by nutrient intake during the second and third trimesters.

Although poor nutrient intake can produce a LBW infant, it is commonly believed that the fetus is protected at the expense of the mother. In some instances, higher requirements are met by increased nutrient absorption; for other nutrients, such as iron and calcium, the mother's stores may be depleted if intake is inadequate.

UNUSUAL DIETARY PATTERNS

Pica affects about 20% of women considered to be at high risk of having premature or LBW infants. These women are from lower socioeconomic groups or have a low educational level; are in poor nutritional health; may be teenaged mothers having clinical problems, such as pregnancy-induced hypertension; or are affected by behavioral/environmental factors, such as alcohol or substance abuse. Pica is more likely to be practiced by black women living in rural areas with a positive childhood and family history of pica. Pica is associated with iron deficiency and has been associated with maternal and perinatal mortality.

Beliefs about cravings and folklore that could influence dietary selections are regional. These beliefs may not be supported by scientific information and may be detrimental. Familiarity with local beliefs is needed to counsel **gravidas** about beliefs that are potentially detrimental to good nutrition during pregnancy. Special dietary restrictions may be practiced based on a food fad, or ethnic, cultural, or religious customs. In addition to assessing the effects of these on nutritional status, an awareness of these practices will allow the dental hygienist to provide guidance about desirable food choices that are within these constraints.

HEALTH CARE

Availability and use of health-care services are related to problems in pregnancy. Inadequate prenatal care leads to more problems for both mother and fetus. Prenatal care is also important to prevent chronic health problems, such as diabetes and hypertension, from affecting the embryo.

AGE

Maternal age can be a factor in the increased number of LBW infants among **primigravidas** under age 18 or over the age of 35. Most females do not complete linear growth and achieve gynecologic maturity until the age of 17. Nutritional requirements are quite high to meet the growth needs for both the adolescent and fetus. Not only are many of these young girls still growing and storing nutrients in their own bodies, but also the majority have an inadequate intake of calcium, iron, vitamin A, niacin, and calories. Intake of calorie-dense foods and erratic eating may preclude adequate intake of required nutrients. The socioeconomic disadvantages of these young mothers may affect their diet as a result of the amount of food available and their uninformed selections. Increased energy requirements are usually met without concentrated effort as a result of the increased appetite.

Pregnancy after the age of 35 or 40 is influenced by the individual's overall health. Maternal risks involve medical conditions, such as diabetes, hypertension, and cardiovascular problems. These conditions are closely supervised to lessen their impact on the fetus. A woman needs to be particularly aware of maintaining her nutritional health if a later pregnancy is anticipated. As the mother's age increases, her baby is more likely to be premature and smaller than average.

WEIGHT

Successful pregnancies depend on ideal preconception weight plus appropriate weight gain during gestation, but weight gain during pregnancy influences the birth weight more than the prepregnancy weight. Ideally, weight adjustments of overweight or underweight women should be made before conception.

DRUGS AND MEDICATIONS

The use of tobacco, alcohol, caffeine, some medications, megadoses of nutrients and illegal drugs may detrimentally affect the fetus. Alcohol can cross the placenta, and alcohol abuse results in fetal alcohol syndrome, discussed in Health Application 13.

ARTIFICIAL SWEETENERS

The debate continues over the use of nonnutritive sweeteners during pregnancy. Saccharin, acesulfame-K, and aspartame or their chemical components can cross the placenta, but may not harm the fetus if used in moderate amounts.

The American Dietetic Association has concluded that artificial sweeteners are safe during pregnancy when used in moderation, however, pregnant women with **phenylketonuria** should not use aspartame.

Factors Affecting Oral Development

In general, the potential arrangement of teeth, their eruption time, pits and fissures on the enamel, and cariogenicity are attributed to heredity. However, nutrition can determine whether teeth achieve their optimum genetic potential.

Calcification of deciduous teeth begins about the fourth month of pregnancy; development of more than 60% of the 52 deciduous and permanent teeth is initiated during gestation (Table 13–1). By the fourth month of pregnancy, the jaw bone is calcified. Critical periods for various stages of tooth development occur at different times. Nutrients supplied by the mother must be available for development of pre-eruptive teeth and soft tissues in the proper sequence.

Severe and irreversible damage results if **nutritional insult** or infection occurs during critical stages, especially to dentin or enamel formation (Table 13–2). After eruption, the tooth has no mechanism to repair itself. Severe nutrient deficiencies can result in malformations such as cleft palate, cleft lip, and shortened mandible. Less severe nutrient deficiencies can reduce the size of the tooth, interfere with tooth formation, delay the time of tooth eruption, and increase susceptibility of the teeth to caries.

When a pregnant woman develops a fever during an infection, the resultant disruption of calcium and phosphorous balance will affect the developing fetal tooth structure. This disruption in tooth structure formation will continue for as long as it takes to regain this balance.

The dentin and enamel of the tooth are dependent on many nutrients: vitamin C for formation of collagen matrix, and calcium, magnesium, phosphorus, and vitamin D for mineralization. Keratin in the enamel is dependent on vitamin A for its synthesis. An inadequate amount of any of these nutrients during the development of the teeth results in an imperfect matrix, with subsequent imperfection of the mineralization (see Table 13–2).

Whether fluoride supplements during pregnancy will prevent dental caries in infants has not been determined. Fluoride passes through the placenta to the fetus, but whether the placenta can filter excess fluoride is unknown. Large amounts of caffeine consumption (e.g., more than 7 cups/day of coffee) during pregnancy and lactation could be responsible for malformations and increased susceptibility to decay of the primary first molars.

Nutritional Requirements for Pregnancy

The RDAs for pregnancy (Table 13–3) indicate advisable nutrient intake for optimum health of mother and fetus. Accelerated growth and metabolism increases most nutrient requirements to some extent. Each vitamin and mineral will not be separately discussed; Table 13–3 shows the increased amounts recommended for each of the nutrients as established by the National Research Council (1989). According to the subcommittee report (IM, 1990), the following mean nutrient intakes are commonly below the 1989 RDAs for pregnant women: calories, vitamins D, E, and B_6, folate, and the minerals iron, zinc, calcium, and magnesium. In addition to low intake of these nutrients, gravidas on vegan diets frequently consume inadequate amounts of vitamin B_{12} and sometimes vitamin D.

ENERGY/CALORIES

During pregnancy, calorie requirements increase to ensure nutrient and energy needs. The RDAs allow an additional 300 calories or 36 to 40 Cal/kg body weight/day during the second and third trimesters. This additional energy is needed to (1) build new tissues (including added maternal tissues and growth of the fetus and placenta), (2) support increased metabolic expenditure, and (3) move the additional weight. Dieting for weight loss is never recommended during pregnancy. Unless the gravida is significantly underweight

TABLE 13–1 *Chronology of Development of the Human Dentition*

Tooth	Hard Tissue Formation Begins	Amount of Enamel Formed at Birth	Enamel Completed	Eruption	Root Completed
Primary Dentition					
Maxillary					
Central incisor	4 mo in utero	Five sixths	1½ mo	7½ mo	1½ yr
Lateral incisor	4½ mo in utero	Two thirds	2½ mo	9 mo	2 yr
Cuspid	5 mo in utero	One third	9 mo	18 mo	3¼ yr
First molar	5 mo in utero	Cusps united	6 mo	14 mo	2½ yr
Second molar	6 mo in utero	Cusp tips still isolated	11 mo	24 mo	3 yr
Mandibular					
Central incisor	4½ mo in utero	Three fifths	2½ mo	6 mo	1½ yr
Lateral incisor	4½ mo in utero	Three fifths	3 mo	7 mo	1½ yr
Cuspid	5 mo in utero	One third	9 mo	16 mo	3¼ yr
First molar	5 mo in utero	Cusps united	5½ mo	12 mo	2¼ yr
Second molar	6 mo in utero	Cusp tips still isolated	10 mo	20 mo	3 yr
Permanent Dentition					
Maxillary					
Central incisor	3–4 mo	—	4–5 yr	7–8 yr	10 yr
Lateral incisor	10–12 mo	—	4–5 yr	8–9 yr	11 yr
Cuspid	4–5 mo	—	6–7 yr	11–12 yr	13–15 yr
First bicuspid	1½–1¾ yr	—	5–6 yr	10–11 yr	12–13 yr
Second bicuspid	2–2¼ yr	—	6–7 yr	10–12 yr	12–14 yr
First molar	at birth	Sometimes a trace	2½–3 yr	6–7 yr	9–10 yr
Second molar	2½–3 yr	—	7–8 yr	12–13 yr	14–16 yr
Mandibular					
Central incisor	3–4 mo	—	4–5 yr	6–7 yr	9 yr
Lateral incisor	3–4 mo	—	4–5 yr	7–8 yr	10 yr
Cuspid	4–5 mo	—	6–7 yr	9–10 yr	12–14 yr
First bicuspid	1¾–2 yr	—	5–6 yr	10–12 yr	12–13 yr
Second bicuspid	2¼–2½ yr	—	6–7 yr	11–12 yr	13–14 yr
First molar	at birth	Sometimes a trace	2½–3 yr	6–7 yr	9–10 yr
Second molar	2½–3 yr	—	7–8 yr	11–13 yr	14–15 yr

Adapted and slightly modified by Massler and Shour from Logan WAG, Kronfeld R: J Am Dent Assoc 1933; 20:420.
From DePaola DP et al. Nutrition in relation to dental medicine. *In* Shils ME et al. (eds): *Modern Nutrition in Health and Disease*, 8th ed. Philadelphia: Lea & Febiger, 1994; 1007-1028.

TABLE 13–2   *Nutrient Deficiencies and Tooth Development*

Nutrient Deficiency	Effect on Tooth and Oral Tissue
Protein	Decreased tooth size; delayed eruption; increased caries susceptibility; dysfunctional salivary glands
Vitamin C	Disturbed collagen matrix of dentin
Vitamin A	Disturbed keratin matrix of enamel; increased enamel hypoplasia; increased caries susceptibility
Vitamin D	Poor calcification; pitting
Calcium, phosphorus	Decreased calcium concentration; hypomineralization
Magnesium	Enamel hypoplasia
Iodine	Delayed tooth eruption
Iron	Increased caries susceptibility
Zinc	Increased caries susceptibility
Fluoride	Increased caries susceptibility

Compiled from information in DePaola DP et al. Nutrition in relation to dental medicine. *In* Shils ME et al. (eds): *Modern Nutrition in Health and Disease,* 8th ed. Philadelphia: Lea & Febiger, 1994; 1007–1028; Nizel AE. Preventing dental caries: The nutritional factors. *Pediatr Clin North Am* 1977; 24;144–155; Shaw JH, Sweeney EA. Oral health. *In* Schneider HA, et al. (eds). *Nutritional Support of Medical Practice.* Philadelphia: Harper & Row, 1983.

before conception, additional calories are probably not needed during the first trimester. Since requirements of other nutrients are also increased, it is more important that foods be chosen wisely, using principally **nutrient-dense** foods (Fig. 13–1). Appropriate weight gain reflects adequacy of energy intake and influences birth weight. When caloric intake is slightly inadequate, physiologic adaptations spare energy for fetal growth. With adequate or generous energy supplies, energy balance is achieved in different ways depending on individual behavioral changes in food intake or energy

expenditures and on adjustments in basal metabolism or fat stores (King et al., 1994).

FAT

Although the Dietary Guidelines for Americans exclude pregnant and lactating women because scientific information confirming the safety of fat restriction on the developing fetus or its benefits to the mother are lacking, it is known that serum cholesterol and triglycerides become significantly elevated during pregnancy. The benefits may vary with type of fats restricted. Polyunsaturated fatty acids lower serum lipids, and omega-3 fatty acids may improve some obstetric complications. Psychomotor and visual development of children may benefit from arachidonic (polyunsaturated fatty acid) and docosahexaenoic acid (omega-3 fatty acid) in the diet.

PROTEIN

Protein is the basic nutrient for growth; therefore an additional 10 to 14 gm of protein, or a total of 60 gm daily, is recommended. This can be accomplished with an additional 2 ounces of meat or meat substitute (14 gm protein), or increasing milk consumption. However, most clients usually consume more than 60 gm protein daily, and additional amounts are not required.

CALCIUM AND VITAMIN D

Vitamin D and the mineral calcium work together in the formation of skeletal tissue and teeth. Inadequate vitamin D intake during pregnancy is associated with infant growth, bone ossification, tooth enamel formation, and neonatal calcium homeostasis. Deficiency is unlikely unless the mother has a low intake of both calcium and vitamin D, and insufficient exposure to sunlight.

Early in pregnancy, hormonal and physiologic adjustments promote increased calcium absorption and retention. This extra calcium is thought to be stored in maternal bone for fetal availability in the third trimester, when fetal bone growth is rapid. Because of the enhanced calcium absorption and utilization, additional calcium supplementation is

TABLE 13–3   *Vitamin-Mineral Recommended Dietary Allowances and Supplements*

Nutrient	Recommended Dietary Allowance (1)			Amount of Supplement Recommended (2)
	Nonpregnant Women	Pregnant Women	Percent Increase*	
Vitamin A	800 mcg RE	800 mcg RE	None	None
Vitamin D†‡	5 mcg	5 mcg	None	None
Vitamin E	8 α-TE	10 α-TE	25	None
Vitamin K	65 mcg	65 mcg	None	None
Vitamin C	60 mg	70 mg	16	50 mg
Thiamin	1.1 mg	1.5 mg	36	None
Riboflavin	1.3 mg	1.6 mg	23	None
Niacin	15 mg NE	17 mg NE	13	None
Vitamin B_6	1.6 mg	2.2 mg	38	2 mg
Folate	180 mcg	400 mcg	122	300 mcg
Vitamin B_{12}	2 mcg	2.2 mcg	10	None
Calcium†§	1,000 mg	1,000 mg	None	None
Phosphorus†§	700 mg	700 mg	None	None
Magnesium†‖	310–320 mg	350–360 mg	11	None
Iron	15 mg	30 mg	100	30 mg
Zinc	12 mg	15 mg	25	15 mg
Iodine	150 mcg	175 mcg	17	None
Selenium	55 mcg	65 mcg	18	None
Copper	1.5-3 mg	None	None	2 mg

*Percent increase for pregnant women above nonpregnancy recommendation.

†From Food and Nutrition Board, National Academy of Science. Dietary Reference Intakes for Calcium, Phosphorus, Magnesium, Vitamin D, and Fluoride. Washington, DC: National Academy Press, 1997.

‡For 14 to 50 year olds.

§For 19 to 50 year olds.

‖For 14 to 50 year olds.

Data adapted from (1) National Research Council, *Recommended Dietary Allowances.* 10th ed. Washington, D.C.: National Academy Press, 1989. (2) Institute of Medicine. *Nutrition During Pregnancy.* Washington, D.C.: National Academy Press, 1990.

felt to be unnecessary. Pregnant women should consume the same amount of calcium as others in her age group.

The recommended 1,000 mg/day of calcium for women over 19 years of age is easily met by three servings of milk or milk products. Pregnant women under 19 years of age may need 4 cups of milk to provide the 1,300 mg/day for adequate intake. Milk may be incorporated into cooking or eaten in different forms, such as cheese, ice cream, or yogurt, for variety (see Table 8–3). A commonly reiterated myth is that a baby will take all the calcium from the mother's teeth. This is a false statement. If a pregnant woman has sufficient calcium in her diet, then problems will not develop. If the diet is deficient in calcium, the calcium requirements of the embryo will be met first and some of the calcium may come from her bones, not from her teeth.

B VITAMINS

Several of the B-vitamin requirements are based on energy intake; usually, their intake increases automatically with intake of additional calories. Adequate intake of several B vitamins is difficult to achieve without careful selection of foods or supplementation.

The RDA for folate (400 mcg) during pregnancy is more than double the nonpregnant allowance. Orofacial clefts and neural tube defects, such as spina bifida and **anencephaly,** have been attributed

FIGURE 13–1 **Sample menu for pregnancy (third trimester). RDA, Recommended Dietary Allowance; RE, Retinol equivalents. (Nutrient data from Nutritionist IV, First Data Bank, San Bruno, CA. From Davis JR, Sherer K.** *Applied Nutrition and Diet Therapy for Nurses,* **2nd ed. Philadelphia: W.B. Saunders, 1994.)**

Sample Menu
Breakfast
1 cup orange juice
1 bagel with 1 oz cream
cheese and
1 packet raisins
1 cup 1% milk
coffee with creamer
Lunch
Tuna salad sandwich
(1 oz tuna with 2 tbsp
mayonnaise, 2 slices
tomato, lettuce slices,
on 2 slices whole
wheat bread)
1 apple
2 fig bar cookies
1 cup 1% milk
Dinner
4 oz lean roast beef with
1/4 cup gravy
1/2 cup brown rice
1/2 cup spinach
1/2 cup three bean salad
2 whole wheat rolls
2 tbsp light tub margarine
1 cup strawberries
1 cup 1% milk
tea
Evening Snack
12 oz diet cola beverage
2 oz peanuts

Nutrient	RDA–Pregnant Third Trimester	Actual	% RDA
Cal		2504 cal	100
Protein		114 gm	190
Carbohydrate		294 gm	94
Fat		107 gm	129
Cholesterol		181 mg	60
Fiber–dietary		35.635 gm	162
Vitamin A		1458 RE	182
Thiamin		1.9 mg	123
Riboflavin		2.6 mg	161
Niacin		26 mg	154
Vitamin B$_6$		1.9 mg	88
Folate		468 mcg	117
Vitamin B$_{12}$		6.8 mcg	310
Pantothenic acid		6.2 mg	113
Biotin		58.9 mcg	91
Vitamin C		220 mg	314
Vitamin D		7.9 mcg	79
Vitamin K		269 mcg	414
Sodium		2807 mg	103
Potassium		4537 mg	227
Calcium		1434 mg	120
Phosphorus		2085 mg	174
Magnesium		591 mg	185
Iron		18.3 mg	61
Zinc		18.7 mg	125
Copper		2.2 mg	97
Manganese		3.3 mg	95
Selenium		0.18 mg	280

^0   ^50   ^100   ^150   ^200

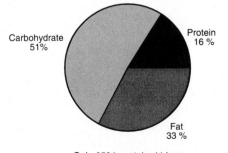

Carbohydrate, Protein, and Fat Distribution

Carbohydrate 51%
Protein 16 %
Fat 33 %

Cal, 2504; protein, 114 gm;
carbohydrate, 294 gm; fat 107 gm

to inadequate periconceptional nutrient intake, especially of folate (Tolarova & Harris, 1995). The role of folate as coenzyme is essential for nucleic acid synthesis. Therefore, a folate deficiency might impair cell growth and replication, causing fetal anomalies. Folate is also required for red blood cell formation, which is increased in pregnancy. Although folate intake is essential, some women take supplements providing as much as eight times the RDA. High intakes may be transferred to the fetus; other nutrients (especially vitamin B_{12}) may be adversely affected by exercise supplementation.

Ideally, attention should be focused on folate intake when a woman is considering a pregnancy since defects related to insufficient folate occur within the first 6 weeks of inception. The requirement for folate is difficult for most women to meet solely from food intake. Absorption from supplements is better than from natural folate in foods (Shaw et al., 1995). Conscientious daily selections of raw fruits and vegetables, especially green leafy vegetables, can help ensure adequate intake. Whole-grain products and folic acid-fortified grains and cereals may also supply significant amounts (see Table 10–6). Because of the critical effects of folic acid during pregnancy, the FDA will require supplementation of all grain products with specific amounts of folic acid by 1998.

IRON

A common problem among nonpregnant women is iron-deficiency anemia, so many women commence pregnancy with diminished iron stores. Increased iron during gestation is needed for production of red blood cells and the placenta, and to compensate for cord and blood loss at delivery. When maternal iron-deficiency anemia is diagnosed upon initiation of prenatal care, it is associated with low dietary energy and iron, inadequate gestional gain, and increased risks of preterm delivery and LBW.

The fetus acts as a parasite in that fetal **erythropoiesis** occurs at the expense of maternal iron stores. Therefore, iron-deficiency anemia is seldom seen in full-term infants. During the last half of pregnancy, iron absorption increases from the normal 10% to 20% to approximately 50% if adequate iron is available. Fetal accumulation of iron occurs principally in the last trimester. Premature infants, having a shortened gestation, have insufficient time to acquire adequate iron and may be born with iron-deficiency anemia; fortunately, iron absorption is significantly increased in premature infants.

Maternal iron deficiency requires that cardiac output increase to maintain adequate oxygen for the maternal and fetal cells. Iron-deficiency anemia therefore places the mother at risk of cardiac arrest and poor prognosis if hemorrhage occurs at delivery.

Approximately 18 to 21 mg of iron are needed daily. Since the average American diet does not provide this amount within the normal caloric requirements, daily iron supplements are usually recommended (IM, 1990; NRC, 1989). Initiation of supplements before gestational week 24 will prevent iron deficiency. If iron supplements are not provided, it may take 2 years after delivery before serum iron levels are normal (IM, 1990).

ZINC

Zinc is critical early in pregnancy during the formation of fetal organs, but requirements are highest in late pregnancy for fetal growth and development. The RDA for zinc is 15 mg during pregnancy. An increase in high-protein foods, especially meats, improves zinc intake.

Vitamin-Mineral Supplements

Vitamin-mineral supplementation is common during pregnancy in the United States. Supplementation should be based on evidence of a benefit as well as a lack of harmful effects. Excessive amounts of many nutrients may have detrimental effects on the fetus (Table 13–4). Food is considered to be the optimal vehicle for providing nutrients; supplements are not routinely recommended and should be used only after assessment of dietary and lifestyle factors to determine the need for nutritional supplements. The supplement composition is then based on the nature of an identified nutritional

TABLE 13–4   *Nutrient Supplementation Associated with Deleterious Fetal Outcomes*

Vitamin A	Pharmacologic use of vitamin A analogues has resulted in major congenital defects (malformation of the cranium, face, heart, thymus, and CNS) and spontaneous abortion, especially during the first trimester
Vitamin D	Excessive intake of vitamin D can result in hyperabsorption of calcium, hypercalcemia, calcification of soft tissues, and mental retardation
Vitamin E	Associated with higher incidence of spontaneous abortions
Vitamin K	Menadione administered parenterally has been associated with hemolytic anemia, hyperbilirubinemia, and kernicterus in the newborn
Vitamin C	Megadoses of vitamin C have been reported to cause vitamin C dependency with symptoms of conditional scurvy observed postpartum
Iodine	Large amounts of iodides have resulted in infants with congenital goiter, hypothyroidism, and mental retardation
Zinc	Large amounts of zinc supplements during the third trimester were implicated in premature delivery and stillbirth
Fluoride	Well water containing 12 to 18 ppm fluoride produced offspring with significant mottling of the deciduous teeth

Data from Worthington-Roberts B. Nutrition deficiencies and excesses: Impact on pregnancy, Part 2. *J Perinatol* 1985; 5(4):12.

need. If the physician recommends a supplement, it should not be used to reduce the woman's motivation to maintain or improve the quality of her diet.

The subcommittee (IM, 1990) concluded that iron is the only known nutrient warranting global supplementation during pregnancy. Consequently, 30 mg of ferrous iron is recommended to provide adequate amounts of iron during the second and third trimesters of pregnancy.

More recent studies have focused on the use of folate and vitamin A supplements. Folate intake does not usually meet the RDA recommendations, but it is hoped that when all grain products are fortified with folate, routine intake of folate from dietary sources will be more appropriate. A folate supplement may be prudent if adequacy of intake is questionable; it should be initiated before conception, if possible, because birth defects from lack of folate intake may occur before the woman realizes she is pregnant.

As a result of several studies showing a relationship between high doses of vitamin A supplements and birth defects, the FDA issued some recommendations for women of childbearing age. Early during pregnancy, as little as 10,000 IU of

vitamin A (preformed from animal sources) may increase the risk of birth defects. Ordinary multivitamins typically contain 5,000 IU, although some brands, especially those sold in health food stores, can contain much more; some capsules containing vitamin A only may contain as much as 25,000 IU. Possible birth defects include malformations of the face, head, heart, and nervous system (Rothman et al., 1995). Women need to limit their intake of preformed vitamin A to about 100% of the Daily Value (5,000 IU). Liver and other animal products and fortified foods and vitamin supplements listing retinyl palmitate and retinyl acetate as ingredients contain preformed vitamin A.

On the other hand, beta-carotene, which the body converts to vitamin A, is much less toxic. Fortified foods that contain beta-carotene and fruits and vegetables that contain natural beta-carotene should be chosen whenever possible.

The increased risks of adolescent pregnancy; carrying more than one fetus; and use of cigarettes, alcohol, or other drugs may warrant nutritional supplementation. The specific nutrient amounts for a daily multivitamin-mineral preparation if supplementation is warranted are shown in Table 13–3.

Dietary Intake and Counseling

Prenatal nutritional care improves outcome by saving lives, averting LBW, and decreasing the costs of care that are consequences of LBW. Although adequate weight gain is the most reliable measurable tool for assessing adequacy of caloric intake, food choices can provide adequate calories yet be deficient in vital nutrients. Nutrient intake therefore deserves more attention than weight gain. For this reason, the Institute of Medicine subcommittee (IM, 1990) has recommended routine assessment of dietary practices for all pregnant women in the United States to determine the need for improved diet or vitamin/mineral supplementation. Most women are highly motivated to make dietary changes during their pregnancy.

Pregnant women may have little or no nutritional knowledge. Nutrition counseling is often unavailable or ignored during pregnancy, yet knowledge is the key to wise food choices. In many cases, low-income expectant mothers have more opportunities to receive nutritional information through established programs such as **WIC,** than do more affluent women through the private sector.

Identification of both poor and desirable food habits and dietary patterns can serve as the foundation for appropriate nutrition counseling and intervention. Identification of nutritional problems, such as pica or fad dieting, or risk factors, such as alcohol abuse, may require special attention. Breastfeeding should also be promoted. Most importantly, it must be determined whether the gravida understands what foods she should be eating.

Dental Hygienist Considerations

ASSESSMENT
- *Physical*—level of education, income status, culture, religion, prenatal health care, medical history (including drugs taken), dental history, oral exam, feelings about weight gain.
- *Dietary*—health and nutritional knowledge and skills; adequacy of intake based on a well-balanced diet using a variety of foods; vegetarianism; food budget; food cravings and aversions; fad diets; beliefs about nutrition during pregnancy; pica, alcohol, and caffeine intake.

INTERVENTIONS
- Become familiar with local nutritional practices and beliefs about pregnancy, since these beliefs are regional.
- Refer clients at risk of inadequate intakes of specific nutrients to a registered dietitian or physician.
- Emphasize consumption of a well-balanced diet to ensure optimal intake of trace elements. This is preferred over routine prenatal supplements.
- Encourage foods high in calcium. Low calcium intake may impair bone mineral deposition, especially in women under 25 years of age. The use of dietary calcium is preferred because these foods also provide other valuable nutrients—protein, riboflavin, and vitamin D.
- Snacking is perfectly normal for pregnant women. Provide information on avoidance of acid attacks and resultant tooth decay by recommending appropriate oral hygiene techniques after snacking and snacking on foods such as nuts, raw vegetables, yogurt, and popcorn.
- If the mother has a strong preference for sweets, the infant's diet will also be high in sugar. Review the pregnant woman's diet for the form and frequency of sugar-containing foods and modify or make substitutions as indicated. This could create a healthier pattern for the pregnant woman and alleviate potential dental problems for the infant.

Nutritional Directions

- Alterations in food choices do not reflect natural instincts for required nutrients. Nutrient needs must be met by deliberate preplanning and informed food choices.

- Illegal drugs are especially harmful to the fetus.
- A dentist or physician may recommend fluoride supplements in areas with a nonfluoridated water supply, but supplementation is generally not recommended in areas where the water is fluoridated.
- Low-fat or skim milk may be used to control weight as well as decrease saturated fat intake and receive equivalent nutrients.
- Although the pregnant client is "eating for two," her normal energy requirements are not double.
- Moderate increases in whole grains, milk, and legumes can provide additional protein requirements as well as other important nutrients, as shown in Figure 13–1 (IM, 1990).
- Vitamin B$_{12}$ (2.0 mcg daily) and vitamin D (10 mcg) supplements are advisable for strict vegetarians (vegans), who exclude all animal products.
- Vitamin D may be a special concern for those with minimal exposure to sunlight. Regular exposure to sunlight and foods fortified with vitamin D (such as milk and cheese) are recommended.
- Powdered milk (⅓ cup) can be added to soups, cooked cereals, mashed potatoes, or casseroles if the gravida has an aversion to milk.
- ℞ Adverse symptoms, such as nausea or constipation, frequently occur from iron supplementation. Rather than discontinue the supplement, take with meals.
- ℞ Absorption of iron supplements is enhanced if taken between meals with liquids other than milk, tea, or coffee.
- ℞ When calcium supplementation is indicated, absorption is enhanced if taken at mealtime.

LACTATION

Breastfeeding is gaining in popularity: in 1993, 56% of mothers breastfed newborns, with 19% still breastfeeding 6 months later. This is an increase of 51% and 18%, respectively, over 1990 (Ross, 1995). The Subcommittee on Nutrition during Lactation recently published *Nutrition During Lactation* (IM, 1991) to help health-care providers understand how nutrition relates to the outcome of lactation and aids in formulating guidelines for clinical application in the United States. The subcommittee concluded that virtually all women are able to produce amounts of milk adequate to provide essential nutrients to support the growth and health of infants.

Breastfeeding has many advantages for the infant and mother:

- Human milk is nutritionally balanced with maximum bioavailability for infants.
- Breast milk has immunologic properties that help reduce infant morbidity (especially certain infectious gastrointestinal and respiratory diseases) and mortality.
- Human milk results in reduced risk of food allergies.
- Breastfeeding promotes infant oral motor and structural development.
- Maternal hormones produced as a result of lactation facilitate contractions of the uterus and control postpartum bleeding.
- Prepregnancy weight is achieved sooner.
- Breastfeeding is generally less expensive than formula feeding.
- Mother-infant bonding is enhanced with breastfeeding.
- Incidence of thumb-sucking and tongue thrusting is lower in breastfed infants.

Nutritional Recommendations for Breastfeeding

For most nutrients, recommendations for lactating women are similar to those for pregnant women. Energy requirements are proportional to the quantity of milk produced. Approximately 85 calories are needed for every 100 mL of milk produced (NRC, 1989), requiring approximately a 500-calorie daily increase. While this may not be fully adequate to cover the needs for milk production, the 2 to 4 kg of fat accumulated during pregnancy is available to supply additional calories. Thus, return to prepregnancy weight is accelerated. The major determinant of milk production is the infant's demand for milk, not maternal energy intake (IM, 1991). Weight loss during lactation has no apparent deleterious effects on milk production.

Carbohydrate intake is important for maintaining lactose synthesis and milk volume. Other nutrients needed in larger quantities than during pregnancy include protein; vitamins A, E, C, thiamin, riboflavin, niacin, and B_{12}; magnesium; zinc; iodine; and selenium (Fig. 13–2). Nutrients most likely to be deficient in the diets of lactating women are calcium, zinc, magnesium, vitamin B_6, and folate (IM, 1991). Calcium supplementation does not appear to affect the calcium concentration of breast milk or alter changes in bone mineral density (Kalkwarf et al., 1997).

The lactating woman requires additional fluids to replace those secreted in the milk. An additional 1,000 mL/day (4 cups) of fluids are needed.

Dietary Patterns for Lactating Women

The dietary pattern of a lactating woman is similar to that of a pregnant woman (see Fig. 13–2). Consumption of 3 cups of milk daily will provide approximately 1,000 mg calcium, or the recommended amount for women over 19 years of age. Other high-calcium foods may also be used. High-protein foods may include about 6 to 8 oz of meat daily, depending on how much milk is consumed. Adequate servings of fresh fruits, vegetables, and grain products will help provide the added caloric requirement.

Many substances consumed by the mother have been thought to affect breast milk. Certain foods, especially strongly flavored foods such as raw onion, garlic, curry, chili peppers, and chocolate, may cause gastrointestinal distress, rash, or irritability in the infant. They need to be omitted only if the infant is affected.

Many non-nutritive substances and drugs may be secreted in breast milk. Alcohol may impair milk flow and is transmitted in breast milk in approximately the same proportions as in the mother's blood. Intake should be limited to less than 0.5 gm/kg daily. Large amounts of coffee intake may adversely affect the iron content of human milk.

Because of the risk of medications being passed into breast milk, all drugs should be used cautiously and only if essential. Medications that are less likely to be secreted into the milk can be prescribed by the physician.

Dietary assessment of routine food intake by a Registered Dietitian is suggested, followed by nutrition counseling regarding foods rich in nutrients deficient in the diet. If dietary changes are not feasible, nutrient supplementation may be recommended, as described by the Institute of Medicine in Table 13–5.

Dental Hygienist Considerations

ASSESSMENT
- *Physical*—socioeconomic status, types of drugs used.
- *Dietary*—adequacy of calorie, nutrient, fluid intake; alcohol and caffeine intake.

INTERVENTIONS
- Encourage lactating women to obtain their nutrients from a well-balanced diet.
- Encourage intake of nutrients from fruits and vegetables, whole-grain breads and cereals, calcium-rich dairy products, and protein-rich and carbohydrate-rich foods.
- Encourage intake of at least 10 to 12 cups of fluid each day.
- For vegan mothers who desire to breast-feed, stress the importance of a balanced diet with appropriate supplements and weaning foods in sufficient quantities.

Sample Menu

Breakfast
1 cup orange juice
1 bagel with 1 oz cream
  cheese and
  1 packet raisins
1 cup 1% milk
coffee with creamer

Lunch
Tuna salad sandwich
  (2 oz tuna with 3 tbsp
  mayonnaise, 2 slices
  tomato, lettuce slices,
  on 2 slices whole
  wheat bread)
1 apple
2 fig bar cookies
1 cup 1% milk

Dinner
3 oz lean roast beef with
  1/4 cup gravy
1 cup brown rice
1/2 cup spinach
1/2 cup three bean salad
2 whole wheat rolls
2 tbsp light tub margarine
1 cup strawberries
1 cup 1% milk
Iced tea

Evening Snack
12 oz cola beverage
1 oz peanuts

Nutrient	RDA–Lactating, first six months	Actual	% RDA
Cal	= = = = = = = = = = = = = = = = =	2688 cal	100
Protein	= = = = = = = = = = = = = = = = = = * = = = = = = = = = = = =	109 gm	168
Carbohydrate	= = = = = = = = = = = = = = = = = *	356 gm	105
Fat	= = = = = = = = = = = = = = = = * = =	101 gm	113
Cholesterol	= = = = = = = = = = =	178 mg	59
Fiber–dietary	= = = = = = = = = = = = = = = = = * = = = = = =	34.180 gm	137
Vitamin A	= = = = = = = = = = = = = = = = = * = =	1476 RE	114
Thiamin	= = = = = = = = = = = = = = = = = * = = =	1.9 mg	119
Riboflavin	= = = = = = = = = = = = = = = = = * = = = = =	2.4 mg	135
Niacin	= = = = = = = = = = = = = = = = = * = = =	24.1 mg	120
Vitamin B₆	= = = = = = = = = = = = = = = = =	2.1 mg	99
Folate	= = = = = = = = = = = = = = = = = * = = = = = = = = =	435 mcg	155
Vitamin B₁₂	= = = = = = = = = = = = = = = = = * =	6.6 mcg	256
Pantothenic acid	= = = = = = = = = = = = = = = = = * = =	6.3 mg	114
Biotin	= = = = = = = = = = = = = = =	54 mcg	83
Vitamin C	= = = = = = = = = = = = = = = = = * = = = = = = = = = = = = = = = = =	220 mg	231
Vitamin D	= = = = = = = = = = = = = =	8.0 mcg	81
Vitamin K	= = = = = = = = = = = = = = = = = * =	269 mcg	414
Sodium	= = = = = = = = = = = = = = = = =	2970 mg	97
Potassium	= = = = = = = = = = = = = = = = = * = = = = = = = = = = = = = = =	4366 mg	184
Calcium	= = = = = = = = = = = = = = = = = * = = =	1418 mg	118
Phosphorus	= = = = = = = = = = = = = = = = = * = = = = = = = = = = = = =	2018 mg	168
Magnesium	= = = = = = = = = = = = = = = = = * = = = = = = = = =	555 mg	156
Iron	= = = = = = = = = = = = = = = = = * = = = =	18.5 mg	123
Zinc	= = = = = = = = = = = = = = =	15.3 mg	80
Copper	= = = = = = = = = = = = = = =	1.9 mg	87
Manganese	= = = = = = = = = = = = = = = =	3.3 mg	93
Selenium	= = = = = = = = = = = = = = = = = * = = = = = = = = = = = = = = = = = = =	0.2 mg	273

^0   ^50   ^100   ^150   ^200

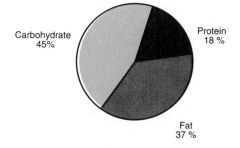

Carbohydrate, Protein, and Fat Distribution

Carbohydrate
45%

Protein
18 %

Fat
37 %

Cal, 2688; protein, 109 gm;
carbohydrate, 356 gm; fat 101 gm

FIGURE 13–2 Sample menu for lactation (first 6 months) RDA, Recommended Dietary Allowance; RE, Retinol equivalents. (Nutrient data from Nutritionist IV, First Data Bank, San Bruno, CA. From Davis JR, Sherer K. *Applied Nutrition and Diet Therapy for Nurses,* 2nd ed. Philadelphia: W.B. Saunders, 1994.)

TABLE 13–5   *Suggested Measures for Improving Nutrient Intake of Women with Restrictive Eating Patterns*

Type of Restrictive Eating Pattern	Corrective Measures
Excessive restriction of food intake, i.e., ingestion of <1,800 Cal of energy/day, which ordinarily leads to unsatisfactory intake of nutrients compared with the amounts needed by lactating women	Encourage increased intake of nutrient-rich foods to achieve an energy intake of at least 1,800 Cal/day; if the mother insists on curbing food intake sharply, promote substitution of foods rich in vitamins, minerals, and protein for those lower in nutritive value; in individual cases, it may be advisable to recommend a balanced multivitamin-mineral supplement; discourage use of liquid weight loss diets and appetite suppressants
Complete vegetarianism, i.e., avoidance of all animal foods, including meat, fish, dairy products, and eggs	Advise intake of a regular source of vitamin B_{12}, such as special vitamin B_{12}-containing plant food products or a 2.6-mcg vitamin B_{12} supplement daily
Avoidance of milk, cheese, or other calcium-rich dairy products	Encourage increased intake of other culturally appropriate dietary calcium sources, such as collard greens for Blacks from the southeastern United States; provide information on the appropriate use of low-lactose dairy products if milk is being avoided because of lactose intolerance; if correction by diet cannot be achieved, it may be advisable to recommend 600 mg of elemental calcium/day taken with meals
Avoidance of vitamin D-fortified foods, such as fortified milk or cereal, combined with limited exposure to ultraviolet light	Recommend 10 mcg of supplemental vitamin D per day

Reprinted with permission from *Nutrition During Lactation.* Copyright 1991 by the National Academy of Sciences. Published by the National Academy Press, Washington, DC.

Nutritional Directions

◆ Breastfeeding will help with weight loss.
◆ Intake of coffee (regular and decaffein-ated), other caffeine-containing beverages and medications, and decaffeinated coffee should be limited (IM, 1991). Encourage fluids such as juice, milk, and water.

ORAL CONTRACEPTIVE AGENTS

Many nutrients (especially folate, vitamin B_6, zinc, and magnesium) are affected by oral contraceptive agents (OCAs). Low-estrogen preparations now being used precipitate fewer changes in vitamin status than earlier preparations. Lower levels of water-soluble vitamins are due to decreased intestinal absorption and increased metabolism. However, vitamin deficiencies have been identified only when the diet was marginal.

Increased amounts of pyridoxine may be indicated because estrogen increases the production of tryptophan, which uses pyridoxine in its metabolism. Depression and impaired glucose tolerance attributed to OCAs may be alleviated with pyridoxine supplementation (10 mg/day) (Dickey, 1991).

Megaloblastic anemia reported in women on OCAs is related to decreased folate absorption. Supplements are not necessary except for high-risk women, in whom other factors, such as deficient diet or disease, could increase chances for a deficiency to develop. To decrease risk of neural tube defects resulting from folate deficiency, clients on OCAs who are planning a pregnancy in the near future may require supplementation of folate for 3 months before becoming pregnant, or they should discontinue the use of OCAs for at least 6 months before conception.

Progestins can cause weight gain related to increased appetite and altered carbohydrate metabolism, and estrogens may lead to an increase in subcutaneous fat and fluid retention.

Use of OCAs is associated with increased risk of heart disease due to changes in serum lipids. The amount and type of progestin and estrogen in the OCA can affect these changes. In general, there is a decrease in high-density lipoprotein (HDL) cholesterol, which is an undesirable affect since HDL is a protective type of cholesterol. Increased total cholesterol, triglyceride, and low-density lipoprotein (LDL) cholesterol levels are undesirable factors. Progestin appears to cause a decrease in HDL cholesterol levels and an elevation of LDL and total cholesterol levels. Since estrogens may increase HDL levels, the net effect on serum lipids is dependent on the ratio of progestin and estrogens. OCAs containing both progestin and estrogen have been shown to have little or no effect on HDL cholesterol levels but may increase fasting triglyceride levels.

NUTRITION UPDATE 13

Fetal Alcohol Syndrome

As little as 2 oz/day of alcohol can cause fetal alcohol syndrome (FAS), a condition characterized by irreversible brain damage and mental retardation. Approximately 10,000 infants are born with FAS each year in the United States (Streissguth et al., 1991). The first trimester is the most vulnerable time for the fetus, because the woman may not even be aware of the pregnancy, especially during the first crucial month. Four to five drinks a day, or at least 45 drinks per month, can produce the full FAS syndrome (Table 13–6), whereas smaller amounts may be associated with adverse effects such as spontaneous abortion, growth

retardation, and subtle behavioral effects without the physical anomalies (IM, 1990).

The FAS child has specific physiologic deformities (Fig. 13–3). It has been hypothesized that zinc deficiency may play a role in the abnormal facial features (IM, 1990). The mental and physical abnormalities cannot be reversed.

Even with adequate nutrition, normal development of fetal organs is jeopardized. Other habits that usually accompany alcohol consumption (e.g., smoking, excessive amounts of coffee the "morning after," poor eating habits with little attention to needed nutrients, and perhaps use of tranquilizers) may also adversely affect the unborn child. Ethanol is a source of energy; thus, chronic alcoholics may have a relatively low intake of protein, essential fats, vitamins, and minerals. Alcohol may impair placental transport of amino acids, calcium, and some vitamins.

Because the brain has a special affinity for alcohol, it is one of the first organs affected. Intellectual impairment is frequently reported in children with FAS. Even at birth, the circumference of the head is small (microcephaly), indicating abnormal brain capacity (i.e., 140 gm in a FAS infant compared to a normal brain weighing 400 gm). Fewer brain cells exist, with damaged cells preventing normal functioning; fewer neurons result in disorganized thought. The thinking ability of the brain is permanently disturbed. The average IQ is 68 (Streissguth et al., 1991). Maladaptive behaviors, such as poor judgment, distractibility, and social interaction problems, are common. Additionally, as a result of fewer total body cells, abnormal weight gain affects normal cell development and growth.

Because of the global adverse effects of alcohol intake, efforts to decrease or stop intake are appropriate. Diet counseling and other efforts to improve food intake, such as referral to a social worker for food or monetary resources, are warranted. The subcommittee has recommended the use of multivitamin-mineral supplements for heavy substance abusers who have difficulty changing their habits to improve nutrient intake (IM, 1990).

TABLE 13–6 *Fetal Alcohol Syndrome*

1. Irreversible mental retardation
2. Head too small (microcephaly)
3. Irritability in infancy and hyperactivity in childhood
4. Less growth in height and weight with more discrepancy in height prenatally and throughout life
5. Eyes
   a. Too close together
   b. Mongolian look; a fold of skin starting at the root of the nose goes to the point where the eyebrow starts and may cover the inner corner of the eye (epicanthus)
   c. Drooping of upper eye lid (ptosis)
   d. Uncontrollable squinting (strabismus)
   e. Nearsightedness (myopia)
6. Nose
   a. Undefined, short, and upturned, remains too short for life
   b. No bridge from the forehead to the nose
   c. Normal pair of ridges with an indentation between them from the bottom of the nose to the upper lip is not seen
7. Ears are poorly formed and incorrectly placed
8. Mouth
   a. Prominent ridges in palate
   b. Cleft lip
   c. Cleft palate
   d. Small teeth with faulty enamel
   e. Small jaws
9. Poor coordination
10. Weak skeletal muscles seen as weakness and floppiness in infants with less ability and strength later in life (hypotonia)
11. Bones and joints underdeveloped
12. Heart—atrial and ventricular membrane wall defects

From Iber FL. The fetal alcohol syndrome. *Nutrition Today* 1980; 15(4):4–11. © by Williams & Wilkins, 1980.

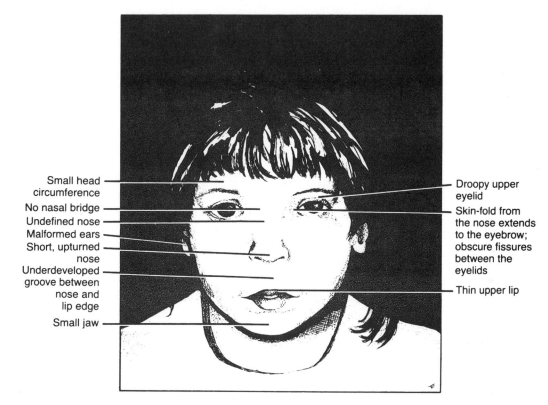

Small head circumference

No nasal bridge

Undefined nose

Malformed ears

Short, upturned nose

Underdeveloped groove between nose and lip edge

Small jaw

Droopy upper eyelid

Skin-fold from the nose extends to the eyebrow; obscure fissures between the eyelids

Thin upper lip

FIGURE 13–3 **Facial anomalies of a child with fetal alcohol syndrome.**

CASE APPLICATION FOR THE DENTAL HYGIENIST

Your regular client, Betty, a 16-year-old, confides to you on her 6-month recall that she is 3 months pregnant. Even though she and her parents have decided to keep the baby, she has not seen a physician yet. She is already about 15 lbs overweight and expresses a concern about the weight she will gain during pregnancy.

Nutritional Assessment

○ Knowledge about nutrition during pregnancy

○ Special dietary restrictions; food fad practices; ethnic, cultural, or religious customs

○ Adequacy of diet, especially calories, protein, calcium, iron, and folate

○ Medications, drug and tobacco use

○ Support of parents, living arrangements, social support

○ Psychological status

Nutritional Diagnosis

Altered nutrition: less than body requirements related to lack of nutritional information and weight concerns.

Nutritional Goals

Client will consume a well-balanced diet (based on the Food Guide Pyramid) and verbalize ways to increase protein, iron, calcium, and folate intake.

Nutritional Implementation

Intervention: Encourage Betty to visit an obstetrician as soon as possible.
Rationale: Fetal outcome is affected by nutrient intake during the pregnancy; birth defects are likely to occur if usual dietary habits are poor or if drug use occurs early in the pregnancy. Inadequate prenatal care leads to more problems for both mother and fetus.

Intervention: Clarify nutritional misconceptions by providing written material and discussing the principal nutrients that need to be increased. Provide the name of a registered dietitian with whom she could discuss these concerns.
Rationale: Nutritional requirements are quite high to meet the growth needs of both the adolescent and fetus because Betty is still growing and storing nutrients in her own body.

Intervention: Encourage her not to worry about weight gain during the pregnancy, but to take care of herself and her baby at this time.
Rationale: Weight gain during pregnancy influences the infant's birth weight more than the prepregnancy weight. Weight loss can be postponed until a later time when nutrient intake is less important.

Intervention: Discuss foods that need to be increased during pregnancy.

Rationale: Most teenagers have an inadequate intake of calories, calcium, iron, vitamin A, and niacin. Adequate intake of calories, protein, calcium, iron, B vitamins, and zinc are essential for a healthy baby and to protect fetal stores.

Intervention: Explain the effects of her nutritional status on oral development of her baby.
Rationale: Nutrition can determine whether teeth achieve their optimum genetic potential.

Intervention: Explain why she should limit her intake of coffee, tea, and especially carbonated beverages containing caffeine.
Rationale: Large amounts of caffeine could be responsible for malformations and increased susceptibility to decay of the primary first molars.

Evaluation

Betty should improve eating habits to consume at least the number of food groups recommended in the Food Guide Pyramid for pregnancy and gain approximately 25 lbs during the pregnancy. Other behaviors, such as decreasing sugar intake, consuming milk and milk products (for calcium intake), and consuming raw fruits and green leafy vegetables (for folate intake), will increase intake of added amounts of nutrients needed during pregnancy.

Student Readiness

1. Plan food intake for 1 day with two snacks for a pregnant woman who has four new carious lesions. What reasons would you give her for restricting sugar intake?
2. Explain what pica is and the type of individuals who may be practicing this behavior.
3. Why is it undesirable to lose weight during pregnancy?
4. List five effects on oral development of the fetus when maternal nutrient intake is inadequate.
5. What is the effect of caffeine on fetal dentition?
6. Which nutrients may be needed if dietary assessment indicates deficient intake that cannot be corrected by changing eating habits?

7. List advantages for breastfeeding, especially oral-motor development.

Case Study

A 32-year-old mother of two children (3 years and 6 months) who is breastfeeding complains of bleeding and sore gums and tongue. She has not returned to the physician since the birth of her youngest child because of lack of time. She has returned to her job as a clerk at a local department store. When questioned about her diet, she reports that she drinks a cup of coffee on her way to work; she usually takes a peanut butter and jelly sandwich and soft drink for lunch; and during the evening she grabs something that is fast and easy to eat such as hot dogs, canned soup, crackers, cookies, chips, or soft drinks. She complains that she is tired and irritable and feels that this is because of the stress imposed on her by the two children and her work.

1. List probable causes of the mother's symptoms.
2. Discuss the added stress of pregnancy and lactation on her nutritional needs.
3. Determine other foods that would be readily available for her to consume, such as cottage cheese, yogurt, nuts, fresh fruit, and raw vegetables.

References

Dickey RD. *Managing Contraceptive Pill Patients.* 6th ed. Durant OK: CIP, 1991.

Institute of Medicine (IM) Subcommittee on Nutritional Status and Weight Gain During Pregnancy. *Nutrition During Lactation.* Washington, D.C.: National Academy Press, 1991.

Institute of Medicine (IM) Subcommittee on Nutritional Status and Weight Gain During Pregnancy. *Nutrition During Pregnancy.* Washington, D.C.: National Academy Press, 1990.

Kalkwarf HJ et al. The effect of calcium supplementation on bone density during lactation and after weaning. *New Engl J Med* 1997; 337(8):523–528.

King JC et al. Energy metabolism during pregnancy: influence of maternal energy status. *Am J Clin Nutr* 1994; 59(Suppl 2S):439S-445S.

National Research Council (NRC). *Recommended Dietary Allowances.* 10th ed. Washington, D.C.: National Academy Press, 1989.

Ross Laboratories. (Unpublished study) Updated breastfeeding trend, 1986–1994, April 3, 1995.

Rothman KJ et al. Teratogenicity of high vitamin A intake. *N Engl J Med* 1995; 333(21):1369–1373.

Shaw GM et al. Risks of orofacial clefts in children born to women using multivitamins containing folic acid periconceptionally. *Lancet* 1995; 346(8972): 393–396.

Streissguth AP, et al. Fetal alcohol syndrome in adolescents and adults. *JAMA* 1991; 265(15):1961–1967.

Tolarova M, Harris J. Reduced recurrence of orofacial clefts after periconceptional supplementation with high-dose folic acid and multivitamins. *Teratology* 1995; 51(2):71–78.

Chapter 14

Other Considerations Affecting Nutrient Intake

GLOSSARY OF TERMS

Nutrient density the amount of a specific nutrient of a food relative to the number of calories it provides

Stable nutrients nutrients of which more than 85% is retained during processing and storage

Basic convenience foods foods having been processed using techniques such as canning, freezing, and drying

Complex convenience foods foods such as soups, or jellies, and jams

Manufactured convenience foods foods that cannot be prepared at home, such as ready-to-eat cereals and carbonated beverages

Food fad catchall term covering all aspects of nutritional nonsense, characterized by exaggerated beliefs about the value of nutrition in health and disease

Food quackery the promotion of nutrition-related products or services having questionable safety and/or effectiveness for the claims made

Organically grown foods foods grown without synthetic pesticides or fertilizers

Organically processed foods foods that have not been treated with additives, preservatives, hormones, antibiotics, dyes, or waxes

Test Your NQ (True/False)

1. Religion can affect food patterns. T/F
2. Adults usually avoid the foods they were raised on. T/F
3. The nutritional content of food is the most important determinant for food choices. T/F
4. Clients spend one-third of their income on food. T/F
5. Fad diets have magical healing qualities. T/F
6. Organic foods are more nutritious. T/F
7. All types of processing are detrimental to the nutritional quality of foods. T/F
8. Fast foods are usually a good source of protein. T/F
9. Food additives can be used to improve the nutritional value of foods. T/F
10. Individual food preferences do not ordinarily influence nutritional adequacy of the diet. T/F

FOOD PATTERNS

In terms of food choices, people are creatures of habit. Patterns throughout societies are quite evident; however, the term *habit* connotes inflexibility. People change their habits for numerous reasons; hence the term *food pattern* is more descriptive of food choices. Many factors are associated with formation of food patterns and preferences. Food patterns are generally developed during childhood and reflect the family's lifestyle as well as its ethnic or cultural, social, religious, geographic, economic, and psychological components. All of these influence one's attitudes, feelings, and beliefs about food. However, the factors that seem to predominate food choices are cultural and economic.

No culture has ever been known to make food choices solely on the basis of nutritional and health values of food. For example, broccoli is one of the most nutritious vegetables (based on nutrient density) available in the United States but is a less popular vegetable; whereas the tomato, the most commonly eaten vegetable, rates sixteenth as

a source of vitamins and minerals. The growing ethnic and cultural diversity of the U.S. population presents new challenges to health professionals in presenting culturally sensitive interventions to improve the health of these people.

Dental hygienists who are aware of economical ways to provide well-balanced meals and recognize that good nutrition can be achieved by utilizing many different types of food will respect a client's need to stretch their food dollar and choose culturally acceptable foods. Advice that takes into consideration a client's needs and food preferences is more likely to be followed.

Cultural Influences

One of the most interesting and visible ways cultural identity is expressed is through the foods a person eats or does not eat. Although milk is the only food used by everybody worldwide, many cultures consider it appropriate only for infants and children.

Children of different cultures, exposed to what adults eat, do not question whether this is what they should be eating. Cultural food patterns establish the foundation for a child's life-long eating customs regarding time and number of meals per day, foods acceptable for specific meals, preparation methods, likes and dislikes, foods suitable for specific members of a group, table manners, the social role of foods and eating, and attitudes toward eating and health. Patterns and attitudes internalized during childhood promote a sense of stability and security for the older individual (Fig. 14–1).

Because so many ethnic groups coexist in the United States, the development of literally thousands of localized patterns has resulted in distinct and discrete patterns of food consumption. These different combinations have remained quite consistent over the past decade. For example, few people in the northern United States would routinely choose grits, and many Southerners would not recognize lentils. Although American diets are diversified, they have become more homogeneous because of transportation, advertising, mobility, new methods of production, changes in income distribution, and appreciation of one another's heritage.

Individual food preferences do not ordinarily influence nutritional adequacy of the diet. Insufficient quantities of basic food groups (milk, fruits, vegetables, cereals, and meats) have the greatest effect on nutritional adequacy rather than specific aversions, such as to turnips or rye bread.

Status and Symbolic Influences

Nutritional value is secondary, especially if a food has established social, religious, or economic status. A food will be regarded differently in various cultures. For example, beef is regarded as a high-status food among some people in the United States, but Hindus from India consider cows sacred and do not eat beef. The status of different foods is influenced by religious beliefs, availability, cost, cultural values, and traditions, or even the endorsement or condemnation of a highly respected person.

Even today in many cultures, men are more highly valued than women. Thus, men of the household may be fed first with the women and children being allowed to eat only after the men are satiated. Consequently, women and children may receive insufficient quantities and a lesser variety of foods.

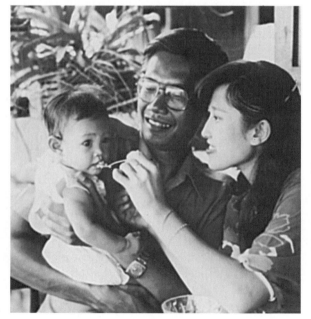

FIGURE 14–1 **Eating habits are established at a very young age. (WHO photo by T. Kelly.)**

Because of symbolic meanings of food, eating becomes associated with sentiments and assumptions about oneself and the world. Foods sometimes become symbolic not only because of religious connotations but because they are often used as rewards. After a child has fallen, a mother may give the child candy to help forget the pain and stop the crying. How many times has a mother been overheard to say, "Just behave yourself, and I'll buy you an ice cream cone when I finish this." Food is also withheld for bad behavior.

WORKING WITH CLIENTS WITH DIFFERENT FOOD PATTERNS

Respect for Other Eating Patterns

Dental hygienists must be prepared to meet the unexpected. Recognizing that eating habits and patterns vary among clients and that characteristic cultural patterns are usually observed among different nationalities and religious groups is important. Of course, people are partial to their own food pattern; however, too many people, including dental hygienists, are convinced that their own beliefs, attitudes, and practices are best and assume that everyone should follow them. It is important when working with clients who have strong cultural ties to be sensitive to their preferences and to avoid being judgmental. An open-minded dental hygienist who avoids cultural biases will be more likely to have clients open up and disclose crucial information that will allow the dental hygienist to help them.

Even when the facts are known, an analysis of the situation may be clouded because of unique individual habits. Information should be obtained regarding food habits by open-ended questions rather than questions that put words into a client's mouth. For example, "Did you have anything to eat this morning?" might elicit a different response than, "What did you have for breakfast this morning?"

Clients sometimes refuse to eat a particular food or to comply with recommended changes because of cultural or religious beliefs. Generally, if these preferences/beliefs are known, an adequate diet can be planned around them, and the client will be more receptive to minor changes in the diet pattern.

Effecting Change

Food preferences and attitudes are more important factors for effecting change. Several basic facts will help in approaching clients from various ethnic groups to promote sound nutritional practices:

1. One can find advantages and faults in each cultural food pattern. These patterns have contributed to the survival of the group in a particular environment. People have a remarkable ability to obtain a nutritious diet out of available foodstuffs. Some eating patterns that appear strange may actually be adaptive by enhancing or preserving nutritional value.

2. Other food patterns are nutritionally superior or at least comparable to "ordinary" American traditions.

3. Each food, food-related behavior, and tradition can be categorized as *beneficial, neutral,* or *potentially harmful.* A food that is beneficial promotes health by contributing necessary nutrients. Neutral foods are not especially beneficial but are not harmful to health. Foods are not usually harmful, but customs that affect nutritional content of the food may be potentially harmful. Tofu, used in Asian cooking, is beneficial because it increases the protein and calcium content of the diet. Efforts should be made to alter only the patterns that affect the nutritional value undesirably. For example, since many water-soluble vitamins are destroyed by heat, the practice of cooking foods (especially vegetables) for long periods of time is discouraged unless the liquids are consumed and/or iron cookware is used. An understanding of ethnic food habits can be used by the dental hygienist to encourage or incorporate beneficial practices into the client's diet.

4. Food patterns are generally deeply ingrained, contribute to psychological stability, and are hard to change. If dietary changes are indicated for health or dental reasons, suggest mini-

mal alterations in the client's normal patterns and, if possible, present the information with options. Additionally, compliance is improved when the client has input into changes in food choices, understands the reason changes are indicated, and feels responsible for following the suggestions.

5. Cultural patterns tend to be used more consistently by older family members. It is not possible to cover the dietary practices of all cultures and religions in this text. Further, individuals from any culture have unique tastes and preferences; therefore, it is important not to stereotype members of cultural groups. It is especially important for dental hygienists to become familiar with patterns common in the local area.

FOOD BUDGETS

When people relocate, established food patterns are transferred to the new location; however, these patterns are retained only if the foods are available in the new location at an affordable price. Therefore, problems arising within various cultural groups are economic rather than the fault of traditional food patterns. Foods from the "old country," which were cheapest at "home," may be very expensive or possibly not available in the new location. Gradually, the diet conforms to the food resources of the new location.

Evidence of malnutrition increases as income level decreases. Despite increasing concern about optimal nutrition, Americans are also anxious about food prices and try to conserve their food dollars. Most people spend only about 20% of their income on food. Of the amount allocated for food, less than 25% pays raw food cost. Purchasing the most nutritious products using available money is a common problem. A general awareness of food costs can be used to assist clients in stretching their food dollar. High-priced foods may not be the most nutritious; palatable, nutritious foods can be provided on a low-cost budget (Table 14–2).

If the amount of calories is not of concern, foods supplying the most nutrients relative to their cost include beef, fresh potatoes, brown rice, wheat

Table 14–1 categorizes foods of different cultures and regions and includes brief descriptions that will help introduce some unique and interesting foods.

Religious Food Restrictions

Religious beliefs affect eating patterns, attaching symbolic meanings to food and drink. Some examples of this are the bread and wine served during the Christian communion service and the Hindu reverence for the cow. These patterns do not usually result in any nutritional problems but could affect one's food patterns and thereby require consideration before making dietary recommendations.

germ, milk, eggs, and peanut butter. On the basis of **nutrient density,** the best buys are spinach, liver, tomatoes, canned tuna, nonfat and low-fat milk, tofu, dry-roasted peanuts, eggs, and fresh carrots (Schaus & Briggs, 1983). In general, more of the food dollar should be spent for fruits, vegetables, grain products, milk, and dry beans; less is needed for meats and high-sugar, high-fat food items (candy, carbonated beverages, chips, and so forth).

The average dollar value of food stamps per household (family of four) is $182 per month (FRAC, 1991). In many instances, food stamp allotments are 4% to 17% short of amounts needed to purchase minimal foodstuffs for adequate nutrition (Crockett et al., 1992). Thus, individuals who depend on food stamps often receive less than adequate nutrition, miss meals, and experience hunger. Prices tend to be higher in small, independent stores. Without transportation, low-income consumers are often limited to shopping in small independent stores more common in inner city areas or to spending more money for travel or delivery services.

Families on food stamps or on a very low food budget need to learn skills in buying and food storage. By utilizing every penny to its fullest, adequate nutrition can be provided on fairly limited budgets. To stretch the food dollar, it is necessary

Text continued on page 316

TABLE 14–1   *Cultural and Regional Foods*

Name of Food	Culture/Region	Type of Food	Description
Adobo	Filipino	Meat	Meat with soy sauce
Ajinomoto	Japanese	Grain	Wheat germ
Anadama	New England	Grain	Cornmeal-molasses yeast bread
Arroz blanco	Puerto Rican	Grain	Enriched white rice
Bacalao	Puerto Rican	Meat	Salted codfish
Bagels	Jewish	Grain	Bread dough, doughnut-shaped, boiled in water and baked
Baklava	Greek	Dessert	Layered pastry made with honey
Bok choy	Asian	Vegetable	Green leafy, stalk-like vegetable
Brioche	French	Grain	Egg-rich cake bread, used as sweet roll or shell for entrees
Bulgur	Middle Eastern	Grain	Granular wheat product with nut-like flavor
Burrito	Mexican	Combination	Sandwich; tortilla filled with beef-bean mixture and fried or baked
Café con leche	Latin American	Beverage	Coffee with milk
Cape Cod turkey	New England	Meat	Codfish balls
Challah	Jewish	Grain	Sabbath or holiday twisted egg-bread
Chayote	Mexican	Vegetable	Squash-like vegetable
Chitterlings	Southern U.S.	Meat	Intestine of young pigs, soaked, boiled, and fried
Chorizo	Mexican	Meat	Sausage
Cilantro	Mexican	Seasoning	Coriander, similar to parsley
Crackling	Southern U.S.	Snack	Crispy pieces of fried pork fat
Croissants	French	Grain	Buttery, flaky, crescent-shaped rolls
Crumpets	English	Grain	Muffin-like product cooked on griddle then toasted
Cush	Montana	Grain	Cornbread mixed with butter and water and fried
Dandelion greens	Southern U.S.	Vegetable	Leaves from dandelion plant
Dolmathes	Greek	Combination	Grape leaves stuffed with beef
Enchiladas	Mexican	Combination	Tortilla filled with meat and cheese
Escargots	French	Meat	Snails
Falafel	Middle Eastern	"Meat"	Vegetarian-type meatball
Fatback	Southern U.S.	Fat	Fat from loin of pig
Feijoada	Brazilian	Meat	Black beans with meat
Feta	Greek	Milk	Soft, salty white cheese from sheep or goat milk
Finnan haddie	Scottish	Milk	Salted, smoked haddock
Frijoles fritos	Mexican	"Meat"	Refried pinto beans
Gazpacho	Spanish	Soup	Cold soup with chopped tomatoes, green peppers, and cucumbers
Gefilte fish	Jewish	Meat	Seasoned fish ground and shaped into balls
Goulash	Hungarian	Meat	Stew seasoned with paprika
Grits	Southern U.S.	Grain	Hulled and coarsely ground corn

Table continued on following page

TABLE 14–1 *Cultural and Regional Foods* (Continued)

Name of Food	Culture/Region	Type of Food	Description
Guava	Cuban	Fruit	Small, yellow or red sweet tropical fruit
Gumbo	Creole	Combination	Well-seasoned okra stew with meat or seafood
Hangtown fry	California	Meat	Fried oysters and eggs
Hoe cake	Southeast U.S.	Grain	Thin corn cake
Hog maw	Southern U.S.	Meat	Stomach of pig
Hoppin' John	Southern U.S.	Combination	Blackeyed peas and rice
Hushpuppies	Southern U.S.	Grain	Fried cornbread
Jalapeños	Latin American	Vegetable	Hot peppers
Jambalaya	Creole	Combination	Well-seasoned combination of seafoods, tomatoes, and rice
Kale	Southern U.S.	Vegetable	Dark green leafy vegetable, similar to spinach
Kasha	Jewish	Grain	Coarsely ground buckwheat, toasted before cooking in liquid
Kelp	Asian	Vegetable	Seaweed
Kibbeh	Middle Eastern	Meat	Fresh raw lamb, ground and seasoned, similar to meat loaf
Kielbasa	Polish	Meat	Sausage
Kimchi	Korean	Vegetable	Peppery fermented combination of pickled cabbage, turnips, radishes, and other vegetables
Kuchen	German	Dessert	Yeast cake
Latkas	Jewish	Grain	Pancakes, sometimes from potatoes
Lard	—	Fat	Shortening-like product from pork
Limpa	Swedish	Grain	Rye bread
Lox	Jewish	Meat	Smoked salmon
Matzo	Jewish	Grain	Unleavened bread
Menudo	Mexican	Meat	Stew made with tripe (cow's stomach)
Minestrone	Italian	Soup	Vegetable soup
Miso	Asian	"Meat"	Fermented soybean paste
Moussaka	Greek	Combination	Meat and eggplant casserole
Mush	Southwest U.S.	Grain	Cooked cereal, usually cornmeal
Pan Dowdy	New England	Dessert	Dumplings and fruit
Papaya	—	Fruit	Large, yellow melon-like tropical fruit
Pasta	Italian	Grain	Macaroni, spaghetti, and noodles in various shapes made from wheat
Pepperoni	Italian	Meat	Hot sausage
Phyllo	Greek	Grain	Paper-thin pastry for making meat, vegetables, cheese and egg dishes, and sweet pastries
Pilaf	Middle Eastern	Grain	Rice enriched with fat and sometimes vegetables, bits of meat, and spices
Poi	Polynesian	Vegetable	Root vegetable, especially taro, cooked and pounded, mixed with water, and sometimes fermented

TABLE 14–1   *Cultural and Regional Foods* (Continued)

Name of Food	Culture/Region	Type of Food	Description
Polenta	Italian	Grain	Cornmeal or cornmeal mush
Polk	Southern U.S.	Vegetable	Dark green leafy vegetable
Potato latkes	Jewish	Vegetable	Potato pancakes
Pot liquor (likker)	Southern U.S.	Vegetable	Liquid from cooking green vegetables or bones
Proscuitto	Italian	Meat	Ready-to-eat, cured, smoked ham
Prickly pear	Native American	Fruit	Fruit of cactus
Pumpernickel	—	Grain	Yeast bread with wheat, corn, rye, and potatoes
Ratatouille	French	Vegetable	Well-seasoned casserole of eggplant, zucchini, tomato, and green pepper
Red-eye gravy	Southern U.S.	Gravy	Fried ham gravy
Sake	Asian	Beverage	Rice wine
Salt pork	Southern U.S.	Fat	Salted pork fat from the belly
Sancocho	Puerto Rican	Combination	Soup with meat and viandas
Sashimi	Japanese	Meat	Raw fish
Sauerbrauten	German	Meat	Pot roast in spicy, aromatic, sweet-and-sour marinade
Scones	English	Grain	Round, flat, unleavened sweetened bread
Scrapple	Pennsylvania Dutch	Combination	Solid mush from cornmeal and the by-products of hog butchering
Shoofly pie	Pennsylvania Dutch	Dessert	Molasses pie
Shoyu	Japanese	Seasoning	Soy sauce
Sofrito	Puerto Rican	Seasoning	Specially seasoned tomato sauce
Sopapillos	Mexican	Grain	Rich fried bread
Spatzle	German	Grain	Small dumplings
Spoonbread	Virginia	Grain	Baked dish with cornmeal
Spumoni	Italian	Dessert	Fruited ice cream
Stollen	German	Dessert	Christmas fruitcake
Strickle sheets	Pennsylvania Dutch	Dessert	Coffee cake
Strudel	German	Dessert	Light pastry, filled with fruit or cheese
Tacos	Mexican	Combination	Fried tortillas, filled with meat, vegetables, and hot sauce
Tamales	Mexican	Grain	Pancake-like leathery bread
Tempura	Japanese	Combination	Deep-fried seafood or vegetables
Teriyaki sauce	Hawaiian	Seasoning	Sweetened soy sauce
Tofu	Asian	"Meat"	Soybean curd
Trotters	Southern U.S.	Meat	Pig's feet
Viandas	Puerto Rican	Vegetable	Starchy tropical vegetables, including plantain, green bananas, and sweet potatoes

From Davis JR, Sherer K. *Applied Nutrition and Diet Therapy for Nurses,* 2nd ed. Philadelphia: W.B. Saunders, 1994.

TABLE 14–2   *Nutritional Bargains From the Basic Food Groups*

Food Group	More Economical	More Expensive
Milk	Skim and 2% milk	Whole milk
	Nonfat dry milk	Whole milk
	Evaporated milk	
Cheese	Cheese in bulk	Grated, sliced, or individually wrapped slices
	Cheese food	Cheese spreads
Ice cream	Ice milk or imitation ice cream	Ice cream and sherbet
Meat	Home-prepared meat	Luncheon meat, hot dogs, canned meat
	Regular hot dogs	All-beef or all-meat hot dogs
	Less tender cuts	More tender cuts
	U.S. Good and Standard grades	U.S. Prime and Choice grades
	Bulk sausage	Sausage patties or links
	Pork or beef liver	Calves liver
	Heart, kidney, tongue	
	Bologna	Specialty luncheon meats
Poultry	Large turkeys	Small turkeys
	Whole chickens	Cut-up chickens or individual parts
Eggs	Grade A eggs	Grade AA eggs
	Grade B eggs for cooking	
Fish	Fresh fish	Shellfish
	Chunk, flaked, or grated tuna	Fancy-pack or solid-pack tuna
	Coho, pink, or chum salmon (lighter in color)	Chinook, king, and sockeye salmon (deeper red in color)
Fruits and vegetables	Locally grown fruits and vegetables in season	Out-of-season fruits and vegetables or those in short supply and exotic vegetables and fruits
	Grades B or C	Grade A or Fancy
	Cut up, pieces, or sliced	Whole
	Diced or short cut	Fancy-cut
	Mixed sizes	All the same size
	Fresh or canned	Frozen
	Plain vegetables	Mixed vegetables or vegetables in sauces
Fresh fruits	Apples	Cantaloupe
	Bananas	Grapes
	Oranges	Honeydew melon
	Tangerines	Peaches
		Plums
Fresh vegetables	Cabbage	Asparagus
	Carrots	Brussels sprouts
	Celery	Cauliflower
	Collard greens	Corn on the cob
	Kale	Mustard greens
	Lettuce	Spinach
	Onions	
	Potatoes	
	Sweet potatoes	

TABLE 14–2   *Nutritional Bargains From the Basic Food Groups* (*Continued*)

Food Group	More Economical	More Expensive
Canned fruits	Applesauce Peaches Citrus juices Other juices	Berries Cherries
Canned vegetables	Beans Beets Carrots Collard greens Corn Kale Mixed vegetables Peas Potatoes Pumpkin Sauerkraut Spinach Tomatoes Turnip greens	Asparagus Mushrooms
Frozen fruit	Concentrated citrus juices Other juices	Cherries Citrus sections Strawberries Other berries
Frozen vegetables	Beans Carrots Collard greens Corn Kale Mixed vegetables Peas Peas and carrots Potatoes Spinach Turnip greens	Asparagus Corn on the cob Vegetables, in pouch Vegetables, in cheese and other sauces
Dried fruits and vegetables	Potatoes	Apricots Dates Peaches
Breads and cereals	Day-old bread White enriched bread Cooked cereal Regular cooking oatmeal Plain rice Long-cooking rice Graham or soda crackers	Fresh bread Rolls, buns Whole grain Ready to eat cereals Quick cooking or instant oatmeal Seasoned rice Parboiled or instant rice Specialty crackers

From Green ML, Harry J. *Nutrition in Contemporary Nursing Practice.* New York: John Wiley & Sons, 1981.

TABLE 14–3   *Meats and Meat Alternates: Cost of 20 gm of Protein from Various Meats and Meat Alternatives**

Food	Cost ($)/ Market Unit	AP† Amount to Provide 20 gm Protein	EP‡ Amount to Provide 20 gm Protein	Cost/20 gm Protein ($)
Dry beans	0.59/lb	½ cup	1½ c	0.13
Beef liver	1.29/lb	3½ oz	3 oz	0.24
Whole fryer	0.99/lb	4 oz	2½ oz	0.25
Eggs (large)	0.97/lb	3.3 ct	3.3 ct	0.27
Whole milk	2.30/gal	2½ cup	2½ cup	0.27
Peanut butter	1.58/lb	5 Tbsp	5 Tbsp	0.27
Bread, white enriched	1.49/24 oz	7 sl	7 sl	0.29
Tuna, canned	$0.64/6.5 oz	3 oz	3 oz	0.30
Ready-to-cook turkey	1.49/lb	3⅓ oz	2⅓ oz	0.31
Frankfurters	0.99/lb	3½ count	3½ count	0.35
Split chicken breasts with bone and skin	1.39/lb	4 oz	2½ oz	0.35
Rump roast, bone-in	1.69/lb	3½ oz	2¼ oz	0.37
Beef, chuck roast, bone-in	1.49/lb	4 oz	3 oz	0.37
Regular ground beef	1.69/lb	4 oz	2⅔ oz	0.42
Pork & beans, canned	0.51/lb	1½ cup	1½ cup	0.43
Chicken wings	1.19/lb	6 oz	3 oz	0.48
Ham, boneless	2.69/lb	3 oz	3 oz	0.50
Beef, round steak, boneless	2.49/lb	3½ oz	3 oz	0.54
Sliced bologna	2.53/lb	6½ oz	6½ oz	0.55
Cured picnic ham, bone-in	1.69/lb	5½ oz	3½ oz	0.58
Processed American cheese	3.58/lb	3¼ oz	3¼ oz	0.73
Perch fillet, frozen	3.99/lb	3½ oz	3 oz	0.87
Center-cut pork chops	3.79/lb	4½ oz	2½ oz	1.07
Sliced bacon	2.79/lb	10 sl	10 sl	1.19
Breaded fish fillets, frozen	4.78/lb	4 fillets	4 ct	2.19

*Prices in Arlington, TX, September 1996.
†AP, as purchased, including weight of bone, skin, fat lost in cooking, and so forth.
‡EP, edible portion, cooked.
ct, count; Tbsp, tablespoon; oz, ounce; lb, pound; sl, slice.
Adapted from Davis JR, Sherer K. *Applied Nutrition and Diet Therapy for Nurses,* 2nd ed. Philadelphia: W.B. Saunders, 1994.

to (1) purchase the least expensive items in each of the basic food groups, (2) rely on minimum servings of meats, (3) utilize meat substitutes (e.g., legumes and peanut butter) frequently, (4) serve larger quantities of grains, cereals, and pasta products, (5) prepare most foods from scratch rather than buying convenience foods, and (6) eliminate most highly processed foods that are expensive or have poor nutrient content (e.g., carbonated beverages and potato chips). Table 14–3 shows the relative cost of 20 gm of protein from various sources.

Referrals for Nutritional Resources

Frequently, special assistance is needed by clients. A variety of nutrition resources is available to help financially, to assist with food budgeting, or to teach basic nutrition and meal planning (Table 14–4). Dental hygienists can identify clients or families with nutritional needs and help them participate in available programs (Table 14–5). One of the best sources is the city or county health department. State and local health departments usually have various programs to provide nutrition services, such as well-baby clinics and family health centers. Health departments and county hospitals are excellent resources for information about various programs available.

The federal government administers several nutrition programs through the Department of Agriculture (USDA) and the Department of Health and Human Services (DHHS). The food stamp program provides coupons to low-income households that meet certain requirements. Food stamps are free to those who qualify. The program is designed to help low-income households purchase nutritious food and adjustments are made annually based on income and household size. Local welfare offices that

administer the program are widely distributed throughout the United States.

The Special Supplemental Food Program for Women, Infants, and Children (WIC) is designed to prevent nutritional problems. The WIC program is available to pregnant and lactating women, infants, and children up to 5 years of age who are considered to be at nutritional risk. Criteria for nutritional risk are evidence of iron deficiency, inadequate weight gain during pregnancy, teenage pregnancy, failure to thrive, poor growth patterns, and inadequate dietary patterns. The WIC program is usually available through county and city health departments. In addition to supplemental foods, health care and nutrition education are provided. Whereas many federal governmental programs are being cut back, studies of the WIC program have shown positive effects on iron status and on growth and development of infants and children, and savings of millions of dollars by decreasing the rate of low-birth-weight and very-low-birth-weight infants (Avruch & Cackley, 1995).

School breakfast and lunch programs provide nutritious meals for children at school. Nutritional standards for the school lunch require that lunch and breakfast must furnish at least one-third and one-fourth of the RDAs for children, respectively.

TABLE 14–4   *Reliable Nutrition Resource Guide*

Type of Information	Title	Resource
General food or nutrition question	Registered dietitian, nutritionist, home economist	Hospital; local or state health department; extension service of a land-grant university
More technical questions	Nutrition professor, registered dietitian	Nutrition or home economics department of a university or college
Questions on food preparation and preservation	Home economist	USDA–County Cooperative Extension Service; gas or electric company
Special diets	Registered dietitian	Hospital; local or state public health departments; volunteer health organization (e.g., a diabetes association)

From Davis JR, Sherer K. *Applied Nutrition and Diet Therapy for Nurses,* 2nd ed. Philadelphia: W.B. Saunders, 1994.

TABLE 14–5 *Referral Chart for Community Nutrition Resources*

Population Group	Risk Factor	Referral Source	Contact
Pregnant and lactating women	Low income	Food stamps	Welfare office
	Anemia, inadequate weight gain, age-related risk factor, inadequate diet, adolescent pregnancy, inadequate health care, or lack of food and nutrition information	WIC Program	City, county, or state health department
		Maternity and Infant Care Project	State health department
		EFNEP	Land-grant universities
		Prenatal education	Prenatal clinic or private health care team
Infants	Low-birth-weight, failure to thrive, or poor growth patterns	WIC Program	City, county, or state health department
		Children and Youth Project	State health department
	Inadequate health care		
Children	Poor growth patterns, inadequate diet, or anemia	WIC Program (up to 5 years of age)	City, county, or state health department
	Low income	Children and Youth Project (up to 18 years of age)	State health department
		Headstart (preschool)	Local community action project
		School lunch	Board of education
		School breakfast	Local community action project
Elderly	Low income	Food stamps	Welfare office
		Congregate meal sites	Social service agency
	Homebound	Meals on Wheels	Social service agency
	Diabetes	American Diabetes Association	Local chapter
	Obesity	Weight reduction groups	(See General Adult section)
	Cardiovascular disease	American Heart Association	Local chapter

Group	Condition/Need	Organization/Program	Contact
General adult	Obesity	Weight Watchers International, Thin Within, Dieters workshop, TOPS, and other weight-reduction groups	Local chapters
	Hyperlipidemia, cardiovascular disease, or hypertension	American Heart Association	Local chapter
	Diabetes	American Diabetes Association	Local chapter
	Low income	Food stamps	Welfare office
	Lack of food and nutrition information	EFNEP	Land-grant universities
	General consumer information for all populations	Community nutrition groups and community cooperatives	Local groups
		American Dietetic Association	(1-800) 366-1655
		Center for Science in the Public Interest	1755 S St, NW Washington, DC 20009
		Nutrition Foundation	888 Seventeenth Street NW Washington, DC 20006
		Society for Nutrition Education	1700 Broadway, Ste 300 Oakland, CA 94612
		U.S. Government Printing Office	Superintendent of Documents Washington, DC 20402

*This is only a partial listing. Program may vary in different parts of the United States.

Adapted from Finkelhor S. Nutrition resources. *Med Clin North Am* 1979; 63(5):1117. From Davis JR, Sherer K. *Applied Nutrition and Diet Therapy for Nurses*, 2nd ed. Philadelphia: W.B. Saunders, 1994.

Free and reduced-price meals are provided based on household income and size. Effective in the 1996–97 school year, meals must provide no more than 30% of calories from fat and less than 10% of calories from saturated fat averaged over a 1-week period. A reduction in sodium and cholesterol and increase in fiber is encouraged.

The Nutrition Program for the Elderly (Title III) provides both group meals and home-delivered ones. The purpose of this program is to improve the nutritional and health status of the elderly through improved access to food. The majority of persons applying for Meals on Wheels are at risk of malnourishment. Besides providing a hot meal to the elderly (containing one-third of the RDAs), a variety of social services is also available.

The Expanded Food and Nutrition Education Program (EFNEP) is designed to help lower socioeconomic groups with all aspects of nutrition. EFNEP is available through county extension services of land-grant universities and assists with meal planning, budgeting, cooking, and other food- and nutrition-related problems. Nutrition aides are low-income homemakers who are trained to visit in homes of low-income clients/families to assist in providing well-balanced meals.

Headstart is a preschool educational program for low-income families. Meals are furnished for the children, and nutrition education is available for parents.

Local chapters of many health-related organizations, listed in the telephone directory, furnish free or inexpensive literature, audiovisual material, and health-oriented programs on various topics. Frequently local churches provide free meals or other help. Referrals can also come from in-hospital sources such as the social worker, dietitian, or nutrition support team. Other referrals are listed in Appendix E.

Dental Hygienist Considerations

• Assist the client in planning a week's menu and grocery shopping list. Assess menus for nutrient adequacy based on the Food Guide Pyramid and food costs; follow this

by praising some of the nutritious/healthy choices made, then suggest some recommendations.
• If calories, sodium, and fat should be restricted, discourage fast-food establishments and/or provide suggestions for appropriate fast-food selections (for example, salads or broiled chicken).

Nutritional Directions

♦ Protein sources are generally the most expensive budget items; however, it is unnecessary to buy choice quality grades for good nutrition.
♦ Discuss guidelines presented in the Basic Principles for Economic Food Purchases to help clients adjust food purchases.

Basic Principles for Economical Food Purchases

♦ Purchase the least expensive items in each basic food group.
♦ Rely on minimal servings of meats.
♦ Utilize meat substitutes (e.g., legumes, nuts, peanut butter, and cheese) several times each week.
♦ Serve larger quantities of grains, cereals, and pasta products.
♦ Prepare most foods from scratch rather than buying convenience items.
♦ Eliminate most highly processed foods that are expensive or have low nutrient content (e.g., carbonated beverages and potato chips).
♦ Plan weekly menus, using the Food Guide Pyramid as a guideline.
♦ Plan menus around seasonal foods or weekly specials advertised in newspapers.
♦ Buy store brands. They are almost always a good buy for the money.
♦ Prepare a shopping list and stick to it. Avoid impulse buying, but be prepared to make substitutions if a similar item is a better buy.
♦ Read labels to determine if similar products are comparable in nutritive value.

♦ Compare unit prices. Generally, the price per ounce is stated, which makes it easier to compare various sizes.

♦ Buy larger sizes (which are usually cheaper) if the food will be eaten before it spoils.

♦ Shop at large supermarkets rather than small operations or convenience stores.

♦ Avoid purchasing snack foods and many sugar-coated breakfast cereals. They are not wise food purchases because of their low nutritive values. The price per ounce is often astonishing.

From Davis JR, Sherer K. *Applied Nutrition and Diet Therapy for Nurses,* 2nd ed. Philadelphia: W.B. Saunders, 1994.

OPTIONAL NUTRITION DURING FOOD PREPARATION

Methods of Preparation

In many instances, cooking enhances palatability, increases digestibility of food, and destroys pathogenic organisms. Cooking affects acceptability as well as nutritional value. Following a few guidelines can help preserve nutrients during cooking (see the Guidelines to Preserve Nutrients During Preparation).

Guidelines to Preserve Nutrients During Preparation

♦ Prepare fresh produce as near to serving time as possible since exposure to air results in deterioration of many nutrients.

♦ Do not soak fruits and vegetables that have been cut. Water-soluble vitamins and some minerals (especially potassium) are leached into the water.

♦ Scrub outer portions of fruits and vegetables rather than pare them. When necessary, pare as thinly as possible.

♦ Utilize parings and portions of vegetables not generally consumable to make soup stock; these are a very rich source of potassium and water-soluble vitamins.

♦ Leave produce whole or in large pieces so less surface area is available for oxidation of nutrients.

♦ Store any fruits or vegetables that have been cut or otherwise processed, such as fruit juice, in air-tight opaque containers. Container size should be appropriate for the amount to be stored to prevent excessive oxidation from air inside the container.

♦ Cook foods just until tender or for the shortest time possible. A covered pan minimizes cooking time because steam increases the temperature inside.

♦ Use the least amount of liquid possible in cooking. Cover the pan to minimize the amount of water necessary. Use leftover liquid, which contains water-soluble vitamins, in gravies and soups.

♦ Serve vegetables as soon as they are cooked.

♦ Do not add baking soda while cooking vegetables.

From Davis JR, Sherer K. *Applied Nutrition and Diet Therapy for Nurses,* 2nd ed. Philadelphia: W.B. Saunders, 1994.

Adding large amounts of fats during the cooking process, as in frying, is discouraged. Specific methods of preparing meats are recommended to lessen natural fat content. Meats cooked to the well-done stage contain less fat. To remove fats during cooking, meats can be boiled, microwaved in a colander or on paper towels, or roasted or broiled on a rack. Cooking increases digestibility of protein in meats.

Cellulose in fresh produce is generally softened by cooking; total volume and bulk of the food is decreased so a greater quantity of these low-calorie foods can be eaten.

A relatively new method of cooking to most Americans is stir-frying, which is an old Asian technique. This method is highly recommended and has the added benefit of being speedy. Bite-sized pieces of food are cooked very briefly over high heat with or without a small amount of vegetable oil. Vegetables retain their nutrient value, color, and crispness.

A microwave oven is another time-saver. Because of the shorter cooking time and smaller quantity of water added, this method is believed to conserve nutrients. However, the vitamin content of foods cooked in a home microwave oven is about the same as those prepared conventionally.

Sanitation Principles

Food carefully chosen for its nutritional value may be adversely affected by how it is handled and prepared before its consumption. Edibles must be handled with care to prevent contamination with food-borne organisms and sometimes must be properly cooked to kill any organisms naturally present. Many foods, especially meat, poultry, and eggs, require sufficiently high temperatures to destroy microorganisms. Over 40 different food-borne pathogens cause between 6.5 and 33 million cases of human illness and up to 9,000 deaths annually in the United States (Buzby & Roberts, 1995).

Processed Foods

Active, mobile lifestyles and an increasing number of women working full-time or part-time outside the home have led to a continued rise in consumption of processed foods. Although growing one's own food and making foods from "scratch" can give consumers control over how food is handled and what is added, this is not feasible for most Americans.

EFFECT OF PROCESSING ON NUTRIENTS

Nutrient content of foods can be affected by the way food is handled—that is, the type of processing to which the food is subjected (i.e., milling, cooking, freezing)—as well as how it is stored. In general, most minerals, carbohydrates, lipids, and proteins, as well as vitamin K and niacin are nutritionally **stable** (those with more than 85% retention during processing and storage). Thiamin, folate, riboflavin, and ascorbic acid are most likely to be seriously depleted by processing and storage as well as the method of preparation of the food. The nutritional value of home-cooked foods is frequently about the same as processed foods. However, highly processed foods are not as nutritious as the fresh form (e.g., potato chips are less nutritious than a baked potato).

Food processing attempts to maintain optimum qualities of color, flavor, texture, and nutritive value. Not everything done to foods by food processors has been good; however, not all processing is detrimental. The milling process removes the bran coat of grains. Removal of the high lipid-containing bran produces a more stable grain, thereby increasing its shelf-life. Nutritionally, however, this results in a reduction of fiber and loss of 70% to 80% of thiamin, riboflavin, vitamin B_6, and other nutrients. Enrichment replaces some nutrients lost in processing but not all of them, as shown in Table 1–5.

Fresh fruits and vegetables have a higher nutritive value and better taste immediately after harvest but rapidly deteriorate if transported long distances or improperly stored. Frozen foods that are packed immediately after harvesting may be higher in nutritive value than their fresh counterparts available in the supermarket.

CONVENIENCE FOODS

Convenience foods are usually popular because they save time in meal preparation, planning, purchasing, and clean-up. The variety of food served is also expanded. However, convenience foods prepared by food manufacturers may cost more because of extra handling and packaging. Convenience foods also require more preservatives. Many convenience foods contain more sodium and fat than the home-cooked product.

Basic convenience foods include peanut butter, pasteurized processed cheese, instant coffee, and frozen orange juice. In general, basic convenience foods, especially vegetables, cost less than fresh ones cooked at home, although this varies with seasonal availability. **Complex convenience foods** generally cost more than foods prepared at home, but this expenditure may be well worth the money in terms of the amount of time needed to prepare that product. **Manufactured convenience foods**

offer many calories and are considered expensive. When items can be purchased in more than one form, such as pizza, more convenient types usually cost more.

FAST FOODS

Fast-food sales have increased dramatically over the last 10 years, becoming an integral part of our fast-paced lifestyle. Spending for meals and snacks away from home has risen substantially since 1965, more than double the amount spent on food eaten at home. Consumers are eating out more as incomes rise and more women enter the work force.

Although some believe that fast food is junk food, this is not always true. Nutritional analyses by fast-food chains and independent studies reveal that their menu items contain rich sources of protein (30% to 50% of the RDAs). Additionally, items are available that (if selected) provide 20% to 30% of the RDAs for thiamin, riboflavin, ascorbic acid, and calcium. When a hamburger or roast beef sandwich is selected, substantial amounts of iron are supplied by the beef.

Most fast-food menus lack a rich source of vitamin A. In many cases, salads have been an added selection because of consumer demand. This provides a source of vitamins A and C as well as dietary fiber; however, the cost may be two to seven times higher than the same foods purchased at supermarkets. Shortages of other nutrients, specifically biotin, folate, pantothenic acid, and copper, are also reported.

Several other problems with fast foods have been of concern: (1) the calorie count of a meal is generally between 900 to 1,800 calories (33% to 66% of the RDA for young men or 45–90% for young women); (2) the sodium content is very high, ranging from 1,000 to 2,515 mg; and (3) the fat content of some fast-food meals can be as high as 51% of calories consumed. The impact of fast foods on nutritional status depends on how frequently they are consumed, the composition of each item selected, and what other foods are eaten during the day. Wise choices are possible when one's own nutritional needs and the nutrient content of menu items are known. Nutritional analysis of many menu items is available from fast-food chains.

Dental Hygienist Considerations

- Stress following the guidelines in Guidelines to Preserve Nutrients During Preparation.

Nutritional Directions

- Products that can be stored at room temperature should be kept in cool, dry areas in airtight containers.
- Regular ground beef is more economical than ground round and total fat content can be significantly reduced by using a low-fat cooking method and by rinsing crumbled ground beef after cooking.

FOOD ADDITIVES

During the 1950s, the Delaney committee investigated food additives. The Delaney clause prohibits use of any food additive if it is found to be carcinogenic in humans or animals. Additives deemed to be harmless were labeled "generally recognized as safe" (GRAS). These substances met certain specifications of safety under what might be called a "grandfather clause"—in other words, they are generally recognized by experts as safe, based on their use in foods for years without any known occurrence of health problems.

In 1960, similar legislation was passed for color additives. Colors currently in use were required to undergo further testing to continue being marketed. Since then, approximately 90 of the original 200 color additives have been classified as safe and continue to be added to foods.

The use of additives is regulated by law. Before a newly proposed additive can be marketed, it must undergo strict testing to establish its safety for the intended purpose. Safety levels of additives have been established by the FDA, limiting both the quantity and how the additive can be used. Currently, additives are specific, well-known substances that meet specifications for purity and have been shown as convincingly as possible to be free from harmful effects in the amounts commonly used.

Almost all food additives (99%) are derived from natural sources or are synthetically produced to be identical to the natural chemical substance. In many instances, the effects of chemicals naturally present in a food are observed, and this chemical is then added to other foods to achieve a similar effect. For instance, calcium propionate in Swiss cheese was observed to retard mold. It was then added to bread to inhibit mold growth.

Currently, additives are as safe as science can make them. They are designed not to be toxic, and most of them would have to be ingested in very large amounts to produce acute symptoms. Of course, allergic reactions to food additives can be experienced by some, just as allergies to specific foods can occur.

The use of food additives makes many foods more readily available by preventing spoilage and keeping food wholesome and appealing. Many are intimidated by the complicated chemical names found on labels. Even the names of vitamins on labels (e.g., thiamin mononitrate) can cause apprehension if unfamiliar. Food additives can have several benefits (Table 14–6):

1. They improve nutritional value. Enrichment and fortification have helped reduce malnutrition in the United States.
2. They prevent oxidation and spoilage. Preservatives retard spoilage caused by mold, air, bacteria, fungi, or yeast and preserve natural color and flavor. Antioxidants prevent oxidation of fats and oils, fruits, and vegetables.
3. They maintain product consistency. Emulsifiers enable particles to mix and prevent separation. Stabilizers and thickeners contribute to a smooth, uniform texture.
4. They provide leavening or control pH. Leavening agents, such as yeast and baking powder, are used to make foods light in texture and baked goods rise.
5. They enhance flavor and appearance. These substances are the most widely used and controversial additives. Included in this category are coloring agents, natural and synthetic flavors, spices, flavor enhancers, and sweeteners. Sugar, corn syrup, and salt are used in the largest amounts. Without these products, foods are less appealing, a factor that influences selections and controls nutrient intake.

Dental Hygienist Considerations

- Stay abreast of local, state, and federal food additive laws.
- Allay clients' fears concerning food additives.

Nutritional Directions

- Food additives are tested before use. They are considered safe, but should be consumed in moderation.

FOOD FADS AND MISINFORMATION

Nutrition is a very popular subject, but even with all the current knowledge, it is no easier to teach today than it was 55 years ago:

More food notions flourish in the United States than in any other civilized country on earth, and most of them are wrong. They thrive in the minds of the same people who talk about their operations; and like all mythology, they are a blend of fear, coincidence, and advertising (Anonymous, 1938).

As consumers' interest in nutrition increases, myths surrounding nutrition continue to confuse. Purveyors of nutritional misinformation capitalize on fears and hopes by exaggerating and oversimplifying health virtues or curative properties of foods. Too few consumers understand the effects of various nutrients on the body and how the body uses these nutrients, thereby opening the door to food faddism or nutrition quackery.

A **food fad** may be based on a food fact or fallacy. People often begin a diet or believe claims for specific foods or supplements on the basis of something they read or hear without investigating

TABLE 14–6   *A Guide to Food Additives*

Functions in Foods	Some Commonly Used Additives	Some Foods in Which Used
Preservatives		
Antioxidants are used to prevent oxidation resulting in rancidity of fats or browning of fruits.	Butylated hydroxyanisole (BHA), tocopherols (vitamin E), citric acid, ascorbic acid.	Vegetable shortenings and oils, potato chips, pudding and pie filling mixes, whipped topping mix, canned and frozen fruits.
Other preservatives are used to control the growth of mold, bacteria, and yeast.	Sodium benzoate, propionic acid, calcium propionate.	Table syrup, bread, cookies, cheese, fruit juices, pie fillings.
For Consistency and Texture		
Emulsifiers make it possible to uniformly disperse tiny particles of globules of one liquid in another liquid.	Mono- and dyglycerides, lecithin, polysorbate 60, propylene glycol, monostearate.	Salad dressing mixes, margarine, cake mixes, whipped topping mix, pudding and pie filling mix, chocolate, bread.
Stabilizers and thickeners aid in maintaining smooth and uniform texture and consistency; provide desired thickness or gel.	Algin derivative, carrageenan, cellulose gum, guar gum, gum arabic, pectin, gelatin.	Instant pudding mixes, ice creams, cream cheese, frozen desserts, chocolate milk, baked goods, salad dressing mixes, frozen whipped toppings, jams and jellies, candies, sauces.
Acid-Bases		
Control the acidity and alkalinity of many foods, may act as buffers or neutralizing agents.	Citric acid, adipic acid, sodium bicarbonate, lactic acid, potassium acid tartrate.	Gelatin desserts, baking powder, baked goods, process cheese, instant soft drink mixes.
Nutrient Supplements		
Mainly vitamins and minerals—are added to improve the nutritive value of foods.	Potassium iodide (iodine), vitamin D, thiamin mononitrate (vitamin B_1), riboflavin (vitamin B_2), ascorbic acid (vitamin C), niacin (a B vitamin), vitamin A, palmitate, ferrous sulfate (iron).	Iodized salt, milk, margarine, enriched or fortified breakfast cereals, enriched macaroni, enriched rice, enriched flour, instant breakfast drink.
Flavors and Flavoring Agents		
Both natural and synthetic types are added to foods to give a wide variety of flavorful products without restrictions of season or geographic locale.	Natural lemon and orange flavors, dried garlic, herbs, spices, hydrolyzed vegetable protein, vanillin and other artificial flavors (mainly fruit flavors).	Pudding and pie filling and gelatin dessert mixes, cake mixes, salad dressing mixes, candies, soft drinks, ice cream, barbeque sauce.

Table continued on following page

TABLE 14–6 *A Guide to Food Additives* (Continued)

Functions in Foods	Some Commonly Used Additives	Some Foods in Which Used
Colorings		
Both natural and synthetic types are used to enhance the appearance of foods. Most colors used today are approved synthetic colors since there are not enough natural colors available.	Carotene, carmel color, beet powder, artificial colors.	Margarine, cheese, soft drink mixes, candies, jams and jellies, fruit-flavored gelatins, pudding and pie filling mixes.
Miscellaneous Additives		
Include anticaking agents; anti-foaming agents; flavor enhancers; humectants; curing agents; seques-trants; and firming, bleaching, and maturing agents; nonnutritive sweeteners.	Sodium silicoaluminate, mono-sodium glutamate (MSG), glycerin, saccharin.	Dessert mixes, soft drink mixes, seasoned coating mixes, salad dressing mixes, flaked coconut, special diet products.

From *Today's Food and Additives.* 1976. General Foods Corporation, 250 North Street, White Plains, NY 10425.

its validity or effectiveness. While some fads are physically harmless, they may create an economic hardship for those with limited income because the foods or supplements may be expensive. Still others are nutritionally inadequate and could lead to serious deficiencies. A fad is frequently harmful because this therapy is substituted for the advice of a physician, thereby delaying medical treatment.

Fad diets are prevalent in the United States as Americans continue to search for a magic formula to lose weight. According to promoters of weight-loss diets, specific foods or food combinations facilitate weight loss, implying that a specific food or combination of foods oxidizes body fat, increases the metabolic rate, or inhibits voluntary food intake. These diets are frequently deficient in essential nutrients. Results of fad diets can be devastating and have even led to death. Other benefits, such as rapid weight loss, may not be long-lasting.

Such diets can be recognized instantly when they promise secret formulas to melt away fat without exercise while eating without limitation and, of course, the immediate result of several pounds lost. Miraculous promises are a good reason to run the other way. Diets that provide adequate nutrients and changes in lifestyle behaviors are desirable and more effective.

Food quackery claims or promises may be due to ignorance, delusion, misconception, or intent to deceive. At a National Health Conference in 1988, quackery was estimated to cost Americans between $10 billion and $40 billion yearly (Grigg, 1988).

The unknowns of medicine and disagreement among reputable scientists regarding interpretation of research findings foster nutritional misinformation. Given the right circumstances, such as confronting a chronic or incurable disease, everyone is potentially capable of exchanging sound judgment and common sense for the promise of a miraculous cure.

Numerous unproven theories abound regarding food allergies and intolerances, from illegitimate diagnostic testing to treatment with diets and supplements, that have not proven effective in scientific studies. Treatments proposed for Candidia hypersensitivity have been of concern to the American Academy of Allergy and Immunology. Candida is present in most healthy people without causing problems; people with diagnosed Candida infections frequently do not manifest the many problems associated with "yeast sensitivity." There is no evidence that the diet proposed for Candidia hypersensitivity (avoidance of sugar, yeast-containing bread products, and alcohols, etc.) will decrease yeast growth or enhance the immune system.

Unconventional procedures for nutritional assessment are numerous. Hair analysis is used to recommend vitamin and mineral supplements. Hair analysis can indicate exposure to toxic heavy metals, but vitamins are not present in hair except in the roots below the skin. Hair grows very slowly and does not reflect current body status. Furthermore, hair mineral content can be affected by shampoos, bleach, dye, and many other factors, including environmental and geographic factors.

Many theories have been proposed regarding the aging process. Nutritional manipulations are used based on these theories to extend a person's life. To date, there are no proven methods to extend the life span. Chelation therapy has been proposed to rejuvenate the cardiovascular system, treat cancer and immune disorders, and retard aging. This treatment has caused kidney damage and may result in people not seeking competent medical treatment.

Herbal medicine should not be regarded as quackery but should be approached with caution. Herbs, including herbal teas, and other plant-based formulations are marketed to prevent and cure numerous conditions. They are marketed as being the only natural means of health care. Several severe health problems, such as cardiovascular disease, cirrhosis, and renal failure, have occurred from use of herbal preparations in the United States. People can reduce the risks of these problems by (1) avoiding herbs if pregnant or nursing (herbs should not be given to infants), (2) not taking large amounts of any single herbal preparation on a daily basis, (3) buying only preparations that list all ingredients on the label (but this is still no guarantee of safety), and (4) avoiding any preparation that contains comfrey.

Frequently a computer-scored questionnaire is used to diagnose nutrient deficiencies. These computers are programmed to recommend supplements for almost everyone, regardless of health problems or the presence/absence of symptoms.

How do unscrupulous health promoters get away with their lies and fake products? Strict laws protect against false advertising and mislabeling, as outlined in Table 14–7 but health food deception and "food terrorism" thrives. The government actively pursues health swindlers, but enforcement agencies lack adequate staff and resources needed to handle all the problems reported.

The First Amendment to the U.S. Constitution protects free speech and a free press; it also protects a person's right to dispense false, misleading, or deceptive health claims. If a food product makes false or misleading claims on its label, the FDA can take action because of mislabeling. For many years, health-related claims on a food product were prohibited by the FDA. Health claims are now permitted on food labels if (1) it is well documented that a particular nutrient can reduce risk, and (2) the benefits of this nutrient are not offset by another ingredient present. (For instance a high-fiber cereal that is high in fat could not be touted as being beneficial to health because of its fat content.)

The Federal Trade Commission can take action if false claims are made in advertising, so claims

TABLE 14–7   *Federal Laws to Protect Consumers*

Laws	Enforcing Agency
Federal Food, Drug, and Cosmetic Act (1938)	Food and Drug Administration (FDA)
Truth in Advertising Act (1938)	Federal Trade Commission (FTC)
Mail Fraud and False Representation Statutes (1948)	U.S. Postal Service

From Davis JR, Sherer K. *Applied Nutrition and Diet Therapy for Nurses*, 2nd ed. Philadelphia: W.B. Saunders, 1994.

made on labels or in promotions are not usually false. However, products can be legally promoted in books and magazine articles and on radio and television talk shows because of protection under the First Amendment.

Evaluating Health Foods

Organically grown and **organically processed foods** have become increasingly popular because of concerns about the effect of chemicals on health and the environment. Legal standards have been established by 26 states for organic food. The Organic Foods Production Act of 1990 calls for national standards to define organic food and assure consumers that food labeled "organic" meets certain prescribed standards. These standards and other problems are still under deliberation. Products sold both in health food and grocery stores labeled as health foods or organic foods imply that all other foods are unhealthy or are not as beneficial to health. Terms are frequently used to imply a meaning different from the officially accepted one, thus misleading users. Standardization of terminology is essential to assure consumers that what they are buying meets their personal definitions, and that all products have been produced according to the regulations.

Despite the fact that numerous studies and reputable scientists have concluded there are no demonstrable nutritional benefits from the consumption of "health foods" instead of conventional foods, health food sales continue to soar, with annual sales in excess of $1 billion. Consumers choose organic foods for many different reasons, such as environmental food safety concerns or esthetic preferences. Many are truly concerned about the use of pesticides. Information about reduced use of pesticides on fresh fruits increases client acceptance of fruit that is imperfect in appearance.

Detecting Fraudulent Claims

Evaluating nutritional information for quackery can be a tedious chore. Dental hygienists and consumers should begin by checking the credentials of the person making a questionable claim. The informa-

tion should be objective, based on scientifically, well-designed studies. Well-documented information written by reliable professionals is usually reported in scientific journals. The questions in the Scrutinizing for Fraudulent Information will help in the evaluation of oral or written claims. If the answer to several of these questions is "yes," stop and investigate further.

Scrutinizing for Fraudulent Information

- Is the information based mainly on testimonials and case histories?
- Is the medical profession or a government agency prosecuting him/her because it does not accept the superior claim?
- Are claims extravagant or emotionally appealing, such as promises of youth, beauty, glamour, long life, or cure of disease?
- Are superlatives such as "amazing" or "exclusive" used frequently to describe the product?
- Are most diseases caused by a bad or faulty diet?
- Does the product contain "biologically active" ingredients?
- Is there danger of being poisoned by food additives and preservatives?
- Are "natural" vitamins better than "synthetic" ones?
- Will the cure be quick, dramatic, or miraculous?
- Is the product good for a wide variety of ailments?
- Is the product or service being offered a "secret remedy" or a "recent discovery" not available from other resources?
- Is the remedy being sold door to door or by a self-styled "health advisor," or promoted by public lecture series or in a popular magazine?
- Are self-diagnosis and treatment being promoted?
- Does the product claim to be approved by the FDA?
- Can treatment only be obtained across the border or ocean?

From Davis JR, Sherer K. *Applied Nutrition and Diet Therapy for Nurses,* 2nd ed. Philadelphia: W.B. Saunders, 1994.

The Role of Dental Hygienists

What role can the dental hygienist play in combating nutrition fads and misinformation? Natalie Van Cleve stated in 1938, when times were different but widespread misinformation on diet was just as prevalent as today:

> It is the duty of all professions active in the field of food and nutrition to cooperate in clarifying any misconceptions of the laity. If the (health care providers) do not know their vitamins, the clients will find a radio announcer who does.

Doctors, dental hygienists, and even dietitians have sometimes promoted nutritional misinformation by failing to apply their knowledge, misunderstanding how nutrients are utilized, or searching for fame and fortune. The dental hygienist is in a unique position to understand the causes of food faddism and to recognize their dangers. Understanding clients and their love of "miracle" answers should help in recognizing the appeal of such misinformation. Secondly, a scientific background permits assessment of potential effects or uselessness of food faddism. Dental hygienists can help clients understand the true essence of nutritional science—the process of nourishing or being nourished—rather than the polypharmacy of supernutrition and organic foods.

Dental Hygienist Considerations

- Assess clients' use of food fads, economic level, and educational level, and the nutrient adequacy of any fad diet undertaken.
- If a client restricts food choices because of a food fad or beliefs in organic food, ensuring nutrient adequacy is more difficult. Therefore, a thorough assessment and evaluation by the dental hygienist and/or a dietitian is needed.
- Clarify any misinformation about the use of organic foods, but respect clients' beliefs and assist them in obtaining economical products that are acceptable to them.
- Help clients choose a variety of foods to ensure a balanced intake and lessen contamination from any one source.

- Provide clients with positive advice based on a broad knowledge base and understanding of nutritional concepts and current research findings.
- Answer any questions about therapies, products, or treatments that a client may be contemplating.
- Speak out to protect the public from misinformation.
- Do not offer proposals or remedies unless they have been demonstrated to be safe and effective.
- If a client is using or contemplating using a food fad or diet you are unfamiliar with, do not hesitate to consult a registered dietitian, home economist, or a nutrition professor.

Nutritional Directions

- Populations that consume large amounts of fruits and vegetables, even with the use of fertilizers and pesticides, have a lower rate of cancer.
- Organic foods cost more money, but are not more nutritious or significantly different in taste.
- Organic produce will not look as attractive and unblemished as traditionally grown produce; organically processed foods will have a shorter shelf life than products containing preservatives.
- Wash produce thoroughly. Some fruits can be scrubbed with a brush under running water.
- In addition to government health agencies already mentioned, numerous health and professional organizations listed in Appendix E provide health information. Other organizations, such as the Better Business Bureau, may also be helpful.

HEALTH APPLICATION 14

Hunger in America

In the United States, hunger may be hidden because those who experience it may not appear to be malnourished. Hunger is often episodic—ranging from several days to a prolonged but low level, including chronic skipping of meals. Hunger can also involve a low-quality diet that is monotonous and may be lacking in nutrients. Hunger, as defined by households in circumstances in which at least some members do not get enough to eat as a result of insufficient resources, represents a public health and public policy concern (Rose et al., 1995). The homeless make up a large percentage of the hungry. A 1987 survey indicated some 600,000 people are homeless (Saal & Douglas, 1992). However, approximately 32 million people in the nation maintain a home, and may even work full-time, but live below poverty level. [Poverty was defined as a yearly income below $14,763 for a family of four in 1993 (Rose et al., 1995)]. The percentage of Americans living in poverty has increased from 12.3% of the population in 1975 to 15.1% of the population in 1993 (Rose et al., 1995).

In the long run, hunger hurts everyone by causing health problems, increased education costs, and less than optimal productivity. Yet this serious health problem is treatable with a simple cure: providing food.

Poverty is a root cause of hunger. Approximately one-third of the monthly income of poverty-level families is spent on food; an average meal for these families costs $0.68 (FRAC, 1991). Meals are often skimpy, and when grocery money runs out, families go to bed without dinner.

Recent cuts in the federal, state, and local budgets have resulted in less availability of financial assistance, placing more people at a greater risk of hunger. Millions of eligible families are unaware of options for obtaining assistance or are declared ineligible from food stamps by onerous regulations.

In 1985, the Physician Task Force on Hunger in America (1985) estimated that hunger afflicted 20 million Americans, or 1 out of every 12. As evidenced by the numbers of people requesting emergency food assistance, the level of hungry people has increased dramatically (FRAC, 1991). FRAC's Community Child-

hood Hunger Identification Project found one in eight American children under age 12 suffers from hunger (some 11.5 million children); millions of other children are at risk of going hungry. It is estimated that some 32,000 children are homeless (Saal & Douglas, 1992) and constitute the fastest growing segment of the homeless population.

Most of the attention has been focused on hunger in children; pregnant women, infants, and the elderly are also vulnerable to adverse effects of hunger. Acute and chronic effects on health and behavior have been observed. Insufficient food intake affects mental and physical health. Growth stunting without muscle wasting is characteristic of homeless children who experience moderate chronic nutritional stress. Hungry children are more likely to suffer from unwanted weight loss, fatigue, irritability, concentration problems, and dizziness, as well as frequent headaches, ear infections, and colds. These problems also result in more absenteeism from school (FRAC, 1991).

Missing a meal such as breakfast can reduce a child's ability to respond to the environment, thereby negatively affecting learning. Apathy, disinterest, irritability and a low tolerance for frustration are common behaviors in hungry children. These hungry children are unable to concentrate in school and are less likely to reach their potential to become fully productive adults.

Prolonged hunger can increase the risk of malnutrition and reduce immune response. Pregnant women are at risk of delivering low-birth-weight infants and developing iron-deficiency anemia; children are also at risk of iron-deficiency anemia.

Federal assistance programs identified in Table 14–5 are already available to address hunger in this country. Full use of these programs, with increased availability and benefits, and increased awareness of programs are good starts. However, many of these programs are not being fully utilized.

The WIC program has proved to be cost effective in improving participants' health and nutritional intake. School breakfast and lunch programs have also proved to be cost-effective. Children participating in both the breakfast and the lunch program were significantly less likely to suffer from problems associated with hunger. Children who receive breakfast at school have fewer absences.

Proper nutrition can decrease money spent on health problems. The dental hygienist can help by referring clients to appropriate resources and agencies and to a social worker for assistance in filling out forms. These embarrassing issues should be discussed matter-of-factly. Clients may benefit by ventilating feelings/beliefs about "handouts" of food. Information should be presented in a positive manner, stating how it will benefit client/family. Most parents desire the best for their children; therefore, stress the benefits children will receive (increased growth, learning, productivity, etc.) by participating. Help clients to recognize that having inadequate funds for food is not a sign of failure, and that asking for help shows strength, courage, and wisdom. In due time, they in turn may be able to help someone else.

Dental hygienists can also help by offering to serve at community food resource centers or food donation drives. Some centers offer dental care utilizing volunteer dental hygienists and dentists.

CASE APPLICATION FOR THE DENTAL HYGIENIST

A client reports that he has found a miracle cure for his advanced periodontal disease. He plans to follow a diet "that will strengthen his gums." This diet eliminates two entire food groups found in the Food Guide Pyramid.

Nutritional Assessment

○ Dietary intake, especially which of the food groups are omitted; nutrients most likely to be lacking
○ Nutrition knowledge
○ Supplements used
○ Economic status
○ Where most meals taken; food preparation

Nutritional Diagnosis

Knowledge deficit related to nutritional requirements.

Nutritional Goals

The client will receive adequate nutrients to maintain oral health status by consuming a well-balanced diet.

Nutritional Implementation

Intervention: Discuss the Food Guide Pyramid—the different groups, numbers of servings needed from each group, portion sizes, and the nutrients provided from each group.
Rationale: Healthy oral structures are dependent on a variety of nutrients that can be obtained by following this guideline.

Intervention: Discuss the nutrients that are deficient in his proposed diet and why those nutrients are important.
Rationale: When essential nutrients are omitted, the body cannot function effectively and its immune response is compromised.

Intervention: Discuss the importance of obtaining the nutrients from foods rather than supplements.
Rationale: Foods are the natural way of obtaining nutrients; when supplements are used, many times they are in proportions that cannot be absorbed or they may interfere with the absorption of other nutrients.

Intervention: Discuss specific foods and oral care that would be helpful in preventing further deterioration.

Rationale: Adequate nutrition and oral self-care promote healing and repair of disease tissue. Maintaining a well-balanced diet will provide the nutrients needed to support a healthy periodontium and resist disease activity.

Evaluation

The client will practice effective oral care and consume a well-balanced diet; as a consequence, his periodontal health will improve.

Student Readiness

1. What ethnic groups are most prevalent in your area?
   - List their dietary problems and some suggestions for altering their diet.
   - Plan a 2-day menu that would fulfill the RDAs and utilize many of their favorite foods or habits.
   - Would a client have any problem being able to follow that menu, such as economic hardship or the local availability of special foods?
   - Does that ethnic group have any predominant dental problems?

2. Other than good foods to eat, what other life-long eating customs are learned as a child?

3. State some reasons why all Caucasians in the United States do not have the same eating patterns.

4. Plan an inexpensive menu for one day, using low-cost foods.

5. A client wants to know about convenience and fast foods. What would you tell him/her?

6. Study the meats at a grocery store. Categorize the types of meats that contain nitrate preservatives. Look at your own daily intake for 3 days and evaluate how frequently you are consuming nitrate-containing foods.

7. Americans are very dependent on commercially prepared frozen foods or purchased foods outside the home. Look at the caloric density of the foods consumed in commercial restaurants and the nature of the diseases that relate to obesity and cardiovascular health. What has consumer demand done to change selections offered in commercial food service establishments?

8. Prepare a rough budget showing how your personal funds are expended on a month-to-month basis. Evaluate the percentage of your own personal income that is earmarked for food prepared at home versus food prepared commercially in a restaurant or convenience items purchased in a grocery store. How well do you spend your own personal food dollar? Make some conclusions about how you could better utilize your dollar to provide optimum nutritional status for you and your family.

9. Compare the cost of three foods from a health food store with the cost of similar items in a supermarket. Which is more economical?

10. Locate an advertisement in a popular magazine or newspaper for a health food product and list merits of the product stated in the ad. Then list information about the product that might have been omitted or should be questioned.

11. Why are food faddism and quackery a problem for the medical profession?

12. Discuss current food fads and how they may have adverse effects.

13. How can one spot a food quack?

14. Discuss the pros and cons of allowing nutritional claims on products.

15. A client states, "I want to follow the '_____' diet because my favorite actor swears by it." How would you respond?

16. Read a nutrition research article from a reputable journal. Utilizing the information provided in this chapter, point out some problems with the validity and applicability of the research. Does the article identify these as problem areas?

CASE STUDY

A young couple with three children, ages 3, 5, and 7, has been living on unemployment insurance payments for 9 months. The mother expresses concerns because of inadequate funds to feed the children. She is worried about their dental health.

1. Prepare a list of social services or federal service agencies in the community that should be contacted to determine whether assistance is available to support the recovery of this couple.

2. What are some nutritional concerns the dental hygienist could address with the client?

3. What are some foods that are nutrient-dense and economical purchases?

4. List some snack foods for the children that are nutritious, economical, and noncariogenic.

5. What methods of food preparation could be suggested to the mother that would preserve the nutritional quality of the food?

References

Anonymous, cited by Wilder RM: Fads, fancies, and fallacies in adult diets. *Sigma Xi O* 1938; 26:73.

Avruch S, Cackley AP. Savings achieved by giving WIC benefits to women prenatally. *Public Health Rep* 1995; 110(1):27–37.

Buzby JC, Roberts T. ERS estimates U.S. food-borne disease. *Food Rev* 1995; 18(2):37–42.

Crockett EG et al. Comparing the cost of a thrifty food plan market basket in three areas of New York state. *J Nutr Ed* 1992; 24(suppl):72S–79S.

Food Research and Action Center (FRAC). *Community Childhood Hunger Identification Project. Executive Summary.* Washington, D.C.: 1991.

Grigg W. Quackery: It costs more than money. *FDA Consumer* 1988; 22(6):30–32.

Physician Task Force on Hunger in America. *Hunger in America—The Growing Epidemic.* Boston MA, Harvard University School of Public Health, 1985.

Rose D et al. Improving federal efforts to assess hunger and food insecurity. *Food Rev* 1995; 18(1):18–23.

Saal NM, Douglas PD. Teaching nutrition survival skills. *J Am Diet Assoc* 1992; 92(5):547.

Schaus EE, Briggs GM. Nutritionally economic foods. *J Nutr Ed* 1983; 15(4):130–131.

Van Cleve N: Food: Facts, fad, and fancy. *Am J Nurs* 1938; 38(3):285.

Chapter 15

Effects of Systemic Disease on Nutritional Status and Oral Health

OBJECTIVES

The Student Will Be Able To:

- Recognize various diseases, conditions, and treatments that usually have oral signs and symptoms.
- Recognize diseases, conditions, and treatments that are likely to affect nutritional intake.
- Discuss appropriate dental hygiene interventions for clients with systemic diseases or conditions with oral manifestations.
- Identify nutritional directions for clients with diseases or conditions with oral manifestations.

GLOSSARY OF TERMS

Anorexia   lack of appetite for food

Megaloblastic anemia   a condition in which the red blood cells are extra-large in size but fewer in number

Polycythemia   a sustained increase in the number of red blood cells which may result in iron-deficiency anemia

Neutropenia   a diminished number of neutrophils in the blood; also called *leukopenia* or *agranulocytosis*

Gastroesophageal reflux   a return of gastric contents into the esophagus, causing a severe burning sensation under the sternum

Hiatal hernia   partial protrusion (herniation) of the stomach through the esophageal opening into the chest cavity

Esophagitis   inflammation of the lower esophagus

Glossopyrosis   pain, burning, itching, and stinging of the mucous membranes of the tongue without apparent lesions

Gluten   a protein found mainly in wheat and to a lesser degree in rye, oat, and barley

Thrombus   blood clot

Ischemia   inadequate blood flow and lack of oxygen due to constriction or obstruction of arteries

Pocketed foods   foods retained in the mouth, especially between gums and cheeks

Varicose veins   unnaturally and permanently distended veins

Prognathism   overgrowth of the mandible

Parotitis   inflammation of the parotid gland

Parkinson's disease   a progressive neurologic condition characterized by involuntary muscle tremors, muscular weakness, rigidity, stooped posture, and a peculiar gait

Epilepsy   a transient disturbance of brain function that results in episodic impairment or loss of consciousness

Early satiety   feelings of fullness after eating a few bites

Odynophagia   pain associated with swallowing

Kaposi's sarcoma   a highly malignant tumor of blood vessel origin that occurs on the skin and oral mucosa

Leukemia   a generalized malignant disease characterized by distorted proliferation and development of white blood cells

Chemotherapy   the treatment of disease by chemical agents

Herpetic   related to the herpes virus

Binges   periods of overeating

Purging   use of laxatives, enemas, emetics, diuretics, or exercise to negate effects of overindulgence

Syrup of ipecac   a cardiotoxic drug used to induce vomiting following accidental ingestion of a chemical or poison

Test Your NQ (True/False)

1. Anorexia, associated with a chronic disease, can result in an increased susceptibility to infection. T/F
2. Antihypertensive, anticholinergic, and antidepressant drugs often cause a decrease in salivary flow. T/F
3. Iron supplements should be recommended to a client who has anemia. T/F
4. It is appropriate for a dental hygienist to give nutritional counseling to a client recently diagnosed with diabetes. T/F
5. A client with a hiatal hernia should be cautioned against eating prior to the appointment to prevent regurgitation. T/F
6. Protein intake should be closely monitored in a client with chronic renal failure. T/F
7. Kaposi's sarcoma is a tumor that occurs frequently in those with epilepsy. T/F
8. Phenytoin (Dilantin) can cause gingival hyperplasia and vitamin deficiencies. T/F
9. A dental hygienist should not confront a client suspected of having an eating disorder but should casually refer him or her to a physician. T/F
10. Bulimics generally have low body weight. T/F

As you have already learned, nutritional deficiencies frequently are evidenced in the oral and perioral areas. Oral lesions can be a reflection of or a marker for disease elsewhere. The oral cavity cannot be isolated from and is not immune to what is occurring in the rest of the body because oral tissues are nourished by the same blood supply that provides oxygen and nutrients to cells throughout the rest of the body. Therefore, oral tissues may reflect changes in its nutrient supply or other metabolic alterations. Oral manifestations are only a single part of the total systemic state.

Oral problems may be caused by a disease process or therapy, or by a nutritional deficiency that results when oral problems related to that condition cause inadequate intake. Systemic diseases or medications usually prescribed for these conditions may cause alterations in the oral cavity, such as oral lesions, xerostomia, or muscular weakness (Table 15–1). These oral alterations may lead to changes in eating patterns which frequently have a general debilitating effect on the entire body. For example, food preferences are affected by one's ability to chew. Those with reduced masticatory efficiency usually choose soft foods, which may not provide adequate amounts of essential nutrients. Therefore, those persons may be at increased risk of nutritional deficiencies as a result of tooth loss, malocclusion, or ill-fitting dentures or partials. The body is dependent on nutrients from foods eaten to regenerate and repair diseased tissues; therefore provisions must be made to provide these nutrients in adequate amounts.

All disease processes result from a combination of factors: the presence of an antagonistic agent (such as bacterial invasion), the susceptibility or resistance of the host (or activation of immune response), and environmental factors. One of the most important factors in one's ability to combat hostile agents is the availability of nutrients acquired from food. Infections can spread rapidly when the immune response is depressed.

The ramifications of a client's systemic health are important to the dental hygienist because they provide cues to possible oral problems; may change treatment goals, priorities, or scheduling; or may influence dietary recommendations provided to the client. Dietary recommendations made by the dental hygienist should take into consideration the systemic health of a client and should not contradict other dietary instructions that may be in place. In other words, dietary counseling for oral health problems must be done in the context of the entire person. Many conditions will require referral to a physician or dietitian.

This chapter presents oral problems frequently caused by systemic health conditions and/or their treatment because these problems typically affect eating patterns. No attempt will be made to cover pathophysiology, and the information given should not be used to diagnose conditions. If the cause of oral signs and symptoms is unknown, the client should be referred to a physician, who can perform a thorough assessment, including diagnostic laboratory evaluation, for accurate diagnosis and treatment.

EFFECTS OF CHRONIC DISEASE ON INTAKE

Anorexia and Appetite

Appetite is associated with enjoyment of food. Most healthy people have a good appetite with no problems eating adequate amounts of food. However, during illness, appetite is decreased because of pain, apathy, **anorexia,** drugs, inactivity, or many other reasons. Persons may become depressed after the diagnosis of a chronic illness, causing mental stress about problems associated with living with or dying as a result of the condition. A modified diet may be prescribed for one with a chronic illness which may adversely affect intake. Because poor food intake may further lessen the desire to eat, sometimes it is unknown whether anorexia is a cause of the illness or an effect of the illness. Anorexia during a simple infection contributes to nutrient deficits. Malnutrition or other stresses such as surgery or other injuries deplete body stores of

vitamin C and other nutrients needed to regenerate and repair cells; the body is thus more susceptible to bacterial or viral invasion. Infections spread easily in these individuals.

Most drugs that affect appetite lead to decreased food intake by suppressing the appetite, but many drugs prescribed for mental health conditions increase appetite and consequently lead to weight gain. As a result of anorexia, less food is consumed, with concomitant decreased intake of calories, protein, vitamins, and other nutrients.

Gustatory and Olfactory Functions

Taste and smell can dramatically affect appetite and food intake. Various conditions alter normal gustatory and olfactory functions (see Table 2–1).

TABLE 15–1 Oral Problems Associated with Systemic Diseases

Condition	Dry Mouth	Taste Alterations	Oral Lesions	↓ Immune Response	→ Masticatory Efficiency	Delayed Wound Healing	Dysphagia	Sore Tongue	↑ Risk of Bleeding	↓ Dental Caries
Anemias										
Iron deficiency	✓	✓	✓	✓		✓		✓		
Plummer-Vinson	✓	✓	✓	✓		✓	✓	✓		
Megaloblastic		✓	✓	✓				✓		
Thalassemia					✓					
Aplastic			✓						✓	
Other Hematologic Diseases										
Polycythemia									✓	
Neutropenia			✓	✓						
Gastrointestinal Problems										
Medications for reflux	✓									
Malabsorptive conditions		✓	✓	✓		✓				
Cardiovascular Conditions										
Cardiovascular accidents					✓	✓	✓	✓		
Antihypertension medications	✓									
Lipid-lowering medications		✓							✓	
Skeletal Anomalies										
Systemic bone disturbances					✓					

Table continued on following page

TABLE 15–1   *Oral Problems Associated with Systemic Diseases*

Condition	Dry Mouth	Taste Alterations	Oral Lesions	↓ Immune Response	↓ Masticatory Efficiency	Delayed Wound Healing	Dysphagia	Sore Tongue	↑ Risk of Bleeding	↑ Dental Caries
Metabolic Problems										
Diabetes mellitus	✓	✓		✓		✓				
Acromegaly					✓					
Hypopituitarism					✓					
Cushing's syndrome					✓					
Hypothyroidism					✓			✓		
Hyperparathyroidism					✓					✓
Renal Disease										
Diminished kidney function			✓		✓	✓			✓	
Neuromuscular Problems										
Parkinson's disease	✓				✓		✓			
Developmental disabilities					✓		✓			
Epilepsy	✓									
Neoplasia										
Cancer		✓								
Kaposi's sarcoma			✓							
Leukemia				✓						
Acquired Immunodeficiency Syndrome										
AIDS	✓		✓	✓					✓	
Mental Health Problems										
Anorexia nervosa/bulimia				✓						✓
Medications for mental illness	✓									

Respiratory infections have a dramatic effect on smell, but fortunately, these have a limited duration.

Numerous medications prescribed for various conditions interfere with the taste and smell of foods. Some drugs deplete the body of nutrients, such as zinc, which leads to reduced taste acuity. Therapies such as radiation therapy may affect taste function.

Reactions to loss of taste and smell are varied: some continue to experience oral satisfaction and overeat, but most severely curtail their eating.

Xerostomia

Disease conditions, drugs, and other therapies can affect oral status and food intake by influencing the amount of saliva secreted. Saliva protects both hard and soft oral tissues, so inadequate amounts may result in many oral problems. Some conditions that cause xerostomia include inflammation of the salivary glands (mumps, tuberculosis), dehydration, Sjögren syndrome, neoplasms (both benign and malignant), and obstruction of salivary ducts or removal of the salivary glands. Fear and anxiety, neuroses, and organic brain disorders can cause xerostomia. Xerostomia can be caused by drugs such as diuretics, anticholinergics, anticonvulsants, antidepressants, tranquilizers, and anti-Parkinson drugs.

Xerostomia can affect nutritional status in several ways: (1) chewing is difficult because a bolus cannot be formed without additional moisture; (2) chewing is painful because the mouth is sore; (3) swallowing is difficult because of loss of lubrication from saliva; and (4) food intake may decrease because of changes in taste perception.

THE ANEMIAS

Typical symptoms of all the anemias are pallor of the skin and oral mucosal and conjunctival tissues and overall weakness as a result of inadequate oxygen-carrying power of the blood. The occurrence and severity of clinical symptoms depends on the degree of anemia and speed of development. The different types of anemia can only be made after evaluation of blood tests.

Iron-Deficiency Anemia

Iron-deficiency anemia can be caused by a deficiency of dietary iron or by excessive bleeding, and may also occur during periods in which iron requirements are high, such as during infancy or pregnancy. Gradual depletion of iron stores may progress to iron-deficiency anemia and levels of iron inadequate to maintain hemoglobin levels to provide oxygen to cells. Food intake is frequently poor because of oral manifestations of the condition. Clients may complain of a burning sensation of the tongue and a dry mouth. Clinical symptoms exhibited include gingival and mucosal pallor and atrophy of the filiform and fungiform papillae that begins at the tip and lateral borders of the tongue and gradually spreads to the entire dorsum of the tongue. As the papillae gradually shrink in size, bald spots appear on the tongue and it becomes smooth, shiny, and red (see Color Plates 14 and 15). Loss of papillae increases susceptibility of the tongue to irritation and inflammatory disease. Leukoplakia, while very rarely seen, may gradually develop in severe cases. Wound healing is delayed, affecting response to dental treatments such as tooth extraction and periodontal or endodontic surgery.

After iron supplements are initiated, glossitis improves rapidly; it may take about 3 weeks for filiform papillae to regenerate.

PLUMMER-VINSON SYNDROME

Plummer-Vinson syndrome is usually observed in middle-aged women with iron-deficiency anemia. Plummer-Vinson is a combination of iron-deficiency anemia, dysphagia, and stomatitis. Erosions and ulcerative lesions are present on the tongue, buccal mucosa, labial mucosa, floor of the mouth, palate, and oropharynx. These painful ulcerations in the pharynx and esophagus are responsible for the dysphagia. There is a high incidence of oral and oropharyngeal carcinomas in clients with Plummer-Vinson syndrome. Angular cheilitis may also be present.

Dental Hygiene Considerations

ASSESSMENT
- *Physical:* burning sensation of the tongue, dry mouth, gingival and mucosal pallor, atrophy of the filiform and fungiform papillae, leukoplakia, dysphagia.
- *Dietary:* adequacy of dietary intake, especially red meats, green vegetables, enriched cereals and bread; use of vitamin/mineral supplements.

INTERVENTIONS
- Encourage iron-rich foods (see Table 11–4); if principally nonheme sources are consumed at a meal, a source of vitamin C will enhance absorption of nonheme iron.

EVALUATION
- Successful outcomes include the client's consuming iron-rich foods and taking the ordered supplement.

Nutritional Directions

- If the iron supplement is liquid, dilute with water or juice and drink with straw to prevent tooth staining.
- Iron stores are replenished very slowly; therapy should be continued for at least a year.

Megaloblastic Anemia

Vitamin B_{12} deficiency can result in a **megaloblastic anemia** called pernicious anemia. This occurs when vitamin B_{12} is deficient in the diet, absorption is inadequate, or requirements are increased. With vitamin B_{12} malabsorption or no dietary source (as occurs in vegans), normal body stores are usually sufficient for 3 to 4 years. Vitamin B_{12} deficiency is most common among strict vegans.

Those with pernicious anemia may initially present with mucosal erythematous macules. The oral mucosa may appear pale or yellowish. Oral changes of vitamin B_{12} deficiency may be the only clinical evidence of the disease preceding significant anemia. They may complain of a painful, sore, burning tongue which may show atrophy of the filiform and fungiform papillae. Glossitis occurs in 50% to 60% and fluctuates in severity. The inflamed tongue is tender and appears glazed and beefy red. Ulcerations and surface erosions are commonly found (see Color Plates 11 and 12). Those with pernicious anemia who smoke cigarettes are likely to develop leukoplakia, in which the tongue becomes covered with thin, white, plaque-like structures.

Replacement therapy with vitamin B_{12} injections will relieve symptoms within 48 hours; evidence of regeneration of tongue papillae may appear within 4 to 7 days and the tongue may be normal in 3 weeks.

Another type of megaloblastic anemia, caused by folic acid deficiency, is frequently associated with poor diets or medications that interfere with folate absorption or metabolism such as phenytoin (Dilantin) or methotrexate. Oral manifestations are similar to those present in pernicious anemia: glossitis, atrophy of the papillae, ulcerations, and glossodynia (Color Plates 9 and 10). Angular cheilitis and fungal infections in the perioral area may also be seen.

Folate replacement is necessary because diet alone is inadequate to replace lost stores. Iron supplements may also be ordered because when folate is deficient, iron usually is also. On the other hand, folate supplementation in one who is deficient in vitamin B_{12} may produce hematologic improvement, whereas neurologic damage from vitamin B_{12} deficiency continues to progress.

Dental Hygiene Considerations

ASSESSMENT
- *Physical:* sex; age; glazed, red, sore tongue; pale skin and oral mucous membranes; shortness of breath; malabsorption, previous gastrointestinal surgeries.
- *Dietary:* dietary intake, especially of dark-green leafy vegetables, animal products, liver, whole-grain breads; alcohol intake.

INTERVENTIONS

- If the client has megaloblastic anemia caused by folate deficiency, encourage rich sources of folate (see Table 10–6).
- If the client is not a vegetarian, encourage intake of foods high in vitamin B_{12} for pernicious anemia (see Table 10–8). If the client is a vegetarian, encourage intake of eggs or dairy products. Dietary intake will help reduce depleted stores.
- Refer the client to a registered dietitian; clients with megaloblastic anemia especially need nutritional counseling because of poor eating habits.

EVALUATION

- Desired outcomes include the client's consuming a well-balanced diet and foods high in folate or vitamin B_{12} (as appropriate) and taking supplements to enhance erythropoiesis.

Nutritional Directions

- ◆ Raw vegetables are a better source of folate than cooked vegetables; heat destroys this vitamin.
- ◆ Daily intake of dietary folate is necessary.
- ◆ Clients with permanent gastric or ileal damage will need monthly intramuscular or oral vitamin B_{12} supplementation for life.
- ◆ Vitamin B_{12} shots are not always indicated for "tired blood."
- ℞ When oral vitamin B_{12} supplements are ordered, take with vitamin C to enhance absorption.
- ℞ Large doses of folate can negate therapeutic effects of anticonvulsants.

Thalassemia

Thalassemia, also called Cooley's anemia, is a genetic condition found in individuals of Mediterranean, southern Asian, or African ancestry. In thalassemia, the red blood cells take on abnormal shapes, are fragile, and rupture easily. Blood transfusions lessen the effects of thalassemia, but a major problem is iron accumulation in the heart and other organs. Nutrient supplementation is of no benefit to these individuals. If transfusions are used frequently, iron-rich foods are avoided. Orally, there are wide spaces between the maxillary incisor teeth, and an open bite caused by protrusion of the maxilla.

Aplastic Anemias

Aplastic anemias occur as a result of exposure to toxic chemicals or drugs, such as antimetabolites used in chemotherapy for cancer, or toxic physical influences, such as radiation therapy, which inhibit bone marrow production of red blood cells, white blood cells, and platelets. Clients usually complain of weakness; pallor of the conjunctiva and oral mucous membranes is present. Other oral manifestations include purpura, gingival hemorrhages, and increased susceptibility to infections. Following irritation and trauma, tissues on the gingivae, buccal mucosa, and palate may become necrotic.

Dental Hygiene Considerations

ASSESSMENT

- *Physical:* race, weight gain/loss pattern; fatigue; pale or yellowish oral mucosa; purpura, gingival inflammation; susceptibility to infections; overdevelopment of maxilla and mandible causing an anterior open bite or deep overbite and inadequate lip closure.
- *Dietary:* appetite, iron and folate intake.

INTERVENTIONS

- Clients should consume a well-balanced diet. Review the number of servings and portion sizes from the Food Guide Pyramid.
- If the client is thalassemic, discuss the need to avoid foods that are iron fortified, such as fortified cereals and breads.
- For thalassemic clients, encourage meticulous oral hygiene and daily home fluoride-treatment because of the oral complica-

tions related to mouth breathing and mal-occlusion.

EVALUATION

- The client consumes a well-balanced diet; caries rate decreases, and gingival inflammation improves.

OTHER HEMATOLOGIC DISORDERS

Polycythemia

In primary **polycythemia,** the increased production of red blood cells in the bone marrow is considered to be a neoplastic condition of unknown origin. Secondary polycythemia is caused by a another condition, such as chronic pulmonary disease (emphysema) or congenital heart disease, or can occur in people living at high altitudes.

Oral changes are principally seen in primary polycythemia and rarely occur in secondary polycythemia. Petechial hemorrhages may be present on the palate and labial mucosa. The oral mucosa, rather than being a normal pink color, become enlarged and edematous, and turn a deep-red-purple color. Any trauma to the oral tissues will cause excessive bleeding.

Neutropenia

Neutropenia may be caused by toxic agents such as antimetabolite drugs acting on the bone marrow, antibiotics, severe vitamin B_{12} or folate deficiency, or a bacterial or viral infection.

Mucous membrane surfaces are invaded by normal oral flora. The first visible manifestations of the condition, ulcerations of the marginal gingivae, may progress to edematous and hyperplastic gingivae. Because of the low white blood cell count, the host is unable to resist this bacterial invasion; large ulcerative and necrotic lesions may develop, with extensive tissue destruction. Extensive generalized bone loss may result in tooth mobility, but periodontitis is not always inevitable. Meticulous oral hygiene is very important in preventing the progressive periodontal disease usually observed.

Dental Hygiene Considerations

ASSESSMENT

- *Physical:* facial and oral mucosal plethora (red appearance due to an excess of blood), painful oral mucosal ulcerations.
- *Dietary:* folate and vitamin B_{12} intake.

INTERVENTIONS

- For polycythemia, consult with the physician to establish the possibility of problems related to bleeding or thrombosis, and the necessity of iron therapy.
- If the client has iron deficiency caused by polycythemia, review iron-rich food sources (see Table 11–4) and tips to enhance absorption (see Fig. 11–6).
- For neutropenia, encourage foods high in folate (see Table 10–6) and vitamin B_{12} (see Table 10–8), if the client's intake is questionable.
- Stress the importance of frequent oral prophylaxis.
- Refer the client to a dietitian for nutritional counseling if eating habits are poor, particularly if the anemia involves a nutrient.

EVALUATION

- Successful outcomes include the client's adherence to a diet that encompasses a variety of foods, concentrating on iron, vitamin B_{12}, or folate; use of supplementation as recommended by a physician or dietitian; frequent dental hygiene recalls and maintenance of good periodontal health.

◆ To ensure adequate iron intake, eat meat, fish, or poultry regularly.

♦ To enhance iron absorption, choose a vitamin C-rich food with a meal and/or eat a small amount of meat with each meal.

GASTROINTESTINAL PROBLEMS

Gastroesophageal Reflux, Hiatal Hernia, and Esophagitis

Heartburn 30 minutes to 1 hour after eating is the most common symptom of **gastroesophageal reflux.** This condition is commonly associated with **hiatal hernia,** pregnancy, and obesity. Normally the lower esophageal sphincter prevents caustic stomach juices from refluxing into the esophagus. Acidity from the stomach, alkalinity, pepsin, or bile may be damaging to the esophageal mucosa and, left untreated, **esophagitis** may result. In addition to discomfort associated with swallowing and eating, clients may complain of **glossopyrosis.**

Clients are normally advised to decrease their intake of foods that precipitate reflux: fatty foods (gravy, pastries, chocolate, fatty meats, cheese, nuts, chips, salad dressing, mayonnaise), caffeine, cola, coffee, alcohol, and onions. Other foods to be avoided are those directly irritating to the esophagus: citrus juices, tomato products, and red peppers. If appropriate, weight loss is recommended. Other suggestions to help reduce pain include eating small, frequent feedings; using antacids to buffer gastric juices; wearing loose-fitting clothing; and sleeping with head and shoulders elevated.

Anticholinergic medications prescribed may interfere with absorption of vitamin B_{12} and folic acid. Observation for oral signs of vitamin deficiency is appropriate for those taking these medications, as they may cause dry mouth.

Dental Hygiene Considerations

ASSESSMENT

● *Physical:* type of medications used, heartburn, bitter taste, visual appraisal of weight, enamel erosion, sensitivity of the dentin.

● *Diet:* adequacy of intake; frequency of intake; caffeine, fat, alcohol intake; knowledge of foods that increase reflux or irritate the esophagus.

INTERVENTIONS

● If weight loss is needed, refer to a dietitian or weight-loss program, such as Weight Watchers or TOPS, for counseling and a nutritionally sound reduction program.

● To reduce risk of regurgitation during dental treatment, the client's head and neck should be positioned above the stomach in the operatory chair; encourage the client not to eat for 2 hours prior to the appointment; omit the use of nitrous oxide.

EVALUATION

● The client plans frequent well-balanced feedings, avoiding foods that cause reflux and irritate the esophagus.

Nutritional Directions

♦ Avoid foods that increase reflux and are irritating: fatty foods, caffeine, cola, coffee, alcohol, onions, citrus juices, tomato products, and red peppers.

♦ Since citrus fruits and tomato products should be avoided, other sources of vitamin C should be selected, including cantaloupe, potatoes, and strawberries.

♦ Heartburn is not caused by inadequate digestion; therefore digestive enzyme tablets are not appropriate.

♦ Eat small meals, evenly distributed throughout the day.

♦ Reduce or eliminate cigarette smoking, which stimulates gastric acid secretion.

Malabsorptive Conditions

Many chronic diseases are associated with poor absorption of nutrients: Crohn's disease, ulcerative colitis, cystic fibrosis, **gluten**-sensitive enteropathy (sprue or celiac disease), and AIDS. Different parts of the gastrointestinal tract are affected in these disorders and their manifestations differ from one individual to another with the same condition.

Oral problems associated with Crohn's disease and ulcerative colitis include oral ulcerations, swelling of the lip, and hypertrophic lesions giving the buccal mucosa a corrugated or cobblestone appearance. Additionally, taste alterations (metallic dysgeusia) and reduction in taste acuity for acidic foods may occur in Crohn's disease. Aphthous ulcerations may be a marker of Crohn's disease, ulcerative colitis, or celiac disease. These clinical signs appear when the disease is in the acute stage and disappear when it is not active.

Diarrhea and malabsorption create deficiencies of nutrients and trace elements in those with these diseases. Nutritional requirements of these individuals are usually increased, yet cramping abdominal pain precipitated by food intake, anorexia, and intolerance to many different food components (gluten, fat, lactose, fiber) inhibits intake. Sufferers are finicky and apprehensive about eating; as a result, they may present with anemia, protein and energy malnutrition, poor wound healing, and suppressed immune response.

Different nutritional modalities are used with these conditions. A diet high in calories and protein with limited fat and fiber, as well as possible lactose restriction, is recommended. Small, frequent feedings are better tolerated and will increase adequacy of intake. Irritating foods are excluded. Extremely hot and cold foods and high-fiber foods are avoided because they increase peristalsis.

Dental Hygiene Considerations

ASSESSMENT
- *Physical:* edema, anemia, weight loss, abdominal pain, diarrhea, fatigue, and emotional stress.
- *Dietary:* iron, folate, vitamin B$_{12}$, and adequate protein and calories.

INTERVENTIONS
- Encourage the client to eat a nutrient-rich, well-balanced diet. Reassess the diet frequently to monitor nutrient adequacy.
- The use of stress management techniques during the appointment can prevent aggravating symptoms associated with the disease.
- Consult with the physician about the client's need for supplemental steroids and prophylactic antibiotics prior to the dental appointment. The physician may also recommend vitamin and mineral supplementation.

EVALUATION
- The client is aware of dietary restrictions and attempts to maintain nutritional status.

Nutritional Directions

- Adequate rest and a relaxed, calm day prior to the prophylaxis will help to avoid aggravating symptoms.
- Multiple nutrient deficiencies are common and can interfere with effectiveness of the prescribed medication, thereby compromising immune function.

CARDIOVASCULAR CONDITIONS

Cardiovascular disease encompasses numerous prevalent chronic heart problems, including hypertension, congestive heart failure, myocardial infarction, cerebrovascular accident, and arteriosclerosis. In contrast to its many ill effects in other sites of the body, cardiovascular disease produces few oral effects and is considered relatively unimportant as a cause of oral problems. These conditions usually do not have any oral manifestations that affect food intake, but medications prescribed may have oral effects. Dietary adjustments may be recommended for these clients which may affect the information the dental hygienist provides.

Cerebrovascular Accident

Arteries afflicted with *atherosclerosis* may gradually lead to *arteriosclerosis*. Atherosclerosis is caused by an accumulation of fatty materials (such as cholesterol) on smooth inner walls of arteries. As this plaque thickens, arteries become progressively narrow and rough, and blood flow, which carries oxygen and nutrients, may be disrupted. Arteriosclerosis is a poorly defined term for atherosclerotic arteries that have lost their elasticity, commonly known as hardening of the arteries. An artery may become blocked from atherosclerosis or **thrombus; ischemia** results in damage to the part of the body supplied by the blocked artery. A cerebral vascular accident (CVA) or stroke results if occlusion occurs in an artery supplying the brain, or if hemorrhaging in the brain occurs.

Dysphagia can occur as a result of CVA. Clients with a brain stem CVA have difficulty handling their own secretions (saliva, mucus) and are more likely to require alternate means of feeding.

Occasionally those who have mini-strokes do not seek medical care. Even though they realize that things are not normal, they may attribute these deficits to the aging process. A dental hygienist may suspect dysphagia in a client who has facial muscle weakness (drooping mouth) or slurred speech; in one with weak oral, neck, or tongue muscles; or in a client who coughs or chokes frequently when taking foods or fluids. Neurologically impaired clients may deny having swallowing problems. Clients suspected of having dysphagia should be referred to a physician.

Normally a speech-language pathologist and registered dietitian work closely with these clients to ensure adequate fluid and nutrient intake. The extent of dietary modification is individualized; the type of dysphagia is diagnosed using a *modified barium swallow* or *videofluoroscopy,* which allows assessment for physiologic and anatomic abnormalities. The client ingests a small amount of liquid barium, barium paste, or a cookie coated with

barium, and the swallowing mechanism is recorded on videotape for review in slow motion. Usually the speech-language pathologist provides swallowing training and recommends specific techniques to facilitate a safe swallow. Various exercises are used to strengthen weakened oral-pharyngeal muscles. Appropriate techniques are used to teach clients to swallow in a safe way, such as thermal stimulation, body and head positioning, food placement in the mouth, and modifying food textures. Clients may receive their nutrition through a tube that provides the feeding directly into the stomach until the swallowing reflex improves.

Liquids are very difficult to control in the mouth, especially in the oral stage of the swallow. The only liquids the client can safely handle orally for a long time may be those that are medium thick (vegetable juice, nectars, eggnog, cream soups, ice cream) or spoon thick (yogurt, pudding).

Foods may need to be restricted to those that are pureed or are soft enough to require little chewing and are easy to control in the mouth. These would include finely chopped meats with gravy or sauce, soft meat salads, cottage cheese, chopped legumes, finely chopped canned and cooked fruits, hot cereal, moistened dry cereal, soft bread without crust or seeds, and cream pies (without coconut or nuts).

Neurologic deficits may cause some to be unaware of the presence of food in the mouth. The mouth should be checked after meals and any **pocketed foods** should be removed with a toothette to decrease chances of unknowing retention of food and increased risk of dental caries. In neurologically affected individuals, sensation may be decreased.

Dental Hygiene Considerations

ASSESSMENT
- *Physical:* slurred speech and inability to effectively communicate; unilateral weakness or paralysis; difficulty chewing and swallowing; loss of oral sensations; lack of tongue control (weak, flabby, and deviates to one side).
- *Dietary:* chewing and swallowing difficulties, dietary inadequacies.

INTERVENTIONS

- Monitor the client's blood pressure at each dental visit.
- Refer to the dietitian when dysphagia exists.
- Antihypertensive drugs may affect types of foods chosen.

EVALUATION

- Desired outcomes include adequate nourishment using modifications according to the client's disability, maintenance of good oral hygiene with no new caries formation, and control of the periodontal condition.

Nutritional Directions

- ◆ Encourage the client or caregiver to maintain adequate oral hygiene, particularly because of limited self-cleansing action on the affected side of the oral cavity.

Hypertension

According to the American Heart Association, blood pressure consistently 140/90 mmHg or high-higher is known as hypertension. Usually, persons with diagnosed hypertension or congestive heart failure will have been told to limit sodium intake to some degree, limit intake of alcohol and caffeine, quit smoking, exercise, lose weight, and reduce stress. One oral sign of uncontrolled hypertension is the presence of **varicose veins** evident under the tongue. When many older individuals are told they must curtail the salt in their diet, their total intake may be substantially curtailed because the food does not taste good.

Diuretics are frequently prescribed for those with congestive heart failure or hypertension to help eliminate excess fluid. These medications also have an effect on the amount of salivary flow, causing xerostomia.

Hyperlipidemia

Persons with other types of heart disease that involve an elevated cholesterol level or increased risk of atherosclerosis will normally have a fat and cholesterol restriction (discussed in Health Appli-

cation 5). Low-fat diets normally result in weight loss, which is beneficial to many. However, for those who are trying to maintain their weight, snacks may be needed. Dental hygienists need to be sure that noncariogenic snacks recommended are not high in fat, such as a light or nonfat cheese or skim milk.

Long-term use of medications prescribed to lower serum lipids may cause malabsorption of fat-soluble vitamins and folic acid. Several may cause gastrointestinal disturbances and affect overall food intake. Clofibrate (Atromid-S) may affect the taste of foods. Those with heart disease may also be taking anticoagulants such as digoxin that may increase risk of bleeding.

Dental Hygiene Considerations

ASSESSMENT

- *Physical:* medications prescribed, xerostomia, varicose veins on lateral side of tongue.
- *Dietary:* dietary recommendations, adequacy of food intake.

INTERVENTIONS

- Since stress is a negative risk factor for most clients with hypertension or heart conditions, the dental hygienist will need to minimize stress and consider the effects of the disease on the proposed dental treatment.
- Generally, hypertension has no typical physiologic symptoms; therefore monitoring blood pressure at each appointment is necessary.
- Refer the client to the dietitian for appropriate dietary guidelines.

EVALUATION

- The client's blood pressure is within a normal range; the client takes prescribed medications and follows recommended dietary guidelines.

Nutritional Directions

- ◆ Most salt substitutes contain potassium and chloride. Remind clients to check with their physician or dietitian for possible excessive dietary potassium.

◆ Help the client determine low-sodium, low-fat, and low-cholesterol foods that are feasible for the client's lifestyle.

℞ Antihypertensive drugs may be responsible for a reduced salivary flow. Fluoride therapy may be necessary.

SKELETAL SYSTEM

Systemic bone disturbances may initially be detected by the following changes in the maxilla or mandible that are noticed during an oral examination: (1) significant increase in size or alteration in contour of the maxilla or mandible; (2) alteration in radiographic pattern; (3) mobility of individual teeth without significant periodontal disease; (4) pain or discomfort in the jaw without obvious dental pathology; (5) increased sensitivity of the teeth without obvious dental or periodontal disease; (6) changes in the occlusion of the teeth; or (7) abnormal sequence of deciduous tooth loss or eruption of permanent molars in young clients. These changes may be caused by osteoporosis, metabolic disturbances such as hyperparathyroidism, or other conditions such as Paget's disease or fibrous dysplasia. For denture-wearing clients with osteoporosis, rapid resorption of the alveolar ridges may lead to continuous loosening of the dentures with resultant oral lesions or the inability to consume foods that require chewing.

In addition to referring the client to a physician for correct diagnosis and treatment, the dental hygienist needs to provide guidance to ensure that the client obtains adequate nutrients in the face of missing teeth, sensitivity to hot or cold foods, or pain when hard foods are chosen.

Dental Hygiene Considerations

ASSESSMENT
● *Physical:* changes involving bone.
● *Dietary:* variety and a well-balanced diet.

INTERVENTIONS
● Encourage consultation with a physician who will evaluate the situation.
● Resorption of the edentulous alveolar ridge requires frequent relining of the mandibular denture to avoid oral lesions and ensure the ability to masticate food.

EVALUATION
● The client seeks medical guidance and adheres to prescribed recommendations.

NUTRITIONAL DIRECTIONS
◆ A combination of sodium fluoride, calcium, and vitamin D may increase bone mass.

METABOLIC PROBLEMS

Diabetes Mellitus

Diabetes mellitus and dietary restrictions are discussed in Health Application 6. Persons with uncontrolled or undiagnosed diabetes may have a characteristic fruity-smelling breath and may complain of increased thirst. These symptoms are associated with elevated blood glucose levels and a level of insulin insufficient to properly metabolize glucose, causing increased urinary glucose excretion accompanied by large fluid losses. Xerostomia is partially responsible for altered taste, general tenderness of the gums, carious lesions, or pain and burning.

Diabetic individuals have a higher percentage of candidal infections. In addition to hyperglycemia, increased glucose levels in the saliva may provide a more available substrate for fungal growth. Xerostomia may also be a factor.

Gingival and periodontal problems are common, although the precise cause is not fully understood (Color Plate 17). Oral lesions usually reflect a reduced resistance to trauma and poor healing. Common oral problems include candidal stomatitis, moderate to severe gingivitis, inflammation and abscesses in periodontal pockets, alveolar bone resorption with increased mobility of the teeth, and gingival recession.

Resistance to infections is lowered and the normal healing process is slow. Minor trauma to the gingiva may result in extensive tissue necrosis with eventual denudation of the underlying bone and the possibility of osteomyelitis. Treatment of oral problems should be reserved until the diabetes is under good control.

Dental Hygiene Considerations

ASSESSMENT
- *Physical:* polyuria, polydipsia, xerostomia, weight loss, weakness, and acetone breath.
- *Dietary:* polyphagia (increased hunger); adherence to prescribed diet.

INTERVENTIONS
- To prevent hypoglycemia during dental treatment, the client must eat at the usual time and take prescribed medications.

EVALUATION
- The client's blood sugar levels are stable and the diabetes is well controlled.

Nutritional Directions

- Read labels carefully for sources of sugar. Foods labeled "sugar-free" may contain sweeteners other than sucrose.
- Because of the risk of periodontal disease, it is imperative to maintain an adequate daily oral hygiene program.
- If the client is taking an oral hypoglycemic agent, the use of aspirin may interfere with its effectiveness.

Acromegaly

Acromegaly is caused by excessive secretion of growth hormone in an adult. **Prognathism,** the main oral manifestation of acromegaly, results in class III malocclusion and possible difficulty with mastication of food. The tongue becomes enlarged and may protrude or develop indentations around its lateral margins as a result of pressing against the teeth (Fig. 15–1).

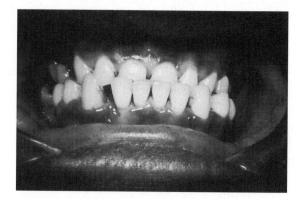

FIGURE 15–1 Acromegaly. (Courtesy of American Dental Association, Chicago, IL.)

Hypopituitarism

In childhood *hypopituitarism,* decreased skeletal growth results in disproportionate retardation of mandibular growth. Childhood hypopituitarism, or decreased production of growth hormone, is usually caused by pressure of a cyst or tumor. Because of normal size teeth erupting into the small mandible and maxilla, proper alignment is not possible. In addition to delayed eruption, malocclusion is the principal oral problem.

Cushing Syndrome

Pharmacologic use of corticosteroids and endogenous secretion of excess cortisol, as seen in Cushing syndrome, result in a state of hypercortisolism. Clients with excess amounts of cortisol will exhibit generalized muscle weakness and loss of muscle mass. Muscles used for mastication and the tongue may undergo similar changes and become hypersensitive. Hyperplastic gingival tissue is another common manifestation.

Hypothyroidism

Hypothyroidism may be related to (1) inadequate consumption of iodine, (2) an inborn error of metabolism, (3) high intake of *goitrogens,* (4) treatment of hyperthyroidism (surgical excision, irradiation, antithyroid drugs), (5) thyroid gland disorder, or (6) deficient secretion of thyrotropin (thyroid stimulating hormone, TSH) by the pituitary gland. Goitrogens are chemicals present in broccoli, kale, kohlrabi, cabbage, rutabagas, turnips, cauliflower, Brussels sprouts, horseradish, and soybeans that inhibit thyroid uptake of iodine. When hypothyroidism occurs at birth or in young children, the child is of short stature and is mentally retarded. The large tongue often protrudes from the mouth, showing indentations on the lateral borders caused by pressure from the teeth (Fig. 15–2). Eruption of the teeth is delayed, causing severe malocclusion; enamel hypoplasia and gingival hyperplasia are common. Proper oral hygiene is difficult and is only one factor in the increased rate of dental caries observed. Dental caries and periodontal problems appear to be related to malocclusion, retention of food debris in the mouth, and heavy calculus at the gingival margin.

When hypothyroidism occurs in the adult, the tongue becomes enlarged and has decreased flexibility. Gingivitis and chronic periodontal disease may be a result of the client's lack of interest in maintaining normal oral hygiene.

Hyperparathyroidism

Hyperparathyroidism results in hypersecretion of parathyroid hormone (PTH), leading to alterations

FIGURE 15–2 **Hypothyroidism. (Courtesy of American Dental Association, Chicago, IL.)**

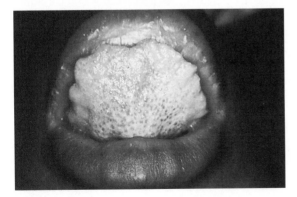

in calcium, phosphorus, and bone metabolism, thus causing calcium resorption from skeletal tissue and decreasing bone integrity. Systemic bone disturbances are reflected in the mouth by jaw enlargement and reduced bone density. Lamina dura around the roots of the teeth may be resorbed. Teeth may become loosened and hypersensitive to percussion or temperature variation.

Renal Disease

The kidney is the primary organ that eliminates significant amounts of waste products; it also has metabolic and endocrine functions that are affected when disease is present. Progressive loss of nephrons in the kidney leads to chronic failure. As kidney function diminishes, complications arise as byproducts accumulate from protein metabolism and alterations occur in electrolyte levels and acid-base balance. Persons with renal disease may be on dialysis while awaiting a kidney transplant.

Nutritional care for these individuals is very tedious. Protein intake is closely controlled while adjusting intake of minerals and electrolytes (such as sodium, potassium, and phosphorus), providing adequate energy intake, and avoiding potentially harmful intake of phosphorus, magnesium, aluminum, and some vitamins. For this reason, nutritional counseling should be left to the registered dietitian.

The oral cavity reflects many signs of systemic involvement. Anorexia is prevalent. Clients complain of a bad taste and have a mouth odor of ammonia, which is due to the build-up of urea in the saliva. **Parotitis,** or glandular enlargement, results in some discomfort.

Nonspecific ulcerations develop as the oral mucosa breaks down. Wound healing is slow because of general loss of tissue resistance and an inability to withstand normal irritative and traumatic insults. Acute necrotizing gingivitis may develop.

Because of calcium-phosphorus imbalances, various changes in bones are observed, a syndrome called *renal osteodystrophy.* This term describes various changes in bones associated with renal failure, such as classic hyperparathyroidism, osteomalacia, osteoporosis, and sometimes osteosclerosis. Decreased bone density leads to tooth mobility and periodontal disease. Fibrocystic lesions in the mandible and maxilla are also seen.

Uremic individuals are at risk of increased bleeding. They are usually anemic and pallor is generalized. The tongue may tingle or become numb.

Dental Hygiene Considerations

ASSESSMENT
- *Physical:* oral manifestations and deteriorating physical status.
- *Dietary:* appetite, prescribed diet, adequacy of oral intake.

INTERVENTIONS
- Consult with the physician prior to treatment.

- Because of the increased occurrence of oral complications, perform a careful and thorough oral examination to detect problems early.
- Refer to a dietitian as needed.

EVALUATION
- The client is able to describe the relationship among the condition, effects of dietary intake, and oral health.

Nutritional Directions

- Meticulous oral hygiene and frequent recalls will prevent or reduce oral infections common with metabolic problems that can lead to difficulties in eating certain foods.
- Chlorhexidine mouth rinses are helpful to minimize possible bacterial and fungal infections.

NEUROMUSCULAR PROBLEMS

Parkinson's Disease

Parkinson's disease affects the oral cavity by causing an abnormal pattern of swallowing, frequently with drooling and tremor of the lips and tongue. Decreased voluntary muscle movement affects muscles used to masticate food. Clients with Parkinson's disease may have many problems associated with feeding and receiving adequate nourishment: (1) mechanical difficulties may interfere with the transfer of food from the plate to the mouth; and (2) oral disturbances may alter normal chewing and swallowing mechanisms. These problems may necessitate a change in the form or consistency of food and/or special eating utensils.

Dysphagia may affect the oral phase of swallow or the pharyngeal stage of swallow. The results include drooling of saliva, holding food in the mouth for extended periods of time, inability to tear food apart and mix it with saliva, and food coating the tongue and palate after the swallow. Because of poor tongue control, a flowing, noncohesive bolus could spill over the base of the tongue, before the swallow reflex is initiated.

Following initiation of the swallow reflex, aspiration may occur when the bolus is able to seep under the epiglottis or from accumulated pharyngeal residue because of reduced peristalsis. Parkinson's clients are frequently *silent aspirators;* these individuals are not aware of food present in the pharynx and may aspirate without choking and coughing.

Medications (levodopa/carbidopa) used to treat Parkinson's disease have been the center of much controversy and research regarding compatibility of the medication and protein. This controversy has not yet been resolved, but intake of large amounts of vitamin B_6 (pyridoxine) decreases effectiveness of the medication. These medications also contribute to xerostomia.

Developmental Disabilities

Many disabilities may impair development of normal feeding reflexes (discussed in chapter 12) and coordination of these reflexes with respiration. These feeding reflexes may be absent or weak and difficult to elicit. Abnormal oral-motor patterns and difficulties associated with feeding may result when structural malformations such as cleft palate, macroglossia, micrognathia, and Pierre Robin syndrome are present. Neuromuscular diseases such as cerebral palsy, muscular dystrophy, Down syndrome, and Prader-Willi syndrome may be factors associated with abnormal oral-motor development. The feeding experience, which is normally pleasurable, becomes a frustrating time-consuming situation for everyone involved in the client's care.

Oral-motor impairment may become evident during the spoon-feeding phase of feeding development. Tongue retraction, tonic bite reflex, tongue thrusting, and persistence of a suckling pattern interfere with placing the spoon in the mouth and result in loss of food from the mouth (Table 15–2). A child with tonic bite reflex may clamp down on a spoon inserted in the mouth and be unable to release the bite. Attempting to free the spoon by pulling is ineffective and may cause continued biting.

For both tongue thrusting and tongue retraction, the tongue is unable to form a bolus and move it to the back of the mouth. Placing food in the mouth can be difficult with a severe tongue thrust and affect the individual's ability to suck, chew, and swallow.

With lip retraction, lips may be unable to remove food from the spoon, and drinking or sucking may be impossible. Sensory defensiveness is associated with a strong emotional reaction to the unwanted tactile stimuli and can result in a severe food intake problem.

Inadequate chewing skills are associated with jaw thrusting, hyperactive or hypoactive gag reflex, abnormal intraoral sensation, poor tongue lateralization, and tongue thrusting.

Oral-motor impairments make providing optimal nutritional care very difficult. Whenever intake of food is limited, either through an oral-motor problem or an inability to self-feed, these persons are at nutritional risk. With extremely severe oral-motor impairment, adequate nutrition cannot be provided with oral feedings and nutrition is provided via nasogastric tubes or gastrostomy feedings. Treatment is facilitated using an interdisciplinary team to determine the best treatment to promote development of feeding skills and provide foods in a form that can be safely handled.

Epilepsy

Epilepsy, or psychomotor seizures, in itself does not usually result in any specific oral or feeding problems. However, the type of treatment, or the use of phenytoin (Dilantin) or phenobarbital may cause problems. Gingival hyperplasia is noted with long-term phenytoin use (Color Plate 18). Several factors may account for this. Phenytoin decreases absorption of folate and vitamin B_{12}, which may lead to vitamin deficiencies. Because many epilep-

TABLE 15–2   *Feeding Problems*

Common Label	Description
Tonic bite reflex	Strong jaw closure when teeth or gums are stimulated
Tongue thrust	Forceful and often repetitive protrusion of an often bunched or thick tongue in response to oral stimulation
Jaw thrust	Forceful opening of the jaw to its maximal extent during eating, drinking, attempts to speak, or general excitement
Tongue retraction	Pulling back the tongue within the oral cavity at presentation of food, spoon, or cup
Lip retraction	Pulling back the lips in a very tight, smile-like pattern at the approach of food, spoon, or cup toward the face
Sensory defensiveness	A strong adverse reaction to sensory input (touch, sound, light)

From Lane SJ, Cloud HH. Feeding problems and intervention: An interdisciplinary approach. *Top Clin Nutr* 1988; 3(3):23–32.

tics do not practice recommended routine hygiene measures, the gingival reaction is compounded.

Calculus deposits, overhanging restorations, and orthodontic treatment are factors that increase the frequency of periodontal involvement. Another factor with both phenytoin and phenobarbital is increased turnover of vitamin D and K, thereby increasing risk of decreased bone density and osteomalacia, especially in children.

Dental Hygiene Considerations

ASSESSMENT
- *Physical:* oral complications related to neuromuscular disorders; medications prescribed, nutrient supplements.
- *Dietary:* adequacy of intake, signs of malnutrition.

INTERVENTIONS
- Carefully assess oral status of clients on anticonvulsants.
- Refer the client to a physician or dietitian if nutrient supplementation is suspected. Some nutrients may interfere with absorption of the prescribed medication.
- To reduce stress and anxiety, keep appointments brief and relaxing. Use of nitrous oxide sedation may be indicated.
- Provide tips for preventing dry mouth and oral problems associated with xerostomia

(see unbox in chapter 18, Recommendations for Clients with Xerostomia).

EVALUATION
- The client's dental health is maintained and prescribed medications are taken.

Nutritional Directions

- ◆ Salivary substitutions and topical fluoride treatments may be recommended for those experiencing xerostomia.
- ◆ Antibacterial rinses are helpful to decrease the chance of bacterial and fungal infections.
- ℞ Clients receiving levodopa or carbidopa should avoid dry skim milk, peas, beans, sweet potatoes, avocados, fortified cereal, oatmeal, wheat germ, yeast, pork and beef organs, tuna, and fresh salmon.
- ℞ Nutritional supplements are not ordinarily recommended for clients taking phenytoin and phenobarbital unless closely monitored by the physician because calcium supplements may decrease bioavailability of both drug and mineral, and pyridoxine and folate supplements may alter response of the medication and result in increased seizure activity.
- ℞ Carbamazepine (Tegretol), another popular anticonvulsant, will cause xerostomia, altered taste, and oral sensitivity.

NEOPLASIA

Tumors cause problems not only in the primary site they invade, but also in regional and remote areas. The manifestations at secondary sites away from the primary lesion may be the presenting feature in some cases. Thus, the mouth and jaw may be involved in generalized malignant disease.

Nutritional requirements for persons with neoplasms are generally increased to maintain lean body mass and immune responses. On the other hand, anorexia is an important symptom of an underlying neoplasm. Thus, oral symptoms or signs may be secondary to malnutrition or nutrient deficiencies. Abnormalities in taste perception have

been noted in some persons with cancer, such as an elevated threshold for sweets and a reduced threshold for bitter flavors. Altered taste sensations may be secondary to a deficiency of zinc. Hormonal factors affect the hypothalamic feeding center to reduce oral intake. **Early satiety** may be related to decreased digestive secretions or impaired gastric emptying.

The location of the tumor itself may also be a factor in reduced food intake, especially when the alimentary tract is affected by the tumor. Intake is reduced in those with cancer of the oral cavity, pharynx, or esophagus because of **odynophagia** or dysphagia. Gastric cancer may lead to reduced gastric capacity or partial gastric outlet obstruction, resulting in early satiety, nausea, and vomiting.

Psychological factors undoubtedly affect appetite. Depression, grief, or anxiety resulting from the disease or its treatment may lead to poor appetite and abnormal eating behaviors.

Kaposi's Sarcoma

Kaposi's sarcoma is characterized by bluish-red cutaneous nodules, usually on the lower extremities, and occurs frequently in immunocompromised persons. Red-purple macular lesions in the mouth may progress to raised, indurated lesions with central areas of necrosis and ulceration. Further, the lesions can cause obstruction of the esophagus, thereby compromising food intake.

Acute Leukemia

Acute **leukemia** is another neoplastic process with many oral manifestations that will detrimentally affect food intake. Gingival tissues are especially susceptible to gingivitis, which appears to be an exaggerated inflammatory response to local irritative stimuli (e.g., calculus, bacterial plaque, and materia alba deposits). Rather than the normal response of chronic marginal gingivitis, the gingivae may become severely inflamed with tissue hyperplasia and areas of ulcerations and necrosis. This is believed to be caused by the body's depressed immune response. Susceptibility to infection is increased and healing responses are delayed. Additionally the gingivae bleed easily.

Cancer Treatments

The primary treatment for cancer is surgical removal of the malignancy. In the case of tumors involving the gastrointestinal tract, the ability to ingest foods orally or adequately digest and absorb nutrients may be affected. Radical surgery in the oropharyngeal area may present problems in chewing and swallowing and decreased taste sensations.

Radiation therapy especially affects the alimentary tract. Early transient effects include general loss of appetite, nausea and vomiting, and diarrhea caused by malabsorption secondary to mucosal damage in the gastrointestinal tract. Food intake is affected because of a loss of taste sensation, xerostomia, difficulty in swallowing, and a burning sensation in the mouth when the larynx or pharynx area is irradiated. Food aversions may be associated with upcoming therapy. Rampant caries and loss of teeth may also become a dietary problem.

Chemotherapy drugs are used to destroy malignant cells without loss of an excessive number of normal cells. Chemotherapy has more widespread effects on the body than either radiation or surgical treatment. Rapid cell turnover rate in the alimentary tract leads to stomatitis, oral ulcerations, and decreased absorptive capacity. As a result, changes in taste sensation and learned food aversions occur.

Dental Hygiene Considerations

ASSESSMENT
- *Physical:* fatigue, caries, adequate weight, weight loss, oral ulcerations, medications.
- *Dietary:* maintaining caloric intake, adequate fluids, food aversions (especially food groups).

INTERVENTIONS
- Use of an antimicrobial rinse (chlorhexidine) may be indicated to reduce inflammation associated with cancer treatment.
- Calcium phosphate solutions are administered to remineralize and strengthen teeth (Dwyer et al., 1991).
- A soft or bland diet may be recommended as oral conditions deem necessary.

EVALUATION
- A dietary recall reveals adequate nutrients and calories with a minimum of fermentable carbohydrates.

Nutritional Directions

- Small, frequent meals are appropriate to provide additional calories and counteract nausea and vomiting.

◆ Meticulous oral hygiene, frequent recalls, and fluoride therapy are essential to curtail the problems associated with poor oral hygiene.

◆ Adequate food and fluid intake will not only improve the physical response to cancer treatment, but also create a more positive psychological outlook.

◆ Discuss the relationship between ferment-

able carbohydrate intake, effects of xerostomia, and caries. Caution against eating hard candy containing fermentable carbohydrates to relieve the xerostomia.

℞ Commonly used chemotherapeutic agents (bleomycin, cyclophosphamide, and methotrexate) generally cause such complications as stomatitis, nausea, vomiting, diarrhea, and anorexia.

ACQUIRED IMMUNODEFICIENCY DISEASE

Human immunodeficiency virus (HIV) debilitates the body's immune system. Following identification of HIV antibodies in the blood, a positive diagnosis of HIV is made. This *retrovirus* causes a dysfunction in the genetic core of T lymphocytes or white blood cells that normally function to resist infection. Retroviruses are characterized by the presence of reverse transcriptase, which interferes with the production of DNA from RNA. Thus, susceptibility to a variety of opportunistic infections (especially *Pneumocystis carinii, Cryptosporidium, Candida, Myocobacterium,* and herpes simplex) as well as certain neoplasms (Kaposi's sarcoma and non-Hodgkin's lymphoma) is increased. These infections can appear in virtually every organ system. Because of the body's inability to fight infections, acquired immunodeficiency syndrome (AIDS) develops.

The course of AIDS is often complicated by profound weight loss, wasting of body tissue, cachexia, multiple nutrient deficiencies, and particularly, protein-energy malnutrition. The cause of malnutrition is multifactorial and may involve inadequate intake, malabsorption, and/or hypermetabolism.

Anorexia may be attributed to respiratory and other infections, fever, dysgeusia, gastrointestinal complications, adverse effects of drugs, and depression. Specific nutritional deficiencies may depress appetite and exacerbate anorectic behavior. Additionally, oral and esophageal pain during eating may decrease intake. Oral candidiasis, which produces pain and inhibits production of saliva, is present in approximately 45% of clients with AIDS (Salik et al., 1987).

Many oral problems in HIV-positive clients have predictive value for development of AIDS. Pharyngeal or esophageal lesions of Kaposi's sarcoma may cause obstruction, whereas **herpetic** or other ulcerations on the tongue and/or throat can cause difficulty in swallowing. The development of thrush may be attributed to a herpes virus, candidiasis (Color Plates 19 and 20), chemotherapy, or drugs such as interferon.

Oral hairy leukoplakia is found predominantly on the lateral margins of the tongue in clients who are HIV positive. These white lesions do not rub off and are occasionally seen on the buccal or labial mucosa. HIV-infected persons frequently have ulcerations that resemble aphthous ulcers. These appear as well-circumscribed ulcers with an erythematous margin. These painful ulcers may become extremely large and necrotic; they may persist for several weeks.

Because HIV-positive clients do not respond normally to standard periodontal therapy, a mild case of gingivitis can progress to severe periodontitis in a few months, resulting in the need for extraction of the affected teeth. Clients with HIV infection may have parotid gland swelling accompanied by xerostomia. Spontaneous oral bleeding may be associated with small purpuric lesions or ecchymoses or gingivitis.

Currently there is no cure for AIDS; numerous medications are used in treating the various illnesses secondary to immunosuppression.

Good nutrition does not cure AIDS, but malnutrition may hasten the progression of the disease and affect outcome. At present, nutritional status is not known to affect the length of time for HIV infections to progress to AIDS. Adequate dietary intake can help maintain strength, comfort, and level of functioning. Providing optimal nutrition influences the functioning of lymphocytes not subject to attack by the HIV and improve resistance to opportunistic infections (Hyman & Kaufman, 1989).

Dental Hygiene Considerations

ASSESSMENT
- *Physical:* weight change, oral infections and malignancies, candidiasis, periodontitis.
- *Dietary:* oral sensitivity, adequate levels of all nutrients.

INTERVENTIONS
- Individualize the care plan and treatment for each AIDS client related to special needs.
- Consult with the physician for the possibility of additional medications to control infection during dental treatment.
- The client should use an antibacterial rinse and antifungal and antiviral agents.

MENTAL HEALTH PROBLEMS
Anorexia Nervosa and Bulimia

Although anorexia nervosa and bulimia are two different conditions, they are symptomatically related (Fig. 15–3). Anorexia nervosa is primarily a disease affecting adolescent girls who have an exaggerated, intense fear of becoming fat. Zealous self-imposed dieting leads to extreme weight loss.

Persons with anorexia nervosa may be described as achievement-oriented perfectionists who seek to rule their life by controlling their body through refusal to eat. These young individuals, generally surrounded with all the evidences of success, become "skeletons only clad with skin" (Bruch, 1978).

Individuals with anorexia nervosa may become excellent gourmet cooks, spending hours planning menus, finding special recipes, and shopping for exotic ingredients. In-depth knowledge of nutritional and caloric value of foods is commonly exhibited by anorexics.

- Refer the client to a dietitian for nutrition therapy.

EVALUATION
- The client exhibits increased attention to oral hygiene care and is maintaining current weight.

Nutritional Directions

- To promote healing and maintenance of oral tissues, encourage attention to nutrient intake. The Dietary Guidelines for Americans recommendation to decrease fat intake is not appropriate for clients with AIDS.
- To add calories and protein: add nuts and dried fruits to hot and cold cereals; use cream instead of milk; add ground meat or poultry, or grated cheese to soups, sauces, casseroles and vegetable dishes; use peanut butter on fruit or crackers; dip vegetables in sour cream mixes; use nutritional supplements or instant breakfast drinks as snacks.

Criteria for a diagnosis of anorexia nervosa include a weight loss equal to or exceeding 15% below expected or original body weight, amenorrhea (for women), and an excessive desire for slimness with a distorted body image (Diagnostic Criteria for Anorexia Nervosa). Dental complications in advanced stages of malnutrition are generally observed in clients with anorexia nervosa.

Diagnostic Criteria for Anorexia Nervosa

- Refusal to maintain body weight at or above a minimally normal weight for age and height (i.e., weight loss leading to maintenance of body weight less than 85% of that expected; or failure to make expected weight gain during period of growth, leading to body weight less than 85% of that expected).
- Intense fear of gaining weight or becoming fat, even though underweight.

PRE-DISEASE/		
Anorexia		Bulimia

EARLY SYMPTOMS · **MIDDLE STAGE SYMPTOMS** · **CRUCIAL STAGE SYMPTOMS**

Anorexia

*Low self-esteem
*Misperception of hunger, satiety and other bodily sensations
*Feelings of lack of control in life
*Distorted body image
*Over-achiever
*Compliant
*Anxiety
*Menstrual cycle stops (Amenorrhea)
*Progressive preoccupation with food and eating
*Isolates self from family and friends
*Perfectionistic behavior
*Compulsive exercise
*Eats alone
*Fights with family about eating (may begin to cook and control family's eating)
*Fatigue
*Increased facial and body hair (Lanugo)
*Decreased scalp hair
*Thin, dry scalp
*Emaciated appearance (At least 25% loss of total body weight)
*Feelings of control over body
*Rigid
*Depression
*Apathy
*Fear of food and gaining weight
*Malnutrition
*Mood swings (Tyranical)
*Diminished capacity to think
*Sensitivity to cold
*Electrolyte imbalance (Weakness)
*Lassitude cardiac arrest
*Denial of problem (See self as fat)
*Joint pain (Difficulty walking and sitting)
*Sleep disturbance
*Fear of food and gaining weight

Bulimia

*Low self-esteem
*Feel that self-worth is dependent on low weight
*Dependent on opposite sex for approval
*Normal weight
*Constant concern with weight and body image
*Experimentation with vomiting, laxatives and diuretics
*Poor impulse control
*Fear of binging/eating getting out of control
*Embarrassment
*Anxiety
*Depression
*Self indulgent behavior
*Eats alone
*Preoccupation with eating and food
*Tiredness, apathy, irritability
*Gastrointestinal disorders
*Elimination of normal activities
*Anemia
*Social isolation/distancing friends and family
*Dishonesty-lying
*Stealing food/money
*Tooth damage (Gum disease)
*Binging/high carbohydrate foods
*Drug and alcohol abuse
*Laxative and diuretic abuse
*Mood swings
*Chronic sore throat
*Difficulties in breathing/swallowing
*Hypokalemia (Abnormally low potassium concentration)
*Electrolyte imbalance
*General ill health/constant physical problems
*Possible rupture of heart or esophagus/peritonitis
*Dehydration
*Irregular heart rhythms
*Suicidal tendencies/attempts

RECOGNITION OF NEED FOR HELP

RECOVERY · **REHABILITATION**

On-going Support

*Trust/openness
*Understanding of personal needs
*Honesty
*Increased assertiveness
*Improved self-image
*Developing optimism
*Respect of family and friends
*More understanding of family
*Full awareness and at ease with life
*Appreciation of spiritual values
*Enjoyment of eating food without guilt
*Acceptance of personal limitations
*Return of regular menstrual cycles
*New interest
*New friends
*Achievement of personal goals in a wide range of activities
*Self-approval (Not dependent on weight)
*Relief from guilt and depression
*Diminished fears
*Resumption of normal eating
*Resumption of normal self-control
*Begin to relax
*Acceptance of illness
*Participation in a treatment program
*Acceptance of a psychiatric treatment plan

The progression of symptoms and recovery signs are based on the most repeated experiences of those with Anorexia and Bulimia. When a patient with Anorexia becomes Bulimic, she will experience symptoms characteristic of both eating disorders. While every symptom in the chart does not occur in every case or in any specific sequence it does portray an average progression pattern. The goals and resultant behavior changes in the recovery process are similar for both eating disorders.

FIGURE 15–3 **Anorexia nervosa-bulimia: a multidimensional profile.**

◆ Disturbance in the way in which one's body weight or shape is perceived, undue influence of body weight or shape on self-evaluation, or denial of the seriousness of the current low body weight.

◆ Amenorrhea in postmenarchal women, that is, the absence of at least three consecutive menstrual cycles. (A woman is considered to have amenorrhea if her menstrual periods occur only after administration of hormones such as estrogen.)

Specific Types

◆ *Restricting type:* During the episode of anorexia nervosa, the person does not regularly engage in binge eating or purging behavior (i.e., self-induced vomiting or the misuse of laxatives, diuretics, or enemas).

◆ *Binge eating/purging type:* During the episode of anorexia nervosa, the person regularly engages in binge eating or purging behavior (i.e., self-induced vomiting or the misuse of laxatives, diuretics, or enemas).

Reprinted with permission, American Psychiatric Association: *Diagnostic and Statistical Manual,* 4th ed. Washington, D.C.: American Psychiatric Association, 1994.

Bulimia occurs more frequently than anorexia nervosa. Bulimia is an eating disorder that is not associated with significant weight loss (Diagnostic Criteria for Bulimia Nervosa). A bulemic might even be normal or slightly overweight and appear healthy. Bulimia is characterized by intentional, although not necessarily controllable, secret **binges** usually followed by **purging.**

Diagnostic Criteria for Bulimia Nervosa

◆ Recurrent episodes of binge eating. An episode of binge eating is characterized by both of the following:
— Eating, in a discrete period of time (i.e., within any 2-hour period), an amount of food that is definitely larger than most people would eat during a similar period of time and under similar circumstances

— A sense of lack of control over eating during the episode (i.e., a feeling that one cannot stop eating or control what or how much one is eating).

◆ Recurrent inappropriate compensatory behavior in order to prevent weight gain, such as self-induced vomiting; misuse of laxatives, diuretics, enemas, or other medications; fasting; or excessive exercise.

◆ Binge eating and inappropriate compensatory behaviors both occur, on average, at least twice a week for 3 months.

◆ Self-evaluation is unduly influenced by body shape and weight.

◆ The disturbance does not occur exclusively during episodes of anorexia nervosa.

Specific Types

◆ *Purging type:* The person regularly engages in self-induced vomiting or the misuse of laxatives, diuretics, or enemas.

◆ *Nonpurging type:* The person uses other inappropriate compensatory behaviors, such as fasting or excessive exercise, but does not regularly engage in self-induced vomiting or the misuse of laxatives, diuretics, or enemas.

Reprinted with permission, American Psychiatric Association: *Diagnostic and Statistical Manual,* 4th ed. Washington, D.C.: American Psychiatric Association, 1994.

Typically bulimia and anorexia nervosa occur for the same reason: fear of becoming fat. However, persons with bulimia try to control this fear by repeatedly restraining eating, but this backfires and leads to binging and purging.

Individuals with bulimia exhibit many of the same characteristics as anorectic persons, but bulimics are more sociable and underneath feel profoundly separated from other people. Usually they appear very mature, but this is a defense mechanism to hide insecurities. Appearance is extremely important.

Bulimics acknowledge their eating behaviors are not normal. They have strong appetites and may binge several times a day, with intakes ranging from 1,200 to 12,500 calories per episode.

Binges may last from minutes to several hours and may be planned or spontaneous, but ordinarily are related to stress. A single binge can cost from $8 to $50 since binging food consists mainly of high-carbohydrate, easily digested junk food (Plehn, 1990). Compulsive stealing, of both food and money to buy food, is another common characteristic.

These binges occur most often in the late afternoon or evening and end with purging. Self-induced vomiting is the main method of purging for white adolescent girls; laxative and or diuretic abuse is used more frequently by black adolescent girls (Emmons, 1992). Vomiting may be induced by sticking a finger or other object down the throat, applying external pressure to the neck, or drinking **syrup of ipecac.** Eventually most bulimics can vomit by merely contracting their abdominal muscles.

In addition to poor overall health status, nutritional effects of bulimia stem from purging and the method employed for purging. Frequent episodes of self-induced vomiting can cause oral cavity trauma; bruises and irritations in the oral cavity may be observed. Frequent vomiting causes erosion of tooth enamel (predominantly on the lingual surfaces of the maxillary teeth), dentinal sensitivity, and enlargement of the parotid glands; these are classic signs of bulimia (Color Plates 21 and 22). Dental hygienists should not falsely assume oral problems result from poor dental hygiene practices; rather, these oral problems develop secondary to frequent vomiting. Another classic sign of bulimia associated with self-induced vomiting is the presence of abrasions and calluses on dorsal surfaces of fingers and hands secondary to friction of the teeth.

Successful outcomes require comprehensive treatment by a multidisciplinary team that addresses individual psychosocial, nutritional, and medical problems. This team usually comprises a psychotherapist and/or psychiatrist, registered dietitian, nurses, social worker, and physician. This pooling of specialties provides more effective treatment as well as a support system for team members when difficult decisions are necessary or progress appears slow.

Mental Illness

A few of the many different types of mental illnesses that occur include schizophrenia, depression, and bipolar disorder or mania. These disorders do not usually display any oral manifestations. However, drugs frequently prescribed to treat the conditions may have side effects that affect oral status. Antipsychotics (e.g., haloperidol, thioridazine, fluoxetine, and thiothixene) used to treat schizophrenia frequently cause xerostomia. Anticholinergic properties of tricyclics, monoamine oxidase inhibitors, and trazodone (Desyrel) used to treat depression also cause dry mouth. Dental caries, mouth ulcers, gum disease, and oral thrush can develop (Brasfield, 1991). Trazodone can also cause a bad taste in the mouth.

Dental Hygiene Considerations

ASSESSMENT
- *Physical:* signs of malnutrition (i.e., thinning hair, always cold, facial hair), trauma to the soft palate from fingernails or sharp objects used to induce vomiting, location of enamel erosion, parotid enlargement, weight.
- *Dietary:* high-carbohydrate diet, very low caloric intake or other unusual dietary habits, obsession with diet or weight.

INTERVENTIONS
- An increased caries rate can be indicative of the high-carbohydrate binging, low pH of saliva from vomiting, and xerostomia.
- Because of the specialized techniques needed to deal with these eating disorders, a dental hygienist must be able to recognize and refer clients with eating disorders to a physician or a local eating disorder facility for assessment and treatment.
- Discuss the specific characteristics observed in the dental assessment with the client.

EVALUATION
- The client is making realistic changes by protecting the hard and soft tissues being plaque-free, and being treated by a multidisciplinary team.

Nutritional Directions

◆ To prevent further damage to the teeth, caution the client against brushing immediately after vomiting; encourage use of a mouthguard during vomiting episodes; and encourage use of daily fluoride and dentinal hypersensitivity products.

◆ Inform the client about various ways to relieve xerostomia and the effect of lack of saliva on hard and soft tissues.

CASE APPLICATION FOR THE DENTAL HYGIENIST

Janie, a 17-year-old cheerleader in high school, came in for her 6-month recall appointment. She complained that "my teeth seem to be wearing down" and "I'm getting holes in my front teeth." Further questioning indicated frequent vomiting to control her weight, because "everyone does it."

Nutritional Assessment

○ Weight changes
○ Oral assessment
○ Food, nutrient, and calorie intake
○ Awareness of the relationship between health and nutritional intake
○ Dietary habits

Nutritional Diagnosis

Consumption of large amounts of high-carbohydrate, low-nutrient foods in a short period of time, several times a week, followed by regurgitation.

Nutritional Goals

Client will avoid fermentable carbohydrates to reduce the incidence of decay.

Nutritional Implementation

Intervention: Conduct an oral examination to note if any of the following complications are present: trauma to the soft palate, erythemic pharyngeal area, enamel erosion, angular cheilosis, salivary gland enlargement and xerostomia.

Rationale: These self-inflicted oral complications can indicate to the dental professional the need to further investigate the possibility of an eating disorder in a client who denies the problem.

Intervention: Discuss effects of frequent vomiting on the oral cavity and appropriate methods to prevent further damage.

Rationale: Not brushing immediately after purging, use of mouthguards during purging, and use of daily fluoride and desensitizing agents are practices Janie is encouraged to adopt to decrease further problems in the oral cavity. Providing such information to the client may be a factor in her reduction of vomiting episodes.

Intervention: Become the dental liaison in the medical/psychological health care team for this client.

Rationale: Because of the complicated issues involved with an eating disorder, several health disciplines are required to treat clients. The dental hygienist plays a crucial role in the overall care of these clients.

Intervention: Discuss specific foods that help to prevent further deterioration of the teeth.

Rationale: Adequate nutrition is essential to support a healthy periodontium and prevents destructive dental activities. Frequent intake of simple carbohydrate foods are factors in the high caries rate.

Evaluation

The client is actively seeking treatment for her eating disorder. She plans to achieve small goals as she works toward improving intake of all nutrients and decreasing episodes of binging and purging to improve her oral hygiene status.

Student Readiness

1. List ways to make a low-fat diet more appealing.
2. Describe several oral manifestations seen in various systemic diseases that create a painful mouth, thereby making eating difficult and less enjoyable.
3. Identify strategies for a client who is experiencing (a) nausea and vomiting; (b) a bitter or metallic taste in the mouth; (c) chewing and swallowing difficulties; (d) stomatitis; and (3) xerostomia.
4. What factors contribute to anorexia in a client with AIDS?
5. What are some of the treatments for cancer and what oral problems can result from these therapies?

CASE STUDY

A new client is seen in the office with complaints of recurrent aphthous ulcers. These ulcers have made it very difficult for him to eat, and he has been losing weight. During an oral examination, candidiasis, hairy leukoplakia, and a flat, bluish, non-symptomatic lesion on the palate, indicative of Kaposi's sarcoma, are noted. HIV/AIDS may be a possible diagnosis.

1. What additional information would you like to obtain from this client?
2. Would this client benefit from nutrition counseling by the dental hygienist? If so, on what areas should the dental hygienist concentrate?
3. What dietary modifications and dental care instructions would you make to this client?
4. Create a list of additional resources or agencies that would be helpful to refer this client to.

References

Brasfield KH. Practical psychopharmacologic considerations in depression. *Nurs Clin North Am* 1991; 26(3):651–653.

Bruch H. *The Golden Cage: The Enigma of Anorexia Nervosa.* New York: Vintage Books, 1978.

Dwyer JT et al. Nutritional support in treatment of oral carcinomas. *Nutr Rev* 1991; 49(11):332–337.

Emmons L. Dieting and purging behavior in black and white high school students. *J Am Diet Assoc* 1992; 92(3):306–311.

Hyman C, Kaufman S. Nutritional impact of acquired immune deficiency syndrome: A unique counseling opportunity. *J Am Diet Assoc* 1989; 89(4):520–527.

Plehn KW. Anorexia nervosa and bulimia: Incidence and diagnosis. *Nurse Pract* 1990; 15(4):22–31.

Salik RM et al. Opportunistic diseases reported in AIDS patients: Frequencies, associations, and trends. *AIDS* 1987; 1:175–182.

Section III

NUTRITIONAL ASPECTS OF ORAL HEALTH

Chapter 16

Nutritional Aspects of Dental Caries: Causes, Prevention, and Treatment

OBJECTIVES

The Student Will Be Able To:

- Explain the roles the tooth, saliva, food, and plaque play as factors in the caries process.
- Identify foods that stimulate salivary flow.
- Suggest anticariogenic food choices to modify a cariogenic diet.
- Describe the characteristics of some foods that are noncariogenic or cariostatic.
- Provide dietary counseling to a client who is at risk for dental decay.

GLOSSARY OF TERMS

Demineralization   the removal or loss of calcium, phosphate, and other minerals from tooth enamel, thereby causing tooth enamel to dissolve

Remineralization   the restoration or return of calcium, phosphates, and other minerals into areas that have been damaged, as by incipient caries, abrasion, or erosion

Fermentable carbohydrate   a carbohydrate that is capable of decreasing the plaque pH to a level where demineralization occurs

Cariostatic   caries-inhibiting

Test Your NQ (True/False)

1. Cariogenic carbohydrates are the sole reason for the development of a carious lesion. T/F
2. Nutrients have a role in the composition and structure of teeth during development. T/F
3. The bicarbonates, phosphates, and proteins in saliva act to dilute and neutralize plaque acids in the mouth. T/F
4. Sucrose, fructose, glucose, and maltose have a relatively equal potential to cause tooth decay. T/F

5. Most sugar alcohols, including sorbitol, mannitol, and xylitol, are cariogenic. T/F
6. For a tooth to demineralize, the plaque pH needs to be 6 or higher when cariogenic foods are consumed. T/F
7. The total quantity of sugar is of greatest importance when assessing the client's diet. T/F
8. A fermentable carbohydrate consumed with a meal is less cariogenic than the same food consumed as a snack. T/F
9. The U.S. RDAs would provide helpful nutrition information for clients trying to reduce dental decay. T/F
10. Providing clients with information about the process of decay leads to desirable dietary and oral behavior changes. T/F

Nutritional status and oral health have a strong interrelationship. Countless research studies have demonstrated the importance of diet in the development, maintenance, and repair of oral tissues. Dental caries is a multifactorial, chronic disease, and it is of no surprise that diet and nutrients play a role (Color Plate 16). Some foods exert a cariogenic effect, while others are cariostatic and offer protection or reduce caries. Nutrients also have both local intraoral and systemic effects, which can be primary or secondary factors in the development of dental decay.

PREVALENCE

Epidemiologic surveys indicate a decline in the incidence of dental decay as compared to the incidence in children born in previous decades (Fig. 16–1). The mean DMFS (decayed, missing filled surface) rate declined from 4.7 in the 1979–1980 survey to 3.07 in the 1986–1987 survey (NIDR 1987, 1989). Not only has this occurred on otherwise immune surfaces (proximal and smooth), but pits and fissures have also had a decreased caries rate (Newbrun, 1992). Unfortunately, reduction of

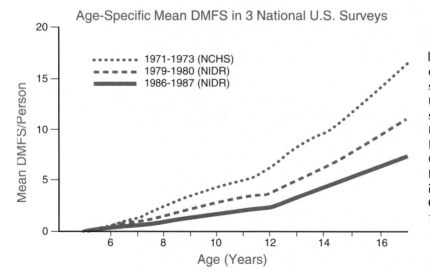

Age-Specific Mean DMFS in 3 National U.S. Surveys

········ 1971-1973 (NCHS)
------ 1979-1980 (NIDR)
—— 1986-1987 (NIDR)

FIGURE 16–1 Age-specific mean decayed, missing, and filled surfaces (DMFS) index in three national United States surveys. (From National Institute of Dental Research: The National Survey of U.S. School Children: 1986–1987. NIH Publication No. 89-2247. Washington DC: United States Government Printing Office, 1989.)

sugar in the diet has not contributed to the decrease in caries. Rather, effective interventions in reducing caries rates have been the promotion of fluoride, frequent dental care, application of sealants, and oral hygiene.

Since sugar consumption, such as in the form of added sugar, "hidden" sugar, and snack foods, in the United States has not declined, the need for dietary advice is imminent. The caries rate increases as the child gets older, and only 15.6% of U.S. teens are caries free by the age of 17 (NIDR, 1989). An increase in dental caries prevalence has also been noted in adults. Data from the National Institute of Dental Research 1985–1986 survey revealed that 2% to 3% of individuals age 60 and over were caries free and 41% were edentulous. The occurrence of caries on the root surfaces of teeth where gingival recession has occurred is common in older adults.

MAJOR FACTORS IN THE DENTAL CARIES PROCESS

No one single parameter is responsible for formation of a carious lesion (Fig. 16–2). It involves a combination of factors: a susceptible tooth surface, a sufficient quantity of cariogenic microorganisms in the mouth, cariogenic carbohydrates, and a particular composition or flow of saliva. All of these must be present simultaneously and for an adequate period of time for decay to occur.

Tooth Structure

Increasing resistance of the tooth against **demineralization** begins in the preeruptive phase. Therefore, it is essential to maintain an adequate intake of nutrients during growth. The most influential nutrients include calcium, phosphorus, vitamins A and D, fluoride, and protein. Indirectly, some simple carbohydrates play a role in caries formation prior to tooth eruption. A child's diet that is high in low-nutrient carbohydrates will likely be deficient in the required nutrients (consider, for example, the child who snacks on cookies, candy, or ice cream throughout the day and is not hungry for the meat, vegetables, fruit, and milk offered at dinner). Other factors, such as genetic or metabolic disturbances, can be responsible for poor tooth formation. Dental anomalies include macrodontia (larger than normal teeth) and enamel hypoplasia (the underdevelopment of the ameloblasts during matrix formation of enamel).

After the tooth erupts, the depth of the natural anatomic pits and fissures and the positions of the teeth will be relevant factors in the occurrence of dental decay. Deep pits and fissures increase susceptibility of the tooth to decay because of the potential for plaque and food to be trapped in these areas. Overlapping and crowding of teeth also offer areas for these materials to collect and ferment, compounded by the difficulty of keeping these areas clean.

Saliva

The impact of essential nutrients is noted during the development of salivary glands, which begins during the fourth week in utero. Of particular importance are vitamin A and protein, which have a role in normal growth, development, and secretion of saliva from the salivary glands.

The protection provided by an adequate salivary flow and saliva's buffering effects will ultimately reduce the destructive capabilities of fermentable carbohydrates on teeth. This fact is recognized in those with xerostomia, who are at high risk of caries development due to decreased salivary production.

Saliva provides protection against caries in several modes. First, saliva acts as a buffer by neutralizing much of the acids produced by plaque as a result of carbohydrate metabolism. Second, normal saliva contains bicarbonates, phosphates, and protein that dilute and neutralize acids to maintain the pH in the mouth. Therefore, after an acidic drink is consumed, the pH of the oral cavity is relatively normalized by the components of saliva.

Particularly important to the prevention of decay is the flow of saliva. An adequate salivary flow enables rapid transport of foods from the mouth, decreasing the length of time harmful bacteria and

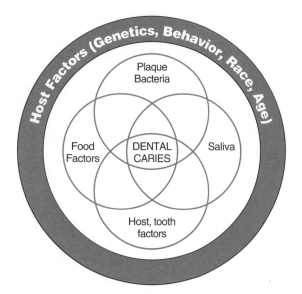

FIGURE 16–2 **Major factors that interact in the dental caries process. (Adapted from United States Department of Health and Human Services, Public Health Service, National Institute of Dental Research: Broadening the Scope. Long Range Research Plan of the 1990's. NIH Publication No. 90-1188. Washington D.C.: United States Government Printing Office, 1990.)**

food particles have to attach to the tooth and cause caries to develop. Consumption of citrus fruits promotes saliva formation by means of their citric acid content, but intake needs to be monitored because of their potential to cause enamel erosion.

Since saliva is saturated with calcium, phosphate, and fluoride ions, the potential for **remineralization** and resistance to enamel dissolution exists. Finally, antimicrobial elements in saliva, such as immunoglobulin IgA, either interfere with adherence of bacteria or compete with bacteria to attach to the tooth surface.

Plaque and Its Bacterial Components

Dental plaque is composed of a mixture of bacteria, polysaccharides, proteins, and lipids. Plaque, by forming a local barrier on enamel, reduces demineralization. However, bacterial acids in plaque have harmful properties that offset the benefit of its barrier effect.

The composition of plaque is altered as it ages and is strongly influenced by the diet. As the sugar intake increases, so does the concentration of acids present in the plaque. It follows that as the amount of acid continues to rise, the pH of the plaque falls. Certain organisms, such as *Lactobacillus acidophilus,* thrive in an acidic environment. They are found in large volumes in carious lesions and in plaque that has often been exposed to carbohydrates (Rugg-Gunn, 1993). *Streptococcus mutans,* a gram-positive, anaerobic, spherical bacterium, is also widely implicated in the initiation of dental caries. Therefore, a low sugar intake will reduce the number of organisms responsible for decay.

Once sugar has been ingested, its metabolism begins within 2 to 3 minutes and can persist for hours. The metabolic products are acetic, butyric, formic, lactic, and proprionic acids. The concentration of the acids escalates as carbohydrate intake continues, whereas the pH of the plaque decreases. Demineralization occurs when the "critical pH" of 5.5 is reached (Rugg-Gunn, 1993). The pH of plaque is eventually neutralized following elimination of cariogenic foods as saliva exerts its protective action.

Dental Hygienist Considerations

ASSESSMENT
- *Physical:* deep pits and fissures, amount of plaque in the oral cavity, composition and flow of saliva.
- *Dietary:* **fermentable carbohydrate** intake (amount and frequency).

INTERVENTIONS
- Encourage the use of sealants in deep pits and fissures to prevent accumulation of plaque.
- Practice meticulous oral hygiene habits, including regular recall visits.
- For clients with a high decay rate, use of chlorhexidine, or other antibacterial agents, can suppress harmful plaque and organisms. Counsel the client regarding the potential of chlorhexidine to stain teeth.

- Caution parents to avoid sharing utensils with children, a practice that allows transfer of the cariogenic microorganism *Streptococcus mutans.*

EVALUATION

- The client's food record reveals intake adequate according to the Food Guide Pyramid, with a low sugar intake, and use of appropriate oral hygiene techniques is demonstrated.
- When questioned, the client is able to discuss risk factors related to caries rate.

Nutritional Directions

- ◆ Eating a variety of foods in moderation will ensure adequate nutrient intake and the development of healthy eating habits will be a factor in tooth development, prevention of dental caries and general good health.
- ◆ Firm, fibrous foods, such as raw fruits and vegetables, chewing gum, and citrus fruits stimulate salivary flow. An increase in the flow rate will have a positive impact on resistance of teeth to decay.

Cariogenic Foods

As discussed above, simple carbohydrates are a factor in the development of caries. The small size of sugar molecules allows plaque to metabolize them rapidly and efficiently. Sucrose is not the only culprit; other mono- and disaccharides, such as sucrose, fructose, glucose, and maltose, all produce similar amounts of cariogenic acids. Each is capable of producing energy for cariogenic bacteria, being involved in plaque formation, and reducing pH through acid production. Lactose is the least cariogenic sugar; galactose may also have low cariogenicity. Natural sugars, such as honey (fructose and glucose), molasses (sucrose and invert sugar), and brown sugar (sugar and molasses), have cariogenic capabilities similar to that of sucrose.

Polysaccharides, starchy foods such as rice, potatoes, and bread, are less cariogenic than mono- and disaccharides. The physical and chemical properties of starches are very different from those of sugars, and render complex carbohydrates less damaging to enamel. Unlike sugar, the large number of glucose units needed to form a starch make it somewhat insoluble. Because starch must be hydrolyzed (split into smaller glucose units) before acid can be produced, the time the starch is in the mouth is not long enough for it to be completely metabolized, and saliva can readily neutralize any acids produced. These unique properties prevent starch from providing a readily available energy source for cariogenic microflora, and therefore it is less likely to produce caries than other carbohydrates (Nizel & Papas, 1989). When starches and sugars are combined (as in pastries or sugar-coated cereals), their potential to produce caries is equal to or greater than that of sucrose. Keep in mind that the cariogenic activity is also related to the form of the starch (discussed later in this chapter).

Fresh fruit is another food group of low cariogenicity because of fruit's low percentage of carbohydrate and high percentage of water. In fact, firm fruits, such as apples, play a protective role by stimulating saliva flow. The high concentration of fruit sugars found in juices is potentially a source of decay. This is clearly demonstrated by baby bottle tooth decay, which occurs in children given unlimited amounts of fruit juice. The sticky nature of dried fruit (such as raisins) also increases the risk of decay. However, each of these foods has high nutritional value and should not be eliminated from the diet.

Cariogenic foods that are a potential risk to dental health are listed in Foods That Cause the pH of Human Interproximal Plaque to Fall Below 5.5. The role of the dental hygienist is to know which foods are cariogenic, create awareness of the potential harm, and offer suggestions for appropriate consumption of sweetened foods.

Foods That Cause the pH of Human Interproximal Plaque to Fall Below 5.5

Apples, dried
Apple drink
Apricots, dried
Bananas

Continued on following page

Beans, baked
Bread, white
Bread, whole-wheat
Caramel
Cereals, non-presweetened
Cereals, presweetened
Cola beverage
Cookies, sugar
Corn flakes
Crackers, soda
Doughnuts, plain
Gelatin, flavored
Milk, whole
Milk, chocolate
Oatmeal, instant cooked
Oats, rolled
Pasta
Peanut butter
Potato chips
Raisins
Rice, cooked
Sponge cake, cream-filled
Wheat flakes

Anticariogenic Properties of Food

SUGAR ALCOHOLS

Sugar alcohols, often used as substitute sweeteners, are viable alternatives to sugar because of their sweet taste and noncariogenicity (see Table 3–1). Sugar alcohols, such as sorbitol and mannitol, are fermented more slowly in the mouth than mono- and disaccharides; therefore, the buffering effects of saliva competently neutralize destructive acids produced by plaque.

Another sugar alcohol, xylitol, is found naturally in plants and is equal to or sweeter than sucrose. Because oral flora do not contain enzymes to ferment xylitol, and metabolizing microorganisms, such as *Streptococcus mutans,* are inhibited, xylitol

is classified as **cariostatic.** Therefore, chewing gums containing xylitol or other sugar alcohols actually inhibit enamel demineralization. This inhibitory effect is enhanced by increased salivary flow, increased oral clearance, and greater buffering capabilities. Compounded by increased mastication, the outcome can be remineralization of incipient decay.

PROTEIN AND FAT

Protein and fat are two nutrient classes that are considered anticariogenic because they do not lower the plaque pH. In general, protein may contribute to the buffering effects of saliva. Both protein and fat may provide a protective layer to make enamel less vulnerable (see Possible Anticariogenic Effects of Fat). Also, consuming foods with fat and protein following a fermentable carbohydrate may raise plaque pH.

Possible Anticariogenic Effects of Fat

- Coats the tooth enamel to make it difficult for food and plaque retention
- Reduces sugar solubility by adversely affecting growth of cariogenic bacteria
- Lubricates food particles to protect them from oral fluids
- Lubricates the tooth surface to protect it from acidic attacks
- Coats the plaque to prevent reduction of fermentable carbohydrates to acids
- Accelerates oral clearance of fermentable carbohydrates
- Reduces carbohydrate intake

These effects are dependent on such factors as the amount and type of fat, food preparation, and food combinations.

Data accumulated from: Bibby BG. Local effects of nutrients. *In* Blix G (ed). *Nutrition and Caries Prevention.* Uppsala: Almquist and Wiksell, 1965, 30–52; Lanke LS. Oral carbohydrate clearance. *In* Blix G (ed). *Nutrition and Caries Prevention.* Uppsala: Almquist and Wiksell, 1965, 53–59; Kabara J. Dietary lipids as anticariogenic agents. *J Environ Pathol Toxicol Oncol,* 1986; 6(3-4);87–113.

PHOSPHORUS AND CALCIUM

Phosphorus and calcium also provide caries-protective qualities. Dispersion of these minerals throughout plaque could provide a buffering effect, reducing plaque pH. Ultimately, this action will curtail demineralization of enamel.

CHEESE AND MILK

Protein, casein, phosphorus, and calcium are all ingredients of other noncariogenic or even cariostatic foods, such as cheese and milk. Despite the fact that lactose is cariogenic (although the least cariogenic of all saccharides), these elements in milk and milk products decrease the risk of dental caries (Fig. 16–3). Cheese, produced from milk, contains several anticariogenic properties and has the potential to reduce demineralization (or enhance remineralization) of tooth enamel.

There is evidence that an increase of salivary flow occurs when hard cheeses are chewed. This provides a neutral environment and increases clearance of carbohydrates from the oral cavity.

Emphasis on following the Food Guide Pyramid's recommendation of two to three servings from the low-fat milk, cheese, and yogurt group would be prudent advice for a dental hygiene client.

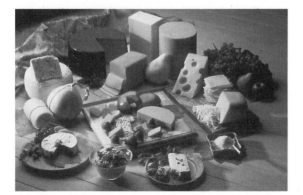

FIGURE 16–3 **Increase intake of milk and milk products to decrease the risk of dental caries. National Dairy Council. Diet and dental caries: An overview.** *Dairy Council Dig* **1994; 65(1):1–6.**

Eating these foods as snacks or at the completion of the meal could provide anticariogenic effects.

OTHER FOODS WITH PROTECTIVE FACTORS

A constituent in chocolate, known as the cocoa factor, has shown anticariogenic properties. The Vipeholm study compared the caries rate of those consuming chocolate with that of those consuming other types of "nonchocolate" candies under similar circumstances. The results indicated a slightly lower caries incidence in those consuming chocolate (Gustaffson, 1954). Glycyrrhizinic acid, the active ingredient in licorice, can also be considered anticariogenic. However, it is contraindicated with some antihypertensive medications; has a staining capability; and can cause sodium retention and increased blood pressure. Foods with these components offer only limited protection against caries; therefore, they are generally not recommended as noncariogenic choices.

Dental Hygienist Considerations

ASSESSMENT
- *Physical:* location and type of dental caries and salivary flow; heart disease; diabetes mellitus.
- *Dietary:* type of carbohydrate and amount of protein and fat.

INTERVENTIONS
- Educate the client about the process of caries and how to prevent demineralization of enamel, including the role diet plays in initiation and progression of decay.
- Using the Dietary Guidelines for Americans and Food Guide Pyramid, evaluate the client's diet for satisfactory nutritional intake and consumption of fermentable carbohydrates.
- Use of topical and systemic fluoride, as well as application of sealants, are factors in increasing tooth resistance.

EVALUATION
- The client assumes responsibility for the diet. Attempts are made to modify dietary

patterns and oral hygiene practices. Consumption of fermentable carbohydrates are followed with oral hygiene care.

Nutritional Directions

◆ Use as little simple sugar in food preparation as possible. Recipes requiring sugar can be reduced to one-half with minor taste and texture changes. For example, a brownie recipe that calls for 1 cup of granulated sugar can be decreased to 1/2 cup of sugar.

◆ Natural sugars (such as honey and molasses) are as cariogenic as refined sugars.

◆ Caution against repeated use of antacids and cough drops that contain sugar.

◆ Chewing gum and mints can be replaced with sugar-free choices.

◆ Increased use of products containing sugar alcohols (such as chewing gum, hard candy, dentifrices, and some medications) can cause diarrhea.

◆ Although sorbitol and mannitol ferment slowly in the mouth, which allows saliva to neutralize the acids produced, frequent use has the potential to cause decay. This is observed especially in a xerostomic client using these products to relieve a dry mouth.

◆ Chewing gums containing xylitol stimulate salivary flow, which reduces caries rate.

◆ High-sugar foods are generally high in fat as well. The Food Guide Pyramid recommends both be used sparingly.

◆ Exercise caution in recommending high-fat foods for their anticariogenic properties to clients with heart disease or diabetes mellitus because of their deleterious effects on these conditions.

◆ Because milk's physical properties are comparable to saliva, increasing low-fat milk intake (two to four 8-oz servings per day) as a saliva substitute may also offer protection against caries for the client with xerostomia. Encourage proper oral hygiene techniques in order to avoid complications associated with exposure to the lactose in the milk, as seen in baby bottle tooth decay.

Other Factors Influencing Cariogenicity

The amount and type of refined carbohydrates are not the only determinants of diet related to caries prevalence and severity. Other considerations include the retentiveness of the carbohydrate, how often teeth are exposed to sugars, and whether the food is eaten with a meal or as a snack. Therefore, some foods thought to have low cariogenic potential (such as cornflakes, crackers, or potato chips) may actually be more acidogenic than simple-carbohydrate foods. It is also important to consider preventive practices, such as regular recalls, appropriate oral hygiene practices, sealants, and use of adequate fluoride, when discussing cariogenicity.

PHYSICAL FORM

How quickly a cariogenic food is cleared from the mouth is a factor related to caries development. A sticky and retentive carbohydrate (such as raisins) will remain in contact with the enamel surface for a longer period than sweetened fluids. Slow oral clearance of the fermentable carbohydrate means longer exposure of the tooth to acid attack.

FREQUENCY OF INTAKE

Closely related to the physical form of a food in caries potential is the frequency of intake of fermentable carbohydrates. Longer periods of exposure to sugar in the oral cavity leads to a greater risk of demineralization and less opportunity for teeth to remineralize. Therefore, two individuals can eat equal amounts of fermentable carbohydrates, but the one who eats more frequently throughout the day has greatest potential for decay. With each exposure, a drop in pH begins within 2 to 3 minutes; at a pH of 5.5 or lower (the critical pH), enamel decalcification occurs. By the end of 40 minutes the pH has risen to its initial value. The classic Stephan curve (Stephan, 1940) shows the pH changes of dental plaque after rinsing with a sugar solution (Fig 16–4). Using a similar scenario, if one subject eats a candy bar within a 5-minute period, the teeth would be exposed to a critical pH for approximately 20 minutes before the pH returned to the original level. If another subject

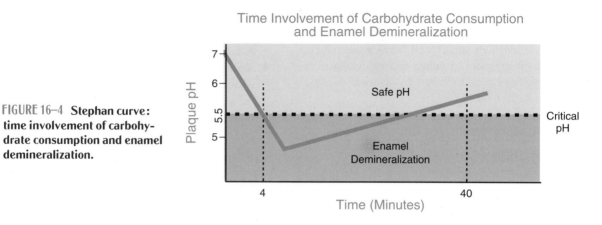

FIGURE 16-4 **Stephan curve: time involvement of carbohydrate consumption and enamel demineralization.**

eats that same candy bar in five bites, but only takes a bite every hour until it is gone, the total acid exposure would be approximately 200 minutes (five bites × 40 minutes = 200 minutes of acid exposure).

Frequent soft drink consumption can also influence caries development despite its rapid oral clearance. Based on Ismail's research, an increase in the DMFS score of up to 179% was observed in individuals who drank three or more sodas between meals each day. Because of soft drinks' popularity as a snack, recommendations should be made to substitute with a soda or flavored water made with a noncariogenic sweetener.

TIME OF DAY

The third consideration is when the cariogenic food is eaten: with a meal or as a snack. Participants in the Vipeholm study who ate foods high in sugar with meals and between meals had a significantly higher decay rate than those who had these foods at mealtime only. Recommendations to eliminate snacks are not always realistic. Children, for example, cannot eat enough food in three meals to get all the nutrients needed. Therefore, snacks are warranted. Foods chosen for snacks should be low in sugar or produce little or no plaque acid (see Foods That Produce Little or No Plaque Acid) and should be followed by oral hygiene practices.

Foods That Produce Little or No Plaque Acid

Cheeses*
    Blue cheese
    Brie
    Aged cheddar
    Gouda
    Monterey jack
    Mozzarella
    Swiss
    Cheese spread
    Cream cheese
    American
Yogurt[†]
Nuts
Licorice
Sugarless chewing gum
Chocolate
Cocoa products

*Remember these natural cheeses are high in fat. Reduced- or low-fat cheeses can be recommended.
[†]Encourage use of low-fat or skim versions.

The location of an acidogenic food within a meal presents yet another consideration. For instance, drinking coffee with sugar following a meal has been determined to lower the plaque pH; whereas consuming cheese after a high-sugar food within a meal prevents the drop of plaque pH that would occur if this high-sugar food were eaten alone. Thus, cariogenic foods create less risk of enamel demineralization if followed by a noncariogenic or cariostatic food.

Dental Hygienist Considerations

ASSESSMENT
- *Physical:* development of caries, degree of plaque formation, and salivary flow.
- *Dietary:* physical form of carbohydrate, time consumed, and frequency of intake.

INTERVENTIONS
- Review diet history for patterns for sugar frequency, form, and amount.
- Further questioning can reveal dietary habits the client failed to recognize as being relevant to dental decay.

EVALUATION
- The client is aware of detrimental habits (e.g., frequent use of chewing gum or mints or leaving a bottle in an infant's mouth) and is making efforts to modify them.

Nutritional Directions

- When consuming fermentable carbohydrates, do so at mealtimes, when possible, to allow other foods to neutralize acids in saliva.
- Foods that require chewing (such as chewing gum, raw fruits and vegetables) are help-ful in increasing salivary flow. This aids in providing additional buffering effects and accelerated removal of harmful foods.
- Noncariogenic snacks include raw fruits and vegetables, low-fat cheese, skim milk, low-fat yogurt, peanuts, popcorn, whole-grain bagels, seeds, pizza, and tacos.
- Encourage the client to read the ingredient list of a food label to assess for sugar content. Inform the client that foods on the ingredient list are listed in order of concentration, therefore, foods having a sugar as the first or second ingredient should be avoided or used in moderation.
- Cariogenic snacks before bedtime should be omitted or followed by careful oral hygiene. The salivary flow is reduced when sleeping; therefore, clearance of plaque acids is limited. Uninterrupted acid production can be harmful for up to 2 hours (Darby & Walsh, 1994).
- Carbohydrate foods that are sticky (such as gumdrops or potato chips) are retained in the mouth longer, creating a greater potential for decay.
- Use of diet products made with an artificial sweetener, such as aspartame, should be done in moderation (two to three products per day). Some clients may not tolerate these products or choose not to use them. Therefore, recommend other acceptable noncariogenic food items and oral hygiene habits.

DENTAL HYGIENE PLAN

Dietary counseling is an essential component of the preventive program. Although all clients would benefit from nutritional counseling, certain populations (Table 16–1) require special attention by the dental hygienist. As mentioned, the quantity of fermentable carbohydrates consumed is of concern. However, the form of the carbohydrate, how often it is consumed, and whether it is eaten with meals or as a snack are more important than the amount consumed.

Assessment

When a dental nutrition care plan is desirable, many factors are to be considered. Anthropometric measures (i.e., height and weight), clinical signs, dental

TABLE 16-1   *Situations Presenting Caries Risk/High But Preventable Groups*

Baby Bottle Tooth Decay
• Parents prior to pregnancy
• Parents during pregnancy
• Parents of young children

Root Caries & Xerostomia
• Elderly
• Periodontal clients

Oral Habits
• Frequent use of hard candy or chewing gum, cough drops, or antacids

and dietary assessment, health and dental history, and laboratory data (if applicable) will be addressed in chapter 19. In addition, assessment should take into account the client's learning style, cultural heritage, and socioeconomic status.

Gathering information about the quality of the client's meal pattern and eating habits is an important step in the assessment of the cariogenic potential of a diet. A *24-hour recall* (Fig. 16–5), which provides data on food intake for one day, can be obtained through an interview by the dental hygienist or the client can be asked to return the completed form at a follow-up appointment. This practical assessment tool is helpful in determining the adequacy of the overall diet as well as the amount of sugar intake and frequency of exposure.

Using the Food Guide Pyramid as a guide, the dental hygienist can assess adequacy of food intake with the cooperation of the client. Actively involve the client in as many steps as possible to enhance motivation and adherence. Have the client circle all the fermentable carbohydrates on the food diary in red. Review the food diary and discuss any oversights with the client as needed. Classify the sugar intake according to its form, its frequency (at least 20 minutes apart), and when it was eaten (Fig. 16–6). More than 2 hours of acid exposure in one day is generally considered high.

Goals

Once all of the facts are gathered, help the client develop realistic goals. These goals need to be flexible to meet the client's needs. Achievement of long-term goals is possible only if the client is able and willing to make behavioral changes, such as altering choices of cariogenic snacks or limiting frequency of cariogenic foods.

Education

Providing current information about detrimental dietary habits is instrumental in determining appropriate goals. Education alone does not guarantee behavioral change. For example, the client may be able to recite the process of decay and list components responsible for caries development, but if several areas of decay are evident at each 6-month recall, then change has not occurred. Individualize dietary advice based on the client's lifestyle rather than request a change in lifestyle to accommodate the recommendations.

The client's assessment and goals are the basis for any recommendations. The dental hygienist should attempt to dispel myths, redirect inaccurate habits, and provide new thoughts. Recommendations to Reduce the Amount of Carbohydrate in the Diet lists additional recommendations to reduce the amount of sugar in the diet.

Recommendations to Reduce the Amount of Carbohydrate in the Diet

Use Sugar Substitutes

◆ These products, however, are generally higher in cost and may not be feasible for low-income families.

◆ Sorbitol ingested in large amounts (30 g or more) can have laxative effects.

◆ One tablespoon of granulated sugar is equivalent to 1½ packets of Equal, ½ teaspoon Sweet 'N Low, or 1¼ packets of Sweet One.

Identify Added Sugar

◆ Read ingredient lists on food labels to identify sugar and other added sugars, such as fructose, honey, corn syrup, high-fructose corn syrup (HFCS), fruit juice, fruit juice concentrate, dextrose, maltose, and hydrogenated starch hydrolysates.

Identify High-Sugar Foods by Reading the Ingredient Label and Nutrition Panel

◆ Ingredients on a food label are listed in order of concentration. If a sugar is listed as one of the first three or four ingredients on a label, it is usually considered a high-sugar food.

◆ A food containing 5 gm or less per serving for sugars on the nutrition label is generally considered a low-sugar food.

◆ Compare some low-fat or nonfat foods that compensate for flavor by increasing sugar or sodium content (such as frozen dairy products).

Reduce Sugar Intake

◆ Purchase fresh fruits or canned and frozen fruits with "no sugar added" or packed "in its own juice."

FIGURE 16–5 **Food diary: the 24-hour recall.**

Food Diary			Day	
Time	Place	Food Eaten	Amount Eaten	How Prepared
Example: 6:00 a.m.	Kitchen	Orange juice Whole wheat bread Diet margarine Egg	1/2 C 2 slices 1 tsp 1	Unsweetened Toasted Tub Fried in oil

Instructions:
1. List EVERYTHING you eat or drink on 3 consecutive and typical days.
2. Use 2 weekdays and 1 weekend day.
3. Include extras such as chewing gum, sugar and cream in coffee, or mustard on a sandwich.

Carbohydrate Intake Analysis				
	Foods Eaten	When Eaten (During, End or Between Meals)	Total Number of Exposures	Total Minutes of Exposure
Sugar in Solution: soft drinks, fruit drinks, sweet sauces, sweetened liquid medicines, nondairy creamers, sugar or honey added to beverages, gelatins, ice cream, pudding, flavored yogurt.				
Retentive sweets: cake, cookies, dried fruits, canned fruit in syrup, jelly, jam, marshmallows, pies, pastries, cereal, muffins, crackers, honey on toast.				
Solid Sweets: candy of all kinds, cough drops, life savers, breath mints, antacid tablets.				
Prevailing form: _____				
Number of end and between meal snacks: _____				

FIGURE 16–6   **Carbohydrate intake analysis.**

◆ Prepare homemade foods rather than commercial products, gradually reducing the amount of sugar in recipes by half.

◆ Substitute spices such as cinnamon, allspice, nutmeg, and ginger to enhance the flavor of reduced-sugar foods.

◆ Slowly reduce the amount of sugar added to such foods as coffee or cereal.

CASE APPLICATION FOR THE DENTAL HYGIENIST

At his 6-month recall, John S. presented with six new areas of decay: three cervical areas and three interproximal areas of the anterior teeth. There is bleeding on probing, indicating a decline in his gingival condition. John admits his busy schedule prevents him from flossing his teeth. He has stopped smoking and replaced it with chewing gum and hard candy since his last appointment. When asked about work, John states that because of the added pressures of his job, he is taking antacids to settle his stomach.

Dietary Assessment

○ Food, nutrient, caloric intake
○ Frequency of eating between meals
○ Eating habits
○ Motivation level
○ Weight changes
○ Knowledge level

Dietary Dental Hygiene Diagnosis

Altered nutrition: frequent intake of chewing gum, hard candy, and antacids at various intervals throughout the day compounded by an increased plaque index are factors in determining the cause of decay.

Dietary Goals

The client will improve his overall nutrient intake and make substitutions or modify the caries-causing habits.

Nutritional Implementation

Intervention: Provide a food record (see Fig. 16–5) with an explanation for its use and instructions emphasizing the inclusion of everything put into his mouth.
Rationale: The food record will provide additional information about John's intake and will reveal habits that he may have neglected to mention, thinking they were not relevant to his dental needs.

Intervention: Review the food record with John to identify aspects that are healthy and those that need revision. Allow John to make the necessary changes.
Rationale: The probability of a client adhering to a recommended regimen is enhanced when the client is actively involved in the

decision-making process. The dental hygienist can suggest possible solutions and direct misguided changes. The client ultimately makes the required changes.

Intervention: Explain the decay process and factors involved, and that his decay is in areas that are usually unaffected.
Rationale: Understanding the total picture of his particular dental status can be motivating for John and may help him to make the changes required.

Intervention: Stress that not only the quantity of fermentable carbohydrates in his diet, but also the spacing and frequency of intake can lead to decay.
Rationale: Each time the client consumes a fermentable carbohydrate, even if it is a small mint, he is decreasing his plaque pH to an acid level for up to 40 minutes. By consuming mints six times throughout the day, the acid production occurs for up to 4 hours.

Intervention: Educate John about the cariogenic potential of antacids and discuss options to avoid or reduce use of antacids.
Rationale: Since one ingredient in antacids is generally a simple carbohydrate, it will have cariogenic potential. Antacids are high in sodium; they can interfere with the absorption of many nutrients. Consuming small, frequent meals, eating slowly, avoiding excessive amounts of caffeine products and alcohol, reducing or eliminating cigarette smoking, and reducing stress are some suggestions to decrease the use of antacids.

Intervention: Recommend fluoride treatments in the office and at home; sealants, if applicable; and optimum oral hygiene practices.
Rationale: Omitting the carbohydrate source is not the only factor involved in the decay process. In John's situation, protecting susceptible tooth surfaces and removing bacteria will also serve to eliminate caries potential.

Evaluation

The client returns for his 6-month recall caries free with a reduction in gingival bleeding. He is still not smoking and uses sugar-free chewing gum and mints on occasion. He has begun an exercise program, which is helping to relieve his stress and therefore has decreased his use of antacids.

Student Readiness

1. Explain the role of firm, fibrous foods in protecting the tooth against decay.
2. List several noncariogenic substitutions for high-sugar snacks.
3. What are the different roles that carbohydrates, protein, and fat play in the decay process?
4. Identify at least four nutritional foods that are contraindicated for the caries-active client.
5. Complete a 24-hour recall. Assess it for nutrient adequacy. Circle the fermentable carbohydrates in red. Determine the number of minutes of acid production. Based on this intake record, create a realistic and appropriate meal pattern. Discuss the rationale for the modifications and substitutions.

CASE STUDY

Carol is a 42-year-old married high school graduate with three teenage children. She is a homemaker and does all the cooking and grocery shopping. Each member of Carol's family continues to have new areas of decay at each recall. The dental hygienist decides to have Carol write down her food consumption from the previous day while waiting for her appointment. Her 24-hour recall revealed:

BREAKFAST: skips

AM SNACK: glazed doughnut, coffee with cream and sugar

LUNCH: grilled cheese sandwich, taco chips, gelatin salad with fruit and whipped cream, coffee with cream and sugar

PM SNACK: candy bar and two or three homemade cookies throughout the afternoon

DINNER: meat loaf, fried potatoes, buttered carrots, roll with margarine

EVENING SNACK: ice cream

1. What other information needs to be obtained before starting the counseling?
2. What dental information does Carol need to have?
3. What dietary recommendations should a dental hygienist suggest? What are some specific substitutions and modifications that can be made?
4. Approximately how many minutes of acid production occurred on the enamel surfaces this day?

CASE STUDY

As a new mother, Barbara wants to take all precautionary measures to prevent her daughter from having rampant dental decay like the neighborhood children. She breast-fed the infant until 9 months of age and refused to allow all sugar-containing foods, including ice cream. The daughter was frequently observed carrying a box of crackers around the house. By age 3, she has six caries.

1. When should dietary counseling have first been initiated for Barbara? Explain.
2. Describe the procedure a dental hygienist will take to counsel Barbara.
3. What suggestions would you recommend to Barbara?

References

American Dietetic Association. Position of the American Dietetic Association: Use of nutritive and nonnutritive sweeteners. *J Am Diet Assoc* 1993; 93(7):816–821.

Bibby BG. Local effects of nutrients, *In* Blix G (ed). *Nutrition and Caries Prevention.* Uppsala, Almquist and Wiksell, 1965, 30–52.

Darby ML, Walsh MM. *Dental Hygiene Theory and Practice.* Philadelphia: W.B. Saunders, 1994.

Gustaffson BE et al. The Vipeholm dental caries study. The effect of different levels of carbohydrate intake on caries activity in 436 individuals observed for 5 years. *Acta Odontol Scand* 1954; 11:232–364.

Kabara J. Dietary lipids as anticariogenic agents. *J Environ Pathol Toxicol Oncol,* 1986; 6(3-4): 87–113.

Lanke LS. Oral carbohydrate clearance. *In* Blix G (ed). *Nutrition and Caries Prevention.* Uppsala, Almquist and Wiksell, 1965, 53–59.

National Dairy Council. Diet and dental caries: An overview. *Dairy Council Dig* 1994; 65(1):1–6.

National Institute of Dental Research. Oral health of United States adults: The national survey of oral health in the United States employed adults and seniors: 1985–86. *In* NIH Publication No. 87-2868. Washington, D.C.: U.S. Government Printing Office, 1987.

National Institute of Dental Research. Oral health of United States children: The national survey of dental caries in United States school children: 1986-87. *In* NIH Publication No. 89-2247. Washington, D.C.: U.S. Government Printing Office, 1989.

Newbrun E. Preventing dental caries: Current and prospective. *J Am Dent Assoc* 1992; 123(5):68–73.

Nizel AE, Papas AS. *Nutrition in Clinical Dentistry.* 3rd ed. Philadelphia: W.B. Saunders, 1989.

Rugg-Gunn AJ. *Nutrition and Dental Health.* New York: Oxford University Press, 1993.

Stephan RM. Changes in hydrogen-ion concentration on tooth surfaces and in carious lesions. *J Am Dent Assoc* 1940; 27:718–723.

Chapter 17

Nutritional Aspects of Gingivitis and Periodontal Disease

LEARNING OBJECTIVES

The Student Will Be Able To:
- Identify the role nutrition plays in periodontal health and disease.
- List the effects of food consistency and composition in periodontal disease.
- Describe the etiologic factors associated with gingivitis and periodontitis.
- Identify the major structures of the periodontium.
- Discuss the components of nutritional counseling for the periodontal client.
- List major differences between full liquid, mechanical soft, bland, and regular diets.

GLOSSARY OF TERMS

Periodontium   the hard and soft tissues that surround and support the teeth: gingiva, alveolar mucosa, cementum, periodontal ligament, and alveolar bone

Supragingival   above the gingival margin

Subgingival   below the gingival margin

Interdental   between the proximal surfaces of adjacent teeth

Fibrosis   the formation of fibrous tissue of the gingiva and other mucous membranes due to chronic inflammation. The tissue may clinically appear to be healthy, concealing the disease.

Purulent   consisting of or containing pus; generally the result of inflammation

Dysphagia   difficulty in swallowing

Test Your NQ (True/False)

1. Supplementation beyond the recommended levels is not effective in controlling or preventing periodontal disease. T/F
2. Firm, fibrous foods physically remove plaque from the gingivae and tooth surface. T/F
3. A deficiency of vitamin C is the cause of gingivitis. T/F
4. A bland and soft diet is a commonly prescribed diet for an ANUG client. T/F
5. An appropriate instruction to a client following periodontal surgery is "Eat whatever foods you can manage." T/F

6. An insulin-dependent diabetic should be referred to a dietitian for nutrition counseling if the diet needs to be modified because of oral discomfort, such as with ANUG or following a periodontal procedure. T/F

7. Cream of chicken soup and ice cream are acceptable on a full liquid diet. T/F

8. A mechanical soft diet is similar to a regular diet except in consistency and texture. T/F

9. It is acceptable for a dental hygienist to recommend an instant breakfast drink or liquid supplement to a periodontal client who is temporarily following a full liquid diet. T/F

10. The dental hygienist should complete the nutrition assessment and provide nutritional counseling immediately following periodontal surgery. T/F

Periodontal disease is a chronic, inflammatory, and infectious disease (Color Plate 24). It can occur in adolescence through the adult years. In fact, periodontal disease is the leading reason for tooth loss over the age of 35.

The involvement of nutrition in periodontal disease is not as clear as it is for dental caries. The predisposing, etiologic, and contributing factors of periodontal disease are diverse; however, the primary initiating agent is bacterial plaque accumulation around teeth and gingivae. Therefore, nutrient deficiencies, excesses, or imbalances do not initiate periodontal disease nor does megadosages of supplements cure or prevent periodontal disease. Indirectly, nutrition may alter development, resistance, and/or repair of the **periodontium,** (Fig. 17–1), which ultimately affects the severity and extent of the disease. In addition, a client's health, medications, and food choices influence the properties of plaque and saliva. The buffering and antimicrobial effects of saliva make it a significant factor in periodontal disease. Therefore, a change in composition or amount of saliva can influence the growth of plaque (refer to discussion of xerostomia in chapter 18).

PHYSICAL EFFECTS OF FOOD ON PERIODONTAL HEALTH

Food Composition

All six classes of nutrients (carbohydrates, protein, fat, vitamins, minerals, and water) have a role in growth, maintenance, and repair in the body. There are at least 50 nutrients that are provided by food, most of which are required for a healthy periodontium. An imbalance of one or more nutrients can be a factor in the disruption of tissue integrity and immune response. Adequate amounts of each is therefore the dietary goal. For instance, normal growth and development of periodontal and oral mucosal tissues depends on sufficient intake of vitamin A (salivary glands, epithelial tissue), vitamin C (collagen, connective tissue), and vitamin B complex (epithelial, connective tissue). Calcification of the alveolus and cementum require amino acids, calcium, phosphorus, vitamin D, and magnesium. Maintenance of oral tissues, as well as the integrity of the host's immune and repair response, requires sufficient amounts of vitamins A, C, and D, protein, carbohydrates, calcium, iron, zinc, and folic acid. Higher calorie ranges are also indicated for increased metabolic needs. Refer to chapters 7 and 8 for more descriptive information on the effects of specific nutrients on the periodontium.

Supragingival plaque formation is influenced by frequent use of mono- and disaccharides in the diet. **Subgingival** plaque appears to be protected from the local effect of sugars.

Nutritional intervention needs to be a component of the treatment plan for periodontal disease

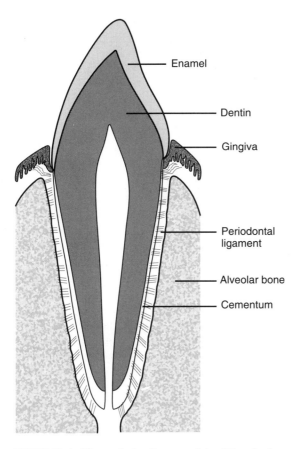

FIGURE 17–1 **The periodontium consists of the gingiva, alveolar bone, cementum, and periodontal ligament.**

since poor nutrition can affect the entire body and thus has an adverse effect on the periodontium. Such systemic factors alone will not cause periodontal problems. In combination with local irritating factors, such as plaque, systemic factors can increase the risk of periodontal disease of a host. A nutrition assessment by the dental hygienist can reveal nutritional deficiencies that should be restored for optimal healing. Referral to a dietitian may be indicated, particularly for medically compromised clients, such as those with diabetes.

Food Consistency

Another factor that affects periodontal health is the texture of food. Chewing firm, coarse, and fibrous foods, such as raw fruits and vegetables, will stimulate salivary flow. The increase in saliva will enhance oral clearance of food, thereby reducing food retention. By decreasing the amount of food debris remaining in the mouth, less debris will accumulate on the teeth. Plaque, however, is not physically removed by eating firm foods. Nizel and Papas (1989) reported that mastication of firm, fibrous foods can also "stimulate and strengthen the periodontal ligament and perhaps may also increase the density of alveolar bone adjacent to the roots." Soft, sticky foods, on the other hand, increase accumulation of food, which enhances bacterial growth.

NUTRITIONAL CONSIDERATIONS FOR PERIODONTAL CLIENTS

Increased nutrients and energy are required by periodontal clients experiencing stress, tissue catabolism, and/or infection. A thorough assessment of the periodontal client, as described in chapter 19, provides the valuable data needed to formulate a nutrition plan.

A medical and social history can indicate whether a client is at risk of nutrient deficiencies because of alcoholism, anorexia, or other health problems. These clients would possibly benefit from nutritional counseling to normalize nutrient levels prior to treatment. Dietary counseling of all periodontal clients will facilitate tissue repair and wound healing, improve resistance to infection, and reduce the number and severity of complications. Optimally, good nutritional status will result in a shorter recovery and a more rapid return to health (see Involvement of Nutrition in Periodontal Disease).

Involvement of Nutrition in Periodontal Disease

- ◆ Growth and development of the periodontium
- ◆ Amount and type of supragingival plaque
- ◆ Inflammation and immune response
- ◆ Integrity of the periodontium
- ◆ Amount and type of saliva
- ◆ Host resistance
- ◆ Repair and healing process

Acute Necrotizing Ulcerative Gingivitis

Acute necrotizing ulcerative gingivitis (ANUG) is generally an acute disease prevalent in young adults. ANUG is characterized by red and shiny marginal labial and lingual gingivae which bleed when probed, cratered interdental papillae, greyish sloughing of the marginal gingiva, foul breath, and metallic taste (Color Plate 23). A fever may also be present. The etiology of ANUG involves bacteria (e.g., *Borrelia vincentii*); systemic factors (e.g., increased susceptibility to infection, as in those with diabetes); local factors (e.g., smoking, poor oral hygiene); and psychological factors (e.g., stress, fatigue) that predispose a client to the disease. It is unknown which contributing factors are the primary causes and which are secondary causes of ANUG.

Nutrient deficiencies, such as protein or vitamin C and/or B complex deficiency, are contributing factors to ANUG because of lowered host resistance. This commonly occurs in a young adult who has poor eating habits, such as high fat and low nutrient intake, and who relies primarily on convenience or fast-food meals. Also, those with ANUG may lose the desire to eat because of pain or they may choose soft foods because they are easier to eat. Excessive alcohol intake and food impacted in the interproximal areas of open contacts are other possible factors related to the condition.

Tissue infection and destruction increase physiologic requirements for all nutrients. When fever is present, a 12% increase in total nutrient and energy intake is recommended for each 1° F above normal body temperature. Also, additional nutrients and energy are necessary for optimal repair and healing of tissue.

NUTRITION MANAGEMENT

Obtaining the client's health, dental, and social history is the first step in nutritional management, followed by an extra- and intraoral examination. Information gathered provides valuable clues as to causes of the disease that need to be altered or eliminated. A 24-hour food recall provides important insights into dietary practices and potential nutrient deficiencies. A 3- to 7-day food record provides a more accurate picture of food intake. This information allows the dental hygienist to make recommendations that are suited to the client's eating behaviors and take into consideration why the client selects certain foods (i.e., food preferences). Staying as close to the client's regular food intake as possible generally results in greater compliance.

The severity of ANUG will determine the initial dietary recommendations. The goal is to provide adequate nutrients, calories, and water. Based on the information obtained, a liquid supplement, such as Carnation Instant Breakfast, Ensure (Ross), or Boost (Mead Johnson), or a multivitamin may be suggested to ensure nutrient and caloric adequacy during acute periods of the disease. As soon as a nutritionally adequate diet is being consumed regularly, nutritional supplements can be eliminated.

Lip and tongue ulcers, extremely painful inflamed gingival tissue, and possibly initial removal of calculus may warrant a *full liquid diet* for 1 to 2 days (Table 17–1). A full-liquid diet consists of transparent and opaque fluids, as well as foods that liquefy at body temperature. Use of the full liquid diet is only temporary, as the nutrient and caloric value of such diets is usually inadequate. As tolerated, the client progresses to a *mechanical soft diet* (Table 17–2). A mechanical soft diet is a regular diet altered in consistency during periods when chewing is difficult. A client's tolerance to consistency will vary; therefore, the dental hygien-

TABLE 17–1 *Full Liquid Diet*

Purpose	The full liquid diet is designed to provide fluids and foods that are or become liquid at body temperature for clients who are unable to chew, swallow, or digest solid foods.
Use	The diet is most often used postoperatively by clients progressing from clear liquids to solid foods. The diet also may be used following oral surgery or plastic surgery of the face or neck area, in the presence of chewing or swallowing dysfunctions, for acutely ill patients, and for patients with esophageal or stomach disorders who cannot tolerate solid foods, owing to stricture or anatomic irregularity.
Modificiations	The full liquid diet consists of foods that are liquid or semiliquid at body temperature. Because milk-based foods constitute a large portion of this diet, clients with lactose intolerance need special consideration. Some clients demonstrate temporary lactose intolerance following surgeries involving the gastrointestinal tract. In these situations, lactose-hydrolyzed milk or lactose-free products may be used. This diet also may be modified for clients with hypercholesterolemia by substituting low-fat dairy products and monounsaturated and polyunsaturated fats for saturated fats. Because of its high concentration of simple carbohydrates, this diet may need to be adjusted for clients with diabetes mellitus and hypoglycemia. Further adjustments to the diet may be necessary (eg. sodium, caffeine) depending on the client.
Related Physiology	Traditionally, the full liquid diet has been used in the progression from clear liquids to solid foods. Whereas many clients do not need this transitional step, this diet may be helpful to those lacking the strength to chew and handle solid foods adequately, as it provides a more even texture and consistency.
Adequacy	The full liquid diet may be inadequate in all nutrients except for calcium, vitamin C, and protein, according to the 1989 Recommended Dietary Allowances. Its nutritional adequacy may be improved with the use of high-protein, high-calorie supplements. If the diet is used longer than 2 to 3 weeks, a liquid vitamin-mineral supplement is recommended. When the diet is used for longer periods and a pureed diet is not appropriate, pureed and thinned potatoes, rice, and pasta may be added to soups to improve the nutrient concentration and provide taste and texture variation.

The following are recommended foods for full liquid diets.

Food Groups	Recommended	May Cause Distress
Beverages	All milk and milk drinks (e.g., eggnogs made from commercial mix); all beverages, including high-protein, high-calorie oral supplements, coffee, tea, and carbonated beverages	None
Breads and cereals	Refined or strained cooked cereals	All others
Desserts	Custard; ice cream; pudding; sherbet; plain or flavored gelatin, fruit pie and frozen pops	All others and any made with coconut, nuts, seeds, or whole fruit
Fats	Butter or fortified margarine; cream, nondairy creamer	None
Fruits	All fruit juices (include one serving of vitamin C-rich juice daily)	All others
Meats and meat substitutes	Eggs in custard; plain or flavored yogurt	Yogurt with seeds or whole fruit pieces; all others
Soups	Broth, bouillon, strained soup	All others
Sweets	Sugar; honey; hard candy; sugar substitute; syrup	All others
Vegetables	All vegetable juices	All others
Miscellaneous	Iodized salt; all mild spices in moderation; flavorings and syrups	Extremes in seasoning, such as hot pepper sauce, chili powder, and highly seasoned meat sauces

Table continued on following page

TABLE 17–1   *Full Liquid Diet* (*Continued*)

The following is a sample menu for the full liquid diet.

▌ Breakfast	▌ Lunch	▌ Dinner
Orange juice (1 cup)	Strained cream of chicken soup (6 oz)	Strained cream of broccoli soup (6 oz)
Farina (1 cup)	Tomato juice (6 oz)	Apple juice (½ cup)
2% milk (1 cup)	Flavored gelatin (½ cup)	2% milk (1 cup)
Custard (½ cup)	Eggnog (1 cup)	Ice cream (½ cup)
Coffee/tea	Coffee/tea	Coffee/tea

▌ Midmorning snack	▌ Midafternoon snack	▌ Evening snack
Milkshake (1 cup)	Vanilla pudding (½ cup)	Milkshake (1 cup)
	Grape juice (½ cup)	

Approximate Nutrient Analysis

Energy (Cal)	2378.7	Sodium (mg)	2,932.1
Protein (g) (12.1% of Cal)	72.2	Zinc (mg)	10.3
Carbohydrate (g) (57.4% of Cal)	341.6	Vitamin A (µg RE)	1,278.8
Total fat (g) (32.3% of Cal)	85.5	Vitamin C (mg)	164.4
Saturated fatty acids (g)	48.4	Thiamin (mg)	1.3
Monounsaturated fatty acids (g)	26.0	Riboflavin (mg)	3.3
Polyunsaturated fatty acids (g)	5.2	Niacin (mg)	8.4
Cholesterol (mg)	577.9	Folate (µg)	277.0
Calcium (mg)	2131.5	Vitamin B_6 (mg)	1.3
Iron (mg)	17.8	Vitamin B_{12} (µg)	6.8
Magnesium (mg)	360.0	Dietary fiber (g)	7.4
Phosphorus (mg)	2,027.2	Water-insoluble fiber (g)	4.9
Potassium (mg)	4,336.8		

©1996, The American Dietetic Association. *Manual of Clinical Dietetics,* 5th ed, used by permission.

ist needs to tailor the dietary information to the client. For instance, a client with ulcerations may need to eliminate nuts and seeds because of the potential for them to get lodged in the ulcer and cause further discomfort. Encourage fluids with meals to make chewing foods easier.

Provide examples of acceptable bland and soothing foods (such as gelatin), while recommending avoidance of spicy and acidic foods (such as citrus fruits and tomatoes) which can irritate the oral mucosa (see Bland Diet). Frequent, small meals (e.g., six small meals one-half the size of a regular meal) are beneficial for a client who is having difficulty eating; intake of a variety of foods from each of the food groups is important. Additional protein intake (in the form of beans, low-fat cottage cheese, or skim milk) will be effective in meeting the increased needs due to fever and infection. Adequate fluid intake is essential.

TABLE 17–2 *Mechanical Soft Diet*

Purpose	The mechanical soft diet is designed to minimize the amount of chewing necessary to ingest food.
Use	The diet is used for clients who have limited chewing or swallowing ability but are able to tolerate a greater variety and texture of foods than the pureed diet offers. Clients who have undergone head and neck surgery, clients with dental problems, and clients with anatomic esophageal strictures are likely to benefit from the mechanical soft diet. The diet also aids clients after surgery of the head, neck, and mouth areas to make the transition to foods of normal consistency.
Modifications	This diet includes foods modified only in texture, such as chopped, ground, and pureed foods, to promote ease of mastication. The foods provided are generally moist and require minimal chewing before swallowing. Raw fruits and vegetables are excluded, as are any foods containing seeds, nuts, and dried fruits. The diet also can be modified to comply with therapeutic diet restrictions.
Related Physiology	The client's acceptance and tolerance of the diet dictate the extent of texture modification. If dysphagia is suspected, a swallowing evaluation should be performed and the diet individualized based on swallowing alterations.
Adequacy	Based on the individual food choice, the diet is adequate in all nutrients according to 1989 Recommended Dietary Allowances.

The following lists recommended foods for the mechanical soft diet.

Food Groups	Recommended	May Cause Distress
Beverages	Milk, malted milk, milkshakes; coffee, tea; carbonated beverages; hot cocoa	Any containing raw eggs
Breads	Soft breads, pancakes, muffins, soft waffles; breads and plain crackers softened in soup or beverage	Any with seeds, dried fruits, or nuts
Cereals	Cooked cereals without added fruit or nuts; plain dry cereals softened in milk	Any with seeds, dried fruits, or nuts
Desserts	Plain custards, puddings; sherbet; ice cream; fruit-flavored ices and frozen pops; fruit whips; fruit-flavored yogurt; flavored gelatin; cakes; soft cookies without fruit or nuts	Any with coconut, seeds, nuts, or whole or dried fruits
Fats	Butter or fortified margarine; cream and cream substitutes; cooking fats and oils; gravies; whipped toppings; salad dressing	All others
Fruits	Canned or cooked chopped fruits without seeds and skin; fruit juices	All others
Meats and meat substitutes	Ground meat and poultry (gravy or sauces may be added to moisten); soft, flaked fish without bones; casseroles made of ground meat, flaked fish, or cheese; cheese sauces; cottage cheese; soft scrambled eggs and egg substitutes	Raw eggs or eggs cooked less than 7 minutes; whole cuts of meat
Potato or substitute	Mashed or creamed potatoes; rice or noodles	All others
Soups	Broth, bouillon, consommé, blended strained soups	Any with pieces of meat or vegetables
Sweets	Clear jelly; honey; sugar; sugar substituttes; syrup	Any with coconut, nuts, or whole or dried fruits
Vegetables	Well cooked, soft vegetables without skin or seeds; vegetable juices	All others
Miscellaneous	Seasonings (e.g. salt and pepper); ground spices; smooth condiments	Nuts, coconuts, seeds, olives

Table continued on following page

TABLE 17–2   *Mechanical Soft Diet* (*Continued*)

The following is a sample menu for the mechanical soft diet.

▌Breakfast	▌Lunch	▌Dinner
Orange juice (½ cup)	Blended vegetable soup (1 cup)	Tomato juice (6 oz)
Cooked cereal (1 cup)	Saltine crackers, softened in soup (4)	Ground chicken (3 oz)
Banana, mashed (½ cup)	Sloppy joes with cooked ground beef (3 oz)	Enriched rice (½ cup)
Muffin, without nuts or fruit (1)	Hamburger bun (1)	Steamed green beans (½ cup)
Margarine (2 tsp)	Canned fruit cocktail (½ cup)	Soft dinner roll (1)
2% milk (1 cup)	Graham crackers (4)	Margarine (2 tsp)
Coffee/tea	2% milk (1 cup)	Low-fat frozen yogurt (½ cup)
	Coffee/tea	Applesauce (½ cup)
		Coffee/tea

Approximate Nutrient Analysis

Energy (Cal)	1,978.0	Phosphorus (mg)	1,341.1
Protein (g)	81.4	Potassium (mg)	3,593.0
(16.5% of Cal)		Sodium (mg)	3,191.1
Carbohydrate (g)	296.2	Zinc (mg)	11.6
(59.9% of Cal)		Vitamin A (µg RE)	800.9
Total fat (g)	55.1	Vitamin C (mg)	120.9
(25.1% of Cal)		Thiamin (mg)	1.7
Saturated fatty acids (g)	18.9	Riboflavin (mg)	2.0
Monounsaturated fatty acids (g)	20.5	Niacin (mg)	21.2
Polyunsaturated fatty acids (g)	11.0	Folate (µg)	231.8
Cholesterol (mg)	161.9	Vitamin B_6 (mg)	2.1
Calcium (mg)	1,027.4	Vitamin B_{12} (µg)	3.4
Iron (mg)	13.1	Dietary fiber (g)	20.3
Magnesium (mg)	352.8	Water-insoluble fiber (g)	12.8

©1996, The American Dietetic Association. *Manual of Clinical Dietetics,* 5th ed, used by permission.

Bland Diet

Purpose: To provide a temporary well-balanced diet for those dental clients with ulcerations.

Foods to Avoid

- Caffeine-containing beverages (coffee, tea, cola, cocoa)
- Alcohol
- Peppermint
- Chocolate
- Black and red pepper
- Chili pepper
- Chili powder
- Acidic foods
- Citrus fruits

Intolerance to these and other foods varies. Those which cause discomfort should be avoided.

Once a regular diet can be reinstated, concentrate efforts on continuing to follow the Dietary Guidelines for Americans and Food Guide Pyramid. Recurrence of ANUG is possible, and preventive guidelines should be encouraged.

Chronic Gingivitis

A progressive inflammatory process that begins in the interdental papillae and advances to the attached gingiva is called chronic gingivitis. The color of the gingiva varies from slight redness to a darker reddish-blue. The gingiva bleeds easily and is either soft and spongy or **fibrotic.** Gingivitis is associated with a large accumulation of plaque on the teeth which is exacerbated by frequent exposure to fermentable carbohydrates and retentive foods.

Gingival disease can be an indication of metabolic disease, such as diabetes mellitus. In combination with local factors, immunocompromise (i.e., AIDS), use of certain medications, hormonal changes (i.e., pregnancy, puberty), and a vitamin C deficiency can be elements in the development of gingivitis. Scurvy, a disease associated with vitamin C deficiency, is rarely seen in the United States because of the availability of fruits, vegetables, and foods fortified with vitamin C; however, alcoholism may result in scurvy. Rebound scurvy occurs as a result of discontinuing large doses of vitamin C. Hemorrhage, bluish-red gingiva, a widened periodontal ligament, and tooth mobility are characteristic oral symptoms of scurvy. Correcting the vitamin C deficiency through appropriate food choices or possible supplementation will improve gingival health.

As seen in ANUG, a lack of nutrients does not cause the gingival inflammation, but may be a predisposing factor in that it disrupts the process of tissue repair. Adequate nutrients can hasten the healing and repair process. Controlling or modifying the etiologic factors can reverse the clinical characteristics. Nutritional intervention for chronic gingivitis involves the same treatment as that for ANUG.

Dental Hygienist Considerations

ASSESSMENT
- *Physical:* inflamed, hemorrhagic, and red labial and lingual gingivae; cratered interdental papillae, greyish sloughing of the marginal gingiva, metallic taste, foul odor, pain, fever, malaise.
- *Dietary:* adequate nutrient, calorie, and fluid intake; alcohol consumption.

INTERVENTIONS
- Explain the extrinsic and intrinsic etiologic factors associated with the type of periodontal disease the client is experiencing.
- Teach appropriate oral hygiene procedures and recommend use of antimicrobial mouth rinses (such as chlorhexidine).
- Explain how fermentable carbohydrates enhance plaque formation by providing substances for bacterial growth; also, how soft and retentive foods cling to the tooth, allowing adherence of plaque.
- Recommendation of liquid supplements (e.g., Ensure [Ross], Boost [Mead Johnson], or Carnation Instant Breakfast) may be necessary. Most of these products contain cariogenic sweeteners; therefore, these should be followed up with appropriate oral hygiene care.
- The methyl red sugar test can be incorporated into nutritional counseling as a practical motivational and educational tool. Its purpose is to determine a low pH (acid environment) in the oral cavity. Plaque is removed from the oral cavity and placed on a porcelain tile. A few drops of methyl red indicator are added to cover the plaque, and sugar is sprinkled on top. A change of color from red to yellow within 10 to 30 minutes indicates a drop in the pH. The client should be taught not only about caries production, but also about sugars that increase bacterial growth and subsequent plaque formation.

EVALUATION
- The client improves the nutritional adequacy of the diet, limiting or avoiding smoking, alcohol, and other associated causes of the periodontal problem.
- Clinical signs and symptoms of the periodontal problems improve.
- Oral hygiene improves with each appointment.

Nutritional Directions

- Progression to a regular diet is dependent on the client's tolerance and comfort. Initially, a liquid diet may be needed; advancement to a soft diet is followed by a regular diet.

- When nutrient requirements are increased because of a periodontal condition, and therapeutic treatment is needed, a multivitamin may be recommended that provides three to five times the RDAs. This can be taken twice a day for the first week and reduced to once a day for the next 2 weeks. Emphasize that once a regular diet with variety is tolerated, the supplement should be discontinued (Nizel & Papas, 1989).

- A proper balance of calcium and phosphorus are associated with bone mineralization. A calcium-to-phosphorus ratio of 1:1 is recommended; however, higher amounts of phosphorus are common. One hypothesis suggests that the inadequate dietary intake of calcium combined with excessive amounts of phosphorus creates a nutritional secondary hyperparathyroidism (NSH). Calcium from bone stores (such as alveolar bone) may contribute calcium to maintain this ratio. Therefore, NSH may be associated with abnormal absorption of the alveolar bone.

- Cooler temperature foods are more soothing when ulcerations are present in the oral cavity.

- Antibiotics (i.e., tetracycline or penicillin) may be prescribed for oral infection to suppress oral microorganisms, such as plaque. Check with the client for possible allergies to the antibiotic prescribed.

Periodontitis

Inflammation affecting the gingivae and other components of the periodontium is referred to as periodontitis. The severity of the gingival inflammation, bone loss, tooth mobility, and periodontal pocket formation varies according to how long the disease has been present and the individual's resistance level. It can be localized or generalized in the mouth with the possibility of **purulent** exudate.

Initiation of periodontitis does not occur unless local irritants are present. As with gingivitis, certain types of food (i.e., soft, retentive, and/or a fermentable carbohydrate) can cause progression of the inflammatory disease by causing more food retention and accumulation of plaque. Systemically, nutritional status determines the immunocompetence of the periodontium. For example, a deficiency of calcium, phosphorus, and vitamin D can contribute to the severity of bone loss (although the deficiency is not the primary cause). Recovery from periodontitis is also enhanced by the positive effect of adequate nutrient reserves and intake on the immune system. Adequate vitamin C reserves, for example, can help ensure wound healing. With the assistance of the dental hygienist, the client can make the dietary adjustments necessary to meet the stresses and increased nutrient requirements of surgery and to ensure optimal wound healing.

NUTRITIONAL MANAGEMENT

The diet regimen recommended for a client with ANUG can be adapted to the needs of a client with periodontitis. Emphasis is placed on maintaining a nutritionally adequate diet; therefore, the Dietary Guidelines for Americans and Food Guide Pyramid are invaluable educational tools. Avoiding retentive foods and fermentable carbohydrates is another aspect on which the dental hygienist should focus. By working toward improving or eliminating the etiologic factors related to periodontitis, the healing process can minimize irreversible damage.

PERIODONTAL SURGERY PREOPERATIVE

PREPARATION   If periodontal surgery is indicated, the body's immunologic competency is important for optimal healing and to prevent or minimize infections. The dental hygienist can assess the client for adequate nutrient reserves prior to the dental procedure. If the recommendations of the Dietary Guidelines and Food Guide Pyramid are met, the client's dietary intake can be considered adequate. Generally, minor periodontal surgical procedures on a healthy client with an adequate intake do not require special dietary modification. On the other hand, surgery on a chronic alcoholic would most likely require preoperative replenishment of several nutrient deficiencies. If the surgery is elective, it may need to be postponed for 1 or 2 weeks to allow nutritional status to be improved. A medically compromised client, such as an alcoholic, might best be served by a dietitian who can appropriately assess and determine energy and other nutrient requirements. Recommendation of a liquid nutritional supplement or multivitamin may be warranted. If the dietitian is unfamiliar with the client's periodontal status, by working closely with the dental hygienist, continuity of care can be established. Further, the dental hygienist can provide the client with a clear understanding of the relationship of nutrition to periodontal status to enhance compliance.

Prior to surgery, the client should be given a diet prescription and a specific list of nutrient-dense foods and beverages to have available during the recovery period. The dental hygienist should consider the extent of the surgery, its potential discomfort, and the client's ability to eat, and instruct the client to make food choices that avoid trauma to the tissues. The client's food preferences and dislikes are other factors to be taken into consideration.

POSTOPERATIVE CARE   Because of blood loss, increased catabolism, tissue regeneration, and host defense activities following periodontal surgery, adequate nutrient intake is required by the client. The requirements for calories, protein, vitamins, minerals, and water may be double the RDA to speed recovery time (Nizel & Papas, 1989).

Dietary intake can be influenced by complications of anorexia, nausea, **dysphagia,** and oral discomfort. Consistency of the diet will depend on the extent of the surgery and symptoms of the client. A liquid diet may be required the first 1 to 2 days. Consideration of any special diet modifications (e.g., low sodium, no concentrated sweets, low fat) and client preferences need to be included. The liquid diet can progress to a mechanical soft diet after 1 or 2 days. A mechanical soft diet may be recommended until the client is able to eat regular foods. The need to follow a mechanical soft diet for 3 to 5 days is usual. A liquid supplement and/or a multivitamin may be recommended to ensure adequate nutrients and to shorten duration of recovery.

CASE APPLICATION FOR THE DENTAL HYGIENIST: THE DENTAL HYGIENE PROCESS IN ACTION

Jenny is a 20-year-old college student. It has been 9 months since her last recall because of her busy school and work schedule. She continues to smoke despite the dental hygienist's encouragement to quit. An oral examination exhibits inflamed gingivae that bleed upon touch and a greyish pseudomembrane covering the marginal gingiva. Jenny complains of severe pain as the dental hygienist probes for pocket depth. The dental hygienist also notices an unusual odor from the client's mouth. A 24-hour recall reveals:

7:30 a.m.   Large coffee with cream and sugar
Pastry

10:00 a.m.   12 oz cola
Potato chips

2:30 p.m.   3 slices pizza
12 oz cola

7:30 p.m.   12-oz can of ravioli
8 oz milk

11:30 p.m.   Hot chocolate
8 sandwich cookies

Dietary Assessment

○ Food, nutrient, caloric intake
○ Eating habits
○ Social history
○ Motivation level
○ Knowledge level

Dietary Dental Hygiene Diagnosis

The client's irregular eating patterns; choices of high-calorie, low-nutrient foods in combination with stress from school and work; and smoking provide several secondary factors to explain the presence of the clinical symptoms of ANUG.

Dietary Goals

Jenny will attempt to discontinue smoking or avoid smoking during periods of acute inflammation. With the help of the dental hygienist, she will review her busy schedule and prioritize events to incorporate a variety of foods, including some choices that are quick to prepare, or more nutritious selections from vending machines.

Nutritional Implementation

Intervention: Question Jenny further on the level of oral discomfort she is experiencing. Determine if a relationship exists between oral health and food choices. Depending on her response, a full liquid diet may initially be suggested, followed by a mechanical soft diet within 1 to 5 days.
Rationale: Oral conditions can interfere with chewing or swallowing. Jenny might be eating too little or omitting foods that are too painful to eat. Consequently, she may be experiencing an eroding nutritional status, which is negatively affecting her oral status. Altering the consistency of her diet can increase the nutrient value since it will facilitate the task of chewing and swallowing. Every client's oral situation is

unique and tolerance levels will vary greatly. The dental hygienist should listen closely to Jenny's response to individualize recommendations to meet her needs.

Intervention: Encourage the client to eat a variety of foods, making choices as similar to her normal eating behaviors as possible.
Rationale: Systemic factors, such as nutrient deficiencies, play a role with influencing the inflammatory response of the gingivae. Explain the role of nutrients in maintaining a healthy periodontium, suggesting food choices that vary slightly from Jenny's regular food intake to enhance compliance. Essential education tools include the use of the Food Guide Pyramid and Dietary Guidelines for Americans. Temporary use of multivitamins may be recommended.

Intervention: Identify the frequency and form of fermentable carbohydrates in her diet, along with the foods that are soft and sticky.
Rationale: Foods and drinks, such as sugar in coffee, pastry, potato chips, and cookies, will influence the formation of plaque. With Jenny's assistance, practical and realistic modifications can be established in her diet that fit in with the demands of her busy lifestyle. The dental hygienist should recognize and expand on the use of milk and milk products (e.g., cheese on pizza and hot chocolate) in her diet.

Intervention: Continue efforts to eliminate smoking. Question Jenny on her decision to smoke. Once an understanding has been reached, a strategy may be developed.
Rationale: Smoking may be a factor in plaque accumulation, as well as inhibit the healing process. The heat, staining, and smoke from cigarettes can lead to unfavorable gingival changes (Hoag & Pawlak, 1990). A local smoking cessation program can be recommended.

Intervention: During an oral examination, note any areas of ulceration.
Rationale: Depending on the client's tolerance, a bland diet may need to be utilized

because of discomfort experienced from highly seasoned or acidic foods. Nuts and seeds should be avoided since they can become lodged in an ulcerated area and lead to pain. Finally, cooler-temperature foods are more soothing.

Evaluation

The client comes to each of her scheduled appointments, with improvement in oral health noted each time. At a 1-month reevaluation appointment, Jenny is (1) consuming a regular diet with variety, (2) eating fermentable carbohydrates only with meals, (3) choosing firm, fibrous foods more frequently, and (4) attending a smoking cessation program. She is also able to verbalize reasons for these lifestyle changes.

Student Readiness

1. List at least four factors that can cause poor nutritional status in a periodontally involved client. Why is it important for this client to concentrate on nutrient intake?

2. Discuss the difference between a clear liquid diet and a full liquid diet. What dental situations benefit from use of each of these diets?

3. Describe a periodontal situation in which small, frequent meals should be recommended. Explain the rationale to a client.

4. What dietary strategies can be offered to the client experiencing oral discomfort?

CASE STUDY

A 43-year-old male comes to his recall appointment with complaints of "sore and bleeding gums, especially after brushing." He is a busy executive and entertains his clients frequently. Consequently, he dines out often and averages two to three alcoholic beverages each day. His medical history is uneventful—no medications or health alerts. An oral examination reveals bleeding on probing with pocket depths generalized at 4 to 6 mm with moderate gingival inflammation.

The dental hygienist asks him to recall everything he has eaten on the previous day. His food consumption is high in fat, calories, and sodium because of heavy reliance on dining out regularly. His diet also lacks variety and is low in nutrient value.

1. List several secondary factors that can be precipitating the periodontal problem. What changes in his lifestyle could be suggested?

2. From the limited information presented, what additional data can the dental hygienist gather in order to help him modify his diet?

3. What vitamins and minerals might be deficient in this client's diet and could cause the progression of his periodontal situation?

4. What diet should be suggested? What is the rationale? Provide a realistic menu for one day on the recommended diet.

References

Hoag PM, Pawlak EA. *Essentials of Periodontics.* 4th ed. Philadelphia: C.V. Mosby, 1990.

Mills JA. Nutrition and periodontics. *Dentistry* 1989; 18–20.

Nizel AE, Papas AA. *Nutrition in Clinical Dentistry.* Philadelphia: W.B. Saunders, 1989.

Schwartz M, Lamster I, Fine J. *Clinical Guide to Periodontics.* Philadelphia: W. B. Saunders, 1995.

Williams RC. Periodontal Disease. *N Engl J Med* 1990; 322(6):373–382.

Chapter 18

Nutritional Aspects of Alterations in the Oral Cavity

LEARNING OBJECTIVES

The Student Will Be Able To:

- Describe the common signs and symptoms of xerostomia and glossitis.
- Determine appropriate dietary recommendations for a client with xerostomia, root caries, and removable appliances.
- Identify dietary guidelines given to new denture patients pre- and postinsertion.
- Explain the process of alveolar osteoporosis.

GLOSSARY OF TERMS

Candidiasis   multiple white patches or a thick white coating on the tongue or mucosa, caused by infection with the fungal organism *Candida albicans*

Edentulous   without teeth or lacking some or all teeth

Trabecular bone   the spongy internal bone

Cortical bone   the compact external part of the skeleton

Test Your NQ (True/False)

1. While charting for caries, the dental hygienist notes several root surface caries and documents xerostomia as the cause. The dental hygienist made the correct assumption. T/F
2. Xerostomia is a consequence of the aging process. T/F
3. Xerostomia can be a contributing factor of malnutrition in an elderly client. T/F
4. Root caries are frequently seen in adolescence. T/F
5. A relationship exists between nutritional status of a client and tooth mobility, missing teeth, and denture performance. T/F
6. Hard, fibrous, nutrient-dense foods are recommended for the first few days after insertion of new dentures to promote healing. T/F
7. Masticatory efficiency, or chewing, is a factor in providing a well-structured, nonatrophic alveolar process. T/F

8. The primary component of alveolar bone is compact cortical bone. T/F
9. Glossitis can be a symptom of a nutrient deficiency. T/F
10. In order to maintain a normal serum calcium level, the body will obtain calcium from the alveolar process when in negative calcium balance. T/F

Following the Dietary Guidelines for Americans and Food Guide Pyramid is practical nutritional advice for optimum general and oral health. A variety of oral conditions can interfere with food intake and therefore influence one's nutritional status. These situations require modifications of eating patterns based on individual needs. The oral health team is in an ideal position to provide dietary advice to the client or to be a valuable member of a multi-disciplinary approach to complicated cases, such as a client with renal disease.

XEROSTOMIA

Good oral health is dependent on adequate salivary flow (see the Functions of Saliva). Xerostomia (salivary gland dysfunction) is characterized by diminished or absent salivary flow or a change in the viscosity of saliva. Consequently, xerostomia has a negative impact on oral tissues and dietary intake.

mon reasons for xerostomia that the dental hygienist should look for in the medical history in order to determine whether the client is at risk. Note that increasing age is not a factor. Salivary flow does not significantly decrease with age in the healthy adult.

Functions of Saliva

◆ Lubricates oral tissues
◆ Assists in chewing, swallowing, and digestion
◆ Removes debris from teeth
◆ Components of saliva have an antibacterial action
◆ Neutralizes, dilutes, and buffers bacterial acids
◆ Aids in remineralization
◆ Affects the rate of plaque accumulation
◆ Influences taste
◆ Allows for ease in talking

Factors Contributing to Xerostomia

◆ Medications
◆ Antineoplastic therapy (chemotherapy and radiation)
◆ Systemic diseases (diabetes, Sjögren syndrome)
◆ Stress and depression
◆ Significant vitamin deficiency (e.g., vitamin A, vitamin C, protein)
◆ Liquid diets, due to lack of mastication
◆ Dehydration

Common complaints of clients experiencing xerostomia include a dry mouth, altered taste (dysgeusia), a burning sensation of the tongue, and difficulty in swallowing and speaking. Discomfort with a removable appliance may be due to the tongue sticking to the prosthesis, an inability to properly retain the appliance, and gingival sores created by an improperly fitting denture. The Factors Contributing to Xerostomia lists com-

Adults most frequently experience xerostomia in relation to taking multiple medications (see the Common Classes of Medications Associated with Xerostomia). Xerostomia can also be a result of one or more chronic diseases. During an oral exam, a dental hygienist should focus on appearance and texture changes of mucosal tissues, for they commonly appear dry, smooth, and shiny. The dental hygienist may also find angular cheilitis, absence of salivary pool, destruction of oral soft and hard tissues if poor oral hygiene exists, and/or oral infections, such as oral **candidiasis.** Atrophy of the papillae and taste buds, present in xerostomia, is a cause of taste alterations. Xerostomia, consequently, results in a variety of oral complications that may compromise a client's nutrient intake (see Consequences of Xerostomia That Influence Nutrient Intake).

Common Classes of Medications Associated with Xerostomia

- Analgesics
- Anticholinergics
- Antidepressants
- Antihistamines
- Antihypertensives
- Anti-inflammatory agents
- Anti-parkinson
- Anti-psychotics
- Bronchodilators
- Decongestants
- Diuretics
- Gastrointestinal agents

Data from Swapp KM. Drugs of the geriatric patient: A dental hygiene perspective. *J Dental Hygiene* 64(7):327, 1990; Soon JA. Effects of drug therapy on oral health of older adults. *J Can Dent Hyg Assoc* 1992; 26(3):118–120; Rhodus NL, Brown J. The association of xerostoma and inadequate intake of older adults. *J. Am Diet Assoc* 1990; 90(12):1688–1692.

Consequences of Xerostomia That Influence Nutrient Intake

- Increased rate of root caries
- Inability to keep mouth moist
- Increased fluid intake
- Sticky or tacky saliva
- Absence of salivary pooling
- Difficulty in chewing and swallowing
- Burning or sensitive oral mucosa
- Dry, crusty, smooth, and/or shiny mucosa
- Low tolerance to spicy and acidic foods
- Ulcerations
- Sore tongue—may be atrophied, fissured, inflamed, edematous

- Angular cheilosis—cracking or burning at the corners of the mouth
- Altered or lack of taste—lack of interest in eating, possible unintentional weight loss
- Difficulty with the use of dentures
- Dental hypersensitivity—hot, cold, sweet
- Dry nose—impairs sense of smell
- Dry throat—difficulty with swallowing
- Food sticking to the hard palate or tongue

An analysis of the diet history of the older adult with xerostomia can reveal deficiencies in fiber, potassium, vitamin B_6, iron, calcium, and zinc (Rhodus & Brown, 1990). A zinc deficiency can be the cause of taste changes and consequent lack of interest in eating. With this information, the dental hygienist can be alert to reduction in appetite, overall dietary adequacy, and weight changes.

Management of Xerostomia

A complete assessment, as described in chapter 19, will allow the dental hygienist to formulate possible and appropriate intervention strategies for xerostomia. Each client's circumstance is unique and therapy must be individualized. Counseling to relieve symptoms of xerostomia can be helpful and effective in minimizing oral discomfort and related conditions. Helpful advice is listed in the Recommendations for Clients with Xerostomia box. Overall, the goals are to protect the oral cavity from the destructive effects of xerostomia and to improve the quality of the diet.

Recommendations for Clients with Xerostomia

- Artificial salivas
- Lip balm to keep lips moist
- Pleasant presentation of food to enhance interest
- Frequent sips of fluids
- Fluids with meals
- Use of a humidifier
- Nutrient-dense, soft, moist foods (e.g., macaroni and cheese, cottage cheese, applesauce)

- Sugar-free items (e.g., gum, hard candy, popsicles)
- Suck on ice chips

- Tart foods to stiulate flow of saliva (e.g., sugar-free lemonade and sour candy, dill pickles)
- Avoid dry spicy and acidic food, commercial mouth washes, alcohol, tobacco, and caffeine

ROOT CARIES

New carious lesions in adults are typically located on the root, below the cemento-enamel junction, in areas of gingival recession. The recession is generally the outcome of periodontal disease or toothbrush abrasion. The cementum is also more susceptible to caries because it is more soluble than enamel and consequently the carious lesion progresses at a faster rate. In combination with poor oral hygiene, xerostomia and ingestion of fermentable carbohydrates create a perfect environment for root caries. Because the population of older adults who have retained their teeth is increasing, root caries are more commonplace.

The microorganism thought to be responsible for the formation of root caries is *Actinomyces* (Rugg-Gunn, 1993). Like streptococci, *Actinomyces* me-

tabolizes carbohydrates to produce an acid; additionally, it promotes formation of plaque. Exposed root surfaces, compounded by limited buffering, diluting, and oral clearance created by xerostomia, allow the bacteria and cariogenic material to accumulate, increasing caries risk. Also implicated in the increased prevalence of root caries are intake of carbohydrates and its frequency. A food record or 24-hour recall from the client may reveal destructive patterns or behaviors that can be modified. For example, it may be discovered that the client snacks continuously throughout the day as opposed to eating three meals, uses sugar-sweetened medications (such as cough syrup), or has a high intake of hard candy to relieve xerostomia. Further recommendations for caries prevention are covered in chapter 16.

DENTITION STATUS

Although a complete dentition is not required for adequate nutrient intake, loss of teeth or the supporting periodontium and improperly fitting dentures are frequently associated with poor food selection and limited chewing ability. Compromised nutritional intake may be an effect of tooth loss, tooth mobility, edentulous status, and discomfort from removable appliances.

It has been estimated that a client with dentures has 20% of the chewing ability of a client with adequate dentition. The client's masticatory efficiency and biting force becomes increasingly difficult with each tooth lost. The number of teeth and to what degree mobility is present will also determine food choices. Soft foods with minimal nutrients are frequent food preferences. Consumption of hard, fibrous foods is avoided because of low masticatory performance, which could also be associated with constipation and other gastrointestinal problems in some elderly persons. Nutrient

intake especially of magnesium, folic acid, and zinc, is found to be significantly below the RDAs. These deficiencies can interfere with maintenance and repair of oral tissues and bone.

During the appointment prior to the placement of a new denture, the client should be given nutritional counseling about the initial days of adaption so that appropriate foods can be available for the adjustment period. Days 1 and 2 of placement may necessitate a liquid diet (see Table 17–1), which does not require chewing or biting. A liquid diet allows the client to master swallowing with the new prostheses (Nizel & Papas, 1989). As tolerated, during the next 2 to 3 days, the client should advance to a soft diet (see Table 17–2), which slowly introduces foods that require limited biting and chewing. As the sore spots heal, the client should add firmer-textured foods, incorporating suggestions provided in the Dietary Suggestions for New Denture Clients. This process is essential for masticatory efficiency and stability of the denture, thus enhancing the client's nutritional status.

Dietary Suggestions for New Denture Clients

- ◆ Cut food into small pieces
- ◆ Lengthen chewing time
- ◆ Evenly distribute food to both sides of mouth
- ◆ Chew in straight up and down motion
- ◆ Adequate nutrient intake
- ◆ Cooked fruits and vegetables
- ◆ Avoid
  Chewing gum
  Sticky foods (e.g., caramels)
  Berries with seeds
  Nuts
  Biting with anterior teeth
  Fermentable carbohydrates

Dental Hygienist Considerations

ASSESSMENT

- ● *Physical:* absence of salivary pool, dryness of soft tissues, mucosal changes, candidiasis, root surface caries, difficulty with speaking and swallowing, ill-fitting denture(s).
- ● *Dietary:* altered taste, difficulty with chewing, lack of interest in eating.

INTERVENTIONS

- ● Recommend a 3-month recall, meticulous oral hygiene, and topical fluoride treatments at home. Self-applied fluoride gels reduce enamel solubility and oral bacteria; indications include root caries and xerostomia.
- ● If the client complains of oral dryness, the dental hygienist can place a mouth mirror or tongue blade on the oral mucosa and watch for stickiness upon removal. Milking the major salivary glands (submandibular, sublingual, and parotid) to observe the amount of saliva produced is another assessment option.
- ● Provide written instructions to reinforce counseling.
- ● Examine the denture for fit. An appointment

to reline or make new dentures may be needed. Explain the significance of a properly fitting denture to the client, including its relationship to a poor-quality diet.

EVALUATION

- ● The client's food record reveals intake of adequate calories that are nutrient dense and contains a variety of foods and textures. The client can also eat comfortably.
- ● The soft and hard tissues of the oral cavity appear healthy. There is improved oral hygiene care.
- ● The client is able to verbalize the problem and discuss ways to continue maintaining the oral cavity.

Nutritional Directions

- ◆ There are more than 400 over-the-counter and prescription medications that indicate xerostomia as one of its side effects. Since drugs are a common cause, review the client's medications to identify drug(s) associated with xerostomia (refer to the Common Classes of Medications Associated with Xerostomia box). It could be suggested that the client contact the physician to request an alternative medication or a reduction in dosage. If the client is unable to reduce the dosage, alternative measures need to be considered.
- ◆ Individualize the counseling according to the client's nutritional needs. Information should be based on the Food Guide Pyramid and Dietary Guidelines for Americans.
- ◆ Changes in taste generally lead to lack of interest in food. Suggestions to improve the appearance and appeal of food can involve colorful combinations of foods. Imagine the lack of appeal of a plate with cauliflower, mashed potatoes, and baked white fish compared to the colorful plate of baked salmon, steamed broccoli, and a baked yam.
- ◆ Since dairy products, especially cheese, are cariostatic, their consumption with or without cariogenic foods can decrease the number of root caries. A lower-fat cheese (5 gm of

fat per ounce or less) and/or smaller portion size is a consideration for many clients.

♦ For successful nutritional intervention, it is important to obtain necessary information prior to the dietary counseling. This should include food preferences, eating patterns, living conditions, economic status, lifestyle, and physical capabilities.

ALVEOLAR OSTEOPOROSIS

Several factors, including a poor calcium intake over a lifetime, create a physiologic negative calcium balance. In order to maintain a normal serum calcium level, the body obtains calcium from other internal sources. It is easily absorbed from **trabecular bone,** the primary component of the alveolar process. It follows that the alveolus may undergo resorption prior to other bones and may be an early indicator of osteoporosis. When osteoporotic change in the alveolus is detected, the dental professional should refer the client to a physician for further evaluation. Pro-

gressive loss of the alveolar ridge can lead to tooth loss.

Chewing is beneficial to the alveolar process by providing sound, well-composed, nonatrophic bone (Rugg-Gunn, 1993). A reduction in masticatory efficiency, as occurs in persons with dentures, increases resorption, resulting in a loss of bone mass or alveolar osteoporosis. As the alveolar ridge reduces in size, it becomes increasingly difficult to provide properly fitting dentures and relined or new dentures are necessary. Management of osteoporosis is described in chapter 8.

GLOSSITIS

Inflammation of the tongue, or glossitis, can prevent nutritional requirements from being met. The tongue is affected by several systemic disorders. Infectious glossitis is caused by a bacterial, fungal, and viral infection or disease. Toxic glossitis is caused by a drug. Psychogenic glossitis is related to psychological stress. Finally, glossitis can be caused by deficiency of many nutrients (such as B vitamins) or an allergic reaction.

Common complaints include a burning sensation, pain and/or tenderness of the tongue. Diminished or lost taste sensation may result from atrophy of the papillae on the dorsum of the tongue. During an oral exam, the dental hygienist may note slight to total atrophy of the filiform and fungiform

papillae. Depending on the degree of atrophy, the tongue will inevitably appear shiny, smooth, and red. The atrophy can be localized or generalized. The tongue size can shrink because of dehydration or be enlarged (macroglossia) as a result of edema. Macroglossia is commonly observed in edentulous mouths.

A thorough assessment of the client will determine the extent and cause of the glossitis. The dental hygienist can individualize dietary instructions with the goal of improving the nutritional quality of the diet. Recommendations would include suggestions to enhance food's taste and appearance, and ideas for soft, nutrient-dense foods (such as tuna salad, cream soups, cottage cheese).

CASE APPLICATION FOR THE DENTAL HYGIENIST: THE DENTAL HYGIENE PROCESS IN ACTION

Mrs. Owen is a 73-year-old client with complete dentition in the maxillary arch and a removable mandibular partial. Canine to canine (teeth 22 to 27) are present, all of which have periodontal involvement, exposing the root surface. Root caries are present on teeth 22 and 26. Examination reveals dry and cracked lips, a lack of a salivary pool, and an ill-fitting prosthesis. The medical history reveals high blood pressure and a 10-year history of antihypertensive drug use. Mrs. Owen complained of difficulty in swallowing dry food, oral dryness, and taste alterations.

While obtaining a 24-hour food recall, the dental hygienist realizes that Mrs. Owen has lost interest in food. She states: "I just don't feel like eating. Food doesn't taste good and I don't feel like cooking for myself." If she eats breakfast, she typically has orange juice and a doughnut, for lunch, she has canned soup, and before bedtime, part of a frozen dinner. A jar of hard candy sits in her living room from which she periodically takes a piece throughout the day, and she is constantly drinking soda for relief of the dryness.

Dietary Assessment

○ Nutrient deficiencies
○ Oral factors affecting nutrient intake
○ Social factors affecting nutrient intake
○ Knowledge level

Dietary Dental Hygiene Diagnosis

Several factors are involved with this client's poor nutrient intake: xerostomia, root caries, an ill-fitting prosthesis, frequent intake of hard candy, lack of variety in food, choice of soft, low-nutrient foods, and social isolation.

Dietary Goals

Mrs. Owen has agreed to gradually improve her overall nutritional status by replacing soft, low-nutrient foods with high-fiber foods and utilizing sugar-free substitutions to prevent root caries.

Nutritional Implementation

Intervention: Enhance intake of calcium-rich foods, such as low-fat milk, yogurt, and cheese.
Rationale: Adequate calcium intake will help to protect the alveolar bone from resorption.

Intervention: Provide education on xerostomia and the effects on the oral cavity and dietary process.
Rationale: An understanding of the cause and effect of xerostomia can help Mrs. Owen to make the necessary changes.

Intervention: Limit the intake of commercial frozen prepared meals and other processed foods high in sodium. Suggest that when the client feels like cooking, she could prepare several meals and freeze them in individual portion sizes.
Rationale: An occasional frozen meal is quick and effortless and a better choice than not eating. However, they are expensive and generally need to be supplemented with other foods for adequate nutrients. Since many are high in sodium, an important factor for Mrs. Owen because of her hypertension, remind her to read labels and to purchase ones that contain less than 500 mg of sodium per serving.

Intervention: Suggest frequent sips of a nutritious beverage (such as milk or juices) or a noncariogenic fluid (such as water or diet soda) throughout the day; saliva substitute; sugar-free choices (such as chewing gum); and tart or sour foods (such as sugar-free lemon drops).
Rationale: High-nutrient or noncariogenic fluids keep the mouth moist to relieve the xerostomia. Tart or sour foods and chewing gum stimulate the flow of saliva.

Intervention: Emphasize the importance of practicing proper oral hygiene techniques and explain the caries and periodontal disease process.
Rationale: Since it has been shown that dentition status is related to nutritional status, it would be to Mrs. Owen's benefit to retain each natural tooth as long as possible. The xerostomia is also a contributing factor to root caries; however, plaque must be present for xerostomia to play a role in their development. Proper daily oral hygiene care will improve her oral status and prevent further complications.

Intervention: Instruct the client on self-applied home fluoride treatments.

Rationale: Topical fluoride application reduce caries risk. The saliva reduction allows the fluoride to have greater clinical benefit for longer periods since there is limited clearance of fluoride (Epstein & Scully, 1992).

Intervention: Dry food, spicy or acidic foods, alcohol, caffeine, and tobacco should be avoided.

Rationale: These choices can worsen the xerostomia or irritate the mucosa.

Intervention: Encourage involvement with a local senior group and/or provide information for food assistance programs for older adults, such as Meals on Wheels.

Rationale: The older adult who lives alone may experience a decreased appetite and lack motivation to prepare appropriate meals. Socializing with others during meals enhances the enjoyment of eating.

Evaluation

Mrs. Owen's mandibular partial has been adjusted. The nutrition goals established with the dental hygienist are gradually being met. She has substituted sugar-free candy for the hard candy, prepares more meals, and has joined the community senior citizen center. She recently began using home fluoride treatments and remains caries free. She appears to be a much happier individual.

Student Readiness

1. To understand what a client with xerostomia experiences, eat several saltine crackers with no fluid and note the dryness of the oral cavity. Imagine this situation indefinitely and its impact on a client's diet. At this point, try an artificial saliva to understand its effect prior to recommending it to a client.

2. Discuss at least two changes that occur in the oral cavity that can change a client's taste sensation. What recommendations can a dental hygienist provide?

3. Prepare an educational program for interdisciplinary health care professionals on recognizing changes in the oral cavity that affect nutrient intake and, ultimately, general health. List at least three health care professionals who would benefit from this knowledge.

References

American Dietetic Association. Position of the American Dietetic Association: Oral health and nutrition. *J Am Diet Assoc* 1996; 96(2):184–189.

Darby ML, Walsh MM. *Dental Hygiene Theory and Practice.* Philadelphia: W.B. Saunders, 1994.

Epstein JB, Scully C. The role of saliva in oral health and the causes and effects of xerostomia. *J Can Dent Assoc* 1992; 58(3):217–221.

Faine MP et al. Dietary and salivary factors associated with root caries. *Special Care Dentistry* 1992; 12(4): 177–182.

Nizel AE, Papas AS. *Nutrition in Clinical Dentistry.* 3rd ed. Philadelphia: W.B. Saunders, 1989.

Papas AS et al. Relationship of diet to root caries. *Am J Clin Nutr* 1995; 61(suppl):423S–429S.

Rhodus NL, Brown J. The association of xerostomia and inadequate intake in older adults. *J Am Diet Assoc* 1990; 90(12):1688–1692.

Rugg-Gunn AJ. *Nutrition and Dental Health.* New York: Oxford Medical Publishing, 1993.

Soon JA. Effects of drug therapy on oral health of older adults. *J Can Dent Hyg Assoc* 1992; 26(3):118–120.

Swapp KM. Drugs of the geriatric patient: A dental hygiene perspective. *J Dental Hygiene* 64(7):326, 1990.

Chapter 19

Nutritional Assessment and Counseling for the Dental Hygiene Client

GLOSSARY OF TERMS

Diet history   a record of a client's dietary intake

Goal   a statement to describe a desired behavior change

Nonjudgmental   remaining neutral in comment and body language and not evaluating a situation in a biased manner

Test Your NQ (True/False)

1. Once the health and dental histories have been reviewed, the dental hygienist has adequate information to begin the dietary counseling with the client. T/F
2. A clinical oral exam is a very sensitive tool for identifying nutritional deficiencies. T/F
3. Using food models when counseling helps the client to learn how to determine portion sizes quickly and accurately. T/F
4. When providing nutritional counseling for a client, the dental hygienist should change the usual intake as little as possible and reinforce positive practices. T/F

5. Results of dietary counseling do not need to be documented or communicated with other dental staff members. T/F

6. Providing a standardized low-carbohydrate menu is sufficient for most clients with a high caries rate. T/F

7. The dental hygienist should circle in red all foods on the food diary that are responsible for causing decay. T/F

8. Once the nutritional counseling session has ended, the client should have enough information and motivation to make the necessary changes. T/F

9. "What type of snacks do you eat?" is an example of an open-ended question. T/F

10. Listening involves interpreting what is said, how it is said, and nonverbal actions seen. T/F

Health is a multidimensional concept, encompassing the interaction of many elements. Dissemination of information does not guarantee that a client will respond by establishing healthier patterns—millions of people start or continue smoking despite countless documentations of health risks. To facilitate positive changes toward a desired health behavior, the health care educator's message must be tailored to meet the client's needs, attitudes, beliefs, and values.

The relationship between nutrition and the oral cavity has already been established in this book, and we know that signs of a nutrient deficiency, excess, or imbalance are detectable in the mouth. Along with radiographs, application of sealants, and fluoride treatments, early diagnosis, treatment, and/or appropriate referrals are components of comprehensive dental hygiene care. However, pre-vention, as opposed to treating the disorder, is the most desirable route. Nutrition is essential for general health, as well as dental health. As a health care professional, one of the dental hygienist's responsibilities is to recognize clients at nutritional risk and provide nutritional counseling. Poor eating habits are widespread among Americans, thus nutritional counseling is justifiable for the majority of clients.

A nutritional assessment involves compiling and comparing data about the client from various sources to provide meaningful evaluation and effective counseling. The evaluation tools to be discussed in this chapter include:

- Health, social and dental, histories
- Clinical evaluations
- Dietary intake evaluation
- Biochemical analysis

EVALUATION OF THE CLIENT

For effective counseling, a comprehensive picture of the client is essential. Gathering only partial information can result in a distorted treatment plan that may be detrimental. The health message will have no meaning for the client. Consider this scenario: a client with rampant caries is told to substitute sugar-free candy for mints. The client agrees to try this until she discovers that sugar-free mints cost more money and are therefore unrealistic given her limited income. The client is unaware of other acceptable alternatives and continues with the mints. This health care professional was missing information essential for making suitable recommendations for the client.

Health History

The health history is designed to identify health-related considerations and medications that can put a client at nutritional risk. The presence of some conditions could interfere with a client's ability to chew, digest, absorb, metabolize, or excrete nutrients, and therefore affect nutritional status. For example, a client taking an antihypertensive medication may experience drug-induced xerostomia and its consequent dental complications.

Additional health-related information can be discovered by reviewing the health history and clarifying statements with the client. Clients may not report valuable information because they (1) perceive it as irrelevant for dental professionals, (2) have forgotten it, (3) are confused by the question, or (4) are apprehensive about their visit to the dental office. For instance, clients frequently neglect to disclose the use of birth control pills, which have several dental and nutrition implications. A few minutes of further questioning by the dental hygienist can save hours of time and effort spent trying to treat the complications. A thorough health history provides the dental hygienist with a strong foundation for developing a plan for dietary counseling (Fig. 19–1).

Screening tools, such as the *Determine Your Oral Health* (Fig. 19–2) and *Determine Your Nutritional Health* checklists (see Fig. 12–5), designed by the Nutrition Screening Initiative for the Elderly, can be used. Obtained during the initial steps of the assessment, they can detect warning signs to be further investigated by the dental hygienist. Additional information on the Nutrition Screening Initiative can be found in chapter 12.

Social History

The purpose of a social history is to identify factors that influence food intake. Personal, environmental, or financial influences can be suggestive of nutritional problems (see the Social Influences on Food Intake). The dental hygienist can obtain much of this information through conversation and further questioning. In addition, by asking a client to describe a "typical day," the dental hygienist can determine routine activities reflective of the client's lifestyle. Understanding reasons for food choices

provides directions for modifying a client's dietary intake.

Social Influences of Food Intake

Examples of factors to be collected by the dental hygienist to further understand the basis of the client's eating practices.

◆ Economic resources

◆ Food preparation and storage facilities

◆ Ethnic or religious group

◆ Eating alone

◆ Frequency of dining out

◆ Responsibility of grocery shopping and food preparation

◆ Motivation level

◆ Education level

◆ Transportation

◆ Physical or mental challenges of an individual

Dental History

Knowing how the client perceives or values a dental situation will assist the dental hygienist in developing strategies for counseling. Such information is part of a dental history (Fig. 19–3). Fluoride history and snacking patterns are also important components.

Medical, social, and dental history forms should be provided prior to the appointment because the client is then more likely to be thorough than if the information has to be filled in while waiting for treatment; alternatively, the client can be interviewed by a member of the dental staff. Ultimately, the dental hygienist must review the information for clarification and need for additional pertinent information.

ASSESSMENT OF NUTRITIONAL STATUS

A thorough assessment will provide the dental hygienist with enough information to determine the nutritional status of the client. An assessment of a healthy client may identify nutritional aspects that can be improved or "fine tuned" for optimal health. For clients experiencing medical or dental compli-

Health History

Name of client _____
Last   First   Middle

Address _____
Number   Street   City   State   Zip

Telephone:(Home) _____ (Business) _____

Date of Birth _____ Emergency Contact _____
Name, Relation and Phone Number

Circle Correct Answer

Y N Have you ever been seen by a physician during the past year?
    For _____

Y N Have you ever been told by a physician that you have a heart murmur?
    Type _____

Y N Females: Do you take oral or subcutaneous contraceptives?
Y N Are you pregnant?
Y N Have you taken steroids in the last two years?
Y N Are you presently under medical care? Are you taking any prescribed or over-the-counter medicine or drugs including aspirin?

Condition	Medication/Dose	Contraindications	PDR Category

Y N Have you ever had surgery, childbirth, hospitalization or serious illness?
    What/When _____

Y N Have you ever had any of the following?
—Rheumatic fever/rheumatic heart disease
—Infectious endocarditis
—Heart trouble (pacemaker/angina)
—Mitral valve prolapse
—Heart attack/congenital heart disease
—Chest pain/discomfort
—Shortness of breath/swelling of ankles
—High or low blood pressure or stroke
—Jaundice, hepatitis, or liver disease
—Kidney trouble
—Organ or tissue transplant
—Thyroid condition/goiter
—Respiratory disorders/tuberculosis/asthma
—Epilepsy/seizures/fainting
—Mental or physical impairment

—Sugar diabetes or family history of
—Fatigue/night sweats/persistent fever
—Excessive thirst or urination (night)
—Lost weight without dieting
—Anemia or blood disorder/diseases
—Serious bleeding or family history of
—Painful or swollen joints/arthritis/spinabifida
—Prosthetic replacement (joints/heart valve:
  pins, plates, surgical wires, screws, implants)
—Sexually transmitted disease
—HIV positive/ARC/AIDS
—Blood transfusion
—Vision or hearing impairment
—Drug/alcohol dependency/use
—Cancer/tumor/growth/radiation therapy
—Other _____

Y N Do the following make you ill or are you allergic to:
—Aspirin or codeine
—Sulfa drugs
—Local or topical anesthetics (Novocaine/Benzocaine)
—Any other substances (e.g. food, clothing, animals, etc.) _____

—Iodine, latex. PABA, bee-sting
—Penicillin or antibiotics
—Barbiturates (sleeping pills)

Do you have any additional health information: Y N _____

FIGURE 19–1 A: Health history. (Courtesy of the Dental Hygiene Program, Raymond Walters College, Cincinnati, OH.)

Figure continued on following page

Name, address & phone of my dentist _____

_____

The name, address & phone of my physician _____

_____

Date of last radiographs: BWS _____ FMS _____ Pan _____ Medical _____

I hereby authorize that the above information is correct to the best of my knowledge. I hereby authorize any physician, hospital, or medical care facility to provide all information on my medical history and treatment to Raymond Walters College Dental Hygiene Clinic. I hereby authorize photocopies of this form to be as valid as the original. I hereby consent to preventive services.

Date _____ Client's Signature/Parent or Guardian _____

Significant Finding	Client Management

Remarks: _____

_____

Date	Blood Pressure	Pulse
Client Signature	Student	Faculty

❖❖❖

Significant Finding	Client Management

Remarks: _____

_____

Date	Blood Pressure	Pulse
Client Signature	Student	Faculty

FIGURE 19–1 *(Continued)* B: See legend on previous page.

cations, the assessment will provide information that will alert the dental hygienist to nutritional factors that can impede responses to dental treatment or recovery (consider a client with anorexia nervosa, whose fragile nutritional status would not make her/him a good candidate for periodontal surgery because of the delayed recovery rate). Overall, assessment provides the basis for the dental hygienist's well-informed recommendations or referrals.

Oral health can affect your nutritional health. A healthy mouth, teeth and gums are needed to eat.

DETERMINE YOUR ORAL HEALTH

If you answered "yes" to "I have tooth or mouth problems that make it hard for me to eat," on the DETERMINE Your Nutritional Health Checklist, answer the questions below.

Check all that apply:

Do you have tooth or mouth problems that make it hard for you to eat, such as loose teeth, ill-fitting dentures, etc. . . . . ____

Is your mouth dry. . . . . ____

Do you have problems with:
- ○ lips (soreness or cracks in corners of your mouth)?. . . . . ____
- ○ tongue (pain/soreness)?. . . . . ____
- ○ sores that do not heal?. . . . . ____
- ○ bleeding or swollen gums?. . . . . ____
- ○ toothaches or sensitivity to hot or cold?. . . . . ____
- ○ pain or clicking in your jaw?. . . . . ____

Have you visited a dentist:
- ○ Within the past 12 months. . . . . ____
- ○ In the last 2 years . . . . ____
- ○ Never been to a dentist . . . . ____

If you have visited a dentist, was the main reason for your visit:
- ○ Regular checkup · ____
- ○ To have a denture made · ____
- ○ To have teeth cleaned · ____
- ○ Bleeding or sore gums · ____
- ○ To have tooth filled · ____
- ○ Loose teeth/loose tooth · ____
- ○ To have tooth pulled or other surgery · · · · · · · · · · · · · · · · · · ____
- ○ Oral or facial pain · ____
- ○ To have a root canal · ____
- ○ Adjustments or repair of denture · ____
- ○ Other · ____

Discuss with your care provider what can be done to correct the problems you have indicated. Also, bring this checklist to your dentist the next time you visit. Remember that warning signs suggest risk, but do not represent diagnosis of any condition.

The Nutrition Screening Initiative
2626 Pennsylvania Avenue, NW, Suite 301
Washington, DC 20037

The Nutrition Screening Initiative is funded in part by a grant from Ross Laboratories, a division of Abbott Laboratories.

21

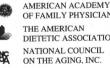

These materials developed and distributed by the Nutrition Screening Initiative, a project of:

AMERICAN ACADEMY OF FAMILY PHYSICIANS

THE AMERICAN DIETETIC ASSOCIATION

NATIONAL COUNCIL ON THE AGING, INC.

FIGURE 19–2 Determine Your Oral Health checklist. (Reprinted with permission by the Nutrition Screening Initiative, a project of the American Academy of Family Physicians, the American Dietetic Association and the National Council on the Aging, Inc., and funded in part by a grant from Ross Products Division, Abbott Laboratories.)

Clinical Observation

Clinical observation begins as soon as the client walks through the door. General appraisal should include posture, gait, overweight, weight loss/gain since previous visit, and physical limitations. Unintentional weight loss, for example, can be in-dicative of numerous disease states or even oral problems.

EXTRAORAL AND INTRAORAL ASSESSMENTS

Visual inspection during an extraoral and intraoral examination will identify abnormal clinical signs.

FIGURE 19–3 **A: Dental history. (Courtesy of the Dental Hygiene Program, Raymond Walters College, Cincinnati, OH.)**

Dental History

Client name _____   Date _____

1. Occupation _____
2. Do you have any pain or sensitivity in your teeth at this time?   YES NO
   If yes, explain
   _____
   _____
3. What was the approximate date of your last dental appointment? _____
   scaling and polishing? _____
4. Did you reside in a fluoridated area from birth to age twelve?   DK YES NO
5. Do you want a fluoride treatment?   DK YES NO
6. Do you expect to keep your teeth a lifetime?   YES NO
7. What type of dental cleaning aids do you use? Frequency?
   a. toothbrush _____
   b. toothpaste _____
   c. dental floss _____
   d. stimulators _____
   e. toothpick _____
   f. water irrigator _____
   g. other _____
8. Do you brush your tongue?   YES NO
9. What do you eat and drink between meals?
   _____
   _____
10. Do you use gum, hard candy, or cough drops?   YES NO
    Sugarless?   YES NO
11. Have you ever had:
    a. canker sores or cold sores?   YES NO
    b. bleeding gums?   YES NO
    c. trench mouth or gum disease   YES NO
    d. teeth sensitive to hot, cold or sweet? YES NO
    e. pain or soreness about your ears or temples?   YES NO
    f. Do you currently have any of these conditions?
       If so, what?   YES NO
    _____

12. Do you ever:
    a. have sinus trouble?   YES NO
    b. clench or grind your teeth?   YES NO
    c. have sore muscles or teeth upon waking?   YES NO
    d. breath through your mouth?   YES NO
    e. use tobacco? What, how much?   YES NO
    _____
    f. have difficulty chewing or swallowing? YES NO
    g. have oral habits (thumb sucking, biting foreign objects)?   YES NO
13. Have you ever had:
    a. periodontal treatment? (when)   YES NO
    _____
    b. orthodontic treatment? (when)   YES NO
    _____
    c. oral surgery? (when)   YES NO
    _____
14. Do you have full or partial dentures? YES NO
    a. do they fit properly?   YES NO
    b. do you remove them at night?   YES NO
15. Have you ever had any serious trouble associated with any previous dental treatment? YES NO
    If yes, explain
    _____
    _____
    _____
16. Are you nervous about dental treatment?
    If yes, explain.   YES NO
    _____
    _____
17. Do you want radiographs?   YES NO
18. Level of education _____
    Are you still in school?   YES NO

Client Education	
First Appointment	Second Appointment
Date:	Date:
Recall (month, year and time interval)_____ Referral(s)_____	

FIGURE 19–3 *(Continued)* **B: Patient education. (Courtesy of the Dental Hygiene Program, Raymond Walters College, Cincinnati, OH.)**

Table 19–1 provides a list of physical signs and symptoms that can indicate an alteration in nutrition. These findings are not a sensitive tool for determining nutrient deficiencies or excesses because they can mirror non-nutritional complications or the possibility of several nutritional difficulties. For example, cheilosis can be the result of a vitamin B complex, iron, or protein deficiency; excess salivation; constantly licking lips; allergies; or environmental exposure. Observations, therefore, are used as an adjunct to supplement other assessment techniques.

Examples of extraoral signs and symptoms for the dental hygienist to document are multiple bruising or pallor of the skin, excessive dryness or pluckability of the hair, dryness of the eyes, and cracked or spoon-shaped fingernails. Intraoral inspection of the integrity of soft tissues, the status of the periodontium, and the presence of plaque and calculus are examples of valuable indicators of the need for nutritional intervention (Fig. 19–4). Data obtained during an extra- and intraoral examination can supply valuable evidence of a nutritional problem that can be confirmed with other assessment procedures.

ANTHROPOMETRIC EVALUATION

Anthropometric evaluation of a client includes measurements of physical characteristics such as height, weight, and change in weight. Indirectly, this information provides an image of body composition of all clients and helps to monitor progress of growth of pregnant women, children, and adolescents. This assessment alone is not sensitive enough to be used to determine nutritional status; however, anthropometric measures may be useful in diagnosis.

Height and weight can be obtained by using a measuring tape and scale, questioning the client, or more practically, visual inspection. Detection of unusual leanness, indicating undernutrition, or notable obesity is the key. As a guide, weights that are more or less than 20% from the norm for height and sex are considered under- or overweight (see Estimating Desired Weight). This formula does not, however, consider variables such as body composition and should not be the only anthropometric measure assessed. Concern arises when weight loss is unintentional. A reduction of 10% of usual weight over a 6-month period is significant and a loss of 20% or greater may indicate a depletion of body mass.

TABLE 19–1 *Nutrition Related Complications of the Oral Cavity*

Nutrient	Deficiency Symptoms
Thiamin (B_1)	Increased sensitivity and burning sensation of oral mucosa; burning tongue; loss of taste and appetite.
Riboflavin (B_2)	Angular cheilosis; blue to purple mucosa; glossitis, magenta tongue, enlarged fungiform papillae, atrophy and inflammation of filliform papillae, burning tongue.
Niacin (B_3)	Glossitis, ulcerations of tongue, atrophy of papillae; cheilosis, thin epithelium; burning of oral mucosa; stomatitis; erythemic marginal and attached gingiva; loss of appetite.
Pyridoxine (B_6)	Cheilosis; glossitis, atrophy and burning of tongue; stomatitis.
Cobalamin (B_{12})	Stomatitis; hemorrhaging, pale to yellow mucosa; glossitis, atrophy and burning of tongue; altered taste; loss of appetite.
Folic Acid	Glossitis with enlargement of fungiform papillae, ulcerations along edge of tongue; gingivitis; erosion and ulcerations on buccal mucosa, pale mucosa.
Biotin	Glossitis, gray mucosa; atrophy of lingual papillae.
Vitamin C	Odontoblast atrophy; porotic dentin formation; gingival inflammation with easy bleeding; deep red to purple gingiva; ulceration and necrosis; slow wound healing; muscle/joint pain; defects in collagen formation.
Vitamin A	Ameloblast atrophy; faulty bone and tooth formation; accelerated periodontal destruction; hypoplasia; xerostomia; cleft lip, keratinization of epithelium; drying and hardening of salivary glands. *Toxicity Symptoms:* Hyperstosis, (hypertrophy of bone), cracking and bleeding lips; thinning of epithelium; erythemic gingiva; and cheilosis
Vitamin D & Calcium	Failure of bones to heal; mild calcification to enamel calcium hypoplasia; loss of alveolar/mandibular bone; delayed dentition; increased caries rate; loss of lamina dura around roots of tooth.
Vitamin K	Gingival hemorrhaging.
Iron	Painful oral cavity; stomatitis; thinned buccal mucosa with ulcerations; pale to gray mucosa, lips, and tongue; angular cheilosis; burning tongue, reddening at lip and margins of tongue.
Zinc	Thickening of epithelium; thickening of tongue with underlying muscle atrophy; impaired taste.
Protein	Smooth, edematous tongue; angular cheilosis; fissures on lower lip; smaller teeth; delayed eruption.

Adapted from Cataldo CB et al. *Nutrition and Diet Therapy.* 3rd ed. New York: West Publishing Co., 1992; Lee M, Stanmeyer W, Weght A. *Nutrition and Dental Health.* Chapel Hill, NC: Health Sciences Consortium, 1982; Palmer C. Dietary and nutritional factors and oral health. *Access/Special Issue* (Special Prevention Issue) 1995; 13–19.

Estimating Desired Weight

Women
100 (lb) + 5 (lb) for every inch over 5 feet
(ex. 5'4" female:
100 + 20 (5 × 4) = 120 ± 10%)
Men
106 (lb) + 6 (lb) for every inch over 5 feet
(ex. 6'3" male:
106 + 90 (15 × 6) = 196 ± 10%)

Laboratory Information

When available, laboratory tests provide another piece of the puzzle in determining nutritional status. Generally, blood and urine samples supply the most data. As with other assessment techniques, a laboratory test alone should not be used to diagnose malnutrition since non-nutritional factors can also influence these data. Interpretation of nutrition-related laboratory tests is generally accomplished by a physician or dietitian. Dental hygienists gener-

Extraoral and Intraoral Examination

Date of Exam _____   Client Name _____

Indicate deviation from normal by placing a check on the line next to the condition or stricture. The lines below or next to each section should be used to describe the deviations. Lines left blank indicate that the condition or structure is within normal limits.

A. General appraisal:
   1___ Posture, gait
   2___ Physical condition (ht., wt., challenged)
   3___ Speech (voice)
   4___ Respiration

   _____
   _____

B. Extraoral exam:
   1___ Head & facial symmetry
   2___ Exposed skin
   3___ TMJ
   4___ Lymph nodes, salivary glands
   5___ Facial muscles

   _____
   _____

C. Intraoral exam:
   1___ Lips
   2___ Vermilion border
   3___ Labial commissure
   4___ Labial mucosa
   5___ Alveolar mucosa
   6___ Labial frenums

   _____
   _____

D. Buccal mucosa:
   1___ Buccal mucosa
   2___ Mucobuccal fold (vestibule)
   3___ Parotid papilla
   4___ Retromolar area
   5___ Pterygomandibular fold

   _____
   _____

E. Hard palate:
   1___ Hard palate
   2___ Incisive papilla
   3___ Palatine raphe & rugae
   4___ Torus
   5___ Maxillary tuberosity

   _____
   _____

F. Soft palate:
   1___ Soft palate
   2___ Uvula
   Pharyngeal area:
   3___ Palatine pillars
   4___ Tonsils
   5___ Oropharynx

   _____
   _____

G. Tongue:
   1___ Papillae
   2___ Dorsal surface
   3___ Lateral borders
   4___ Ventral surface

   _____
   _____

H. Sublingual area:
   1___ Floor of mouth
   2___ Lingual frenum
   3___ Sublingual folds
   4___ Sublingual caruncle

   _____
   _____

I. Alveolar ridge or alveolus:
   1___ Maxillary
   2___ Mandibular
   3___ Exostosis
   4___ Torus

   _____
   _____

FIGURE 19–4 A: Extraoral and intraoral examination. (Courtesy of the Dental Hygiene Program, Raymond Walters College, Cincinnati, OH.)

Periodontal Assessment

Gingival Assessment:

Color:	pink	erythematous	magenta	pigmented	keratinized
Papillary contour:	pointed	flat	blunted	cratered	edematous bulbous
Marginal contour:	normal	rolled	enlarged	receded	irregular
Texture:	stippled	smooth	glossy	hyperkeratosis	
Consistency:	firm	edematous	fibrotic		
Attached gingiva:	adequate	inadequate	mucogingival involvement (1 mm or less)		
Exudate:	none	suppuration			

Gingivitis:

	Localized				Generalized		
	slight	moderate	severe		slight	moderate	severe
	papillary	marginal	diffuse		papillary	marginal	diffuse

Location: _____

Oral hygiene plaque amount :

	Localized				Generalized		
	slight	moderate	severe		slight	moderate	severe

Location:_____

Materia alba:	none	present		
Stain type:	intrinsic	extrinsic	color: _____	
Quantity:	light	moderate	heavy	

Calculus class:

Supragingival:	light	moderate	heavy	Location:_____
Subgingival:	light	moderate	heavy	Location: _____

Periodontitis: *(early 5 mm; moderate 6-7 mm; advanced 8+mm; total attachment loss)*

	Localized				Generalized		
	slight	moderate	severe		slight	moderate	severe

Location: _____

Radiographic interpretation:

	Horizontal bone loss				Vertical bone loss		
	early	moderate	advanced		early	moderate	advanced

Location: _____   Location: _____

Angles class: Right: M: ____ C: ____   Left: M: ____ C: ____

Anterior: overbite: normal moderate severe overjet: ____ mm

edge to edge   openbite   crossbite _____   midline off-center

Posterior: end to end ____ crossbite ____ openbite ____

FIGURE 19–4 *(Continued)* B: Periodontal assessment. (Courtesy of the Dental Hygiene Program, Raymond Walters College, Cincinnati, OH.)

ally do not have access to this information and therefore it is not commonly used in a nutritional dental assessment.

Dental Hygienist Considerations

ASSESSMENT

- *Physical:* deviations from normal anatomy, particularly of the head and neck area; diseases or conditions; emotional state; abnormal anthropometric measurements; if accessible, laboratory tests.
- *Dietary:* medications responsible for difficulties in eating; conditions that interfere with obtaining adequate nutrients (e.g., financial status, ability to shop or prepare food).

INTERVENTIONS

- To be an effective nutritional counselor, it is important for the dental hygienist to understand the eating habits of local ethnic or religious groups.
- Questioning the client about mode of transport and mobility in the community may reveal difficulties in food procurement related to immobility or isolation.
- Have the client describe past dental experiences to gauge knowledge level as well as perception of and attitude toward dentistry.
- Information about a client's history of fluoride exposure will provide valuable indicators for the assessment. Additional questions can include: "Were you raised in an area with fluoridated water?" "Did you take fluoride supplements growing up?" "How often does/did the dentist provide fluoride treatments?" "Were fluoride treatments given at school?" "Have you used fluoridated rinses or gels at home?"
- Observations of the client's attentiveness, anxiety level, motivation, previous dental treatment, and present oral conditions provide direction when initiating a nutritional treatment plan.
- Questions and comments made by the client reflect existing knowledge and understanding of information presented, as well as their

needs and desires. A dental hygienist should practice active listening skills in order to gain valuable material needed in the assessment.
- While interviewing, maintain verbal and nonverbal neutrality in response to the client's statements.

EVALUATION

- Once the various histories and other information about the client have been obtained and the clinical examination performed, the dental hygienist should have gained an understanding of the client's needs.

Determining Diet History

In order to further assess the client's nutritional status, the evaluation process should include screening a **diet history,** the goal of which is to determine usual dietary habits so as to individualize recommendations and minimally modify the diet. Reviewing the intake of the parent, guardian, and/or caregiver is necessary in order to understand the food choices of a child or adolescent. Explain the need for a nutritional assessment prior to distributing the diet history form. Once the form has been completed, additional questioning may be necessary to clarify the information provided by the client. Asking about food preparation, whether foods chosen are nonfat or dietetic, and use of beverages or condiments is common. Also, use of food models and measuring devices easily and precisely identify the client's usual serving sizes. Table 19–2 is a list of appropriate questions the dental hygienist can utilize in gathering accurate information.

The diet history is evaluated according to the Food Guide Pyramid and Dietary Guidelines for Americans for adequacy and variety of nutrients. An analysis of daily carbohydrate exposures will identify the cariogenic potential of the diet. Practical tools used to gain data on dietary intake include the 24-hour recall, food frequency questionnaire, and the 3- to 7-day food diary.

TWENTY-FOUR-HOUR RECALL

The 24-hour recall allows the dental hygienist to collect data on food consumed during a single day.

TABLE 19–2 *Checklist for Food Records*

Type of Food	Did You Specify
All	☐ Amount eaten? By cup, tablespoon, or teaspoon. By size, giving dimensions (length, width, thickness, or diameter)? By number, for standard-size items? By weight?
Cereals	☐ Size of servings? Brand name? Additions, such as milk, sugar, or fruit? Instant or ready-to-eat type?
Baked Goods	☐ Homemade or commercial? From scratch or mix? Topping or frosting? Portion size? Number eaten? Low fat?
Fruits and Juices	☐ Cooked, raw, or dried? Peeled? Fresh, frozen, or canned? Sweetened? Size of serving?
Vegetables	☐ Cooked or raw? Fresh, frozen, or canned? Sauces, other additons? Serving size?
Milk Products	☐ Percent fat? Made with sweetener? Regular, lowfat, or nonfat? Powder or liquid?
Meat, Fish, Poultry	☐ Type of cut? Oil or water packed? Fat, skin removed? Preparation method? Additions? Cooked weight or dimensions of amount eaten?
Eggs	☐ Added fat? Egg substitutes? Quantity? Preparation method?
Mixed Dishes	☐ Homemade or commercial? From scratch or mix? Brand? Major ingredients and proportions? Cooking method?
Soups	☐ Homemade or commercial? Brand? Broth or milk base? Type of milk? Principal ingredients?
Fats and Oils	☐ Stick, tub, diet, whipped, liquid or nonfat margarine? Brand? Major oil? Type of shortening? Homemade or commercial salad dressing? Low calorie or nonfat? Creamy?
Beverages	☐ Brand? Sweetened? Diet? Decaffeinated? Alcohol content? Additions? Amount?
Snacks	☐ Brand? Size, weight, or number eaten?
Restaurant Meals	☐ Type: fast food, ethnic, seafood, steak? How often?
Vitamin or Mineral Supplements	☐ Type? Reasons? Amount?

Use this list to help clarify and increase accuracy of a Food Diary.

From Aronson V. Checklist for Food Records. *Guidebook for Nutrition Counselors,* Copyright © 1990 by Allyn and Bacon. Reprinted/adapted by permission.

The information is most accurate when interviewing the client, or the parent/guardian of a child, and requesting intake from the previous day. This requires little time and is easy to obtain. The client is generally able to recreate the dietary intake from the preceding day with minimal effort. Snacking patterns and spacing of meals may also be revealed in a 24-hour recall. Another advantage is that it allows a general analysis of basic nutrient adequacy, variety, and cariogenicity.

An account of the previous day may not be optimal, however, because that day may not be typical. For example, the client may have been extremely busy the day before and ate only one meal, instead of the usual three meals and two snacks. Requesting recall of a typical day may also result in unreliable estimates, as the client is more likely to supply information about the best nutrition day. It is an option, however, for obtaining a typical day's intake when the past 24 hours were atypical. Another limitation is that some clients have difficulty recollecting the previous day's food intake. Take a minute to write down what you ate yesterday to understand how arduous this task can be and how easy it is to omit snacks and other foods of lesser importance.

FOOD FREQUENCY QUESTIONNAIRE

Another dietary evaluation tool is the food frequency questionnaire. The purpose of this checklist is to determine how often a client consumes specific foods. A list of foods is provided to the client with instructions to circle the number of times per day or week the food is chosen (Table 19–3). It requires limited explanation and little time; therefore, the client can fill out the questionnaire while waiting for the appointment. The data gained allow for a survey of food group consumption and carbohydrate intake.

The food frequency questionnaire is not specific and does not register enough data to evaluate nutrient content. It also relies on the client's memory, and the client can easily improve the choices and supply the healthiest alternatives.

A food frequency questionnaire can be used to supplement the 24-hour recall to increase the reliability of the information collected. A client, for instance, may have had a glass of milk the day before; however, the food frequency questionnaire indicates this is unusual. The dental hygienist may not have concentrated on dairy products with only the 24-hour recall, but in combination with the food frequency questionnaire, it becomes a component of the nutritional counseling.

FOOD DIARY

The client (or parent/guardian) may also be asked to record food and drink consumption for 3 to 7 days, including a weekend day, to evaluate intake. Figure 16–5 is an example of 1 day of a food diary. Verbal and written instructions for its use can be given at the prophylaxis appointment (see the How To Keep Your Food Record). The client can return the diary at the follow-up appointment. Overall, this is the most effective method of obtaining dietary information because the greater quantity of data is more likely representative of actual intake. An analysis of nutrient and sugar intake will therefore be more legitimate. In addition, the client becomes actively involved when recording the information and may actually see eating patterns emerge that were obscure to them.

How to Keep Your Food Record

1. Record foods as quickly after eating as possible.

2. Record days when not sick or dieting.
3. Record all meals, snacks for each day, including one weekend day.
4. Write down portion sizes. (Examples: 3 oz. fish, 1 cup of cereal, ½ cup of milk, or 1 tsp. of vegetable oil).
5. How was your food prepared. (Examples, baked, broiled, fried, or grilled).
6. Write down added sugar, creamer, sauces, gravies, and condiments (mayonnaise or mustard), as well as the amount.
7. For combination dishes such as casseroles, soups, chili or pasta, record all the ingredients and the amounts accurately, as well as the portion eaten.
8. Record brand names, such as Cheerios or Promise Margarine.
9. Enter the time of consumption.
10. Include miscellaneous foods, such as mints, gum, and cough drops.

Unfortunately, client compliance is a deterring factor. Requesting records for too many days may decrease cooperation. The validity of the food diary is threatened by the client's underestimating food intake by neglecting to record all foods or accurate portion sizes. The client can also easily adjust the food diary to reflect "perfect" eating patterns. Emphasizing that this is not a test, but an instrument to identify healthy practices and areas for improvement of health and/or dental status may increase the legitimacy of recording. The dental hygienist can concentrate on applying the data or may be able to dispel myths and misinformation that surface from the food diary. Finally, it is important to keep in mind that the food diary represents food consumed only in that period of time and does not always reflect usual intake.

The dental hygienist and other members of the dental team can cooperatively establish the most practical and realistic approach for determining food intake in their setting. Along with other components of assessment, the dental hygienist can generally evaluate the nutritional status of the client

TABLE 19–3 *Food Frequency Checklist*

The following questions will help show your (your child's) normal eating behavior. This information will allow the dental health team to thoroughly evaluate your (your child's) dental status. Please mark how often you (or your child) ate or drank each of these items in the past week.

Food Item	Never	1–3 Times per Month	1–3 Times per Week	5 or More Times per Week	1–2 Times per Day	3–4 Times per Day	5 or More Times per Day
Fruit & Juices							
Vegetables, other than starchy choices							
Potatoes & other starchy choices							
Milk & Yogurt							
Meat, Fish, Poultry, Eggs							
Cheese							
Cereals (Cold & Hot)							
Cookies, Cake, Pies, Pastries							
Candy							
Soda							
Diet Soda							
Gum							
Sugarfree Gum							
Alcohol							

Source: Thompson FE, Byers TB. Dietary assessment resource manual. *Journal of Nutrition*, 1994, Nov. 124 (II Suppl), page 2297S.

and be knowledgeable about the role of food habits on oral status.

INTERVENTIONS

- When interviewing a client for a 24-hour recall, a practical first question might be, "What was the first thing eaten?" (do not assume breakfast was eaten). Other questions commonly used are: "Do you use gum, mints, or cough drops? Snacks?" "How often do you brush?" and "How much water do you drink?"

- Allow as much participation by the client as possible, encouraging the client to make his/her own decisions and prescribe his/her own dietary modifications. Active involvement in problem solving is more effective in changing client habits and making the client more accountable for his/her actions.

- Nutritional analysis of food intake, even if it is a computer printout, cannot be used exclusively for diagnosing a deficiency or replacing nutritional counseling. Many programs do not have complete or current data, nor do they consider other factors, such as overcooking. Thus, nutrient intakes may not be accurately estimated. Because nutritional analysis provides only an approximation of nutrient content, it should be used only as an assessment tool and a guide in counseling.

EVALUATION

- The client participates in the nutrition assessment process, asking appropriate questions and making statements that reflect understanding.

IDENTIFICATION OF DIETARY STATUS

Once all of the information is collected, the dental hygienist can begin to identify nutritional status and cariogenicity of the client's dietary intake and help the client establish goals. (Determining the cariogenic potential of the diet is described in chapter 16.) A thorough understanding of the nutrients in each group of the Food Guide Pyramid will help the dental hygienist to identify nutrients that may be deficient or excessive. A commonly omitted food group is the dairy group, which if evaluated would alert the dental hygienist to possible deficiencies of calcium, vitamin D, protein, and riboflavin. If such deficiencies are found, the dental hygienist could concentrate on helping the client to find suitable food choices that are enjoyed and are accessible and affordable. Preferably, choices to replenish these nutrients would be from the dairy group or other food groups rather than supplements.

Several methodologies are available to evaluate a dietary intake. A form produced by the Penn State Nutrition Center provides an interesting and simple approach to evaluating a 24-hour recall or each day of a 3- to 7-day food record (Fig. 19–5). The foods from the 24-hour recall are transferred to the appropriate food categories with the assistance of the client. It is helpful to have the parent/guardian present when counseling a child or adolescent, however, letting the child or adolescent participate as much as possible. Adequacy of intake is easily determined by the client and ideas for modifications or substitutions can follow. For a 3- to 7-day food record, the dental hygienist can separate foods into appropriate food groups for each day. The client can be responsible for one day. The number of servings consumed from each group are totalled. Average intakes are determined by dividing the totals by the number of days in the diary, and the averages compared to the Food Guide Pyramid. As described in chapter 16, the client should be encouraged to circle each carbohydrate exposure in red and distinguish each as to form, frequency, and time eaten (i.e., with a meal or as a snack), in order to evaluate the cariogenic potential of the diet.

Combination foods can be problematic for the client because of the numerous ingredients and difficulties of assigning different components into the appropriate food groups. Each ingredient is considered separately and placed in the appropriate food group with servings. A 1-cup serving of spaghetti and meatballs, for example, generally is

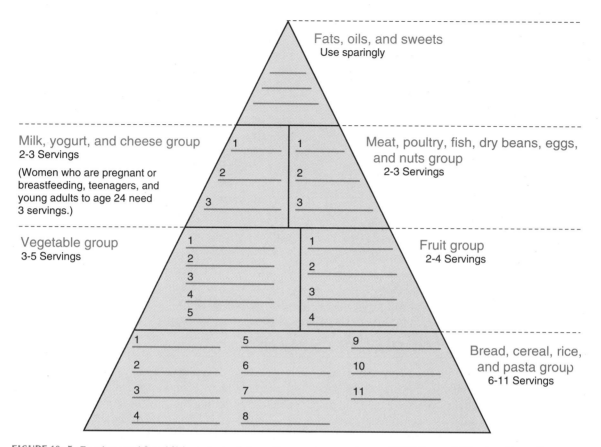

FIGURE 19–5   **Food record for children, teen girls, active women, and men. (1993 Pyramid Packet, Penn State Nutrition Center, 417 East Calder Way, University Park, PA 16801-5663; (814) 865-6323.)**

categorized as two bread/starch servings (spaghetti), one meat serving (meatballs), one fat serving (if oil is present in spaghetti sauce or meatballs are fried), and one vegetable serving (tomato sauce).

These types of approaches to determining dietary intake are adequate and practical for most dental clients. The primary goal of a dietary assessment in dentistry is to identify those clients with oral concerns related to eating and correct these habits to prevent dental disease. If a more thorough assessment is required, the client should be referred to a dietitian.

Computer dietary analysis software packages are available that provide data about the client's dietary intake. Several packages are specifically

designed for the dental office. Some computer programs can sort Mrs. R's 24-hour diet recall in descending order from highest grams of sugar to the lowest (Fig 19–6). The dental hygienist can clarify these figures for the client by converting them to teaspoons of sugar per food product. For example, the soda has 38.4 gm of sugar in a 12-oz serving and we know that 1 teaspoon contains 4 gm of sugar. The amount of sugar in 12 oz is divided by the number of grams of sugar in 1 teaspoon to determine the sugar content of the soda. The soda contains 9.6 teaspoons of sugar ($38.4 \div 4 = 9.6$). Other nutrients that can be determined include calories, vitamins, minerals, protein, fiber, fat, and cholesterol. A printout of the comparison to the RDA, dietary goals, and exchanges will provide a useful and "eye-opening" supplement to the nutritional counseling session (Fig. 19–7).

Use of a computer is limited by the cost of the hardware and software and the time factor. Not all software is reliable and accurate. Before relying on the data, randomly compare the nutrient content of several foods to U.S.D.A. nutrient data or the manufacturer's information. Most importantly, use computer feedback to supplement nutrition counseling, not replace it.

FORMATION OF NUTRITION TREATMENT PLAN

Following evaluation of the data, the results can be shared with the client and parent/guardian, if appropriate. Both the dental hygienist and client can begin to establish an individualized dietary prescription and course of action. It is important to involve the client in as many processes as possible to enhance adherence. When assisting the client in preparing an altered meal pattern, several strategies need to be considered. As discussed earlier in the chapter, accommodating factors that affect food intake, whenever possible, will be advantageous.

The goal is client adherence so that oral health is improved. Other important considerations are food preferences, food habits, food allergies, and special diets. Compliance is more likely if changes are minimal or deviate as little as possible from the client's normal pattern of eating. Other results indicated by the assessment should be verified by the client. For instance, if a client's intake seems deficient in fruits, further questioning may reveal that no fruit was available during the days of recording because of the client's inability to go to

FIGURE 19–6 Mrs. R. sorted on sugar intake—computer-generated analysis. (Nutrient data from Nutritionist IV software. First Data Bank, San Bruno, CA.)

Item	Food Name	Serving	Portion	Sugar
693	COLA-TYPE-SODA	12.00	FL OZS	38.40 Gm (19%)
1782	CANDY-SNICKERS BAR	1.000	ITEM	27.80 Gm (14%)
235	BANANAS-RAW-PEELED	1.000	ITEM	17.80 Gm (9%)
291	PEARS-RAW-BARTLET-UNPEELED	1.000	ITEM	17.40 Gm (9%)
454	PIE-APPLE-HOME REC	1.000	SLICE	15.50 Gm (8%)
370	CEREAL-RAISIN BRAN-RALSTON	1.000	CUP	14.90 Gm (8%)
278	ORANGE JUICE-FROZ-DILUTED	0.500	CUP	13.00 Gm (7%)
561	SUGAR-WHITE-GRANULATED	1.000	TBSP	11.60 Gm (6%)
50	MILK-WHOLE-3.3% FAT-FLUID	1.000	CUP	11.20 Gm (6%)
436	DOUGHNUTS-CAKE-PLAIN	2.000	ITEMS	8.460 Gm (4%)
1780	CANDY-LIFE SAVERS	6.000	ITEMS	7.980 Gm (4%)
561	SUGAR-WHITE-GRANULATED	2.000	TSPS	7.733 Gm (4%)
651	POTATO-MASH-RAW-PREP/MILK	0.500	CUP	4.095 Gm (2%)
590	BROCCOLI-FROZ-BOIL-DRAIN	1.000	CUP	2.500 Gm (1%)
113	MARGARINE-REG-HARD-STICK	1.000	ITEM	0.000 Gm (0%)
731	COFFEE-BREWED	16.00	FL OZS	0.000 Gm (0%)
733	TEA-BREWED	8.000	FL OZS	0.000 Gm (0%)
28	CREAM-COFFEE-TABLE-LIGHT	2.000	TSPS	- Gm (-%)
843	GRAVY-CHICKEN-CANNED	1.000	TBSP	- Gm (-%)
210	CHICKEN-BREAST-FRIED/FLOUR	1.000	ITEM	- Gm (-%)
1906	SANDWICH-HAM/CHEESE	1.000	ITEM	- Gm (-%)
710	SOUP-TOMATO-CAN-MILK	1.000	CUP	- Gm (-%)
1389	CORN CHIPS	1.000	SERVING	- Gm (-%)
868	BEER-BUDWEISER	12.00	FL OZS	- Gm (-%)

Mrs. R. Sorted on Sugar

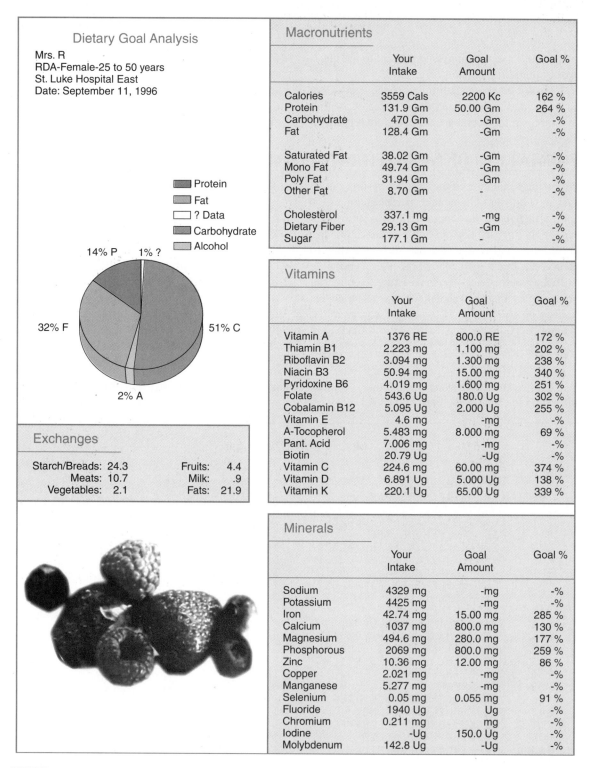

Dietary Goal Analysis

Mrs. R
RDA-Female-25 to 50 years
St. Luke Hospital East
Date: September 11, 1996

Legend:
- Protein
- Fat
- ? Data
- Carbohydrate
- Alcohol

Pie chart: 14% P, 1% ?, 51% C, 32% F, 2% A

Macronutrients

	Your Intake	Goal Amount	Goal %
Calories	3559 Cals	2200 Kc	162 %
Protein	131.9 Gm	50.00 Gm	264 %
Carbohydrate	470 Gm	-Gm	-%
Fat	128.4 Gm	-Gm	-%
Saturated Fat	38.02 Gm	-Gm	-%
Mono Fat	49.74 Gm	-Gm	-%
Poly Fat	31.94 Gm	-Gm	-%
Other Fat	8.70 Gm	-	-%
Cholesterol	337.1 mg	-mg	-%
Dietary Fiber	29.13 Gm	-Gm	-%
Sugar	177.1 Gm	-	-%

Vitamins

	Your Intake	Goal Amount	Goal %
Vitamin A	1376 RE	800.0 RE	172 %
Thiamin B1	2.223 mg	1.100 mg	202 %
Riboflavin B2	3.094 mg	1.300 mg	238 %
Niacin B3	50.94 mg	15.00 mg	340 %
Pyridoxine B6	4.019 mg	1.600 mg	251 %
Folate	543.6 Ug	180.0 Ug	302 %
Cobalamin B12	5.095 Ug	2.000 Ug	255 %
Vitamin E	4.6 mg	-mg	-%
A-Tocopherol	5.483 mg	8.000 mg	69 %
Pant. Acid	7.006 mg	-mg	-%
Biotin	20.79 Ug	-Ug	-%
Vitamin C	224.6 mg	60.00 mg	374 %
Vitamin D	6.891 Ug	5.000 Ug	138 %
Vitamin K	220.1 Ug	65.00 Ug	339 %

Exchanges

Starch/Breads:	24.3	Fruits:	4.4
Meats:	10.7	Milk:	.9
Vegetables:	2.1	Fats:	21.9

Minerals

	Your Intake	Goal Amount	Goal %
Sodium	4329 mg	-mg	-%
Potassium	4425 mg	-mg	-%
Iron	42.74 mg	15.00 mg	285 %
Calcium	1037 mg	800.0 mg	130 %
Magnesium	494.6 mg	280.0 mg	177 %
Phosphorous	2069 mg	800.0 mg	259 %
Zinc	10.36 mg	12.00 mg	86 %
Copper	2.021 mg	-mg	-%
Manganese	5.277 mg	-mg	-%
Selenium	0.05 mg	0.055 mg	91 %
Fluoride	1940 Ug	Ug	-%
Chromium	0.211 mg	mg	-%
Iodine	-Ug	150.0 Ug	-%
Molybdenum	142.8 Ug	-Ug	-%

FIGURE 19–7 **Dietary goal analysis. (Nutrient data from Nutritionist IV v. 4.0 software First Data Bank, San Bruno, CA.)**

the grocery store. Thus this deficiency would be interpreted by the dental hygienist as atypical.

Integration and Implementation

The purpose of nutritional counseling is to motivate and encourage the client to initiate positive changes in behavior and to continue healthful practices. Obtaining knowledge and changing a personal habit requires that a client internalize and accept that modifying a specific behavior is beneficial to himself/herself. There is a large gap between gaining information and applying this information because of difficulties in changing eating patterns. The client and dental hygienist work together to bridge the gap. Knowledge alone does not determine desired behavior. For instance, providing a sheet with a textbook diet or a list of nutrition "do's and don'ts" is very unlikely to effect change. These written guidelines are not meaningful because they do not account for each client's individuality and unique nutritional needs, and for the difficulty in changing established eating patterns. Consider the client who accurately describes the Food Guide Pyramid, but continues to omit vegetables. This client is knowledgeable but does not change behavior; therefore, learning is not effective.

Accordingly, effective nutritional counseling involves the client and dental hygienist working together to define the diet-dental problem and formulate solutions. A counseling session controlled by the dental hygienist who points out each negative behavior is not conducive to learning. The dental hygienist's responsibility is to supply accurate information and guide the client in making healthful decisions toward improving the diet-dental situation. It is the client's responsibility to make changes in food patterns, but the dental hygienist can offer some acceptable suggestions.

SETTING GOALS

Resistance to change, despite knowledge, is a very natural response of an individual. Consider the dental health professional who encourages clients to floss, yet he/she does not floss regularly. The

Exercise to Understand Resistance to Change provides an exercise to further understanding. Establishing a **goal** is an important aspect of changing behaviors because it sets a concrete standard for change. A meaningful and attainable goal will give the client something to strive for. The goal chosen should be difficult enough to be challenging, but not so difficult as to seem impossible. Occasionally behaviors may need to be prioritized; one that causes the most oral problems is addressed first. Perhaps frequent use of cough drops has led to an increased caries rate. The dental hygienist should emphasize the reason this behavior is detrimental and guide the client in establishing goals to decrease use of or eliminate cough drops from the diet. This may include referring the client to an appropriate physician to determine what is causing the sore throat or cough, or explaining to the client why the mouth is so dry.

Exercise to Understand Resistance to Change

Procedure: Fold your arms in front of you. Do not glance down to identify which arm rests on top of the other. Quickly unfold your arms and refold them the opposite way. For example, if the right arm was initially on top, it should be under the left arm after the switch.

Note the awkwardness. Does this reflect a change in an established behavior? If even this slight physical change lends to some resistance, think of the implications for more substantial behavioral changes asked of the client.

Adapted from Newstrom, Newstrom JW, Scannell EE. *Games Trainers Play.* New York: McGraw-Hill, Inc. 1980.

A goal needs to be measurable or observable. "Eat one vegetable each day" is a very specific goal that can readily be measured. However, "Improve oral health" is vague and difficult to observe; this goal should be more specific. Finally, creating goals for multiple behavior changes at one time will seem overwhelming. Gradual changes in behavior are more successful and can be accomplished by breaking goals into smaller steps. The dental hygienist can work with the client to initially select and develop a realistic goal. Once established, the goal should be modified as needs change. For example, "Eat one vegetable every other day" may be more appropriate for someone eating no vegetables at all than "Eat three to five servings each day as recommended." The latter example may prove to be too difficult, and the client may just give up. Successfully achieving smaller steps motivates one toward larger changes. Once smaller steps are accomplished, the client can modify the goal to eating one vegetable every day and eventually work toward eating three to five vegetables per day.

MENU CREATION

Once the client has a grasp of the dietary need and has direction as how to accomplish it, he/she should create a realistic menu for a day (Fig. 19–8). The dental hygienist assists the client in establishing a menu that follows the principles discussed, including nutritionally adequate and noncariogenic foods. It should vary as little as possible from the original intake and include foods the client likes. Many times the client will suggest an ideal intake, modeling the Food Guide Pyramid. The dental hygienist can intervene and suggest more practical options to improve long-term compliance. For instance, most persons know it is unwise to eat at fast-food establishments frequently, but it is unrealistic to say "never eat there." Particularly if the client eats fast food several times each week, the dental hygienist can help the client determine the best food selections available.

The feedback given by the client to formulate a diet will be one indicator the dental hygienist can use to determine if learning has taken place. The client who provides an ideal menu reflects knowledge-based skills, but this is a signal for the dental hygienist to redirect the client toward more workable modifications.

FOLLOW-UP

A follow-up appointment to monitor the client's progress can be scheduled separately or in conjunc-

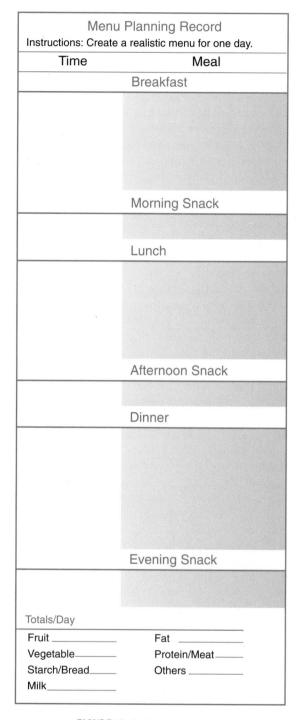

FIGURE 19–8 **Menu planning.**

tion with another dental appointment. Primary approaches for the dental hygienist include support for continued change, establishing challenging goals or revising existing goals, and/or clarifying information. Reviewing a new food record with the client will promote feedback of progress, particularly when compared to the original. Rather than expressing disappointment over not meeting a goal, pointing out the positive behaviors, no matter how small, is more motivating for the client.

REVIEW

The dental hygienist concludes the session by summarizing the pertinent points and giving the client a sense of accomplishment and direction after leaving the appointment. Providing a work phone number and encouraging the client to call with questions will also help the client recognize your concern.

Evaluation

Evaluation is an ongoing process that takes place in all stages of assessment and counseling. The dental hygienist will need to continuously revise the nutritional assessment and counseling, making appropriate changes as needed (Fig. 19–9).

FACILITATIVE COMMUNICATION SKILLS

Intertwined with implementing an effective nutrition care plan are the interpersonal communication skills of the dental hygienist. An atmosphere of sincerity, trust, and empathy should be established to help the client relax and feel more comfortable in revealing accurate information and be more cooperative in working toward a goal. Good rapport is the foundation; without it, very little is accomplished (Fig. 19–10). Formulating **nonjudgmental** and noncritical responses encourages a client to provide accurate accounts of food intake without the threat of being reprimanded. If a client's food record reveals donuts and soda for breakfast, it would be judgmental for the dental hygienist to say, "I can't believe you eat that for breakfast!" Instead, a noncommittal verbal and nonverbal acknowledgement of the food, such as "Is this usual?", would elicit a more accurate reply. Phrases that discount a client's feelings do not promote the warm and caring atmosphere that is essential for good rapport. Phrases such as, "You're making a mountain out of a molehill," "Don't be ridiculous," or "It is good, but . . . ," are guaranteed to inhibit the client's participation.

Listening

Listening to the client is an important and distinguishing feature of effective communication that the dental hygienist must practice. Listening involves more than hearing. It includes interpreting what is said, how it is said, and nonverbal actions observed. Active listening is difficult and requires the full attention of the listener. It can actually save time, however, since the dental hygienist will have a better understanding of a situation.

Impediments to careful listening include interrupting, preparing a response while the other person is speaking, distracting mannerisms, daydreaming, and finishing the speaker's sentences. Awareness of personal barriers to listening allows the dental hygienist to focus on establishing appropriate alternatives for more effective communication.

To improve listening skills, the dental hygienist can practice being attentive by shutting out external distractions or not interrupting (e.g., decreasing the number of questions asked, not taking the subject in another direction). The client feels more comfortable and important when he/she is being heard.

Nonverbal Actions

Facial expressions, eye contact, body movements, personal distance, head-nodding, and vocal cues are nonverbal behaviors that substitute or enhance verbal behavior. Positive nonverbal actions increase the effectiveness of communication and create a comfortable atmosphere for the client. Eye contact, for example, is a significant interaction between the dental hygienist and client. Good eye

	Dental Hygienist	Client	Dental Hygienist and Client
Prior to Counseling	Obtain health, social, dental histories Explain purpose of nutrition counseling Explain diet history form Use questions to clarify and obtain more information Clinically assess client Evaluate Document pertinent information	Provide accurate information Ask questions as needed Complete diet history	
Counseling Session	Present results of analysis Acquire client's interpretation of diet-dental situation *Reinforce healthy points *Educate weak areas Point out concerns from assessment and verify with client Note positive habits, deficiencies, excesses Determine average intake- Total number servings from each group Number days in diary	Restate problem as he/she understands it Ask questions and comment as needed	Define problem Classify each food into food groups Compare to food guide pyramid and dietary guidelines Circle fermentable carbohydrate foods in red, if applicable *Determine form, frequency, time of day for each Establish goals
	Review principles of caries prevention, if applicable Evaluate Summarize main points of session Document pertinent information		Plan a realistic meal pattern
Follow-Up Session	Evaluate progress Reinforce positive changes in behavior *Clarify information from counseling session *Offer support for unresolved areas Monitor and report effects on dental health Document pertinent information	Complete new food reccord Provide feedback of progress *Ask questions *Explain difficulties, successes	Establish new goals

FIGURE 19–9 **Responsibilities.**

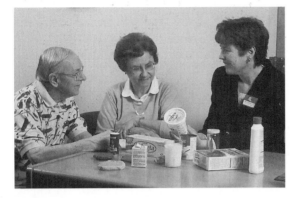

FIGURE 19–10 Counseling. (Courtesy of the St. Luke Hospitals of North Kentucky.)

contact communicates interest, understanding, and warmth, whereas, a lack of eye contact or staring can be interpreted as indifference or preoccupation. Eye contact and other nonverbal signals can communicate what cannot be verbalized.

Questioning

Asking open-ended questions encourages the client to expand on the answers, which can include much more information about food choices than anticipated. "What is your evening routine?" will evoke greater response than a question with a yes or no reply, such as "Do you snack in the evening?"

Dental Hygienist Considerations

INTERVENTIONS
- Avoid scheduling the nutritional counseling after a long or difficult dental appointment.
- The operatory causes anxiety for many clients; choose a quiet and private location for nutritional counseling so that the client feels more relaxed and less apprehensive.
- The room designated for nutritional counseling should be equipped with educational material such as pertinent literature, posters, flannel boards, food packages, food models, and measuring utensils to enhance the learning experience.
- Resist the temptation to create an ideal diet prescription and solve all nutritional problems for the client. Help clients to adapt and develop a less than perfect menu plan that will more likely be followed routinely.
- When appropriate, request that a family member or friend participate with the client in the counseling session, especially a person who is responsible for the cooking and food shopping. Assistance is also warranted when a physical or mental impairment interferes with the client's understanding.
- Explain to the client you will be making notes of what is being discussed so that you will not forget important information.

EVALUATION
- The client follows the changes in food choices agreed to in the nutritional counseling session. Upon evaluation at the follow-up visit, the client has continued with the first goals and has advanced to implement other more difficult suggestions.

Nutritional Directions

◆ Establishing good eating habits is a wise investment toward lifelong positive health and dental status. Prevention, alleviation, or postponing the onset of a disease is possible with good nutrition.

CASE APPLICATION FOR THE DENTAL HYGIENIST

As 70-year-old Mr. B walks into the operatory, it is noted that he continues to lose weight and has less energy than at his previous 4-month recall. His health history reveals no significant findings except one daily medication to control hypertension. The social history unveils that his wife has been deceased for 2 years and his limited income makes it difficult to purchase the foods he needs. He complains of a loose-fitting maxillary denture and xerostomia.

Nutritional Assessment

○ Medical, dental, and social history
○ "Determine Your Nutritional Health" and "Determine Your Oral Health" checklists
○ Extra- and intraoral examination
○ Anthropometric evaluation for weight changes
○ Three-day food record

Nutritional Diagnosis

Social and oral factors are affecting not only the desire, but the ability to obtain adequate nutrients.

Nutritional Goals

The client will seek support from suggested referrals and begin to improve his caloric intake and variety of food.

Nutritional Implementation

Intervention: Have Mr. B complete the "Determine Your Nutritional Health" (see Fig. 12–5) and "Determine Your Oral Health" (see Fig. 19–1) checklists.
Rationale: These screening tools will help identify areas of health risk, along with a number of components that interfere with the ability to obtain adequate food, such as Mr. B's limited income or oral pain. Referrals to federal, state, or community services (e.g., food stamps or congregate meal programs) can be made on the basis of information gathered.

Intervention: Examine the oral cavity for any deviation from normal, as well as the fit of the maxillary denture.
Rationale: Ill-fitting dentures can be a result of weight loss, which can be responsible for

creating sore spots. The presence of oral infections can decrease the ability and desire to eat, ultimately affecting nutrition status. Identifying such areas can allow for treatment and education on prevention.

Intervention: Provide instruction for completing a 3-day food record.
Rationale: This component will complete the assessment process. Determining typical eating habits and patterns, as well as variety of foods, will give direction to the nutritional counseling. Look for the possibility of soft foods, convenience foods, many fermentable carbohydrates, limited variety, low calories, and/or one meal per day.

Intervention: Educate Mr. B regarding basic information about nutrient needs and the relationship between diet and health status.
Rationale: Depression over a spouse's death and/or dining alone are two factors that decrease the desire to eat in older Americans. Referral to a community-based senior citizen program may provide support and companionship needed to improve his desire to eat.

Intervention: Explain to Mr. B that frequent consumption of acid-containing beverages (e.g., sodas, citrus juices) as well as use of sugar alcohols can put him at high risk for caries.
Rationale: Clients with xerostomia have limited cleansing and buffering capabilities. Therefore, even foods that are generally non-cariogenic for those with an adequate saliva flow can be detrimental for those who do not. Suggest rinsing with water to dilute the effects of citrus juices.

Intervention: Provide positive feedback on even small changes Mr. B makes.
Rationale: An older adult may be more resistant to modifications in well-established habits. Small goals may be more realistic. Allow him to make the goals based on the information presented to him. Recognize that any change is a sign of effort. Follow-up on his progress will be

important to establish new goals or modify those that need it.

Evaluation

At a return visit, Mr. B's new 24-hour recall reveals adequate caloric intake and improvement in variety of food choices. He has slowly begun to gain back some of his weight. He has sought the support of various local senior citizen groups. His denture has been repaired, and he presents a healthy oral cavity.

Student Readiness

1. Examine your own health, social, and dental histories and identify health-related factors that a dental hygienist would find useful in developing a dietary plan. Interview another student to obtain the health, social, and dental histories. What questions were effective in clarifying or obtaining additional pertinent information?

2. Select and explain at least two reasons why a dental hygienist should conduct a nutritional assessment for clients.

3. Describe the components needed for an assessment of a client's nutritional status and explain the rationale of each.

4. The following 24-hour recall was obtained by a dental hygienist. What questions need to be asked to get a more accurate estimate of the client's intake?

BREAKFAST: Bagel and cream cheese, coffee

LUNCH: Hamburger, french fries, soda

SNACK: Candy bar

DINNER: Roast beef, potatoes, salad, corn

5. Explain why the following question asked during a nutritional counseling session is undesirable. Reword the question to enhance effectiveness. "Do you realize that omitting fruits and vegetables from your day could lead to a deficiency in vitamins A and C?"

6. Establish a nutrition goal that you can realistically apply this week and have a partner evaluate. Review progress with the partner at the conclusion of the week. Would you do anything differently to increase the likelihood of accomplishing the goal?

Case Study

The dental hygienist has reviewed Jim S's medical, dental, and social histories at the prophylaxis appointment, indicating no significant changes. Jim presents observable weight gain since the last 6-month recall and three new areas of decay. He has no idea how the areas of decay occurred. A 3-day food record is explained and a nutritional counseling session is established following his restorative treatment. At the restorative appointment, the client forgot to bring his completed food record. The dental hygienist attributed this to a lack of interest. A 24-hour recall is obtained and the session is conducted in the operatory.

1. Prioritize the diet and dental information that Jim S needs.

2. Explain why and how a nutritional counseling session could be beneficial to Jim.

3. What questions should be asked prior to and during the counseling session to gain additional information?

4. State several reasons why the counseling session may not be effective to motivate behavior change. How could these situations be modified to enhance motivation?

References

American Dietetic Association. Position of the American Dietetic Association: Nutrition education for the public. *J Am Diet Assoc* 1990; 90(1):107–110.

Cataldo CB et al. *Nutrition and Diet Therapy.* 3rd ed. New York: West Publishing Co., 1992.

Darby ML, Walsh MM. *Dental Hygiene Theory and Practice.* Philadelphia: W.B. Saunders, 1994.

DeBlase CB. *Dental Health Education.* Philadelphia: Lea & Febiger, 1991.

Nizel A, Papas A. *Nutrition in Clinical Dentistry.* 3rd ed. Philadelphia: W.B. Saunders, 1989.

NSI Technical Review Committee. Appropriate and effective use of the NSI checklist and screens. *J Am Diet Assoc* 1995; 95(6):647–648.

Nutrition Screening Initiative Survey. Washington, D.C.: Peter D. Hart Research Associates, 1990.

Nutritionist IV for Windows. Version 4. First Data Bank Division. San Mateo, CA: The Hearst Corporation, 1995.

Slagter AP et al. Masticatory ability, denture quality, and oral conditions in edentulous subjects. *J Prosthet Dent* 1992; 68:299–307.

Thompson FE, Byers TB. Dietary assessment resource manual. *J Nutr* 1994 (11 suppl) 124.

Appendices

A. Median Heights and Weights and Recommended Energy Intake

B. Synopsis of Mineral Elements

C. Sources for Reliable Nutrition Information

D. Recommended Journals and Newsletters

E. Answers to NQ

F. Dietary Reference Intakes, 1997

Appendix A

Median Heights and Weights and Recommended Energy Intake

Category	Age (years) or Condition	Weight (kg)	Weight (lb)	Height (in)	Height (cm)	REE (cal/day)	Multiples of REE	Average Energy Allowance (cal)* Per kg	Average Energy Allowance (cal)* Per day†
Infants	0.0–0.5	6	13	60	24	320		108	650
	0.5–1.0	9	20	71	28	500		98	850
Children	1–3	13	29	90	35	740		102	1,300
	4–6	20	44	112	44	950		90	1,800
	7–10	28	62	132	52	1,130		70	2,000
Males	11–14	45	99	157	62	1,440	1.70	55	2,500
	15–18	66	145	176	69	1,760	1.67	45	3,000
	19–24	72	160	177	70	1,780	1.67	40	2,900
	25–50	79	174	176	70	1,800	1.60	37	2,900
	51+	77	170	173	68	1,530	1.50	30	2,300
Females	11–14	46	101	157	62	1,310	1.67	47	2,200
	15–18	55	120	163	64	1,370	1.60	40	2,200
	19–24	58	128	164	65	1,350	1.60	38	2,200
	25–50	63	138	163	64	1,380	1.55	36	2,200
	51+	65	143	160	63	1,280	1.50	30	1,900
Pregnant	1st trimester								+0
	2nd trimester								+300
	3rd trimester								+300
Lactating	1st 6 months								+500
	2nd 6 months								+500

*In the range of light to moderate activity, the coefficient of variation is ± 20%.

†Figure is rounded.

Reprinted with permission from RECOMMENDED DIETARY ALLOWANCES: 10th EDITION. Copyright 1989 by the National Academy of Sciences. Courtesy of the National Academy Press, Washington, D.C.

Appendix B

Synopsis of Mineral Elements

Mineral	Physiologic Roles	Hyper- and Hypo- States	Food Sources	Recommended Amounts
Calcium	Structural part of bones and teeth Blood clotting Transmission of nerve impulses Muscle activity Membrane permeability Cofactor for enzyme function	*Hyper:* Renal calculi Calcification of soft tissues Inhibits absorption of iron and zinc *Hypo:* Rickets Osteoporosis Tetany	Milk and other dairy products Dark green leafy vegetables Salmon; sardines Fortified orange juice	Infants 0–0.5: 210 mg* 0.5–1: 270 mg Children 1–3: 500 mg* 4–8: 800 mg* Males and females: 9–18 1,300 mg 19–50: 1,000 mg 51 and over: 1,200 mg* Pregnancy and lactation: same as for the particular age group
Phosphorus†	Structural part of bones and teeth Energy storage Component of DNA and RNA Metabolism of fats, carbohydrates, and proteins	*Hyper:* Tetany Convulsions Renal insufficiency *Hypo:* Increased calcium excretion, bone loss Muscle weakness	Milk and dairy products Meats Whole grains Legumes Nuts	Infants 0–0.5: 100 mg* 0.5–1: 275 mg* Children 1–3: 460 mg Males and females: 4–8: 500 mg 9–18: 1,250 mg over 19: 700 mg Pregnancy and lactation: same as for particular age group
Magnesium†	Cardiovascular function Structural part of bones and teeth Enzyme function Muscle and nerve function	*Hyper:* Weakness *Hypo:* Neuromuscular dysfunction Personality changes Muscle spasm Convulsions Hyperexcitability, tremors, anorexia, apathy Decreased tendon reflexes Cardiac arrhythmias	Whole-grain products Nuts Beans Green leafy vegetables Bananas	Infants 0–0.5: 30 mg* 0.5–1: 75 mg* Children 1–3: 80 mg 4–8: 130 mg 9–13: 240 mg Males 14–18: 410 mg 19–30: 400 mg 31 and over: 420 mg Females 14–18: 360 mg 19–30: 310 mg 31 and over: 320 mg Pregnancy: 18 and under: 400 mg 19–30 yrs: 350 mg 31–50 yrs: 360 mg Lactation: 18 and under: 360 mg 19–30 yrs: 310 mg 31–50 yrs: 320 mg

Mineral	Physiologic Roles	Hyper- and Hypo- States	Food Sources	Recommended Amounts
Sulfur	Structural proteins in cartilage, tendons, and bone matrix; keratin in hair and nails Part of amino acids and vitamins Acid–base balance Neutralizes toxins	*Hyper:* None *Hypo:* None	Protein foods	None
Iron	Transports oxygen Catalyzes oxidative reactions Energy metabolism Synthesis of collagen Conversion of beta-carotene to vitamin A Formation of purines Removal of lipids Detoxification of drugs Production of antibodies	*Hyper:* Hemochromatosis Hemosiderosis *Hypo:* Microcytic, hypochromic anemia	Liver Meats, egg yolk Dark green vegetables Enriched breads and cereals	Infants 0–0.5: 6 mg 0.5–1: 10 mg Children 1–10: 10 mg Males 11–18: 12 mg 19 and over: 10 mg Females 11–50: 15 mg over 51: 10 mg Pregnancy: 30 mg Lactation: 15 mg
Copper	Red blood cell formation Connective tissue Cofactor in enzyme functions for protein metabolism and oxidative reactions	*Hyper:* Nausea *Hypo:* Anemia Decreased skin and hair pigmentation Failure to grow Disturbances in bone development	Shellfish Liver Nuts Sesame and sunflower seeds Legumes Cocoa	ESADDI: Infants 0–0.5: 0.4– 0.6 mg 0.5–1: 0.6–0.7 mg Children 1–3: 0.7–1 mg 4–6: 1–1.5 mg 7–10: 1–2 mg 11: 1.5–2.5 mg Adults: 1.5–3 mg
Zinc	Cofactor for over 120 enzymes affecting growth and replication, sexual maturation, fertility and reproduction, night vision, immune responses, and taste and appetite	*Hyper:* Vomiting, diarrhea Epigastric pain Lethargy and fatigue Renal damage Pancreatitis *Hypo:* Growth failure Hypogonadism Wound healing Impaired taste Poor appetite Infections	Meats Eggs Crustaceans Leafy and root vegetables	Infants 0–1: 5 mg Children 1–10: 10 mg Males over 11: 15 mg Females over 11: 12 mg Pregnancy: 15 mg Lactation: 16–19 mg

Table continued on following page

Synopsis of Mineral Elements (*Continued*)

Mineral	Physiologic Roles	Hyper- and Hypo- States	Food Sources	Recommended Amounts
Manganese	Part of enzymes Bone development Insulin production	*Hyper:* Unknown from food intake *Hypo:* Unknown	Whole-grain products Legumes Leafy vegetables Tea Meats Milk Eggs	ESADDI: Infants 0–0.5: 0.3–0.6 mg 0.5–: 0.6–1 mg Children 1–3: 1–1.5 mg 4–6: 1.5–2 mg 7–10: 2–3 mg 11+: 2–5 mg Adults: 2–5 mg
Iodine	Part of thyroid hormone Regulates basal metabolic rate	*Hyper:* Enlargement of thyroid gland Thyroiditis, hypo-thyroidism Goiter and hyper-thyroidism *Hypo:* Goiter Poor growth Cretinism Congenital anomalies, stillbirths	Iodized salt Saltwater fish	Infants 0–0.5: 40 mcg 0.5–1: 60 mcg Children 1–3: 70 mcg 4–6: 90 mcg 7–10: 120 mcg Males and females over 10: 150 mcg Pregnancy: 175 mcg Lactation: 200 mcg
Molybdenum	Enzyme cofactor	*Hyper:* Unknown *Hypo:* Unknown	Legumes Whole grains Organ meats Milk	ESADDI: Infants 0–0.5: 15–30 mcg 0.5–1: 20–40 mcg Children 1–3: 25–50 mcg 4–6: 30–75 mcg 7–10: 50–150 mcg over 11 and adults: 75–250 mcg
Fluoride†	Structural component of bones and teeth, increasing hardness	*Hyper:* Mottling of tooth enamel Fluorosis Bone deformities *Hypo:* Increased risk of dental caries	Seafood Fluoridated water	Infants 0–0.5: 0.01 mg* 0.5–1: 0.5 mg* Children 1–3: 0.7 mg* 4–8: 1.1 mg* 9–13: 2.0 mg* Males 14–18: 3.2 mg* 19 and over: 3.8 mg* Females 14–18: 2.9 mg* 19 and over: 3.1 mg* Pregnancy and lactation: same as for particular age group*

Mineral	Physiologic Roles	Hyper- and Hypo- States	Food Sources	Recommended Amounts
Selenium	Cofactor of anti-oxidant enzymes	*Hyper:* Nausea and vomiting Hair loss Liver disease *Hypo:* Muscle pain and weakness Heart disease	Seafood Liver Meats Dairy products Vegetables--varies with soil	Infants 0–0.5: 10 mcg 0.5–1: 15 mcg Children 1–6: 20 mcg 7–10: 30 mcg Males 11–14: 40 mcg 15–18: 50 mcg over 19: 70 mcg Females 11–14: 45 mcg 15–18: 50 mcg over 19: 55 mcg Pregnancy: 65 mcg Lactation: 75 mcg
Chromium	Cofactor for insulin Involved in carbo-hydrate and lipid metabolism	*Hyper:* Unknown *Hypo:* Possibly decreased glucose tolerance	Meats Whole-grain products Brewer's yeast	ESADDI: Infants 0–0.5: 10–40 mcg 0.5–1: 20–60 mcg Children 1–3: 20–80 mcg 4–6: 30–120 mcg 7–10: 50–200 mcg 11+ and adults: 50–200 mcg
Cobalt	Component of vita-min B_{12}	*Hyper:* Unknown *Hypo:* Associated vita-min B_{12} deficiency	Vitamin B_{12} sources	None

From Davis JR, Scherer K. *Applied Nutrition and Diet Therapy for Nurses,* 2nd ed. Philadelphia: WB Saunders, 1994.

*Adequate intake (AI). The observed average or experimentally set intake by a defined population or subgroup that appears to sustain a defined nutritional status, such as growth rate, normal circulating nutrient values, or other functional indicators of health. AI is utilized if sufficient scientific evidence is not available to derive an estimated average requirement (EAR). For healthy breast-fed infants, AI is the mean intake. All other life-stage groups should be covered at the AI value. The AI is not equivalent to a RDA.

Appendix C

Sources for Reliable Nutrition Information

American Association of Dental Research
1111 14th St. N.W., Ste. 1000
Washington, D.C. 20005

American Cancer Society
1599 Clifton Road, N.E.
Atlanta, GA 30329-4251

American Cleft Palate-Craniofacial Association
1218 Grandview Ave.
Pittsburgh, PA 15211

American Council on Science & Health
1995 Broadway, 2nd floor
New York, NY 10023-5860

American Dental Association
211 E. Chicago Avenue
Chicago, IL 60611

American Dental Hygienists Association
444 N. Michigan Ave, Ste. 3400
Chicago, IL 60611

American Diabetes Association
National Center
1660 Duke St.
P.O. Box 25757
Alexandria, VA 22314

American Dietetic Association
216 West Jackson Blvd, Ste. 800
Chicago, IL 60606-6995
(800) 366-1655 (National Center for Nutrition
and Dietetics consumer hotline)

American Heart Association, National Center
7272 Greenville Ave.
Dallas, TX 75231-4596

American Institute for Cancer Research
1759 R Street, N.W.
Washington, D.C. 20009-2012

American Medical Association
Department of Foods and Nutrition
515 North State St.
Chicago, IL 60610

American Red Cross, National Headquarters
431 18th Street, N.W.
Washington, D.C. 20006

American Public Health Association
1015 Fifteenth Street, N.W.
Washington, D.C. 20005

American Society for Geriatric Dentistry
211 E. Chicago Ave, 17th Floor
Chicago, IL 60611

Cancer Information Service
Office of Cancer Communication
NCI/NIH, Bldg. 31, 10A07
31 Center Dr. M5C2580
Bethesda, MD 20892-2580

Centers for Disease Control & Prevention
U.S. Department of Health & Human Services
1600 Clifton Rd., N.E.
Atlanta, GA 30333

Center for Nutrition Policy & Promotion
1120 20th St., N.W., Ste. 200
Washington, D.C. 20036

Center for Science in the Public Interest (CSPI)
1875 Connecticut Ave., N.W., No. 300
Washington, D.C. 20009-5728

Community Nutrition Institute
2001 S Street N.W., Ste. 530
Washington, D.C. 20009

Food and Consumer Service
Special Nutrition Programs
U.S. Department of Agriculture
3101 Park Center Dr.
Alexandria, VA 22302

Food and Drug Administration
U.S. Department of Health & Human Services
5000 Fishers Lane
Rockville, MD 20857

Food and Nutrition Information Center
National Agricultural Library Bldg.
U.S. Department of Agriculture
Beltsville, MD 20705

Food Nutrition and Consumer Service
Child Nutrition Division
Homeless Children Nutrition Program
U.S. Department of Agriculture
3101 Park Center Dr., Rm. 1017
Alexandria, VA 22302

Food Research and Action Center (FRAC)
1875 Connecticut Avenue, N.W., Ste. 540
Washington, D.C. 20009

Healthy Mother Coalition
Directory of Educational Materials
U.S. Dept of Health and Human Services
200 Independence Ave., S.W.
Room 750-G
Washington, D.C. 20201

International Food Information Council
1100 Connecticut Avenue N.W., Ste. 430
Washington, D.C. 20036

International Life Science Institute
Office of Education and Public Affairs
1126 16th St., N.W., No. 300
Washington, D.C. 20036

Metropolitan Life Insurance Company
Health and Welfare Division
One Madison Ave.
New York, NY 10010

National Association of Nutrition
and Aging Services Programs
2675 44th Street, S.W., Ste. 305
Grand Rapids, MI 49509

National Center for Education in Maternal
and Child Health
2000 15 St. N., Ste. 701
Arlington, VA 22201-2617

National Council Against Health Fraud
P.O. Box 1276
Loma Linda, CA 92354

National Dairy Council
10255 W. Higgins Rd, Ste. 900
Rosemont, IL 60018-5616

National Foundation/March of Dimes
1275 Mamaroneck Ave.
White Plains, NY 10605

National Institute on Aging
Administration on Aging
U.S. Department of Health & Human Services
330 Independence Ave., S.W.
Washington, D.C. 20201

National Institutes of Health
Information Services
Bldg. 31-A, Rm. 4A-21
Bethesda, MD 20892

National Live Stock and Meat Board
Nutrition Research Department
444 North Michigan Ave.
Chicago, IL 60611

National Cancer Institute
U.S. Department of Health & Human Services
9000 Rockville Pike
Bethesda, MD 20892

National Cholesterol Education Program
National Heart, Lung, and Blood Institute C-200
National Institutes of Health
Bethesda, MD 20892

National Institute of Dental Research
U.S. Department of Health & Human Services
NIH Bldg. 31, Rm. 2C39
9000 Rockville Pike
Bethesda, MD 20892

National Screening Association
1010 Wisconsin Avenue, NW, Ste. 800
Washington, D.C. 20007

President's Council on Physical Fitness and Sports
Director of Information
U.S. Department of Health & Human Services
405 Fifth Street N.W., Ste. 7103
Washington, D.C. 20001

U.S. Department of Agriculture
200 Independence Ave., S.W.
Washington, D.C. 20201

U.S. Department of Health & Human Services
2000 Independence Ave., S.W.
Washington, D.C. 20201

Appendix D

Recommended Journals and Newsletters

American Journal of Clinical Nutrition

American Journal of Dentistry

American Journal of Public Health

British Dental Journal

Caries Research

Clinical Preventive Dentistry

Compendium Continuing Education Dentistry

Contemporary Nutrition (General Mills)

Dental Update

Dietetic Currents (Ross Laboratories)

Dairy Council Digest (National Dairy Council)

Diabetes Care

Diabetes Forecast

Diabetes Talk

FDA Consumer

Journal of the American College of Nutrition

Journal of the American Dietetic Association

Journal of the American Medical Association

Journal of Dental Education

Journal of Dental Research

Journal of Nutrition Education

Nutrition and the MD

Appendix E

Answers To NQ

Chapter 1

1. False. No single food contains all the essential nutrients in the amounts needed for optimal health.
2. False. Sugar consumption is associated with dental caries; however, many other factors, such as oral hygiene practices and fluoride, are also important.
3. True.
4. False. RDAs are based upon a healthy person's nutrient needs and stands for recommended dietary allowances.
5. True.
6. False. Three to five servings are recommended for vegetables and two to four servings for fruit.
7. True.
8. False. Sugar is implicated in dental caries but not in other major diseases, such as hypertension, cardiovascular disease, or diabetes mellitus.
9. True.
10. False. The nutrients that provide energy are carbohydrate, fats, and protein.

Chapter 2

1. True.
2. False. This is the hydrolysis of lipids or fat; carbohydrate yields monosaccharides.
3. False. Absorption occurs primarily in the small intestine.
4. False. Long-chain triglycerides enter the lymphatic system; short-chain and medium-chain triglycerides enter the portal circulation.
5. True.
6. False. Most enzymes end in "-ase" (e.g., lactase).
7. True.
8. False. Villi are located in the small intestine.
9. True.
10. True.

Chapter 3

1. False. The FDA has labeled raw sugar as unfit for direct use as a food or a food ingredient because of the impurities it contains.
2. True.
3. False. Oral bacteria are unable to metabolize xylitol, which is a calorie-containing sugar alcohol.
4. False. The desire for sweetness is not considered an acquired taste because newborn infants exhibit a preference for it.
5. True.
6. True.
7. False. Excessive caloric intake leads to obesity, whether from carbohydrates, proteins, fats, or alcohol.
8. False. Sucrose is table sugar.
9. False. Many other factors, including the consumption of other fermentable carbohydrates, contribute to the development of caries.
10. True.

Chapter 4

1. True.
2. False. The breed of hen determines the color of eggshell, and color is not related to its nutritional value.
3. False. Gelatin does not contain all the EAAs.
4. False. The protein requirement is at least equal to that of the young adult and may be increased.
5. False. Adequate amounts of protein are needed for the development of healthy teeth but increasing protein beyond the RDA will not have any effect on tooth enamel.
6. True.
7. True.
8. False. It is both a protein- and calorie-deficiency disorder.

9. False. In addition to foods from plants, dairy products are consumed. Eggs are excluded.
10. True.

Chapter 5

1. False. It is the overall average of fat intake that is important; foods, such as margarine and oils, are 100% fat but can be used safely in the diet.
2. False. Many manufacturers have responded by eliminating tropical oils from processed foods. Americans currently consume less than 2% of calories from tropical oils.
3. True.
4. True.
5. False. Bananas contain a trace of fat; avocados are 88% fat. However, they are both plant products, so they do not contain any cholesterol.
6. False. All fats produce 9 Cal/gm.
7. True.
8. False. Even though they are nutritious foods, for most Americans, their use should be limited because of their high fat content.
9. True.
10. True.

Chapter 6

1. True.
2. True.
3. False. BMR stands for basal metabolic rate, the amount of energy needed to maintain involuntary physiologic functions.
4. True.
5. True.
6. False. Hunger is the physiologic drive to eat, while appetite implies a desire for specific types of food.
7. False. Fats are stored by the body for energy, but they must first be converted into a form the body can use. Glycogen stores, which are dependent on carbohydrate intake, are readily available for energy.
8. True.
9. True.
10. False. Only fats, carbohydrate, protein, and alcohol provide energy.

Chapter 7

1. True.
2. True.
3. True.
4. True.
5. False. Retinol is obtained from animal foods; beta-carotene is found in fruits and vegetables.
6. True.
7. True.
8. False. A deficiency of vitamin D causes rickets.
9. False. Vitamin K is essential for blood clotting; vitamin D functions in the regulation of blood calcium and phosphorus levels.
10. True.

Chapter 8

1. True.
2. False. Many nutrients work together in building strong healthy bones, including protein, calcium, phosphorus, magnesium, fluoride, and vitamins C and D.
3. False. Dolomite is produced from animal bone that has accumulated lead, and can cause lead poisoning with prolonged use.
4. True.
5. False. Based on the RDA, teenagers need 1,200 mg of calcium. To obtain adequate amounts of calcium, 4 cups of milk is recommended for teenagers (300 mg calcium/cup × 4 + 1,200 mg calcium).
6. False. Fluoridation of community water supplies is the most effective method of preventing dental caries.
7. False. Calcium supplements by themselves probably are not beneficial to women over 30 years of age.
8. True.
9. False. Caffeine decreases calcium absorption.
10. False. Bottled waters vary in fluoride content.

Chapter 9

1. True.
2. True.

3. True.

4. False. Alzheimer's disease and aluminum toxicity are two different conditions.

5. True.

6. False. Unrefined foods generally provide more trace minerals.

7. False. Aluminum is cariostatic, especially in combination with fluoride.

8. True.

9. False. Sugar is not a good source of any nutrients except calories; sugar consumption results in increased insulin levels, affecting the chromium requirement.

10. False. Selenium supplements are not recommended because selenium can be toxic.

Chapter 10

1. True.

2. False. Vitamin D is called the sunshine vitamin because the sun facilitates the body's production of vitamin D; vitamin B_6 is also called pyridoxine, pyridoxal, and pyridoxamine.

3. False. Beriberi is caused by a thiamin deficiency; niacin deficiency causes pellagra.

4. True.

5. False. Flushing and intestinal disturbances are symptoms of niacin toxicity. No toxicity symptoms have been observed for riboflavin.

6. True.

7. True.

8. False. Liver, leafy vegetables, legumes, grapefruit, and oranges are rich sources of folate.

9. True.

10. True.

Chapter 11

1. True.

2. True.

3. True.

4. True.

5. True.

6. False. The minimum requirement for sodium is 500 mg/day for adults, but no RDA has been established for sodium.

7. True.

8. False. Potassium is principally within the cells (intracellular).

9. True.

10. False. Oral pallor is a sign of iron-deficiency anemia.

Chapter 12

1. True.

2. True.

3. False. Solid foods are introduced between 4 and 6 months of age, not at 6 weeks.

4. False. It is one of the last because of the high-frequency of allergies.

5. False. Denture wearers need to learn to swallow liquids, then chew soft foods, and last, bite and pulverize regular foods.

6. True.

7. False. Intake is lower because of menopause.

8. True.

9. False. Toxicity or nutrient imbalances may occur.

10. True.

Chapter 13

1. False. These do not reflect natural instincts for required nutrients.

2. True.

3. False. If the diet is deficient in calcium, the fetal calcium requirements will be met first, but some of the calcium may come from her bones, not from her teeth.

4. False. Although she is "eating for two," normal energy requirements are not doubled. An additional 300 calories are recommended during the second and third trimesters.

5. False. Weight gain is individualized for each woman.

6. False. Iron and possibly folate are usually the nutrients needing supplementation.

7. True.

8. False. Breast milk is normally thin and is nutritionally adequate.

9. False. The more often an infant nurses, the more milk is produced. Milk production is most active during infant sucking.

10. True.

Chapter 14

1. True.
2. False. Patterns and attitudes internalized during childhood promote a sense of stability and security for the older client.
3. False. No culture has ever been known to make food choices solely on the basis of nutritional values of food. The factors that seem to predominate in food choices are cultural and economic.
4. False. Only about one-fifth of the American food dollar is spent on food.
5. False. Fad diets may be physically harmless, but they may not be based on sound nutritional principles.
6. False. There are no demonstrable nutritional benefits from the use of organically grown foods.
7. False. Although some food processing is detrimental to the nutritive value of foods, the goal of food processing is to maintain optimum qualities of color, flavor, texture, and nutritive value.
8. True.
9. True.
10. True.

Chapter 15

1. True.
2. True.
3. False. Supplements for anemia should not be prescribed without the results of blood testing to determine the type of anemia. High intakes of iron could possibly complicate the situation.
4. False. Because of the various considerations involved in constructing a meal pattern for a diabetic, it is imperative that the client be referred to a physician and dietitian.
5. True.
6. True.
7. False. Kaposi's sarcoma is a tumor that occurs frequently in immunocompromised individuals.
8. True.
9. False. Although the eating disorder client should be referred to a physician or an eating disorder program, it is the responsibility of the dental

hygienist to approach the client with the objective findings.
10. False. Bulimics are generally of normal weight or sometimes slightly above recommended body weight.

Chapter 16

1. False. A combination of diet, host, environment, and saliva are necessary for initiation of dental decay.
2. True.
3. True.
4. True.
5. False. Sugar alcohols are fermented slowly by oral bacteria, thus they are noncariogenic. In fact, xylitol is cariostatic due to its ability to inhibit production of *Streptococcus mutans*.
6. False. An acid environment is required to demineralize a tooth; therefore, a cariogenic food will cause the plaque pH to fall below 5.5. Foods that allow plaque pH to rise above 6 are considered noncariogenic.
7. False. It is one factor to consider, along with the frequency of intake, the physical form, and the spacing of food within a day.
8. True.
9. False. Though the RDAs provide a lot of factual information, it is too overwhelming for most clients. The Food Pyramid and Dietary Guidelines for Americans provide practical and general nutrition information that will be a factor in preventing dental decay and improving overall health.
10. False. Information alone does not guarantee a behavioral change.

Chapter 17

1. True.
2. False. Indirectly, firm, fibrous foods reduce the amount of bacterial plaque by stimulating salivary flow, which will promote oral clearance of food and thus lessen food retention.
3. False. A nutrient deficiency can be a contributing factor to gingivitis, but local irritants (plaque and calculus) must be present. The inflammation can

be exaggerated by a nutrient deficiency, as well as by reduced resistance and recovery time.

4. True.

5. False. A client may interpret this advice as condoning ice cream, gelatin, and chicken noodle soup, which would not provide enough nutrients or calories for quick recovery. The dental hygienist should provide a specific list of nutrient-dense foods for the client to purchase prior to the periodontal surgery.

6. True.

7. False. Clear liquids are foods and fluids that are relatively transparent to light in color, such as gelatin and apple juice. These fluids are readily digested and absorbed.

8. True.

9. True.

10. False. If surgery is indicated for a periodontal client, optimally, the nutritional assessment and counseling should be done prior to the procedure to increase nutrient reserves that will expedite the recovery period.

Chapter 18

1. False. Though root surface caries can be a complication of xerostomia, there are other possible causes to consider, such as frequent intake of hard candy. Also, a complete and thorough assessment of the client is essential. No single factor is adequate to diagnose the presence, extent, or cause of xerostomia. An inaccurate evaluation can lead to inappropriate recommendations.

2. False. Although xerostomia is a common complaint in an older adult, the changes in saliva in a healthy geriatric individual are minimal. It has been strongly associated with multiple factors, such as use of medications, one or more systemic diseases, or radiation, all of which are common to this population.

3. True.

4. False. Root caries appear on the root surface, in areas of gingival recession. This condition is seen more often in older adults who have experienced periodontal disease or toothbrush trauma.

5. True.

6. False. It is important to have nutrient-dense foods available, but in different consistencies. A liquid

diet, progressing to a soft diet and then to a regular diet will allow the client to adjust to swallowing, chewing, and biting with the new appliance.

7. True.

8. False. Spongy trabecular bone is the major component of alveolar bone.

9. True.

10. True.

Chapter 19

1. False. Though the health and dental histories provide valuable information, they are not enough to determine the client's nutritional status. Other evaluation tools include clinical and dietary intake.

2. False. Clinical oral exams detect physical signs and symptoms of many nutrient deficiencies. However, deficiencies generally do not appear until an advanced state exists. An oral exam, therefore, should be used as an adjunct in identifying potential nutritional deficiencies.

3. True.

4. True.

5. False. It is imperative that dietary counseling be documented and other staff members be informed about the nutritional counseling for consistency and reinforcement of the information at future appointments.

6. False. Changing a dietary habit is difficult and requires a menu plan tailored to meet the client's needs. A thorough assessment will identify many factors that should be considered. Active involvement of the client in establishing a meal pattern enhances compliance.

7. False. The dental hygienist is responsible for providing information and guiding the client to make healthier decisions. Active participation, problem solving, and decision making allow for greater compliance.

8. False. Changing food habits is very difficult. The first attempt established by the dental hygienist and client may not have been successful and other alternatives may need to be established. Therefore, follow-up is an essential component of the nutritional counseling process.

9. True.

10. True.

Appendix F

Dietary Reference Intakes, 1997

Life-Stage Group	Calcium AI[a] (mg/day)	Phosphorus RDA[b] (mg/day)	Phosphorus AI (mg/day)	Magnesium RDA (mg/day)	Magnesium AI (mg/day)	Vitamin D AI[c,d] (µg/day)	Fluoride AI (mg/day)
Infants							
0 to 6 months	210		100		30	5	0.01
6 to 12 months	270		275		75	5	0.3
Children							
1 through 3 years	500	460		80		5	0.7
4 through 8 years	800	500		130		5	1.1
Males							
9 through 13 years	1,300	1,250		240		5	2.0
14 through 18 years	1,300	1,250		410		5	3.2
19 through 30 years	1,000	700		400		5	3.8
31 through 50 years	1,000	700		420		5	3.8
51 through 70 years	1,200	700		420		10	3.8
>70 years	1,200	700		420		15	3.8
Females							
9 through 13 years	1,300	1,250		240		5	2.0
14 through 18 years	1,300	1,250		360		5	2.9
19 through 30 years	1,000	700		310		5	3.1
31 through 50 years	1,000	700		320		5	3.1
51 through 70 years	1,200	700		320		10	3.1
>70 years	1,200	700		320		15	3.1
Pregnancy							
≤18 years	1,300	1,250		400		5	2.9
19 through 30 years	1,000	700		350		5	3.1
31 through 50 years	1,000	700		360		5	3.1
Lactation							
≤18 years	1,300	1,250		360		5	2.9
19 through 30 years	1,000	700		310		5	3.1
31 through 50 years	1,000	700		320		5	3.1

[a]AI = Adequate Intake. The observed average or experimentally set intake by a defined population or subgroup that appears to sustain a defined nutritional status, such as growth rate, normal circulating nutrient values, or other functional indicators of health. AI is utilized if sufficient scientific evidence is not available to derive an EAR. For healthy breastfed infants, AI is the mean intake. All other life-stage groups should be covered at the AI value. The AI is not equivalent to a RDA.

[b]RDA = Recommended Dietary Allowance. The intake that meets the nutrient need of almost all (97–98 percent) individuals in a group.

[c]As cholecalciferol. 1 µg cholecalciferol = 40 IU vitamin D.

[d]In the absence of adequate exposure to sunlight.

Source: Reprinted with permission from *Recommended Dietary Allowances: 10th Edition.* Copyright 1989 by the National Academy of Sciences. Courtesy of the National Academy Press, Washington, D.C.

Index

Note: Page numbers in *italic* refer to illustrations; those followed by t refer to tables.

Index

No Newer edition as of 1/27/04
Dm